PHYSIOLOGY OF SPORT AND EXERCISE

Jack H. Wilmore, PhD
Margie Gurley Seay Centennial Professor
Department of Kinesiology and Health Education
University of Texas at Austin

David L. Costill, PhD
John and Janice Fisher Chair in Exercise Science
Director of Human Performance Laboratory
Ball State University
Muncie, Indiana

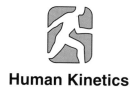

Human Kinetics

Library of Congress Cataloging-in-Publication Data

Wilmore, Jack H., 1938-
    Physiology of sport and exercise / Jack H. Wilmore, David L.
Costill.
       p.   cm.
    Includes index.
    ISBN 0-87322-693-3
    1. Exercise--Physiological aspects. 2. Sports--Physiological
aspects. I. Costill, David L. II. Title.
QP301.W6749   1994
612'.044--dc20   94-3913
                                 CIP

ISBN: 0-87322-693-3

Editorial Director: Sue Mauck
Writer: Lori K. Garrett
Developmental Editor: Lori K. Garrett
Assistant Editors: Julie C. Lancaster, Dawn Roselund, Jackie Blakley, Anna Curry, Ed Giles, and John Wentworth
Copyeditor: Thomas Plummer
Proofreader: Pam Johnson
Production Director: Ernie Noa
Text Designer: Keith Blomberg
Photo Editor: Karen Maier
Typesetter: Julie Overholt
Layout Artists: Denise Lowry, Denise Peters, and Tara Welsch
Illustrator: Thomas-Bradley Illustration & Design
Medical Illustrator: Beth Young
Cover Designer: Keith Blomberg
Cover Photographer: John Kelly
Printer: Bang Printing
Binder: Dekker

Printed in the United States of America   10 9 8 7 6 5 4

Human Kinetics
P.O. Box 5076, Champaign, IL 61825-5076
1-800-747-4457
http://www.hkusa.com

Canada: Human Kinetics, Box 24040, Windsor, ON N8Y 4Y9
1-800-465-7301 (in Canada only)

Europe: Human Kinetics, P.O. Box IW14, Leeds LS16 6TR, United Kingdom
(44) 1132 781708

Australia: Human Kinetics, 2 Ingrid Street, Clapham 5062, South Australia
(08) 371 3755

New Zealand: Human Kinetics, P.O. Box 105-231, Auckland 1
(09) 523 3462

To those who have had the greatest impact on my life: to my lovely wife, Dottie, and our three wonderful daughters, Wendy, Kristi, and Melissa, for their patience, understanding, and love; to Mom and Dad for their love, sacrifice, direction, and encouragement; to my students, who are a continual source of joy and inspiration; and to my Lord, Jesus Christ, who is always there providing for every one of my needs.

Jack H. Wilmore

To my mother and father:
Helen Frances Costill
1914-1993
Bruce Calvin Costill
1911-1972

David L. Costill

Acknowledgments

We would like to thank Rainer Martens for accepting the challenge of trying something new and different and for putting up with a couple of old dogs who were resistant to trying any new tricks. Rainer and the staff at Human Kinetics have been supportive of our many demands and have been extremely dedicated to publishing a quality product. Special recognition must go to Sue Mauck, Editorial Director, who kept this project on a tight timeline, and to Julie Lancaster, for her endless hours of editorial assistance. But most importantly, Lori Garrett, our Developmental Editor, was the glue that held everything together. Lori had to deal with us almost daily and is largely responsible for taking our ideas and putting them into a rational and logical flow. She made us work hard, but no harder than she did, to make this book come alive. Lori, we owe you a great big thanks!

We appreciate the efforts of Jim Pivarnik, Jack Ewing, Art Weltman, and Bill Kraemer, who read the initial manuscripts and gave us important feedback that was incorporated into this final product. Special thanks also go to Vic Convertino, Ed Coyle, Bob Malina, and Matt Vukovich for reading and reacting to chapters, keeping us focused and on target.

Finally, we thank our families, who put up with our many long hours of isolation while we were writing, rewriting, editing, and finally proofing this book. Their patience and support can never be repaid.

Jack H. Wilmore
David L. Costill

Contents

Preface

Your body is an amazingly complex machine. All of its various cells and tissues communicate with each other, and their activities are precisely coordinated. When you think of the numerous processes occurring within your body at any given time, it is truly remarkable that all of the body systems function so well together. Even as you sit reading this, your heart pumps blood throughout your body, your intestines digest and absorb nutrients, your kidneys clear waste products, your lungs bring in oxygen, and your muscles hold this book while your brain concentrates on reading. Although you may feel at rest, your body is physiologically quite active. Imagine, then, how much more active all of your body systems become when you engage in active movement. As your physical activity increases, so does your muscles' physiological activity. Active muscles require more nutrients, more oxygen, more metabolic activity, and thus more efficient clearance of waste products. How does your body respond to the high physiological demands of physical activity?

That is the key question when you study the physiology of sport and exercise, and we answer it in this book. *Physiology of Sport and Exercise* introduces you to the fields of sport and exercise physiology. Our goal is to build upon your foundation of knowledge constructed through basic coursework in human anatomy and physiology by applying the principles you've learned to how the body performs and responds to physical activity.

We begin in chapter 1 with a historical overview of sport and exercise physiology as they have emerged from the parent disciplines of anatomy and physiology, and we explain basic principles that will be used throughout the text. In each of Parts A through C, we review selected physiological systems, focusing on their responses to acute bouts of exercise and finally considering how these systems adapt to long-term exposure to exercise—training. In Part A we focus on how the muscular and nervous systems coordinate to produce body movement. In Part B we address how the basic energy systems provide the energy needed for movement and the role of the endocrine system in regulating metabolism. In Part C we look at the cardiovascular and respiratory systems—how they transport nutrients and oxygen to the active muscles and waste products away from them during physical activity.

We change perspective in Part D to examine the impact of the external environment on physical performance. We consider the body's response to heat and cold, then we examine the impact of low atmospheric pressure that is experienced at altitude, and high atmospheric pressure that is experienced during diving. We conclude by considering the effects of a unique environment—one of little gravity—that is experienced during space travel.

In Part E we shift our attention to how athletes can optimize physical performance. We evaluate the effects of different amounts of training. Moving on, we explore the use of ergogenic aids—substances purported to improve athletic ability. We continue by examining athletes' special dietary needs and how nutrition can be used to enhance performance. Finally, we consider the importance of appropriate body weight for performance.

In Part F we examine unique considerations for specific populations of athletes. We look first at the processes of growth and development and how they affect the performance capabilities of young athletes. We evaluate changes that occur in physical performance as we age and explore the ways that physical activity can prolong our youthfulness. Finally, we examine gender issues and special physiological concerns of female athletes.

In Part G, the final part of the book, we turn our attention to the application of sport and exercise physiology for the prevention and treatment of various diseases and the use of exercise for rehabilitation. We focus on cardiovascular disease, obesity, and diabetes, then we close the book with a discussion of prescribing exercise to maintain health and fitness.

Physiology of Sport and Exercise offers a novel approach to the study of sport and exercise physiology. It is designed for the student reader, with the goal of making your learning easy and enjoyable. This text is comprehensive, but we don't want you to be overwhelmed by either its size or its scope. We have included special features to help you progress through the book. For example, each part is color-coded: Every chapter within a given part has a box of the same color appearing at the edge of its pages. A glance at the table of contents reveals which color corresponds to which text part and what chapters are included in that part. Then, by scanning the colored edges of the pages while the book is closed, you can easily locate the part you're seeking and identify the individual chapters within it.

Once you turn to a part, you will find brief text that describes the contents of that part's chapters. Each chapter then begins with a brief overview and a chapter outline with page numbers to help you locate material. Within a chapter, Key Points are placed in blue boxes for quick reference. Key terms are highlighted in the text in blue, are listed at the end of the chapter, and

are defined in the glossary at the end of the book. Review boxes scattered throughout each chapter summarize the major points presented.

At the chapter's end, the key terms are listed so you can check your vocabulary comprehension. Study questions allow you to test your knowledge of the chapter's contents. References, numbered throughout the text, also appear here, as do several selected readings, which provide additional information about any topics of special interest within that chapter. Finally, at the end of the book you will find a comprehensive glossary that includes definitions of all key terms, a thorough index, and, inside the back cover, a table of conversions and metric equivalents for easy reference.

Many of you will read this book only because it is a required text for a required course. But we hope that the information will entice you to continue to study in this relatively new and exciting area. We plan at the very least to further your interest and understanding of your body's marvelous abilities to perform physical work, to adapt to stressful situations, and to improve its physiological capacities. What you learn here is practical not only for anyone who pursues a career in exercise or sport science but also for anyone who wants to be active, healthy, and fit.

PHYSIOLOGY
OF SPORT
AND EXERCISE

Chapter 1

An Introduction to Exercise and Sport Physiology

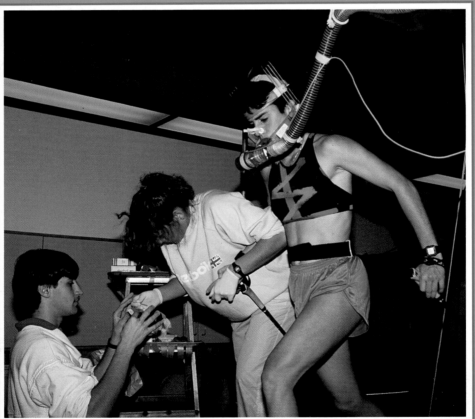

Chapter Overview

The human body is an amazing machine! As you sit reading this chapter, countless perfectly coordinated events are occurring simultaneously in your body. These events allow complex functions, such as hearing, seeing, breathing, and information processing, to continue without your conscious effort. If you stand up, walk out the door, and jog around the block, almost all your body's systems will be called into action, enabling you to successfully shift from rest to exercise. If you continue this routine daily for weeks or months and gradually increase the duration and intensity of your jogging, your body will adapt so you can perform better.

For centuries, scientists have studied how the human body works. During the past several centuries, a small but growing group of scientists have focused their studies on how the body's functioning, or physiology, is altered during physical activity and sport. This chapter will introduce you to exercise and sport physiology, presenting a historical overview then explaining some basic concepts that form a foundation for the chapters that follow.

Much of the history of exercise physiology in the United States can be traced to the effort of a Kansas farm boy, David Bruce (D.B.) Dill, whose interest in physiology first led him to study the composition of crocodile blood. Fortunately for us, this young scientist redirected his research to humans when he became the first director of the Harvard Fatigue Laboratory, established in 1927. Throughout his life he was intrigued by the physiology and adaptability of many animals who survive extreme environmental conditions, but he is best remembered for his research on human responses to exercise, heat, high altitude, and other environmental factors. Dr. Dill always served as one of the human "guinea pigs" in these studies. During the Harvard Fatigue Laboratory's 20-year existence, he and his co-workers produced 330 scientific papers along with a classic book entitled *Life, Heat, and Altitude*.[3]

After the Harvard Fatigue Laboratory closed its doors in 1947, he began a second career as deputy director of medical research for the Army Chemical Corps, a position he held until his retirement from that post in 1961. Dr. Dill was then 70 years old—an age he considered too young for retirement—so he moved his exercise research to Indiana University, where he served as a senior physiologist until 1966. In 1967 he obtained funding to establish the Desert Research Laboratory at the University of Nevada at Las Vegas. Dr. Dill used this laboratory as a base for his studies on human tolerance to exercise in the desert and at high altitude. He continued his research and writing until his final retirement at age 93, the same year he produced his last publication, a book entitled *The Hot Life of Man and Beast*.[4] Dr. Dill once bragged to me [DLC] that he was the only scientist to have retired four times.

As the busy executive goes out for her morning jog or the point guard directs his team down the basketball court on a fast break, their bodies must make many adjustments that require a series of complex interactions involving most body systems. Consider a few examples:

- The skeletal system provides the basic framework through which muscles act.
- The cardiovascular system delivers nutrients to the body's various cells and removes waste products.
- The cardiovascular and respiratory systems together provide oxygen to the cells and remove carbon dioxide.
- The integumentary system (skin) helps maintain body temperature by allowing exchange of heat between the body and its surroundings.
- The urinary system helps maintain fluid and electrolyte balance and provides long-term regulation of blood pressure.
- The nervous and endocrine systems coordinate and direct all this activity to meet the body's needs.

Adjustments occur even at the cellular level. For example, to enable muscles to contract, various enzymes are activated and energy is generated.

Physical activity is a complicated process. Scientists must examine each adjustment that the body makes by observing these events both singly and collectively. In this chapter, we will discuss how they approach this task.

The Focus of Exercise and Sport Physiology

Exercise and sport physiology have evolved from anatomy and physiology. Anatomy is the study of an organism's structure, or morphology. From anatomy, we learn the basic structure of various body parts and their interrelationships. Physiology is the study of body function. In physiology, we study how our organ systems, tissues, and cells work and how their functions are integrated to regulate our internal environments. Because physiology focuses on the functions of structures, we can't easily discuss physiology without understanding anatomy.

Exercise physiology is the study of how our bodies' structures and functions are altered when we are exposed to acute and chronic bouts of exercise. Sport physiology further applies the concepts of exercise physiology to training the athlete and enhancing the athlete's sport performance. Thus sport physiology is derived from exercise physiology.

> ## KEY POINT
>
> **Exercise physiology has evolved from its parent discipline, physiology. It is concerned with the study of how the body adapts physiologically to the acute stress of exercise, or physical activity, and the chronic stress of physical training. Sport physiology has evolved from exercise physiology. It applies exercise physiology to problems unique to sport.**

Let's consider an example to help us distinguish between these two closely related branches of physiology. In exercise physiology, through considerable research, we now better understand how our bodies derive energy from the foods we eat to permit muscle actions to initiate and sustain movement. We have learned that fat is our major energy source when we are at rest and during low-intensity exercise, but that our bodies use proportionately more carbohydrate as exercise intensity increases, until carbohydrate becomes our primary energy source. Prolonged high-intensity exercise can substantially reduce our bodies' carbohydrate stores, which can contribute to exhaustion.

Sport physiology then takes this information and, realizing that the body has limited carbohydrate energy stores, attempts to find ways to

- increase the body's carbohydrate storage capacity (carbohydrate loading),
- decrease the rate at which the body utilizes carbohydrate during physical performance (carbohydrate sparing), and
- improve the athlete's diet both before and during competition to minimize the risk of depleting carbohydrate stores.

The area of sport nutrition, a subdiscipline of sport physiology, is one of the most rapidly growing areas of research in this field.

As another example, exercise physiology has uncovered an important sequence of events that occur when the body is trained beyond its ability to adapt, a condition known as overtraining. Sport physiology has applied this information to both the design and the evaluation of training programs to reduce the risk of overtraining.

But sport physiology is not merely applied exercise physiology. Because exercise physiology also has its own applications, it is often hard to clearly distinguish the two. For this reason, exercise and sport physiology are often considered together, as they are in this text. Now let's look at how exercise physiology, the parent discipline of sport physiology, has evolved through the years.

A Historical Perspective

As a beginning student of exercise physiology, you might be tempted to think that the information in this book is new and is the final word on each topic. Contributions of contemporary exercise physiologists might seem to present new ideas never before treated to the rigors of science, but this is not the case. Rather, the information we'll explore represents the lifelong efforts of many outstanding scientists who have helped piece together the puzzle of human movement. Often, the thoughts and theories of today's physiological detectives were shaped by the efforts of scientists who are long forgotten. What we consider as original or new is most often an assimilation of previous findings or the application of basic science to problems in exercise physiology. To help you appreciate this, let's briefly reflect on the history and people that have shaped the field of exercise physiology.

The Beginnings of Anatomy and Physiology

Although the ancient Greeks made a fair start at studying the function of the human body, not until the 1500s were any truly significant contributions made to understanding both the structure and function of the human body. Anatomy was the forerunner of physiology. A landmark text by Andreas Vesalius, entitled *Fabrica Humani Corporis* [*Structure of the Human Body*], published in 1543, changed the direction of future studies. Though Vesalius's book focused primarily on anatomical descriptions of various organs, the book occasionally attempted to explain their functions as well. British historian Sir Michael Foster said, "This book is the beginning, not only of modern anatomy, but of modern physiology. It ended, for all time, the long reign of fourteen centuries of precedent and began in a true sense the renaissance of medicine."[6]

Most early attempts at explaining physiology were either incorrect or so vague that they could be considered only speculation. Attempts to explain how a muscle generates force, for example, were usually limited to a description of its change in size and shape during action because observations were limited to what could be seen with the eye. From such observations, Hieronymus Fabricius (ca. 1574) suggested that a muscle's contractile power resided in its fibrous tendons, not in its "flesh." Anatomists didn't discover the existence of individual muscle fibers until Dutch scientist Anton van Leeuwenhoek introduced the microscope (around 1660). But how these fibers shortened and created force remained a mystery until the middle of the present century, when the intricate workings of muscle proteins could be studied by electron microscopy.

The Emergence of Exercise Physiology

Exercise physiology is a relative newcomer to the world of science. Before the late 19th century, physiologists' major goal was to gain information of clinical value. The body's response to exercise received almost no attention. Although the value of regular physical activity was well known in the mid-1800s, the physiology of muscular activity gained little attention until the latter part of that century.

The first published textbook on exercise physiology was written by Fernand LaGrange in 1889, entitled *Physiology of Bodily Exercise*.[9] Considering the small amount of research on exercise that had been conducted at that time, it is intriguing to read the author's accounts of such topics as "Muscular Work," "Fatigue," "Habituation to Work," and "The Office of the Brain in Exercise." This early attempt to explain the body's response to exercise was, in many ways, limited to a lot of rambling theory and little fact. Although some basic concepts of exercise biochemistry were emerging at that time, LaGrange was quick to admit that many details were still in the formative stages. For example, he stated that ". . . vital combustion (energy metabolism) has become very complicated of late; we may say that it is somewhat perplexed, and that it is difficult to give in a few words a clear and concise summary of it. It is a chapter of physiology which is being rewritten, and we cannot at this moment formulate our conclusions."[9]

The first published textbook on exercise physiology was an 1889 work by Fernand LaGrange entitled *Physiology of Bodily Exercise*.

During the late 1800s, many theories were proposed to explain the source of energy for muscle contraction. Muscles were known to generate much heat during exercise, so some theories suggested that this heat was used directly or indirectly to cause muscle fibers to shorten. After the turn of the century, Walter Fletcher and Sir Frederick Gowland Hopkins observed a close relationship between muscle action and lactate formation.[5] This observation led to the realization that energy for muscle action is derived from the breakdown of muscle glycogen to lactic acid (chapter 5), though the details of this reaction remained obscure.

Because the energy demands for muscle action are high, this tissue served as an ideal model to help unravel the mysteries of cellular metabolism. In 1921, Archibald (A.V.) Hill (see Figure 1.1) was awarded the Nobel prize for his findings on energy metabolism. At that time, biochemistry was in its infancy, though rapidly gaining recognition through the research efforts of such Nobel laureates as Albert Szent Gorgyi, Otto Meyerhof, August Krogh, and Hans Krebs, who were all actively studying how living cells generate energy.

Although much of Hill's research was conducted with isolated frog muscle, he also conducted some of the first physiological studies on runners. Such studies were possible through the technical contributions of John (J.S.) Haldane, who developed the methods and equipment needed to measure oxygen use during exercise. These and other investigators provided the basic framework for our understanding of whole-body energy production, which became the focus of considerable research during the middle of this century and is incorporated into computer-based systems used to measure oxygen uptake in exercise physiology laboratories today.

The Harvard Fatigue Laboratory

No laboratory has had more impact on the field of exercise physiology than the Harvard Fatigue Laboratory (HFL), founded in 1927. Creation of this laboratory is credited to the insightful planning of world famous biochemist Lawrence J. Henderson, who rec-

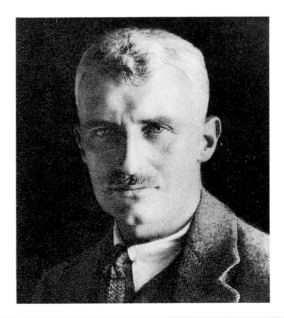

Figure 1.1 1921 Nobel prize winner Archibald (A.V.) Hill (1927).

ognized the importance of studying the physiology of human movement with special interest in the effects of environmental stress (such as heat and altitude). Henderson did not want to head the research program himself, so he appointed a young biochemist from Stanford University, David Bruce (D.B.) Dill (see Figure 1.2), as the first director.

Despite little experience in applied human physiology, Dill's creative thinking and ability to surround himself with young, talented scientists created an environment that would lay the foundation for modern exercise and environmental physiology. For example, HFL personnel examined the physiology of endurance exercise and described the physical requirements for success in events such as distance running. Some of the most outstanding HFL investigations were not conducted in the laboratory, but in the Nevada desert, the Mississippi delta, and on White Mountain in California (altitude 13,000 ft, or 3,962 m). These and other studies provided the foundation for future investigations on the effects of the environment on physical performance and human physiology.

In its earlier years, the HFL focused primarily on general problems of exercise, nutrition, and health. For example, studies on exercise and aging were first conducted in 1939 by Sid Robinson (see Figure 1.3), a student in the HFL. Based on his studies of subjects ages 6 to 91 years, Robinson described the effect of aging on maximal heart rate and oxygen uptake. But with the onset of World War II, the HFL took a different direction. Henderson and Dill realized the HFL's

potential contribution to the war effort. They and other HFL personnel were instrumental in forming new laboratories for the Army, Navy, and Army Air Corps. They also published the methodologies necessary for relevant military research; those methods are still in use throughout the world.

Today's exercise physiology students would be amazed by the technology used in the early days of the HFL and the time and energy committed to early research. What is now accomplished in mere seconds with the aid of computers and automatic analyzers demanded days of effort by HFL personnel. Measurements of oxygen uptake during exercise, for example, required collecting samples of expired air that were analyzed for oxygen and carbon dioxide using a manually operated chemical analyzer (see Figure 1.4). The analysis of a single 1-min sample of air required 20 to 30 min of effort by one or more laboratory personnel. Today, such measurements are made almost instantaneously, with little effort by laboratory personnel. We must marvel at the dedication of the HFL's pioneers of knowledge.

The Harvard Fatigue Laboratory was an intellectual center that attracted young physiologists from many places. Scholars from 15 countries worked in the HFL between 1927 and its closure in 1947. Most went on to develop their own laboratories and to become noteworthy international figures in exercise physiology. Thus, the HFL planted seeds of intellect around the world that resulted in an explosion of knowledge and interest in this new field.

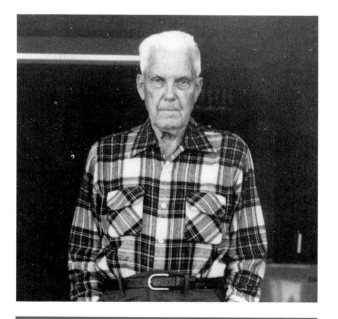

Figure 1.2   David Bruce (D.B.) Dill in the Desert Research Institute (ca. 1985).

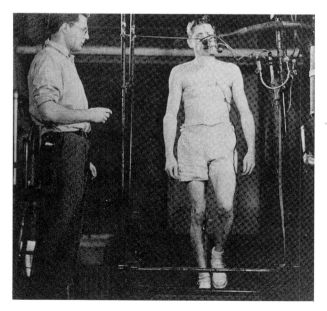

Figure 1.3   Sid Robinson (right) on the treadmill in the Harvard Fatigue Laboratory (1938).

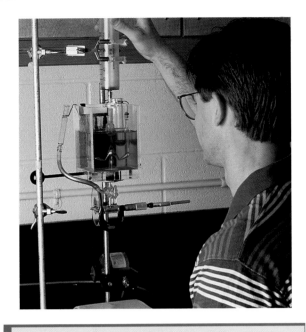

Figure 1.4   The Per Scholander gas analyzer.

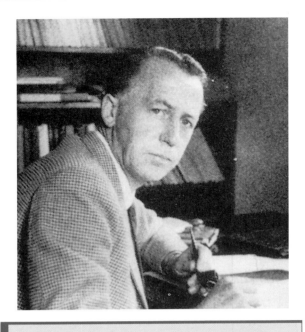

Figure 1.5   Erik Hohwü-Christensen was the first physiology professor at the College of Physical Education at Gymnastik-och Idrottshogskolan.

KEY POINT

The Harvard Fatigue Laboratory became the mecca of exercise physiology in the late 1920s until its closure in 1947. Founded by biochemist L.J. Henderson and directed by D.B. Dill, this laboratory trained most of those who became world leaders in exercise physiology through the 1950s and 1960s. Most contemporary exercise physiologists can trace their roots back to the Harvard Fatigue Laboratory.

The Scandinavian Influence

Early contacts between D.B. Dill and August Krogh, a Danish Nobel prize winner, led to the coming of three exceptional Danish physiologists to the Harvard Fatigue Laboratory in the 1930s. Krogh encouraged Erik Hohwü-Christensen, Erling Asmussen, and Marius Nielsen to spend time at Harvard studying exercise in the heat and at high altitude. After returning to Scandinavia, each man established a separate line of research. Asmussen and Nielsen became professors at the University of Copenhagen. Asmussen studied the mechanical properties of muscle and Nielsen studied body temperature control. Both remained active at the University of Copenhagen's August Krogh Institute until their retirements.

In 1941, Hohwü-Christensen (see Figure 1.5) moved to Stockholm to become the first physiology professor at the College of Physical Education at Gymnastik-och Idrottshogskolan (GIH). In the late 1930s he teamed with Ole Hansen to conduct and publish a series of five studies of carbohydrate and fat metabolism during exercise. These studies still are cited frequently and are considered among the first and most important sport nutrition studies. Hohwü-Christensen introduced Per-Olof Åstrand to the field of exercise physiology. Åstrand, who conducted numerous studies related to physical fitness and endurance capacity during the 1950s and 1960s, became the director of GIH after Hohwü-Christensen retired in 1960. Åstrand and Hohwü-Christensen were also the mentors of Bengt Saltin, one of today's leading contributors to our understanding of muscle metabolism during exercise.

In addition to their work at the Gymnastik-och Idrottshogskolan, both Hohwü-Christensen and Åstrand interacted with physiologists at the Karolinska Institute in Stockholm who studied clinical applications of exercise. It is hard to single out the most exceptional contributions from this institute, but Jonas Bergstrom's reintroduction of the biopsy needle (ca. 1966) to sample muscle tissue was a pivotal point in the study of human muscle biochemistry and muscle nutrition. This technique, which involves withdrawing a tiny sample of muscle tissue through a small incision, was first introduced in the early 1900s to study muscular dystrophy. The needle biopsy enabled physiologists to conduct histological and biochemical studies of human muscle before, during, and after exercise.

Other invasive studies of blood circulation have subsequently been conducted by physiologists at GIH and at the Karolinska Institute. Just as the Harvard Fatigue Laboratory had been the mecca of exercise physiology research between 1927 and 1947, the Scandinavian laboratories have been equally noteworthy since. Many leading investigations during the past 20 years were collaborations between American and Scandinavian exercise physiologists. (For a more detailed listing of the Scandinavian contributions to exercise physiology, consult Åstrand's review.[1])

Contemporary Exercise and Sport Physiology

Many advancements in exercise physiology must be credited to improvements in technology. For example, in the 1960s development of electronic analyzers to measure respiratory gases made studying energy metabolism much easier and more productive than before. This technology and radiotelemetry (which uses radio-transmitted signals), used to monitor heart rate and body temperature during exercise, were developed as a result of the U.S. space program. Although such instruments took the labor out of research, they did

---

Exercise Physiology and Other Fields

Physiology has always been the basis for clinical medicine. In the same manner, exercise physiology has provided essential knowledge for many other areas, such as physical education, physical fitness, and health promotion. Although physical educators such as Dudley Sargent, J.H. McCurdy, and others studied the effects of physical training on strength and endurance, Peter Karpovich, a Russian immigrant who had been briefly associated with the Harvard Fatigue Laboratory, must be credited with introducing physiology to physical education in the United States. Karpovich established his own research facility and taught physiology at Springfield College (Massachusetts) from 1927 until his death in 1968. Although he made numerous contributions to physical education and exercise physiology research, he is best remembered for the outstanding students he advised.

Another Springfield faculty member, swim coach T.K. Cureton (see Figure 1.6), created an exercise physiology laboratory at the University of Illinois in 1941. He continued his research and taught many of today's leaders in physical fitness and exercise physiology until his retirement in 1971. Physical fitness programs developed by Cureton and his students and Kenneth Cooper's 1968 book, *Aerobics*, established a physiological rationale for using exercise to promote a healthy lifestyle.[2]

Although there was some awareness as early as the mid-1800s of a need for regular physical activity to maintain optimal health, this idea did not gain popular acceptance until the late 1960s. Subsequent research continues to support the importance of exercise in resisting the physical decline associated with aging.

Awareness of the need for physical activity has alerted the public to the importance of preventive medicine and the establishment of wellness programs. Though exercise physiology cannot be given credit for the current wellness movement, it provided the basic knowledge and justification for the inclusion of exercise as an integral component of a healthy lifestyle and laid the foundation for the science of exercise prescription in both sickness and health.

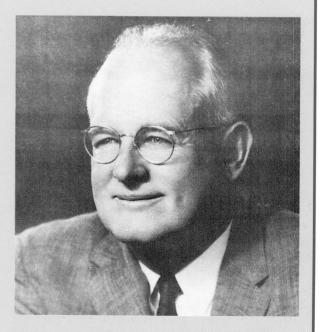

Figure 1.6 Thomas (T.K.) Cureton directed the exercise physiology laboratory at the University of Illinois at Urbana-Champaign from 1941 to 1971.

not alter the direction of scientific inquiry. Until the late 1960s, most exercise physiology studies focused on the whole body's response to exercise. The majority of investigations were measurements of such variables as oxygen uptake, heart rate, body temperature, and sweat rate. Cellular responses to exercise received little attention.

At about the time Bergstrom reintroduced the needle biopsy procedure, a new breed of exercise physiologists, well trained as biochemists, emerged. In Stockholm, Bengt Saltin (see Figure 1.7) realized the value of this procedure for studying muscle structure and biochemistry. He first collaborated with Bergstrom in the late 1960s to study the effects of diet on muscle endurance and muscle nutrition. About the same time, Reggie Edgerton (University of California, Los Angeles) and Phil Gollnick (Washington State University) were using rats to study the characteristics of individual muscle fibers and their responses to training. Saltin combined his knowledge of the biopsy procedure with Gollnick's biochemical talents. These researchers were responsible for many early studies on human muscle fiber characteristics and use during exercise. Although many biochemists have used exercise to study metabolism, few have had more impact on the current direction of human exercise physiology than Bergstrom, Saltin, and Gollnick.

Now that we have an understanding of the historical basis for the discipline of exercise physiology, from which sport physiology emerged, we can explore the scope of exercise and sport physiology.

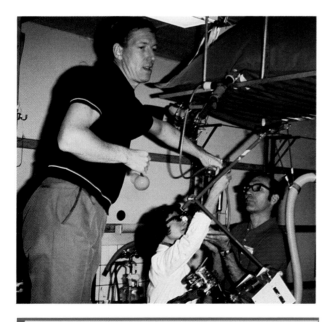

Figure 1.7   (From left) Bengt Saltin, Anne Britt (technician), and Phil Gollnick conducting research at the Gymnastik-och Idrottshogskolan (1972).

Athletes have served as subjects in exercise physiology studies since the early days at the Harvard Fatigue Laboratory. Most often, these athletes were used to assess the upper limits of human strength and endurance and to ascertain the characteristics needed for record-setting performances. Some attempts have been made to use the technology and knowledge derived from exercise physiology to predict performance, to prescribe training, or to identify athletes with exceptional potential. In most cases, however, these applications of physiological testing are of little more than academic interest because few laboratory or field tests can accurately assess all the qualities required to become a champion.

The Acute Physiological Responses to Exercise

When you begin your study of exercise and sport physiology, you must first learn how your body responds to an individual bout of exercise, such as running on a treadmill. This response is called an acute response. You can then better understand the chronic adaptations your body makes when it is challenged with repeated bouts of exercise, such as changes in your cardiovascular function following 6 months of endurance training. In the following sections, we address basic concerns, concepts, and principles associated with both acute responses to exercise and chronic adaptations to training. This material is vital to your understanding of much of the material in later chapters.

How are physiological responses to exercise determined? Neither the highly skilled athlete nor the recreational jogger perform their daily runs in environments that permit extensive physiological monitoring. Few selected physiological variables can be monitored during exercise in the field, but some can be assessed accurately without disrupting performance. For example, radiotelemetry and miniature tape recorders can be used during activity to monitor

- heart activity (heart rate and electrocardiogram),
- respiration rate,
- skin and deep body temperature, and
- muscle activity (electromyogram).

Recent developments even allow direct monitoring of oxygen consumption during free-ranging activity outside the confines of the research laboratory. Unfortunately, most often participants must be evaluated in the laboratory where they can be studied more thoroughly and under tightly controlled conditions.

Factors to Consider During Monitoring

Many factors can alter your body's acute response to a bout of exercise. For example, environmental conditions must be carefully controlled. Factors such as the temperature and humidity of the laboratory and the amount of light and noise in the test area can markedly affect your body's response, both at rest and during exercise. Even the time and size of your last meal must be controlled.

To illustrate this, Table 1.1 shows how varying environmental factors can alter heart rate at rest and during running on a treadmill at 14 kph (9 mph). The subject's heart rate response during exercise differed by 25 beats per minute when the temperature was increased from 21 °C to 35 °C (70 °F to 95 °F). Most physiological variables normally assessed during exercise are similarly influenced by environmental fluctuations. Whether comparing a person's test results from different days or comparing one person's results to another's, these factors must be carefully controlled.

Table 1.1   Variations in Heart Rate Response to Running at 14 kph on a Treadmill With Environmental Alterations

Environmental factor	Heart rate, beats per min	
	Rest	Exercise
Temperature (50% humidity)		
21 °C (70 °F)	60	165
35 °C (95 °F)	70	190
Humidity (21 °C)		
50%	60	165
90%	65	175
Noise level (21 °C, 50% humidity)		
Low	60	165
High	70	165
Food intake (21 °C, 50% humidity)		
Small meal 3 hr before exercising	60	165
Large meal 30 min before exercising	70	175

KEY POINT

Conditions under which research participants are monitored, both at rest and during exercise, must be carefully controlled. Environmental factors, such as temperature, humidity, altitude, and noise, can affect the magnitude of response of all basic physiological systems. Likewise, diurnal and menstrual cycles must be controlled for.

Physiological responses, both at rest and during exercise, also vary throughout the day. The term diurnal variation refers to fluctuations that occur during a normal 24-hr day. Table 1.2 illustrates this variation for heart rate when at rest, during various levels of exercise, and during recovery. Deep body (rectal) temperature shows similar fluctuations throughout the day. As seen in Table 1.2, tests of the same person in the morning on one day and in the afternoon on the next can produce quite different results. Test times must be standardized to control for this diurnal effect.

At least one other cycle must also be considered. The normal 28-day menstrual cycle often involves considerable variations in

- body weight,
- total body water,
- body temperature,
- metabolic rate,
- heart rate, and
- stroke volume (the amount of blood leaving the heart with each contraction).

These variables must be controlled for when testing women. Testing should always be conducted at the same point in the menstrual cycle.

Use of Ergometers

When physiological responses to exercise are assessed in a laboratory study, the participant's physical effort

Table 1.2   An Example of Diurnal Variations in Heart Rate at Rest and During Exercise

Condition	Time of day					
	2 a.m.	6 a.m.	10 a.m.	2 p.m.	6 p.m.	10 p.m.
	Heart rate, beats per minute					
Resting	65	69	73	74	72	69
Light exercise	100	103	109	109	105	104
Moderate exercise	130	131	138	139	135	134
Maximal exercise	179	179	183	184	181	181
Recovery, 3-min	118	122	129	128	128	125

Data from Reilly and Brooks (1990).

must be controlled to provide a constant and known rate of work. This is generally accomplished by using ergometers. An ergometer (ergo = work; meter = measure) is an exercise device that allows the amount and rate of a person's physical work to be controlled (standardized) and measured. Let's consider some examples.

Cycle Ergometers

For many years the cycle ergometer was the primary testing device in use. It is still used extensively in both research and clinical settings today, although the trend in the United States has been toward more widespread use of treadmills. Cycle ergometers can be used by a person either in the normal upright position (see Figure 1.8) or in the supine position.

Cycle ergometers are generally based on one of four types of resistance:

1. Mechanical friction
2. Electrical resistance
3. Air resistance
4. Hydraulic fluid resistance

With mechanical friction devices, a belt encompassing a flywheel is tightened or loosened to adjust the resistance against which you pedal. Your power output depends on your pedal rate—the faster you pedal, the greater your power output. To maintain the same power output throughout the test, you must maintain the same pedal rate, so pedal rate must be constantly monitored.

With electrical resistance devices, also known as electrically braked cycle ergometers, resistance is provided by an electrical conductor that moves through a magnetic or electromagnetic field. The strength of the magnetic field determines the resistance to pedaling. The resistance increases automatically as your pedal rate decreases, and decreases as your pedal rate increases, to provide a constant power output.

Air resistance cycle ergometers (see Figure 1.9) are quite popular, although more for training purposes than for laboratory testing. In these devices, the flywheel of a standard mechanically braked ergometer is replaced by a wheel that contains a series of fan blades arranged like spokes. The fan blades displace air as the wheel turns, so the resistance encountered is directly proportional to the pedaling rate.

Cycle ergometers that use hydraulic fluid to vary resistance can produce constant power outputs independent of pedal rate. As you pedal the ergometer, hydraulic fluid is forced through an opening. Varying the size of this opening allows variation of the resistance against which you pedal. The larger the opening, the easier the fluid can flow and the less resistance you experience.

Cycle ergometers offer some advantages over other ergometric devices. Your upper body remains relatively immobile when you use a cycle ergometer, allowing more accurate determination of blood pressure and easier blood sampling during exercise. Furthermore, the rate of work when you pedal does not depend on your body weight. This is important when investigating physiological responses to a standard rate

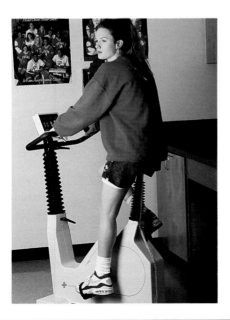

Figure 1.8 A cycle ergometer.

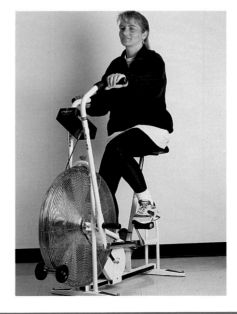

Figure 1.9 An air-braked cycle ergometer.

of work (power output). As an example, if you lost 15 lb, data derived from treadmill testing could not be compared to data obtained before your weight loss, because physiological responses to a set speed and grade on the treadmill vary with body weight. After the weight loss, you would do less physical work than before at the same speed and grade. With the cycle ergometer, weight loss does not have as great an effect on your physiological response to a standardized power output.

KEY POINT

Cycle ergometers are the most appropriate devices for evaluating changes in submaximal physiological function before and after training in people whose weights have changed. Resistance on a cycle ergometer is independent of body weight, but the work performed on a treadmill is directly related to it.

Cycle ergometers also have disadvantages. If you don't cycle regularly, your leg muscles will likely fatigue before your body does. In addition, peak (maximal) values for some physiological variables obtained on a cycle ergometer are frequently lower than comparable values obtained on a treadmill. This may be due to local leg fatigue, blood pooling in the legs (less blood returns to the heart), or the use of less muscle mass during cycling than during treadmill exercise.

Treadmills

Treadmills (see Figure 1.10) are now the ergometers of choice for an increasing number of researchers and clinicians, particularly in the United States. With these devices, a motor and pulley system drives a large belt on which you can either walk or run. Belt length and width must accommodate your body size and stride length. It is nearly impossible to test elite athletes on treadmills that are too narrow or too short.

Treadmills offer a number of advantages. Unlike most cycle ergometers, the rate of work on a treadmill need not be monitored closely—if you don't maintain the belt speed, you are carried off the back of the device. Treadmill walking is a very natural activity, so individuals normally adjust to the skill required within 1 to 2 min. Also, average people almost always achieve their highest physiological values on the treadmill, although some athletes achieve higher values on ergometers that more closely match their mode of training or competition.

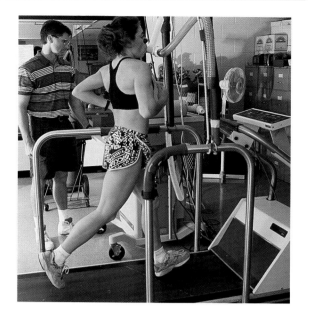

Figure 1.10   A treadmill.

KEY POINT

Treadmills generally produce higher peak values for almost all assessed physiological variables, such as heart rate, ventilation, and oxygen uptake.

Treadmills also have certain disadvantages. They are generally more expensive than cycle ergometers. They are also bulky, require electrical power, and are not very portable. Accurate measurement of blood pressure during treadmill exercise can be difficult because the noise associated with normal treadmill operation makes hearing through a stethoscope difficult. Also, obtaining accurate blood pressure measurements becomes difficult when treadmill speed requires jogging. Obtaining blood samples from a person who is on a treadmill is also difficult.

Other Ergometers

Other ergometers allow athletes who compete in specific sports or events to be tested in a manner that closely approximates their training and competition. For example, arm ergometers, shown in Figure 1.11a, are used to test athletes or nonathletes who primarily use their arms and shoulders in physical activity (such as swimmers). The rowing ergometer, seen in Figure 1.11b, was devised to test competitive oarsmen.

Valuable research data have been obtained by instrumenting swimmers and monitoring them during swimming in a pool. However, the problems associated

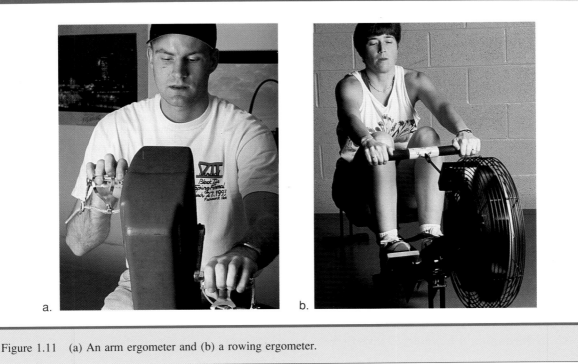

a.

b.

Figure 1.11   (a) An arm ergometer and (b) a rowing ergometer.

with turns and constant movement led investigators to try tethered swimming, in which the swimmer is attached to a harness connected to a rope, a series of pulleys, and a pan containing weights. This arrangement is depicted in Figure 1.12a. The swimmer swims at a pace that maintains a constant body position in the pool. As weights are added to the pan, the swimmer must swim faster (work harder) to maintain position.

Although important data have come from tethered swimming, the swimmer's technique is not at all similar to that used in free swimming. The swimming flume, seen in Figure 1.12b, allows swimmers to more closely simulate their natural swimming strokes. The swimming flume operates by propeller pumps that circulate water past the swimmer, who attempts to maintain body position in the flume. The pump circulation

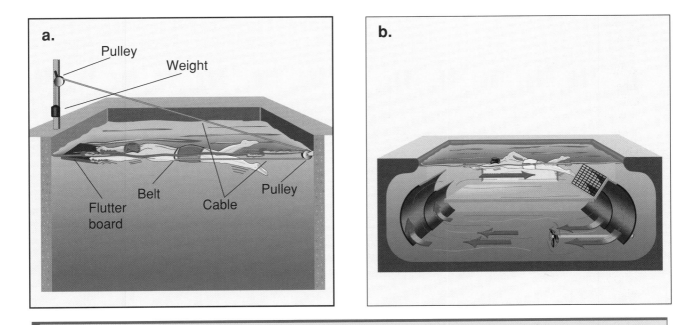

a.

Pulley

Weight

Belt

Pulley

Cable

Flutter board

b.

Figure 1.12   (a) Tethered swimming and (b) a swimming flume.

can be increased or decreased to vary the speed at which the swimmer must swim. The swimming flume, unfortunately very expensive, has at least partially resolved the problems with tethered swimming and has created new opportunities to investigate the sport.

Specificity of Exercise Testing

When choosing an ergometer for testing, the concept of test specificity is particularly important with highly trained athletes, as has been illustrated by two research

---

IN REVIEW ...

1. A major area of interest for exercise physiologists is the body's acute responses to individual bouts of exercise.
2. When researchers assess acute responses, environmental conditions, such as temperature, humidity, light, and noise, must be carefully controlled so that variations in these factors do not alter the body's responses.
3. Diurnal (daily) cycles and the menstrual cycle must also be considered. Testing should be conducted at the same time of day and at the same point in the menstrual cycle.
4. An ergometer is a device that allows the amount and rate of physical work to be measured under standardized conditions.
5. Cycle ergometers allow easier blood pressure assessment and blood sampling because the upper body remains relatively immobile. Results on these devices also are not greatly affected by changes in body weight.
6. Treadmills ensure that the rate of work remains relatively constant because a person cannot stay on the treadmill if the work rate is not maintained. Treadmill walking is also a very natural activity. But the results depend on body weight, and measuring physiological change is more difficult than on a cycle ergometer. Maximum physiological values are generally higher when tested on the treadmill.
7. Tethered swimming has provided valuable information about physiological responses, but swimmers' movements are not very natural with this method. The swimming flume, however, allows free swimming and provides results that can be applied to competitive and recreational swimming.
8. When assessing the body's responses to exercise, it is essential that the mode of testing be carefully matched to the type of activity a person usually performs.

---

studies.[8,10] In both studies, improvements in aerobic endurance after 10 weeks of swim training were monitored. Subjects performed maximal treadmill running and tethered swimming, both before and after training. Endurance as measured by the tethered swimming test increased by 11% to 18%, but treadmill endurance capacity did not change. If the treadmill alone had been used for testing, the researchers would have concluded that swim training had no influence on cardiorespiratory endurance capacity!

Chronic Physiological Adaptations to Training

When examining the acute response to exercise, we are concerned with the body's immediate response to an individual exercise bout. The other major area of interest in exercise and sport physiology is how the body responds over time to the stress of repeated exercise bouts. When you perform regular exercise over a period of weeks, your body adapts. The physiological adaptations that occur with chronic exposure to exercise improve both your exercise capacity and your efficiency. With resistance training, your muscles become stronger. With aerobic training, your heart and lungs become more efficient and your endurance capacity increases. These adaptations are highly specific to the type of training you do.

Basic Training Principles

In following chapters, we will discuss in detail specific physiological adaptations that result from chronic exercise, or training. Several principles can be applied to all forms of physical training. Each will be discussed as it applies to specific types of training later in this text. For now, let's examine basic training principles.

The Principle of Individuality

We were not all created with the same capacity to adapt to exercise training. Heredity plays a major role in determining how quickly and to what degree your body adapts to a training program. Except for identical twins, no two people have exactly the same genetic characteristics, so individuals are unlikely to show precisely the same adaptations to a given training program. Variations in cellular growth rates, metabolism, and neural and endocrine regulation also lead to tremendous individual variation. Such individual variation might explain why some people show great improvement after participating in a given program while others experience little or no change after following the same program. For these reasons, any training program must take into account the specific needs and abilities of the individuals for whom it is designed. This is the principle of individuality.

The Principle of Specificity

Training adaptations are highly specific to the type of activity and to the volume and intensity of the exercise performed. To improve muscular power, for example, the shot-putter would not emphasize distance running, or slow, low-intensity resistance training. Similarly, the distance runner wouldn't concentrate on sprint-type interval training. This is likely the reason why athletes who train for strength and power, such as weight lifters, often have great strength but don't have better aerobic endurance than untrained people. By the principle of specificity, the training program must stress the physiological systems that are critical for optimal performance in the given sport in order to achieve specific training adaptations.

The Principle of Disuse

Most athletes would agree that regular physical exercise improves your muscles' capacity to generate more energy and to resist fatigue. Likewise, endurance training improves your ability to perform more work for longer periods. But if you stop training, your state of fitness will drop to a level that only meets the demands of daily use. Any gains you achieved with training will be lost. This principle of disuse leads to the popular phrase, "Use it or lose it." A training program must include a maintenance plan. In chapter 13 we will examine specific physiological changes that occur when the training stimulus stops.

The Principle of Progressive Overload

Two important concepts, overload and progressive training, form the foundation of all training. According to the principle of progressive overload, all training programs must include these components. For example, to gain strength, the muscles must be overloaded, which means they must be loaded beyond the point to which they are normally loaded. Progressive resistance training implies that as the muscles become stronger, a proportionately greater resistance is required to stimulate further strength increases.

As an example, consider a young man who can perform only 10 repetitions of a bench-press before reaching fatigue, using 68 kg (150 lb) of weight. With a week or two of resistance training, he should be able to increase to 14 or 15 repetitions with the same weight. He then adds 2.3 kg (5 lb) to the bar, and his repetitions drop to 8 or 10. As he continues to train, the repetitions continue to increase, and within another week or two,

he is ready to add an additional 2.3 kg (5 lb). Thus there is a progressive increase in the amount of weight lifted. Similarly, with anaerobic and aerobic training, training volume (intensity and duration) can be increased progressively.

■ IN REVIEW . . . ■

1. A major area of concern for exercise physiologists is how the body adapts to chronic exposure to exercise, or training.
2. According to the principle of individuality, each person must be recognized as unique, and such individual variation must be allowed for when designing training programs. Different people will respond to a given training program in different ways.
3. According to the principle of specificity, to maximize the benefits, training must be specifically matched to the type of activity the person normally engages in. An athlete involved in a sport that requires tremendous strength, such as weight lifting, would not expect great strength gains from endurance running.
4. According to the principle of disuse, training benefits are lost if training is either discontinued or reduced too abruptly. To avoid this, all training programs must include a maintenance program.
5. According to the principle of progressive overload, training must involve working the body (muscles, cardiovascular system) harder than normal; as the body adapts, training progresses to a higher work level.

Types of Training Programs

Now that we understand the basic principles underlying training, we can briefly review several types of training programs. Let's examine

- resistance training,
- interval training,
- continuous training, and
- circuit training.

Resistance Training

Resistance training is specifically designed to increase strength, power, and muscular endurance. When designing a resistance training program, you must first consider the muscle groups you wish to train, then select resistance exercises accordingly. For each exer-

Table 1.3 Two-Arm Curl Resistance Training Program

Set 1	Resistance	100 lb
	Repetitions	10
Set 2	Resistance	90 lb
	Repetitions	10
Set 3	Resistance	80 lb
	Repetitions	10

cise, the workout is broken down into sets, repetitions, and resistance. Consider the example in Table 1.3, using the two-arm curl with a barbell. This program is designed for three sets, performing 10 repetitions in each set. For the first set, the resistance is 100% of the maximum weight that can be lifted only 10 times. This is referred to as the 10-repetition maximum or 10-RM. In our example, the 10-RM is 100 lb. A resistance of 90% of the 10-RM (90 lb) is used for the second set, and 80% of the 10-RM (80 lb) is used for the third set. We will consider more details about resistance training programs in chapter 4.

Interval Training

With interval training, short to moderate periods of work are alternated with short to moderate periods of rest or reduced activity. The concept has a firm physiological foundation. Researchers have demonstrated that athletes can perform considerably more work if they break the work into short intense bouts, allowing periods of rest or reduced activity between consecutive work bouts. Consider the example of a middle-distance runner's interval training program shown in Table 1.4. These two sets can be written as follows:

> Set 1: 6 × 400 m at 75 s (75-s jog)
> Set 2: 6 × 800 m at 180 s (180-s jog/walk)

Referring to the table, we see that for the first set you would run six repetitions (work intervals) of 400 m each, completing each work interval in 75 s, then recover with slow jogging for 75 s between work intervals. For the second set, you would run six repetitions of 800 m each, completing the work interval in 180 s, and recover with slow jogging or walking for 180 s between work intervals.

Interval training can be used in almost any sport or activity, but it is used most often in track, cross-country, and swimming. Interval procedures can be adapted to other activities by selecting the form or mode of training and manipulating the primary variables to fit the sport and athlete. Fox and Mathews have identified the major variables that must be individually adjusted for each athlete:[7]

- Rate and distance of the work interval (load and duration for resistance training)
- Number of repetitions and sets during each training session
- Duration of the rest (recovery) interval
- Type of activity during the rest interval
- Frequency of training per week

Continuous Training

As the name implies, continuous training involves continuous activity without rest intervals. This varies from high-intensity continuous activity of moderate duration to low-intensity activity of extended duration. Let's differentiate these types of training.

High-Intensity Continuous Training. High-intensity continuous training is performed at work intensities that represent 85% to 95% of the athlete's maximal heart rate (HR max). For example, a middle distance runner may run 8 km (5 mi), averaging a 3 min · km^{-1} (5 min · mi^{-1}) pace, with an average heart rate of 180 beats per minute (assuming a HR max of 200 beats per minute).

High-intensity continuous training is very effective for training endurance athletes without requiring high work levels that are stressful and uncomfortable. Training at a constant near-competition pace enhances a runner's ability to maintain an even pace during a race and typically results in the best race times. Furthermore, serious runners need to regularly train or race at or near their race paces to develop leg speed, leg strength, and muscular endurance. Unfortunately, the demands of such a training program are extraordinary, particularly when extended over weeks and months. Slower paced variations should be introduced periodically, such as once or twice per week, to give the athlete some relief from exhaustive, high-intensity, continuous training.

Table 1.4 Sample Interval Training Program for a Middle-Distance Runner

Set	Repetitions	Distance	Interval time	Recovery time	Recovery activity
1	6	400 m	75 s	75 s	Jog
2	6	800 m	180 s	180 s	Jog/walk

LSD Training.   Long, slow distance, or LSD, training became extremely popular during the late 1960s. With this type of training, the athlete performs at a relatively low intensity, for example at 60% to 80% of HR max. Heart rates seldom get above 160 beats per minute for the young athlete or over 140 beats per minute for the older athlete. The main objective is distance rather than speed. Endurance runners can train 24 to 48 km (15 to 30 mi) each day using LSD techniques, with weekly totals of 160 to 320 km (100 to 200 mi). The pace is considerably slower than the maximum pace the runner can sustain. For example, if you can run at a 3 min · km^{-1} (5 min · mi^{-1}) pace, you would train at a 4 to 5 min · km^{-1} (7 to 8 min · mi^{-1}) pace. This training is much more tolerable than high-intensity continuous training because LSD training places considerably less stress on the cardiovascular and respiratory systems. However, the extreme distances can result in significant muscle and joint discomfort and actual injury.

LSD training is probably the most common endurance conditioning used by

- people who want to stay in condition for health-related purposes,
- the athlete who participates in team sports and endurance-trains only for general conditioning, and
- the athlete who wants to maintain endurance conditioning during the off-season.

For these purposes, the pace is kept at 60% to 80% of HR max, but the distance is reduced. For example, runners might decrease to 5 to 8 km (3 to 5 mi).

LSD training is an excellent approach to general endurance conditioning because it is effective and can be performed at a comfortable rate of work. For the middle-aged or older person trying to attain or maintain acceptable physical fitness, LSD training is also the least risky and most judicious way to train. Very high intensity exercise in older individuals is potentially dangerous, and sprint- or burst-types of activities should not be encouraged.

Fartlek Training.   Fartlek training, or speed play, is a form of continuous exercise with a hint of interval training. It was developed in Sweden in the 1930s and is used primarily by distance runners. Fartlek runs are normally performed for 45 min or longer, during which runners can vary their pace from high speed to jogging as desired. This is free-form training, where fun is the main goal and distance and time are not considered. Fartlek training is normally performed in the countryside where there are a variety of hills. Athletes can run whatever course and speed they prefer, although their speed should periodically reach high-intensity levels. To supplement either high-intensity continuous training or interval training, many coaches have used Fartlek training because it provides variety.

Circuit Training

In circuit training, you perform a series of selected exercises or activities in a given sequence, called a circuit. A circuit usually has 6 to 10 stations. You perform a specific exercise at each station, such as push-ups or barbell curls, then proceed to the next station. You should progress through the circuit as rapidly as possible. Improvement is apparent when you can complete the circuit in less time or when you can do more work at each station, or both. Also, because you run between stations, cardiovascular conditioning increases as the stations are moved farther apart.

When circuit training merges with traditional resistance training, the result is referred to as circuit resistance training. Traditional resistance training is usually performed slowly and methodically, with very short work intervals and very long rest intervals. With circuit resistance training, you typically work at 40% to 60% of your maximum strength for periods of about 30 s, with 15-s rest intervals between work periods, although work and rest intervals can be altered. As an example, at the first station you complete as many repetitions as possible in 30 s, take a 15-s rest during which you move to the next station, and then start your next 30-s work period. This usually continues until you complete six to eight stations in the circuit. Two to three sets are normally prescribed.

Circuit resistance training provides modest increases in aerobic endurance capacity and major increases in

- strength,
- muscular endurance, and
- flexibility.

It also can significantly alter your body composition, increasing your muscle mass and decreasing your body's fat content.

Research Methodology

Throughout this book, we will discuss research studies that have led to our current understanding of how the body functions during physical activity and how this functioning is altered by training. To more easily interpret these studies, you should first understand some basic points about research methodology. Let's consider two areas.

Research Design

In this text, we will primarily refer to two basic types of research design: cross-sectional and longitudinal. With a cross-sectional research design, a large cross

1. Resistance training increases strength, power, and muscular endurance. The workout is designed around sets, repetitions, and resistance.
2. Interval training involves alternating periods of work with periods of rest or reduced activity. It allows more work to be performed overall, because some recovery occurs during the workout.
3. Continuous training is a nonstop workout with no rest intervals. High-intensity continuous training is performed at high intensities (85% to 95% of HR max) and is very effective for endurance training without requiring highly stressful and uncomfortable work levels. Long, slow distance (LSD) training uses relatively low-intensity work (60% to 80% of HR max) performed for a very long distance or duration, which places less stress on the cardiovascular and respiratory systems but can cause joint and muscle discomfort or injury.
4. Fartlek training (speed play), used primarily by distance runners, is continuous training done in an interval fashion. Runners can vary their pace at will from high speed to slow jogging. Runs are normally performed for 45 min or longer.
5. Circuit training involves a series of stations forming a circuit through which a person progresses as rapidly as possible. A different activity is performed at each station. Most circuit training allows modest increases in aerobic endurance and major increases in strength, muscular endurance, and flexibility. Cardiovascular conditioning can be enhanced by increasing the speed through the circuit and by placing stations farther apart.

- Don't run any miles per week
- Run 48 km (30 mi) per week
- Run 97 km (60 mi) per week
- Run 145 km (90 mi) per week

You would then compare the results from each group, basing your conclusions on how much running was done. This approach has been used in past studies, and scientists did find that the greater the weekly mileage, the higher the HDL-C level; this suggests a positive health benefit related to running distance.

Using the longitudinal approach to test the same question, you could design a study in which untrained people would be recruited to participate in a 12-month distance running program. You could, for example, recruit 40 people willing to begin running, then randomly assign 20 to a training group and the remaining 20 to a control group. Both groups would be followed for 12 months. Blood samples would be tested at the beginning of the study, then at 3-month intervals, concluding at 12 months when the program ends.

With this design, both the running group and the control group are followed over the entire period of the study, and you can determine changes in their HDL-C levels across each period. The control group acts as a comparison group to make certain that any changes observed in the running group are due solely to the training program and not to any other factors, such as the time of the year, or aging. Actual studies using this design to study changes in HDL-C with distance running have been conducted, but their results have not been as clear as the results of the cross-sectional studies.

However, a longitudinal research design is best suited to studying this problem. Too many factors that may taint results can influence cross-sectional designs. For example, genetic factors might interact so that those who run high mileage are also those who have high HDL-C levels. Also, different populations might follow different diets, but in a longitudinal study, diet and other variables can be more easily controlled. However, longitudinal studies are not always possible and cross-sectional studies provide some insight into these questions.

section of the population is tested at one specific time and the differences between individual groups within that population are used to estimate change in any given physiological variable across time. With a longitudinal research design, participants are tested one or more times after initial testing to measure their changes over time.

The differences between these two approaches are best understood through an example. Let's say that you want to determine if distance running increases the concentration of HDL-cholesterol (HDL-C) in the blood. HDL-C is the desirable form of cholesterol—increased concentrations of it reduce the risk for heart disease. Using the cross-sectional approach, you could, for example, test a large number of people who fall into the following categories:

KEY POINT

Longitudinal research studies are generally the most accurate for studying a given problem or issue. However, it is not always possible to use a longitudinal study, so cross-sectional studies must sometimes be used.

Research Settings

Research can be conducted either in the laboratory or in the field. Laboratory tests are usually more accurate because more specialized equipment can be used and conditions can be carefully controlled. As an example, the direct laboratory measurement of maximal oxygen uptake ($\dot{V}O_2 \text{ max}$) is considered the most accurate estimate of cardiorespiratory endurance capacity. However, some field tests, such as the 1.5-mi (2.4-km) run, are used to predict or estimate $\dot{V}O_2 \text{ max}$. The field test is not totally accurate, but it provides a reasonable estimate of $\dot{V}O_2 \text{ max}$, it is inexpensive to conduct, and you can test many people in a short time. To have your $\dot{V}O_2 \text{ max}$ measured directly, you would need to go to a university or clinical facility such as a hospital, but you could easily have your $\dot{V}O_2 \text{ max}$ estimated from your time for the 1.5-mi run.

Sometimes the field test is the most appropriate. For example, during early research on blood doping—when blood is removed from an athlete, stored, and later reinfused (see chapter 14) —all research was conducted in the laboratory. The resulting data were very accurate because they were collected under tightly controlled conditions. But they really didn't determine whether blood doping improves performance. Only later, when studies were designed that combined laboratory tests with field tests of actual racing performance, were we able to see the influence of blood doping.

IN REVIEW . . .

1. Cross-sectional research involves collecting data once from a diverse population, then making comparisons based on groups in that population.
2. Longitudinal research involves following participants over an extended period of time, collecting data at intervals to note individual changes with time. It is the more accurate design, but cannot always be done, in which case a cross-sectional design can provide some insight.
3. Research can be conducted in the laboratory or in the field. Laboratory research allows careful control of most variables and use of elaborate and very accurate equipment. Field research is less controllable and fewer equipment options are available, but participants' activity is often more natural in the field than in a laboratory. Each setting has advantages and drawbacks, and often research is conducted in both settings to get an accurate picture.

In Closing . . .

In this chapter we uncovered the roots of exercise and sport physiology. We learned that the current state of knowledge in these fields builds on the past and is merely a bridge to the future—many questions remain unanswered. We examined the two primary areas of concern for today's researcher: acute responses to exercise bouts and chronic adaptations to long-term training. We discussed basic training principles and various types of training, concluding with an overview of the most common types of research.

In Part A, we begin examining physical activity like exercise physiologists do, as we explore the essentials of movement. In the next chapter, we will examine the structure and function of skeletal muscle, how it produces movement, and how it responds during exercise.

Key Terms

acute response
chronic adaptation
circuit resistance training
circuit training
continuous training
cross-sectional research design
cycle ergometer
diurnal variation
ergometer
exercise physiology
Fartlek training (speed play)
high-intensity continuous training
interval training
longitudinal research design
long, slow distance (LSD) training
principle of disuse
principle of individuality
principle of progressive overload
principle of specificity
resistance training
sport physiology
swimming flume
test specificity
tethered swimming
treadmill

Study Questions

1. What is exercise physiology? What is sport physiology?
2. Describe the evolution of exercise physiology from the early studies of anatomy. Who were some of the key figures in the development of this field?
3. Name the originator of the Harvard Fatigue Laboratory. Who was the first director of this laboratory?
4. What were some of the areas of research emphasized by the Harvard Fatigue Laboratory personnel?
5. Name the three Scandinavian physiologists who conducted research in the Harvard Fatigue Laboratory.

6. Who was responsible for introducing the muscle biopsy needle to the study of exercise physiology? Name the physiologists who collaborated in describing the muscle fiber characteristics in humans.

7. Provide an illustration of what is meant by studying acute responses to a single bout of exercise and chronic adaptations to exercise training.

8. What are several environmental conditions that could affect your response to an acute bout of exercise? What is meant by diurnal variation? Why is it important when testing to control for environmental and diurnal conditions? Give several examples.

9. What is an ergometer? Give examples of two ergometers and explain their principle of operation.

10. What would be the appropriate ergometer to use when testing a cyclist? A distance runner? A swimmer?

11. Define the principle of individuality and provide an example.

12. Define the principle of specificity and provide an example.

13. Define the principle of disuse and provide an example.

14. Define the principle of progressive overload and provide an example.

15. Describe the major components of a resistance training program. Do the same for an interval training program.

References

1. Åstrand, P.-O. (1991). Influence of Scandinavian scientists in exercise physiology. *Scandinavian Journal of Medicine and Science in Sports*, **1**, 3-9.

2. Cooper, K.H. (1968). *Aerobics*. New York: Evans.

3. Dill, D.B. (1938). *Life, heat, and altitude*. Cambridge, MA: Harvard University Press.

4. Dill, D.B. (1985). *The hot life of man and beast*. Springfield, IL: Charles C Thomas.

5. Fletcher, W.M., & Hopkins, F.G. (1907). Lactic acid in amphibian muscle. *Journal of Physiology*, **35**, 247-254.

6. Foster, M. (1970). *Lectures on the history of physiology*. New York: Dover.

7. Fox, E.L., & Mathews, D.K. (1974). *Interval training conditioning for sports and general fitness*. Philadelphia: Saunders.

8. Gergley, T.J., McArdle, W.D., DeJesus, P., Toner, M.M., Jacobowitz, S., & Spina, R.J. (1984). Specificity of arm training on aerobic power during swimming and running. *Medicine and Science in Sports and Exercise*, **16**, 349-354.

9. LaGrange, F. (1889). *Physiology of bodily exercise*. London: Kegan Paul International, Ltd.

10. Magel, J.R., Foglia, G.F., McArdle, W.D., Gutin, B., Pechar, G.S., & Katch, F.I. (1975). Specificity of swim training on maximum oxygen uptake. *Journal of Applied Physiology*, **38**, 151-155.

Selected Readings

Åstrand, P.-O., & Rodahl, K. (1986). *Textbook of work physiology* (3rd ed.). New York: McGraw-Hill.

Bainbridge, F.A. (1931). *The physiology of muscular exercise*. London: Longmans, Green.

Bang, O., Boje, O., & Nielsen, M. (1936). Contributions to the physiology of severe muscular work. *Scandinavica Archives of Physiology*, **74**(Suppl.), 1-208.

Beecher, C.E. (1858). *Physiology and calisthenics*. New York: Harper & Brothers.

Bergstrom, J. (1962). Muscle electrolytes in man. *Scandinavian Journal of Clinical Investigation*, **14**(Suppl.), 1-110.

Brooks, G.A., & Fahey, T.D. (1984). *Exercise physiology: Human bioenergetics and its applications*. New York: Wiley.

Consolazio, C.F., Johnson, R.E., & Pecora, L.J. (1963). *Physiological measurements of metabolic functions in man*. New York: McGraw-Hill.

Costill, D.L. (1985). Practical problems in exercise physiology research. *Research Quarterly*, **56**, 378-384.

Fox, E.L., Bowers, R.W., & Foss, M.L. (1993). *The physiological basis for exercise and sport* (5th ed.). Philadelphia: Saunders.

Hill, A.V. (1923). Muscular exercise, lactic acid, and the supply utilization of oxygen. *Quarterly Journal of Medicine*, **16**, 135-171.

Hill, A.V. (1927). *Muscular movement in man: The factors governing speed and recovery from fatigue*. London: McGraw-Hill.

Hill, A.V. (1970). *First and last experiments in muscle mechanics*. Cambridge, England: Cambridge University Press.

MacDougall, J.D., Wenger, H.A., & Green, H.J. (1991). *Physiological testing of the high performance athlete* (2nd ed.). Champaign, IL: Human Kinetics.

McArdle, W.D., Katch, F.I., & Katch, V.L. (1991). *Exercise physiology: Energy, nutrition, and human performance* (3rd ed.). Philadelphia: Lea & Febiger.

McCurdy, J.H., & Larson, L. (1939). *The physiology of exercise*. Philadelphia: Lea & Febiger.

Reilly, T., & Brooks, G.A. (1990). Selective persistence of circadian rhythms in physiological responses to exercise. *Chronobiology International*, **7**, 59-67.

Robinson, S. (1938). Experimental studies of physical fitness in relation to age. *Arbeitsphysiologie*, **10**, 251-327.

Sargent, D.A. (1906). *Physical education*. Boston: Ginn.

Sargent, D.A. (1921). The physical test of a man. *American Physical Education Review*, **26**, 188-194.

Strømme, S.B., Ingjer, F., & Meen, H.D. (1977). Assessment of maximal aerobic power in specifically trained athletes. *Journal of Applied Physiology*, **42**, 833-837.

PART A

Essentials of Movement

In the introductory chapter, we explored the foundations of exercise and sport physiology. We defined these two fields of study, gained a historical perspective of their development, and established basic concepts that underlie the remainder of this book. With this foundation, we can begin our quest to understand how the human body performs physical activity. We start our journey in chapter 2, Muscular Control During Exercise, where we will focus on skeletal muscle, examining the structure and function of muscle fibers and how they produce body movement. We will learn how muscle fiber types differ and why these differences are important to specific types of activity. In chapter 3, Neurological Control of Movement, we will discuss how the nervous system coordinates muscle action by integrating sensory information coming in from all parts of the body, then signaling the appropriate muscles to act. Finally, in chapter 4, Neuromuscular Adaptations to Resistance Training, we will learn how the muscular system and nervous system adapt when they are subjected to several weeks or months of resistance training. We will examine changes in individual muscle fibers and neural control, how these changes improve performance in resistance activities, and how to design a resistance training program to maximize the benefits.

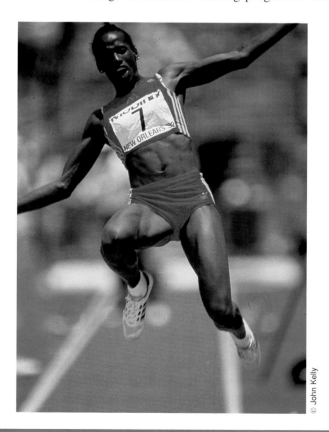

© John Kelly

Chapter 2
Muscular Control of Movement

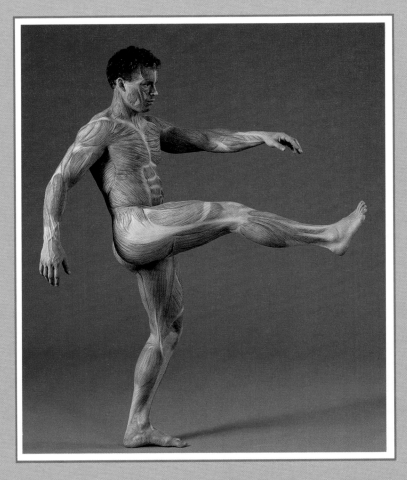

Chapter Overview

All human movement, from the blinking of an eye to the running of a marathon, depends on the proper functioning of skeletal muscle. Whether it is the strained effort of a sumo wrestler or the graceful pirouette of a ballerina, physical activity can be accomplished only through muscle force.

In this chapter we will examine the nature of skeletal muscle. We will begin by reviewing basic anatomy and physiology, examining muscle at both the gross and the microscopic levels. Then we will discuss how muscle functions during exercise and how the force needed to create movement is generated.

Chapter Outline

Nine-year-old Jeremy Schill weighed only 65 lb, but that didn't stop him from lifting the rear of the family's 4,100-lb car off his father's chest! The car had slipped off the jack while Rique Schill was working underneath it, pinning him under the rear axle. When Jeremy realized that his father was slowly suffocating, the third-grader lifted the car enough to enable his father to breathe and to allow his mother to place another jack under the rear bumper.

When our hearts beat, when a meal we've eaten moves through our intestines, and when we move any part of our bodies, muscle is involved. The myriad functions of the muscular system are performed by only three types of muscle:

1. Smooth
2. Cardiac
3. Skeletal

Smooth muscle is called involuntary muscle, because it is not directly under our conscious control. It is found in the walls of most blood vessels, allowing them to constrict or dilate to regulate blood flow. It is also found in the walls of most internal organs, allowing them to contract and relax, perhaps to move food along the digestive tract, to expel urine, or to give birth to a child.

Cardiac muscle is found only in the heart, comprising most of the heart's structure. It shares some characteristics with skeletal muscle but, like smooth muscle, it is not under conscious control. Cardiac muscle controls itself, with some mere fine-tuning by the nervous and endocrine systems. Cardiac muscle is discussed fully in chapter 8.

We usually pay attention only to those muscles we can consciously control. These are the skeletal, or voluntary, muscles, so named because most attach to and move the skeleton. We know many of these muscles by their names—deltoid, pectorals, biceps—but the human body contains over 215 pairs of skeletal muscles. The thumb alone is controlled by nine separate muscles!

Exercise requires movement of the body, which is accomplished through the action of skeletal muscles. Because this is an exercise and sport physiology book, our primary interest is the structure and function of skeletal muscle. However, although the anatomical structures of smooth, cardiac, and skeletal muscle differ somewhat, their principles of action are similar.

The Structure and Function of Skeletal Muscle

When we think of muscles, we tend to think of each muscle as a single unit. This is natural because a skeletal muscle seems to act as a single entity. But skeletal muscles are far more complex than that.

If you were to dissect a muscle, you would first cut through the outer connective tissue covering. This is the epimysium. It surrounds the entire muscle, holding it together. Once you cut through the epimysium, you would see small bundles of fibers wrapped in a connective tissue sheath. These bundles are called fasciculi. The connective tissue sheath surrounding each fasciculus is the perimysium.

Finally, by cutting through the perimysium and using a magnifier, you could see the muscle fibers, which are the individual muscle cells. Each muscle fiber is also covered by a sheath of connective tissue, called the endomysium.

KEY POINT

A single muscle cell is known as a muscle fiber.

Now that we know how muscle fibers fit into the whole muscle, let's look at them more closely.

The Muscle Fiber

Muscle fibers range in diameter from 10 to 80 micrometers (μm), nearly invisible to the naked eye. Most extend the entire length of the muscle. This means that a muscle fiber in the thigh may be more than 35 cm (14 in.) long! The number of muscle fibers per whole muscle varies considerably depending on the muscle's size and function.

The Sarcolemma

If you looked closely at an individual muscle fiber, you would see that it is surrounded by a plasma membrane, called the sarcolemma. At the end of each muscle fiber, its sarcolemma fuses with the tendon, which inserts into the bone. Tendons are made of fibrous cords of connective tissue that transmit the force generated by muscle fibers to the bones, thereby creating motion. So typically each individual muscle fiber is ultimately attached to bone via the tendon.

The Sarcoplasm

Inside the sarcolemma, with the aid of a microscope you could see that a muscle fiber contains successively smaller subunits, as shown in Figure 2.1. The largest of these are myofibrils, which we will discuss separately. For now, consider myofibrils to be rod-like structures running the length of the muscle fibers. A gelatin-like substance fills the spaces between the myofibrils. This is the sarcoplasm. It is the fluid part of the muscle fiber—its cytoplasm. The sarcoplasm mainly contains dissolved proteins, minerals, glycogen, fats, and the necessary organelles. It differs from the cytoplasm of most cells because it contains a large quantity of stored glycogen, as well as the oxygen-binding compound, myoglobin, which is quite similar to hemoglobin.

The Transverse Tubules.   The sarcoplasm also houses an extensive network of transverse tubules (T tubules), which are extensions of the sarcolemma (plasma membrane) that pass laterally through the muscle fiber. These tubules are interconnected as they pass among the myofibrils, allowing nerve impulses received by the sarcolemma to be transmitted rapidly to individual myofibrils. Tubules also provide pathways into the inner parts of the muscle fiber for substances carried in the extracellular fluids, such as glucose, oxygen, and ions.

The Sarcoplasmic Reticulum.   A longitudinal network of tubules, known as the sarcoplasmic reticulum (SR), is also found within the muscle fiber. These membranous channels parallel the myofibrils and loop around them. The sarcoplasmic reticulum serves as a storage site for calcium, which is essential for muscle contraction.

▬ IN REVIEW . . . ▬

1. An individual muscle cell is called a muscle fiber.
2. A muscle fiber is enclosed by a plasma membrane called the sarcolemma.
3. The cytoplasm of a muscle fiber is called the sarcoplasm.
4. The extensive tubule network found in the sarcoplasm includes T tubules, which allow communication and transport of substances throughout the muscle fiber, and the sarcoplasmic reticulum, which stores calcium.

Figure 2.2 depicts the T tubules and the sarcoplasmic reticulum. We will discuss their functions in more detail when we discuss the process of muscle action.

The Myofibril

Each individual muscle fiber contains several hundred to several thousand myofibrils. These are the contractile elements of skeletal muscle. Myofibrils appear as long strands of still smaller subunits—the sarcomeres.

Striations and the Sarcomere

Under a light microscope, skeletal muscle fibers have a distinctive striped appearance. Because of these markings, or striations, skeletal muscle is also called striated muscle. This is also seen in cardiac muscle, so it, too, can be considered striated muscle.

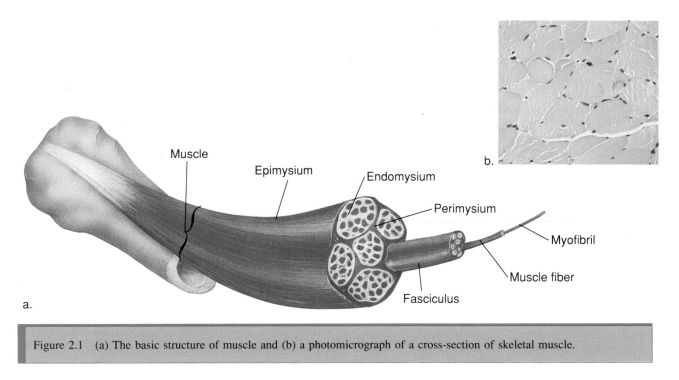

b.

Muscle
Epimysium
Endomysium
Perimysium
Myofibril
Muscle fiber
Fasciculus

a.

Figure 2.1   (a) The basic structure of muscle and (b) a photomicrograph of a cross-section of skeletal muscle.

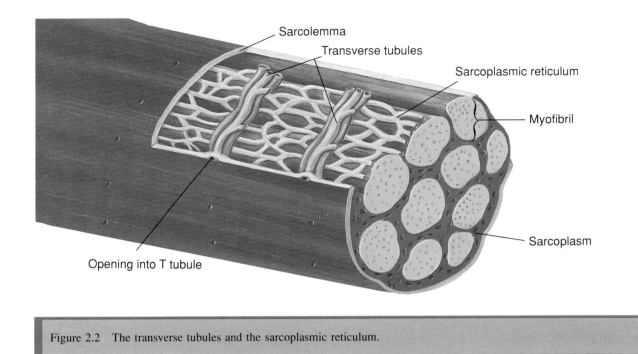

Sarcolemma

Transverse tubules

Sarcoplasmic reticulum

Myofibril

Sarcoplasm

Opening into T tubule

Figure 2.2   The transverse tubules and the sarcoplasmic reticulum.

Refer to Figure 2.3, showing myofibrils. You can clearly see the striations. Note that dark regions, known as A bands, alternate with light regions, known as I bands. Each dark A band has a lighter region in its center, the H zone, which is visible only when the myofibril is relaxed. Now refer to the light I bands. These are interrupted by a dark stripe known as the Z disk.

A sarcomere is the basic functional unit of a myofibril. Each myofibril is composed of numerous sarcomeres joined end to end at the Z disks. Each sarcomere includes what is found between each pair of Z disks, in this sequence:

- An I band (light zone)
- An A band (dark zone)
- An H zone (in the middle of the A band)
- The rest of the A band
- A second I band

KEY POINT

The sarcomere is the smallest functional unit of a muscle.

If you look at an individual myofibril through an electron microscope, you can differentiate two types of small protein filaments that are responsible for muscle action. The thinner filaments are actin, and the thicker ones are myosin. Approximately 3,000 actin and 1,500 myosin filaments lie side by side within each myofibril. The striations seen in muscle fibers result from alignment of these filaments, as illustrated in Figure 2.4. The light I band indicates the region of the sarcomere where there are only thin actin filaments. The dark A

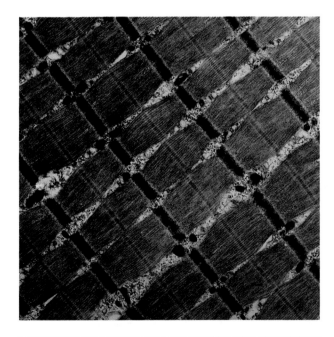

Figure 2.3   An electron micrograph of myofibrils. Note the presence of striations.

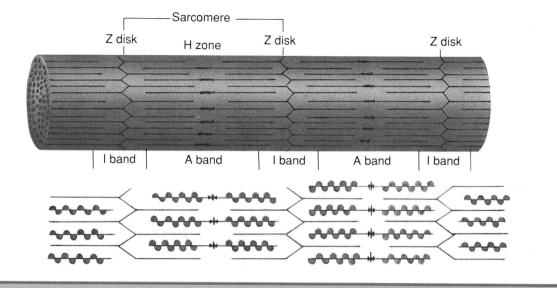

Figure 2.4   The basic functional unit of a myofibril is the sarcomere, which contains a specialized arrangement of actin and myosin filaments.

band represents the region that contains both thick myosin filaments and thin actin filaments. The H zone is the central portion of the A band that appears only when the sarcomere is in a resting state. It is occupied only by the thick filaments. The absence of the actin filaments causes the H zone to appear lighter than the adjacent A band. The H zone is visible only when the sarcomere is relaxed, because the sarcomere shortens during contraction and the actin filaments are pulled into this zone, giving it the same appearance as the rest of the A band.

Myosin Filaments.   Although we just told you that each myofibril contains about 3,000 actin filaments and 1,500 myosin filaments, those numbers are misleading. About two thirds of all skeletal muscle protein is myosin. Recall that myosin filaments are thick. Each myosin filament typically is formed by about 200 myosin molecules lined up end to end and side by side.

Each myosin molecule is composed of two protein strands twisted together (see Figure 2.5). One end of each strand is folded into a globular head, called the myosin head. Each filament contains several such heads, which protrude from the myosin filament to form cross-bridges that interact during muscle action with specialized active sites on the actin filaments.

Actin Filaments.   Each actin filament has one end inserted into a Z disk, with the opposite end extending toward the center of the sarcomere, lying in the space between the myosin filaments. Each actin filament contains an active site to which a myosin head can bind.

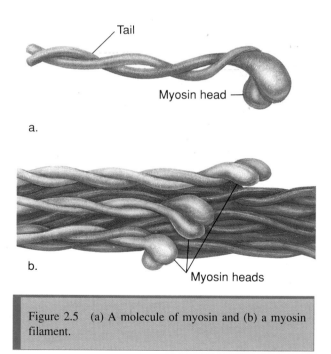

Figure 2.5   (a) A molecule of myosin and (b) a myosin filament.

Each thin filament, though referred to simply as an actin filament, is actually composed of three different protein molecules:

1. Actin
2. Tropomyosin
3. Troponin

Actin forms the backbone of the filament. Individual actin molecules are globular and join together to form strands of actin molecules. Two strands then twist into a helical pattern, much like two strands of pearls twisted together.

Tropomyosin is a tube-shaped protein that twists around the actin strands, fitting in the groove between them. Troponin is a more complex protein that is attached at regular intervals to both the actin strands and the tropomyosin. This arrangement is depicted in Figure 2.6. Tropomyosin and troponin work together in an intricate manner along with calcium ions to maintain relaxation or initiate action of the myofibril, which we will discuss later in this chapter.

■■■   IN REVIEW . . .   ■■■

1. Myofibrils are composed of sarcomeres, the smallest functional units of a muscle.
2. A sarcomere is composed of filaments of two proteins, which are responsible for muscle contraction.
3. Myosin is a thick filament, folded into a globular head at one end.
4. An actin filament is composed of actin, tropomyosin, and troponin. One end of each actin filament is attached to a Z disk.

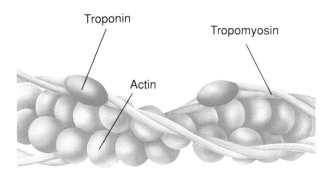

Troponin

Tropomyosin

Actin

Figure 2.6   An actin filament, composed of molecules of actin, tropomyosin, and troponin.

Muscle Fiber Action

Each muscle fiber is innervated by a single motor nerve, ending near the middle of the muscle fiber. A single motor nerve and all the muscle fibers it supplies are collectively termed a motor unit. The synapse between a motor nerve and a muscle fiber is referred to as a neuromuscular junction. This is where communication between the nervous and muscular systems occurs. Let's examine this process.

■■   KEY POINT   ■■

A motor unit consists of a single motor neuron and all the muscle fibers it supplies.

The Motor Impulse

The events that trigger a muscle fiber to act are complex. The process, depicted in Figure 2.7, is initiated by a motor nerve impulse. The neural impulse arrives at the nerve's endings, called axon terminals, which are located very close to the sarcolemma. When the impulse arrives, these nerve endings secrete a neurotransmitter substance called acetylcholine (ACh) that binds to receptors on the sarcolemma (see Figure 2.7a). If enough ACh binds to the receptors, an electrical charge will be transmitted the full length of the muscle fiber. This is known as firing, or generating, an action potential. An action potential must be generated in the muscle cell before it can act. These neural events are discussed more fully in chapter 3.

The Role of Calcium

In addition to depolarizing the fiber membrane, the electrical impulse travels through the fiber's network of tubules (T tubules and sarcoplasmic reticulum) to the interior of the cell. The arrival of an electrical charge causes the SR to release large quantities of stored calcium ions into the sarcoplasm (see Figure 2.7b).

In the resting state, tropomyosin molecules are believed to lie on top of the active sites on the actin filaments, preventing binding of the myosin heads. Once calcium ions are released from the sarcoplasmic reticulum, they bind with the troponin on the actin filaments. Troponin, with its strong affinity for calcium ions, is believed to then initiate the action process by lifting the tropomyosin molecules off of the active sites on the actin filaments. This is shown in Figure 2.7c. Because tropomyosin normally hides the active sites, it blocks the attraction between the myosin cross-bridge and actin filament. However, once the tropomyosin has been lifted off of the active sites by troponin and calcium, the myosin heads can attach to the active sites on the actin filaments.

The Sliding Filament Theory

How do muscle fibers shorten? The explanation for this phenomenon is termed the sliding filament theory.

When a myosin cross-bridge attaches to an actin filament, the two filaments slide past one another. The myosin heads and cross-bridges are thought to undergo a conformational change at the instant that they attach to the active sites on the actin filaments. The arm of the cross-bridge and the myosin head experience a strong intermolecular attraction that causes the head

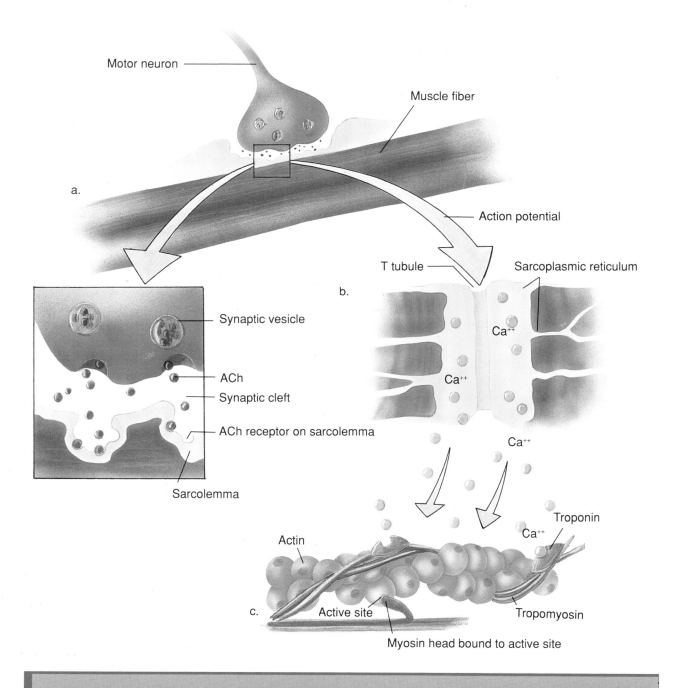

Figure 2.7 The sequence of events leading to muscle action. (a) A motor neuron releases acetylcholine (ACh), which binds to receptors on the sarcolemma. If enough ACh binds, an action potential is generated in the muscle fiber. (b) The action potential triggers Ca^{++} release from the sarcoplasmic reticulum into the sarcoplasm. (c) The Ca^{++} binds to troponin on the actin filament, and the troponin pulls tropomyosin off the active sites, allowing myosin heads to attach to the actin filament.

to tilt toward the arm and to drag the actin and myosin filaments in opposite directions (see Figure 2.8). This tilting of the head is referred to as the power stroke.

Immediately after the myosin head tilts, it breaks away from the active site, rotates back to its original position, and attaches to a new active site further along the actin filament. Repeated attachments and power strokes cause the filaments to slide past one another, giving rise to the term sliding filament theory. This process continues until the ends of the myosin filaments reach the Z disks. During this sliding (contraction), the actin filaments are brought closer to each other and protrude into the H zone, ultimately overlapping. When this occurs, the H zone is no longer visible.

The Energy for Muscle Action

Muscle action is an active process requiring energy. In addition to the binding site for actin, a myosin head contains a binding site for ATP (adenosine triphosphate). The myosin molecule must bind with ATP for muscle action to occur because ATP supplies the needed energy.

The enzyme ATPase, which is located on the myosin head, splits the ATP to yield ADP (adenosine diphosphate), P_i, and energy. The energy released from this breakdown of ATP is used to bind the myosin head to the actin filament. Thus, ATP is the chemical source of energy for muscle action. We will discuss this in much more detail in chapter 5.

The End of Muscle Action

Muscle action continues until the calcium is depleted. Calcium is then pumped back into the sarcoplasmic reticulum, where it is stored until a new nerve impulse

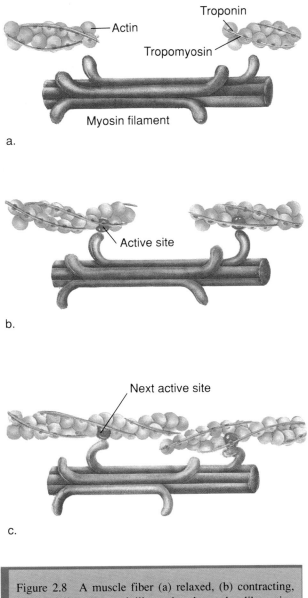

a.

b.

c.

Figure 2.8　A muscle fiber (a) relaxed, (b) contracting, and (c) fully contracted, illustrating the ratchet-like action responsible for the sliding of actin and myosin filaments.

IN REVIEW . . .

1. Muscle action is initiated by a motor nerve impulse. The motor nerve releases ACh, which opens up ion gates in the muscle cell membrane, allowing sodium to enter the muscle cell (depolarization). If the cell is sufficiently depolarized, an action potential is fired and muscle action occurs.
2. The action potential travels along the sarcolemma, then through the tubule system, and eventually causes stored calcium to be released from the sarcoplasmic reticulum.
3. Calcium binds with troponin, and then troponin lifts the tropomyosin molecules off of the active sites on the actin filament, opening these sites for binding with the myosin head.
4. Once it binds with the actin active site, the myosin head tilts, pulling the actin filament so that the two slide across each other. The tilting of the myosin head is the power stroke.
5. Energy is required before muscle action can occur. The myosin head binds to ATP, and ATPase found on the head splits ATP into ADP and P_i, releasing energy to fuel the contraction.
6. Muscle action ends when calcium is actively pumped out of the sarcoplasm back into the sarcoplasmic reticulum for storage. This process, leading to relaxation, also requires energy supplied by ATP.

arrives at the muscle fiber membrane. Calcium is returned to the sarcoplasmic reticulum by an active calcium-pumping system. This is another energy-demanding process, again relying on ATP. Thus energy is required for both the action and relaxation phases.

When the calcium is removed, troponin and tropomyosin are deactivated. This blocks the linking of the myosin cross-bridges and actin filaments and stops the use of ATP. As a result, the myosin and actin filaments return to their original relaxed state.

Skeletal Muscle and Exercise

Now that we have reviewed the overall structure of muscles and the process by which myofibrils act, we

---

The Muscle Biopsy Needle

It was once difficult to examine human muscle tissue from a live specimen. Would you want someone cutting into your body to surgically remove some muscle? Most early muscle research used muscle from laboratory animals. But technological advances now allow us to obtain samples of muscle tissue from human subjects, even during exercise.

Samples are removed by muscle biopsy, which involves removing a very small piece for analysis from the belly of a muscle. The area from which the biopsy is taken is first deadened with a local anesthetic, then a small incision (approximately 1/4 in.) is made with a scalpel through the skin, subcutaneous tissue, and fascia. A hollow needle is then inserted to the appropriate depth into the belly of the muscle (see Figure 2.9a). A small plunger is pushed through the center of the needle to snip off a very small sample of muscle.

The biopsy needle is withdrawn, and the sample, weighing 10 g to 100 g, is removed (see Figure 2.9b), cleaned of blood, mounted, and quickly frozen. It is then thinly sliced, stained, and examined under a microscope. Figure 2.9a illustrates the use of a biopsy needle to obtain a sample from the leg muscle of an elite female runner; Figure 2.9b shows a close-up view of a muscle biopsy needle.

This method allows us to study muscle fibers and gauge the effects of acute exercise and chronic training on their composition. Microscopic and biochemical analyses of the samples aid our understanding of the muscle's machinery for energy production.

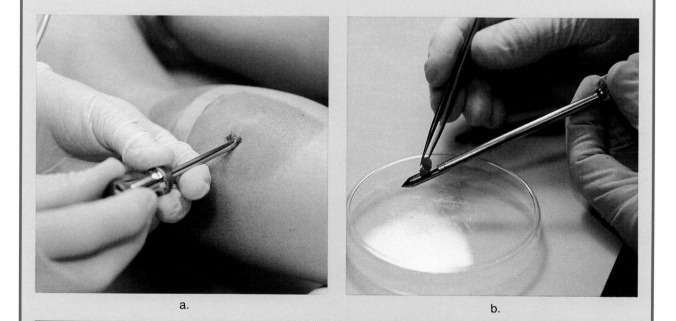

a.

b.

Figure 2.9   (a) A muscle biopsy needle is inserted into the belly of the muscle to remove a sample of muscle tissue; (b) the muscle sample that's removed can then be studied.

are ready to look more specifically at muscle function-ing during exercise. Your endurance and speed during exercise depend largely on your muscles' ability to produce energy and force. Let's examine how muscles accomplish this task.

Slow-Twitch and Fast-Twitch Muscle Fibers

Not all muscle fibers are alike. A single skeletal muscle contains two major fiber types: slow-twitch (ST) and fast-twitch (FT). Slow-twitch fibers take approxi-mately 110 ms to reach peak tension when stimulated. Fast-twitch fibers, on the other hand, can reach peak tension in about 50 ms.

Though only one type of ST fiber has been identi-fied, FT fibers can be further classified. The two major types of FT fibers are fast-twitch type a (FT_a) and fast-twitch type b (FT_b). Figure 2.10 is a micrograph of human muscle in which thinly sliced (10 μm) cross sections of a muscle sample have been chemically stained to differentiate the fiber types. The ST fibers are stained black, FT_a fibers are unstained, and FT_b fibers appear gray. Although not apparent in this figure, a third subtype of fast-twitch fibers has also been iden-tified: type c (FT_c).

The differences between the FT_a, FT_b, and FT_c fibers are not fully understood, but FT_a fibers are be-lieved to be the most frequently recruited. Only ST fibers are recruited more frequently than FT_a fibers.

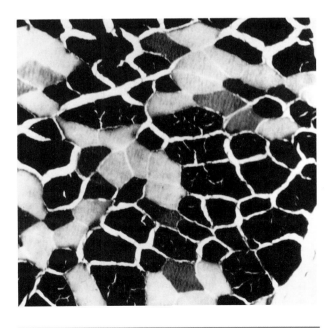

Figure 2.10 A photomicrograph showing slow-twitch (ST) and fast-twitch (FT) muscle fibers.

FT_c fibers are the least often used. On the average, most muscles are composed of roughly 50% ST fibers and 25% FT_a fibers. The remaining 25% are mostly FT_b, with FT_c fibers making up only 1% to 3% of the muscle. Because knowledge about them is limited, we will not discuss FT_c fibers further. The exact percent-ages of these fiber types in various muscles vary greatly, so the numbers listed here are averages.

Characteristics of ST and FT Fibers

Knowing that there are different muscle fiber types, we need to understand their significance. What roles do they play in physical activity? To answer this, let's first examine how the fiber types differ.

ATPase. The ST and FT fiber types derive their names from the difference in their speed of action. This differ-ence results primarily from different forms of myosin ATPase. Recall that myosin ATPase is the enzyme that splits ATP to release energy to drive contraction or allow relaxation. ST fibers have a slow form of myosin ATPase, whereas FT fibers have a fast form. In response to neural stimulation, ATP is split more rapidly in FT fibers than in ST fibers. As a result, the FT fibers have energy for contraction available more quickly than the ST fibers.

The system used to classify muscle fibers employs a chemical stain applied to a thin slice of tissue. This staining technique acts on the ATPase in the fibers. Thus the ST, FT_a, and FT_b fibers stain differently, as we saw in Figure 2.10. This technique makes it appear that each muscle fiber has only one type of ATPase, but fibers can have a mixture of ATPase types. Some have a predomi-nance of ST-ATPase, but others have mostly FT-ATPase. Their appearance in a stained slide preparation should be viewed as a continuum, rather than as absolutely dis-tinct types.

Table 2.1 summarizes the characteristics of the dif-ferent muscle fiber types. The table also includes alterna-tive names that are used in other classification systems to refer to the muscle fiber types.

Sarcoplasmic Reticulum. FT fibers have a more highly developed sarcoplasmic reticulum than do ST fi-bers. Thus, FT fibers are more adept at delivering calcium into the muscle cell when stimulated. This ability is thought to contribute to the faster speed of action of FT fibers.

Motor Units. Recall that a motor unit is a single motor neuron and the muscle fibers it innervates. The neuron appears to determine whether the fibers are ST or FT. The motor neuron in a ST motor unit has a small cell body and innervates a cluster of 10 to 180 muscle fibers. In contrast, a FT motor unit has a larger cell body and more axons and innervates from 300 to 800 muscle fibers.

Table 2.1   Classification of Muscle Fiber Types

System 1 System 2 System 3	Fiber classification		
	Slow-twitch Type I SO	Fast-twitch a Type IIa FOG	Fast-twitch b Type IIb FG
Characteristic			
Oxidative capacity	High	Moderately high	Low
Glycolytic capacity	Low	High	Highest
Contractile speed	Slow	Fast	Fast
Fatigue resistance	High	Moderate	Low
Motor unit strength	Low	High	High

Note. In this text we use System 1 to classify muscle fiber types. Other systems are also often used. System 2 classifies ST fibers as Type I and FT fibers as Type IIa and Type IIb. System 3 classifies the fiber types based on the fibers' contraction speed and primary mode of energy production. ST fibers are referred to as SO (slow oxidative) fibers, FT_a fibers are FOG (fast oxidative glycolytic) fibers, and FT_b are considered FG (fast glycolytic) fibers.

Such an arrangement of the motor units means that when a single ST motor neuron stimulates its fibers, far fewer muscle fibers contract than when a single FT motor neuron stimulates its fibers. Consequently, FT motor fibers reach peak tension faster and generate relatively more force than ST fibers do. However, the strength of individual ST and FT fibers is not dramatically different.[1]

KEY POINT

The difference in force development between FT and ST motor units is due to the number of muscle fibers per motor unit, not the force generated by each fiber.

Distribution of Fiber Types

As mentioned earlier, the percentages of ST and FT fibers are not the same in all the muscles of the body. Generally, a person's arm and leg muscles have similar fiber compositions. Studies have shown that people with a predominance of ST fibers in their leg muscles will likely have a high percentage of ST fibers in their arm muscles as well. A similar relationship exists for FT fibers. There are some exceptions, however. The soleus muscle (deep to the gastrocnemius in the calf), for example, is almost completely composed of ST fibers in everyone.

Fiber Type and Exercise

We've looked at various ways in which ST and FT fibers differ. Based on these differences, you might expect that these fiber types would also have different functions when you are physically active. Indeed, this is the case.

ST Fibers.   In general, slow-twitch muscle fibers have a high level of aerobic endurance. Let's define this term. Aerobic means "in the presence of oxygen," so oxidation is an aerobic process. ST fibers are very efficient at producing ATP from the oxidation of carbohydrate and fat.

Recall that ATP is required to produce the energy needed for muscle fiber action and relaxation. As long as oxidation occurs, ST fibers continue producing ATP, allowing the fibers to remain active. The ability to maintain muscular activity for a prolonged period is known as muscular endurance, so ST fibers have high aerobic endurance. Because of this, they are recruited most often during low-intensity endurance events, such as marathon running or channel swimming.

FT Fibers.   Fast-twitch muscle fibers, on the other hand, have relatively poor aerobic endurance. They are better suited to perform anaerobically (without oxygen) than the ST fibers. This means their ATP is formed through anaerobic pathways, not oxidation. (These pathways will be discussed in detail in chapter 5.)

FT_a motor units generate considerably more force than ST motor units, but they fatigue easily because of their limited endurance. Thus, FT_a fibers appear to be used mainly during short, high-intensity endurance events such as the mile run or the 400-m swim.

Although the significance of the FT_b fibers is not fully understood, they apparently are not easily turned on by the nervous system. Because of this, they are used rather infrequently in normal, low-intensity activity, but are predominantly used in highly explosive events such as the 100-m dash and the 50-m sprint swim. Characteristics of the various fiber types are summarized in Table 2.2.

Table 2.2 Structural and Functional Characteristics of Muscle Fiber Types

Characteristic	Fiber type		
	ST	FT_a	FT_b
Fibers per motor neuron	10-180	300-800	300-800
Motor neuron size	Small	Large	Large
Nerve conduction velocity	Slow	Fast	Fast
Contraction speed (ms)	110	50	50
Type of myosin ATPase	Slow	Fast	Fast
Sarcoplasmic reticulum development	Low	High	High
Motor unit force	Low	High	High
Aerobic capacity (oxidative)	High	Moderate	Low
Anaerobic capacity (glycolytic)	Low	High	High

Determination of Fiber Type

The slow- and fast-twitch characteristics of muscle fibers appear to be determined early in life, perhaps within the first few years. Studies with identical twins have shown that muscle fiber composition is genetically determined, changing little from childhood to middle age. These studies reveal that identical twins have nearly identical fiber compositions, whereas fraternal twins differ in their fiber profiles. The genes we inherit from our parents determine which motor neurons innervate our individual muscle fibers. After innervation is established, our muscle fibers differentiate (become specialized) according to the type of neuron that stimulates them.

But this can change with time. As we age, our muscles tend to lose FT fibers, which increases the percentage of ST fibers.

Muscle Fiber Recruitment

When a motor neuron stimulates a muscle fiber, a minimum amount of stimulation, called the threshold, is required to elicit a response. If the stimulation is less than this threshold, no muscle action occurs. But with any stimulation equal to or exceeding the threshold, maximal action occurs in the muscle fiber. This is known as the all-or-none response. Because all muscle fibers in a single motor unit receive the same neural stimulation, all of the fibers in the motor unit act maximally any time the threshold is met. Thus the motor unit also exhibits an all-or-none response.

More force is produced by activating more muscle fibers. When little force is needed, only a few fibers are stimulated to act. Recall from our earlier discussion that FT motor units contain more muscle fibers than ST motor units. Skeletal muscle action involves selective recruitment of ST or FT muscle fibers, depending on the requirements of the activity being performed. In the early 1970s, Gollnick et al. demonstrated that,

IN REVIEW . . .

1. Most skeletal muscles contain both ST and FT fibers.
2. The different fiber types have different ATPases. The ATPase in the FT fibers acts faster, providing energy for muscle action more quickly than the ATPase in ST fibers.
3. FT fibers have a more highly developed sarcoplasmic reticulum, enhancing the delivery of calcium needed for muscle action.
4. Motor neurons supplying FT motor units are larger and supply more fibers than do neurons for ST motor units. Thus FT motor units have more fibers to contract and can produce more force than ST motor units.
5. The proportions of ST and FT fibers in an individual's arm and leg muscles are usually quite similar.
6. ST fibers have high aerobic endurance and are well suited to low-intensity endurance activities.
7. FT fibers are better for anaerobic activity. FT_a fibers are well utilized in explosive bouts of exercise. FT_b fibers are not well understood, but it is known that they are not easily recruited into activity.

indeed, this selective recruitment is determined not by the speed of action, but by the level of force demanded of the muscle.[5,6]

Figure 2.11 illustrates the relationship between force development and the recruitment of ST, FT_a, and FT_b fibers. During low-intensity exercise such as walking, most of the muscle force is generated by ST fibers. As the muscle tension requirements increase at higher exercise intensities such as jogging, FT_a fibers are added to the work force. Finally, in events where maximal strength is needed, such as sprint running, FT_b fibers are also activated.

However, even during maximal efforts, the nervous system does not recruit 100% of the available fibers. Despite your desire to produce more force, only a fraction of your muscle fibers are stimulated at any specific time. This prevents damage to your muscles and tendons. If you could contract all the fibers in your muscle at the same instant, the force generated would likely tear the muscle or its tendon.

During events that last several hours, you must exercise at a submaximal pace, and the tension in your muscles is relatively low. As a result, the nervous system tends to recruit those muscle fibers best adapted to endurance activity: the ST and some FT_a fibers. As the exercise continues, these fibers become depleted of their primary fuel supply (glycogen), and the nervous system must recruit more FT_a fibers to maintain muscle tension. Finally, when the ST and FT_a fibers become exhausted, the FT_b fibers are called upon in your effort to continue exercising.

This may explain why fatigue seems to come in stages during events like the marathon, a 26.2-mile run. It also likely explains why it takes great conscious effort to maintain a given pace near the finish of the event. This conscious effort results in the activation of muscle fibers that are not easily recruited. Such information is of practical importance to our understanding of the specific requirements of training and performance. We will discuss this further in chapters 4 and 7.

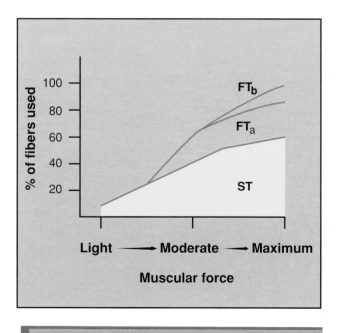

Figure 2.11   The ramplike recruitment of slow-twitch and fast-twitch muscle fibers.

IN REVIEW . . .

1. Motor units give all-or-none responses. For a unit to be recruited into activity, the motor nerve impulse must meet or exceed the threshold. When this occurs, all muscle fibers in the motor unit act maximally. If the threshold is not met, no fibers in that unit act.
2. More force is produced by activating more motor units, and thus more muscle fibers.
3. In low-intensity activity, most muscle force is generated by ST fibers. As the resistance increases, FT_a fibers are recruited, and if maximal strength is needed the FT_b fibers are activated. The same pattern of recruitment is followed during events of long duration.

Fiber Type and Athletic Success

Knowledge of the composition and use of muscle fibers suggests that athletes who have a high percentage of ST fibers might have an advantage in prolonged endurance events, whereas those with a predominance of FT fibers could be better suited for short-term and explosive activities. Can it be that the proportions of an athlete's various muscle fiber types determine athletic success?

The muscle fiber makeup of successful athletes from a variety of athletic events is shown in Table 2.3. Compare the runners. As anticipated, the leg muscles of distance runners, who rely on endurance, have a predominance of ST fibers. Studies of elite male and female distance runners revealed that, in many, the gastrocnemius (calf) muscles contain more than 90% ST fibers. Also, although muscle fiber cross-sectional area varies markedly among elite distance runners, ST fibers in their leg muscles average about 22% more cross-sectional area than FT fibers.

In contrast, the gastrocnemius muscles are composed principally of FT fibers in sprinters, who rely on speed and strength. Though swimmers tend to have higher percentages of ST fibers (60% to 65%) in their muscles than untrained subjects (45% to 55%), fiber type differences between good and elite swimmers are not apparent.[2,3,4]

World champions in the marathon have been reported to possess 93% to 99% ST fibers in their gastrocnemius muscles. World-class sprinters, however, have only about 25% ST fibers in this muscle.

The fiber composition of muscles in distance runners and sprinters is markedly different. However, it

Table 2.3 Percentages and Cross-Sectional Areas of Slow-Twitch (ST) and Fast-Twitch (FT) Fibers in Selected Muscles of Male (M) and Female (F) Athletes

Athlete	Gender	Muscle	% ST	% FT	Cross-sectional area (μm^2) ST	FT
Sprint runners	M	Gastrocnemius	24	76	5,878	6,034
	F	Gastrocnemius	27	73	3,752	3,930
Distance runners	M	Gastrocnemius	79	21	8,342	6,485
	F	Gastrocnemius	69	31	4,441	4,128
Cyclists	M	Vastus lateralis	57	43	6,333	6,116
	F	Vastus lateralis	51	49	5,487	5,216
Swimmers	M	Posterior deltoid	67	33	—	—
Weight lifters	M	Gastrocnemius	44	56	5,060	8,910
	M	Deltoid	53	47	5,010	8,450
Triathletes	M	Posterior deltoid	60	40	—	—
	M	Vastus lateralis	63	37	—	—
	M	Gastrocnemius	59	41	—	—
Canoeists	M	Posterior deltoid	71	29	4,920	7,040
Shot-putters	M	Gastrocnemius	38	62	6,367	6,441
Nonathletes	M	Vastus lateralis	47	53	4,722	4,709
	F	Gastrocnemius	52	48	3,501	3,141

may be a bit risky to think we can select champion distance runners and sprinters solely on the basis of predominant muscle fiber type. Other factors, such as cardiovascular function and muscle size, also contribute to success in such events of endurance, speed, and strength. Thus fiber composition alone is not a reliable predictor of athletic success.

Use of Muscles

We have examined the different muscle fiber types. We understand that, when stimulated, all fibers in a motor unit act at the same time and that different fiber types are recruited in stages, depending on the nature of an activity. Now we can move back to the gross level, turning our attention to how whole muscles work to produce movement.

The more than 215 pairs of skeletal muscles in the body vary widely in size, shape, and use. Every coordinated movement requires the application of muscle force. This is accomplished by

- agonists or prime movers, muscles primarily responsible for the movement;
- antagonists, muscles that oppose the prime movers; and
- synergists, muscles that assist the prime movers.

As illustrated in Figure 2.12, the smooth flexion of the elbow requires shortening of the brachialis and biceps brachii muscles (agonists) and the relaxation of the triceps brachii (antagonist). The brachioradialis

muscle (synergist) assists the brachialis and biceps brachii in their flexion of the joint.

The agonists produce most of the force needed for any particular movement. The muscles act on the bones to which they are attached, pulling them toward each other. Synergists assist this action and sometimes are involved in fine-tuning the direction of movement. The antagonists play a protective role. Think of the quadriceps (front) and hamstrings (back) in your thigh. When your hamstrings (agonists) contract forcefully, your quadriceps (antagonists) also contract slightly, opposing the motion of the hamstrings. This prevents overstretching of your quadriceps by the strong contraction of the hamstrings and allows more controlled thigh movement. This opposing action between agonists and antagonists also produces muscle tone.

Types of Muscle Action

Muscle movement can generally be categorized into three types of actions:

1. Concentric
2. Static
3. Eccentric

In many activities, such as running and jumping, all three types of actions may occur in the execution of a smooth, coordinated movement. For the sake of clarity, though, we will examine each type separately.

Concentric Action. A muscle's principal action, shortening, is referred to as a concentric action. This is shown in Figure 2.13a. We are most familiar with this type of

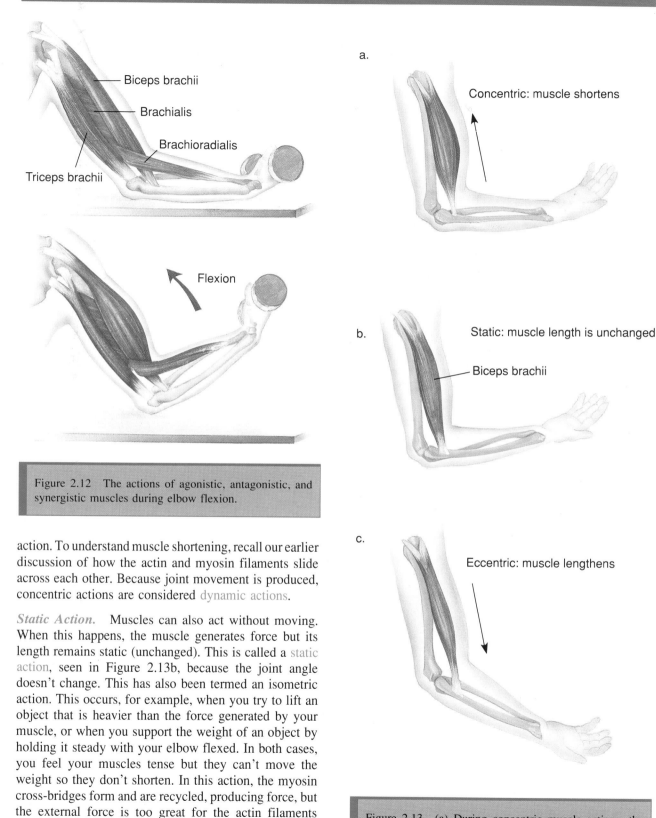

Figure 2.12 The actions of agonistic, antagonistic, and synergistic muscles during elbow flexion.

action. To understand muscle shortening, recall our earlier discussion of how the actin and myosin filaments slide across each other. Because joint movement is produced, concentric actions are considered dynamic actions.

Static Action. Muscles can also act without moving. When this happens, the muscle generates force but its length remains static (unchanged). This is called a static action, seen in Figure 2.13b, because the joint angle doesn't change. This has also been termed an isometric action. This occurs, for example, when you try to lift an object that is heavier than the force generated by your muscle, or when you support the weight of an object by holding it steady with your elbow flexed. In both cases, you feel your muscles tense but they can't move the weight so they don't shorten. In this action, the myosin cross-bridges form and are recycled, producing force, but the external force is too great for the actin filaments to be moved. They remain in their normal position, so shortening can't occur. If enough motor units can be recruited to produce sufficient force to overcome the resistance, a static action can become a dynamic one.

Eccentric Action. Muscles may even exert force while lengthening. This movement is an eccentric action, shown

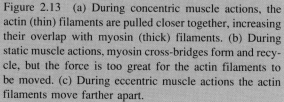

Figure 2.13 (a) During concentric muscle actions, the actin (thin) filaments are pulled closer together, increasing their overlap with myosin (thick) filaments. (b) During static muscle actions, myosin cross-bridges form and recycle, but the force is too great for the actin filaments to be moved. (c) During eccentric muscle actions the actin filaments move farther apart.

in Figure 2.13c. Because joint movement occurs, this is also a dynamic action. An example of this is the action of the biceps brachii when your elbow is extended to lower a heavy weight. In this case, the actin filaments are pulled farther away from the center of the sarcomere, essentially stretching it.

Generation of Force

Your muscles' strength reflects their ability to produce force. If you have the strength to bench-press 300 lb, your muscles are capable of producing enough force to overcome a load of 300 lb. Even when unloaded (not trying to lift a weight), your muscles must still generate enough force to move the bones to which they are attached. The development of this muscle force depends on the following:

- The number of motor units activated
- The type of motor units activated
- The size of the muscle
- The muscle's initial length when activated
- The angle of the joint
- The muscle's speed of action

Let's examine these components.

Motor Units and Muscle Size.   We previously discussed motor units. To recap, more force can be generated when more motor units are activated. FT motor units generate more force than ST motor units because each FT unit has more muscle fibers than a ST unit.

In a similar manner, larger muscles, having more muscle fibers, can produce more force than smaller muscles.

Muscle Length.   Muscles and their connective tissues (fasciae and tendons) have the property of elasticity. When stretched, this elasticity results in stored energy. During subsequent muscle activity, this stored energy is released, increasing the amount of force.

In the intact body, muscle length is restricted by the anatomical arrangement and attachment of muscle to bone. When attached to the skeleton, a muscle at resting length is normally under slight tension because it is moderately stretched. If a muscle were freed from its attachments, it would assume a relaxed, somewhat shorter length.

Measurements indicate that maximal force can be generated in a muscle when the muscle is first stretched to a length approximately 20% greater than its resting length. When the muscle is stretched to this length, the combination of stored energy and the force of muscle action is optimized, resulting in maximal force production.

Increasing or decreasing the muscle length beyond 20% reduces force development. For example, if the muscle is stretched to twice its resting length, the force it produces will be nearly zero. Energy is still stored in the muscle because of the stretching. In fact, more stretching means more stored energy.

But another factor must be considered. The force created by muscle fibers during muscle action depends on the number of cross-bridges in contact with the actin filaments at any given time. The more that are in contact at once, the more forceful the muscle action. When muscle fibers are overstretched, the actin and myosin filaments are pulled farther apart. The decreased overlap between these filaments results in fewer cross-bridges binding to create force.

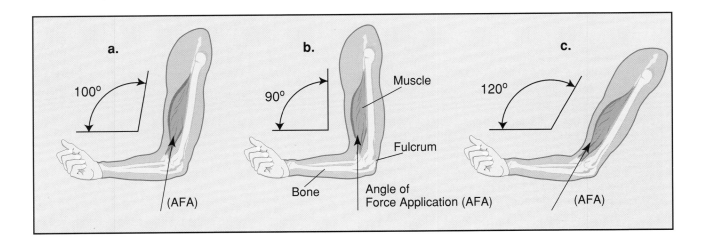

Figure 2.14   Each joint has an optimum angle of force application (AFA). (a) For the biceps brachii acting across the elbow, the optimum angle is 100°. (b) Decreasing or (c) increasing the joint angle alters the angle of force application and reduces the force transferred from the muscle to the bone.

Angle of the Joint.   Because muscles exert their force through skeletal levers, understanding the physical arrangement of these muscle-pulleys and bone-levers is crucial to understanding movement. Consider the biceps brachii. The tendon attachment for the biceps is only one tenth the distance from the elbow fulcrum to the weighted resistance held in the hand. Thus, to hold a 10-lb weight, the muscle must exert 10 times (100 lb) as much force.

The force generated in the muscle is transferred to the bone through the muscle's insertion (tendon). As with muscle length, an optimum joint angle will maximize the amount of force transmitted to the bone. This angle depends on the relative positions of the tendinous insertion on the bone and the load being moved. In our example of the biceps brachii, the best joint angle for application of the needed 100 lb of force is 100°. More or less flexion of the elbow joint will alter the angle at which the force is applied, reducing the amount of force transferred to the bone. This is illustrated in Figure 2.14.

Speed of Action.   The ability to develop force also depends on the speed of muscle action. During concentric (shortening) actions, maximal force development decreases progressively at higher speeds. Think of when you try to lift a very heavy object. You tend to do it slowly, maximizing the force you can apply to it. If you grab it and quickly try to lift it you will likely fail, if not injure yourself. However, with eccentric (lengthening) actions, the opposite is true. Fast eccentric actions allow maximal application of force.

These relationships are depicted in Figure 2.15. Eccentric actions are shown on the left and concentric on the right. Note that the units are meters per second, so the higher the number, the faster the muscle action (moving 0.8 m in 1 s is faster than moving only 0.2 m in the same time).

IN REVIEW . . .

1. Muscles involved in a movement can be classed as
   - agonists (prime movers),
   - antagonists (opponents), or
   - synergists (assistants).
2. The three main types of muscle action are
   - concentric, in which the muscle shortens;
   - static, in which the muscle acts but the joint angle is unchanged; and
   - eccentric, in which the muscle lengthens.
3. Force production can be increased by recruiting more motor units.
4. Force production can be maximized if the muscle is stretched 20% prior to action. At this point, the amount of energy stored and the number of linked actin-myosin cross-bridges are optimum.
5. All joints have an optimal angle at which the muscles crossing the joint function to produce maximum force. This angle varies with the relative position of the muscle's insertion on the bone and the load placed on the muscle.
6. Speed of action also affects the amount of force produced. For concentric action, maximum force can be achieved with slower contractions. The closer you get to zero velocity (static) the more force can be generated. With eccentric actions, however, faster movement allows more force production.

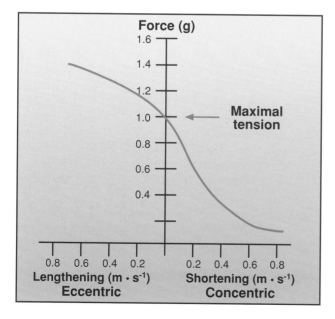

Figure 2.15   The relationship between muscle length and force production. Adapted from Åstrand and Rodahl (1985).

In Closing . . .

In this chapter, we reviewed the components of skeletal muscle. We considered the differences in fiber types and their impact on physical performance. We learned how muscles generate force and produce movement by pulling on bones. Now that we understand how movement is produced, it is time to turn our attention to how it is coordinated. In the next chapter, we will focus on the neurological control of movement.

Key Terms

ATP
actin
concentric action
dynamic action
eccentric action
endomysium
epimysium
fasciculus
fast-twitch fiber
motor unit
muscle fiber
myofibril
myosin
myosin cross-bridge

perimysium
power stroke
sarcolemma
sarcomere
sarcoplasm
sarcoplasmic reticulum
sliding filament theory
slow-twitch fiber
static action
transverse tubules
  (T tubules)
tropomyosin
troponin

Study Questions

1. List and define the components of a muscle fiber.
2. List the components of a motor unit.
3. What is the role of calcium in the muscle action process?
4. Describe the sliding filament theory. How do muscle fibers shorten?
5. What are the basic characteristics of slow- and fast-twitch muscle fibers?
6. What is the role of genetics in determining the proportions of muscle fiber types and the potential for success in selected activities?
7. Describe the relationship between muscle force development and the recruitment of slow- and fast-twitch fibers.
8. What is the pattern of muscle fiber recruitment during (a) high jumping, (b) running a 10-km race, and (c) running a marathon?
9. Differentiate and give examples of concentric, static, and eccentric actions.
10. What is the optimal length of a muscle for maximal force development?
11. What is the relationship between maximal force development and the speed of shortening (concentric) and lengthening (eccentric) actions?

References

1. Close, R. (1967). Properties of motor units in fast and slow skeletal muscles of the rat. *Journal of Physiology* (London), **193**, 45-55.

2. Costill, D.L., Daniels, J., Evans, W., Fink, W., Krahenbuhl, G., & Saltin, B. (1976). Skeletal muscle enzymes and fiber composition in male and female track athletes. *Journal of Applied Physiology*, **40**, 149-154.

3. Costill, D.L., Fink, W.J., Flynn, M., & Kirwan, J. (1987). Muscle fiber composition and enzyme activities in elite female distance runners. *International Journal of Sports Medicine*, **8**, 103-106.

4. Costill, D.L., Fink, W.J., & Pollock, M.L. (1976). Muscle fiber composition and enzyme activities of elite distance runners. *Medicine and Science in Sports*, **8**, 96-100.

5. Gollnick, P.D., & Hodgson, D.R. (1986). The identification of fiber types in skeletal muscle: A continual dilemma. *Exercise and Sport Sciences Reviews*, **14**, 81-104.

6. Gollnick, P.D., Piehl, K., & Saltin, B. (1974). Selective glycogen depletion pattern in human muscle fibers after exercise of varying intensity and at varying pedal rates. *Journal of Physiology*, **241**, 45-47.

Selected Readings

Blomstrand, E., & Ekblom, B. (1982). The needle biopsy technique for fibre type determination in human skeletal muscle—A methodological study. *Acta Physiologica Scandinavica*, **116**, 437-442.

Brobeck, J.R. (Ed.) (1979). *Best and Taylor's physiological basis of medical practice* (10th ed). Baltimore: Williams & Wilkins.

Brooke, M.H., & Kaiser, K.K. (1970). Muscle fiber types: How many and what kind? *Archives of Neurology*, **23**, 369-379.

Buchthal, F., & Schmalbruch, H. (1970). Contraction times and fiber types in intact muscle. *Acta Physiologica Scandinavica*, **79**, 435-452.

Burke, R.E. & Edgerton, V.R. (1975). Motor unit properties and selective involvement in movement, *Exercise and Sports Sciences Reviews*, **3**, 31-81.

Edington, D.W., & Edgerton, V.R. (1976). *The biology of physical activity* (pp. 51-72). Boston: Houghton Mifflin.

Essen-Gustavsson, B., & Borges, O. (1986). Histochemical and metabolic characteristics of human skeletal muscle in relation to age. *Acta Physiologica Scandinavica*, **126**, 107-114.

Essen-Gustavsson, B., & Henriksson, J. (1984). Enzyme levels in pools of microdissected human muscle fibres of identified type. *Acta Physiologica Scandinavica*, **120**, 505-515.

Gordon, T., & Pattullo, M.C. (1993). Plasticity of muscle fiber and motor unit types. *Exercise and Sport Sciences Reviews*, **21**, 331-362.

Karlsson, J. (1977). Skeletal muscle fibres and muscle enzyme activities in monozygous and dizygous twins of both sexes. *Acta Physiologica Scandinavica*, **100**, 385-392.

Komi, P.V., & Karlsson, J. (1979). Physical performance, skeletal muscle enzyme activities, and fibre types in monozygous and dizygous twins of both sexes. *Acta Physiologica Scandinavica*, (Suppl. 462), 1-28.

Lexell, J., & Taylor, C.C. (1989). Variability in muscle fibre areas in whole human quadriceps muscle: How to reduce sampling errors in biopsy techniques. *Clinical Physiology*, **9**, 333-343.

Lexell, J., Taylor, C., & Sjöström, M. (1985). Analysis of sampling errors in biopsy techniques using data from whole muscle cross sections. *Journal of Applied Physiology*, **59**, 1228-1235.

MacLaren, D.P.M., Gibson, H., Parry-Billings, M., & Edwards, R.H.T. (1989). A review of metabolic and physiological factors in fatigue. *Exercise and Sport Sciences Reviews*, **17**, 29-66.

Roy, R.R., Baldwin, K.M., & Edgerton, V.R. (1991). The plasticity of skeletal muscle: Effects of neuromuscular activity. *Exercise and Sport Sciences Reviews*, **19**, 269-312.

Simoneau, J.-A., & Bouchard, C. (1989). Human variation in skeletal muscle fiber-type proportion and enzyme activities. *American Journal of Physiology*, **257**, E567-E572.

Wickiewicz, T.L., Roy, R.R., Powell, P.L., Perrine, J.J., & Edgerton, V.R. (1984). Muscle architecture and force-velocity relationships in humans. *Journal of Applied Physiology*, **57**, 435-443.

Chapter 3
Neurological Control
of Movement

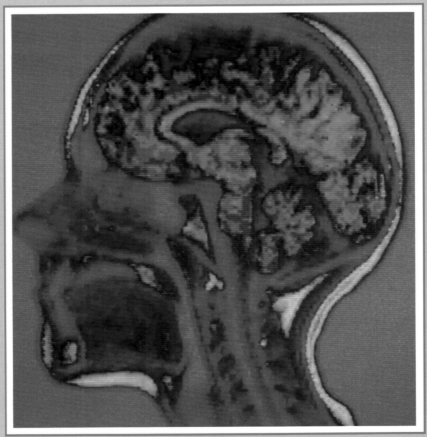

© Dan McCoy/Rainbow

Chapter Overview

In chapter 2, we discussed how muscles, by generating force, pull on the bones to which they are attached to produce movement. This movement would not be possible without the nervous system. Just as the skeleton remains motionless without the application of force by the muscles, the muscles themselves cannot move unless activated by the nervous system. It plans, initiates, and coordinates all human movement. This role of the nervous system—controlling body movement—will be our focus in this chapter.

Chapter Outline

In 1959, at age 15, Jimmie Huega was the youngest male ever to make the U.S. Ski Team. He raced internationally for 10 years, competing on the 1964 and 1968 Olympic teams and on the 1962 and 1966 World Championship teams. In 1964, Huega and teammate Billy Kidd made history by winning the first U.S. Olympic medals in men's alpine skiing. In 1967, Huega won a World Cup in the giant slalom, finishing third in the world for the entire season. He remains the only American male to win the Arlberg-Kandahar at Garmisch, Germany, one of the oldest and most prestigious alpine ski races.

After competing in the 1968 Olympics, troubled by unknown physical ailments, Huega retired from the U.S. Ski Team. In 1970, he was diagnosed with multiple sclerosis (MS), a neurological disorder. At that time people with MS were advised that physical activity would exacerbate their condition, so he was advised to live a quiet and tranquil life. Huega followed that advice and began feeling unhealthy, unmotivated, and less energetic. He began to deteriorate physically and mentally.

Six years later Huega decided to defy medical convention. He developed a cardiovascular endurance exercise program and began stretching and strengthening exercises. He established realistic goals for his personal wellness program. With this program, Huega regained his health within the constraints of MS. In 1984, inspired by his own success, he created the Jimmie Huega Center, a nonprofit organization based in Avon, Colorado. Since then, more than 800 people with MS have gone through the center's medical program.

All physiological activity in the human body can be influenced by the nervous system. Nerves provide the wiring through which electrical impulses are received from and sent to virtually all parts of the body. The brain acts as a computer, integrating all incoming information, selecting an appropriate response, then instructing the involved body parts to take appropriate action. Thus the nervous system forms a vital link, allowing communication and coordination of interaction between the various tissues in the body as well as with the outside world.

Our discussion in this chapter will center on neural control of voluntary movement. But you must remember that virtually any physiological function that can affect athletic performance is to some extent regulated and monitored by the nervous system. The material we are about to cover, although it might seem complex, considers only a tiny fraction of the nervous system's extensive involvement in performing physical activity.

The Structure and Function of the Nervous System

The nervous system is one of your body's most complex systems. Many of its functions are not yet fully understood. For these reasons, and because this book is concerned only with specific functions of the nervous system, we will not go into as much detail about the nervous system as a whole as you did in introductory anatomy and physiology. Rather, we will first look at an overview of the nervous system, then focus on specific topics relevant to sport and exercise. We will begin our discussion by closely examining the basic units of the nervous system: the neurons.

The Neuron

Individual nerve fibers (nerve cells), depicted in Figure 3.1, are called neurons. A typical neuron is composed of three regions:

1. The cell body, or soma
2. The dendrites
3. The axon

The cell body contains the nucleus. Radiating out from the cell body are the cell processes: the dendrites and the axon. On the side toward the axon, the cell body tapers into a cone-shaped region known as the axon hillock. It has an important role in impulse conduction, which we will discuss later.

Most neurons contain many dendrites. These are the neuron's receivers. Most impulses coming into the nerve, from sensory stimuli or from adjacent neurons, typically enter the neuron via the dendrites. These processes then carry the impulses toward the cell body.

In contrast, most neurons have only one axon. The axon is the neuron's transmitter. It conducts impulses away from the cell body. Near its end, an axon splits

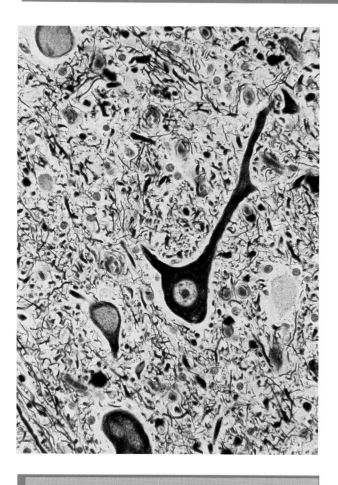

Figure 3.1   A photomicrograph of neurons.

into numerous branches. These are the axon terminals, or terminal fibrils. The tips of these terminals are dilated into tiny bulbs known as the synaptic knobs. These knobs house numerous vesicles (sacs) filled with chemicals, known as neurotransmitters, that are used for communication between a neuron and another cell. (This will be discussed later in more detail.)

The Nerve Impulse

A nerve impulse—an electrical charge—is the signal that passes from one neuron to the next and finally to an end organ, such as a group of muscle fibers, or back to the central nervous system. For simplicity, you can think of the nerve impulse traveling through a neuron much as electricity travels through the electrical wires in your home. Let's look at how this electrical impulse is generated and how it travels through a neuron.

Resting Membrane Potential

The cell membrane of a neuron at rest has a negative electrical potential of about −70 mV. That means if

you were to insert a voltmeter probe inside the cell, the electrical charges found there and the charges found outside the cell would differ by 70 mV, and the inside would be negative relative to the outside. This potential difference is known as the resting membrane potential, or the RMP. It is caused by a separation of charges across the membrane. When the charges across the membrane differ, the membrane is said to be polarized.

The neuron has a high concentration of potassium ions (K^+) on the inside and a high concentration of sodium ions (Na^+) on the outside because the sodium-potassium pump actively moves sodium out of the cell and potassium into it. That seems to imply that the charges are balanced across the membrane, but the sodium-potassium pump moves three Na^+ out of the cell for each two K^+ it brings in. Also, the cell membrane is much more permeable to potassium ions than to sodium ions, so the K^+ can move freely. To establish equilibrium, the K^+ will move to an area of lower concentration, so some of it moves to the outside. The Na^+ cannot move in this manner. The end result is that more positively charged ions are outside of the cell than inside, creating the potential difference across the membrane. Maintenance of a constant resting membrane potential of −70 mV is primarily a function of the sodium-potassium pump.

Depolarization and Hyperpolarization

If the inside of the cell becomes less negative relative to the outside, the potential difference across the membrane will decrease. The membrane will be less polarized. When this happens, the membrane is said to be depolarized. Thus depolarization occurs any time the charge difference becomes less than the RMP of −70 mV, moving closer to zero. This typically results from a change in the membrane's Na^+ permeability.

The opposite can also occur. If the charge difference across the membrane increases, moving from the RMP to an even more negative number, then the membrane becomes more polarized. This is known as hyperpolarization.

Changes in the membrane potential are actually signals used to receive, transmit, and integrate information within and between cells. These signals are of two types, graded potentials and action potentials. Both are electrical currents created by the movement of ions. Let's look at them now.

Graded Potentials

Graded potentials are localized changes in the membrane potential. These can be either depolarizations or hyperpolarizations. The membrane contains ion channels that have ion gates acting as doorways into and out of the neuron. These gates are usually closed, preventing ion flow, but they open with stimulation, allowing ions to move from the outside to the inside or vice versa. This ion flow alters the charge separation, changing the polarization of the membrane.

Graded potentials are triggered by a change in the neuron's local environment. Depending on the location and type of neuron involved, the ion gates may open in response to the transmission of an impulse from another neuron or in response to sensory stimuli such as changes in chemical concentrations, temperature, or pressure.

Recall that most neuron receptors are located on the dendrites (though some are on the cell body), yet the impulse is always transmitted from the axon terminals at the opposite end of the cell. For a neuron to transmit an impulse, the impulse must travel almost the entire length of the neuron. Although a graded potential may result in depolarization of the cell membrane, this is usually just a local event, and the depolarization does not spread very far along the neuron. To travel the full distance, an impulse must generate an action potential.

KEY POINT

Nerve impulses typically pass from the dendrites to the cell body, and from the cell body along the length of the axon to its terminal fibrils.

Action Potentials

An action potential is a rapid and substantial depolarization of the neuron's membrane. It usually lasts only about 1 ms. Typically, the membrane potential changes from the RMP of −70 mV to a value of +30 mV, then rapidly returns to its resting value. How does this marked change in membrane potential occur?

Threshold and the All-Or-None Principle.   All action potentials begin as graded potentials. When enough stimulation occurs to cause a depolarization of at least 15 to 20 mV, an action potential results. That means if the membrane depolarizes from the RMP of −70 mV to a value of −50 to −55 mV, the cell will experience an action potential. The minimum depolarization required to produce an action potential is called the threshold. Any depolarization less than the threshold value of 15 to 20 mV will not result in an action potential. For example, if the membrane potential changes from the RMP of −70 mV to −60 mV, the change is only 10 mV and doesn't meet the threshold; thus no action potential occurs. But any time depolarization reaches or exceeds the threshold, an action potential will result. This is the all-or-none principle.

Sequence of Events in an Action Potential.   For each action potential, the following sequence of events, depicted in Figure 3.2, occurs:

1. *Increased Na+ permeability.* The stimulus opens the membrane's Na+ gates, and when threshold is reached, the membrane's Na+ permeability increases several hundredfold. Sodium ions flood into the cell. During this initial phase, the amount of sodium entering the cell exceeds the amount of potassium leaving the cell, causing the inside of the cell to become positively charged relative to the outside. The voltage change (depolarization) is typically from −70 mV to +30 mV, as seen in Figure 3.2b.

2. *Decreased Na+ permeability.* The initial Na+ influx is very brief. As the membrane potential passes 0, movement of more positive charge into the cell is resisted. Also, the sodium gates close very quickly, so the initial sodium influx is short-lived.

3. *Repolarization.* In response to the increased positive charge inside the cell, the K+ gates open. Because potassium ions are positively charged, they move toward the more negative area outside. As this movement occurs, the outside of the cell once again builds up a more positive charge than the inside, and the voltage returns to the RMP of −70 mV. This final step is repolarization, shown in Figure 3.2d.

After repolarization is completed, one final event must occur before the neuron has truly returned to its normal resting state. During an action potential, Na+ enters the cell. Then to reverse the depolarization, K+ leaves the cell. Thus Na+ concentration is high inside the cell, and K+ concentration is high outside the cell—opposite from the resting state. To reverse this, once repolarization is completed the sodium-potassium pump is activated and the ions are returned to the correct side of the membrane. This is shown in Figure 3.2e.

Propagation of the Action Potential

Now that we understand how a neural impulse, in the form of an action potential, is generated, we can look at how the impulse is propagated, or how it travels through the neuron. Two characteristics of the neuron become particularly important when considering how quickly an impulse can pass through the axon: myelination and diameter.

The Myelin Sheath.   The axons of most motor neurons are myelinated, meaning they are covered with a sheath formed by myelin, a fatty substance that insulates the cell membrane. In the peripheral nervous system, this sheath is formed by Schwann cells.

The sheath is not continuous. As it spans the length of the axon, the myelin sheath exhibits gaps between

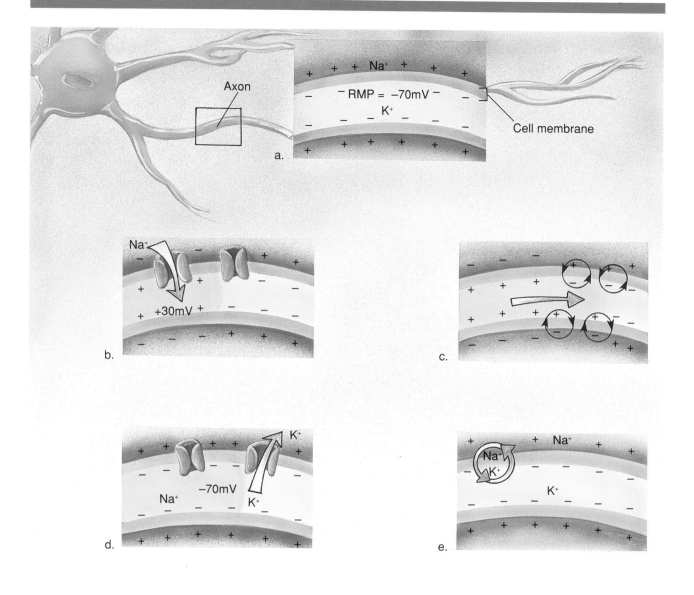

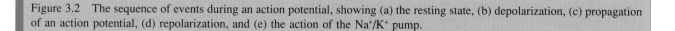

Figure 3.2   The sequence of events during an action potential, showing (a) the resting state, (b) depolarization, (c) propagation of an action potential, (d) repolarization, and (e) the action of the Na⁺/K⁺ pump.

adjacent Schwann cells, leaving the axon uninsulated at those points. These gaps are referred to as nodes of Ranvier. The action potential appears to jump from one node to the next as it traverses a myelinated fiber. This is referred to as saltatory conduction, a much faster rate of conduction than in unmyelinated fibers.

Myelination of motor neurons occurs over the first several years of life, partly explaining why children need time to develop coordinated movement. Individuals affected by certain neurological diseases, such as multiple sclerosis, experience degeneration of the myelin sheath and a subsequent loss of coordination.

The velocity of nerve impulse transmission in large myelinated fibers can approach 120 m · s⁻¹ (more than 250 mph), 5 to 50 times faster than in unmyelinated fibers of the same size.

Diameter of the Neuron.   The velocity of nerve impulse transmission is also determined by the neuron's size. Neurons of larger diameter conduct nerve impulses faster than neurons of smaller diameter because larger neurons present less resistance to local current flow.

The Synapse

For a neuron to communicate with another neuron, an action potential must occur. Once the action potential is fired, the nerve impulse travels the full length of the axon, ultimately reaching the axon terminals. How does the nerve impulse move from the neuron in which it starts to another neuron?

Neurons communicate with each other across synapses. A synapse is the site of impulse transmission from one neuron to another. The most common type of synapse is the chemical synapse, which will be our focus.

As seen in Figure 3.3, a synapse between two neurons includes

- the axon terminals of the neuron carrying the impulse,

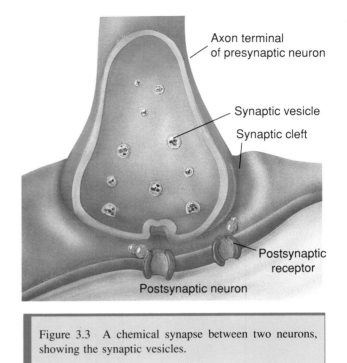

Figure 3.3   A chemical synapse between two neurons, showing the synaptic vesicles.

- receptors on the second neuron, and
- the space between these structures.

The neuron sending the impulse across the synapse is called the presynaptic neuron, so axon terminals are presynaptic terminals. Similarly, the neuron receiving the impulse on the opposite side of the synapse is called the postsynaptic neuron, and it has postsynaptic receptors. The axon terminals and postsynaptic receptors are not physically in contact with each other. A narrow gap, the synaptic cleft, separates them.

A nerve impulse can be transmitted across a synapse only in one direction: from the axon terminals of the presynaptic neuron to the postsynaptic receptors usually on the dendrites of the postsynaptic neuron. Impulses can also go directly to receptors on the cell body: About 5% to 20% of the axon terminals are adjacent to the cell body instead of the dendrites.[2]

The presynaptic terminals of the axon contain a large number of sac-like structures, called synaptic vesicles. These sacs contain neurotransmitter chemicals. When the impulse reaches the presynaptic terminals, the synaptic vesicles respond by dumping their chemicals into the synaptic cleft. These neurotransmitters then diffuse across the synaptic cleft to the postsynaptic neuron's receptors. The postsynaptic receptors bind the neurotransmitter once it diffuses across the synaptic cleft. When this binding occurs, the impulse has been transmitted successfully to the next neuron and can be transmitted onward.

The Neuromuscular Junction

Whereas neurons communicate with other neurons at synapses, a motor neuron communicates with a muscle fiber at a site known as a neuromuscular junction. The function of the neuromuscular junction is essentially the same as a synapse. In fact, the proximal part of the neuromuscular junction is the same: It starts with the axon terminals of the motor neuron, which release neurotransmitters into the space between two cells. However, in the neuromuscular junction, the axon terminals are expanded into flat disks called motor end-plates.

In the neuromuscular junction, the impulse is received by a muscle fiber. Refer to Figure 3.4. Where the axon terminals approach the muscle fiber, you see that the fiber is invaginated. The cavity thus formed is called the synaptic gutter. As with synapses, the space between the neuron and the muscle fiber is the synaptic cleft.

Neurotransmitters released from the motor axon terminals diffuse across the synaptic cleft and bind to receptors on the muscle fiber's sarcolemma (membrane). This binding typically causes depolarization by opening sodium ion channels, allowing more sodium to enter the muscle fiber. As always, if the depolarization

reaches threshold, an action potential is fired. It spreads across the sarcolemma, and the muscle fiber contracts.

Now we know how the impulse is transmitted between two cells. But to understand what happens once the impulse is transmitted, we must first examine the chemical signals that accomplish transmission. Let's turn our attention to neurotransmitters.

Neurotransmitters

More than 40 neurotransmitters have been identified. These can be categorized as either (a) small-molecule, rapid-acting neurotransmitters, or (b) neuropeptide, slow-acting neurotransmitters. These are outlined in Table 3.1. The small-molecule, rapidly acting transmitters, which are responsible for most neural transmissions, will be our main concern.

Acetylcholine and norepinephrine are the two major neurotransmitters involved in regulating our physiological responses to exercise. Acetylcholine is the primary neurotransmitter for the motor neurons that innervate skeletal muscle and many parasympathetic neurons. It is generally an excitatory neurotransmitter, but it can have inhibitory effects at some parasympathetic nerve endings such as in the heart. Norepinephrine is the neurotransmitter for some sympathetic neurons, and it, too, can be either excitatory or inhibitory, depending on the receptors involved.

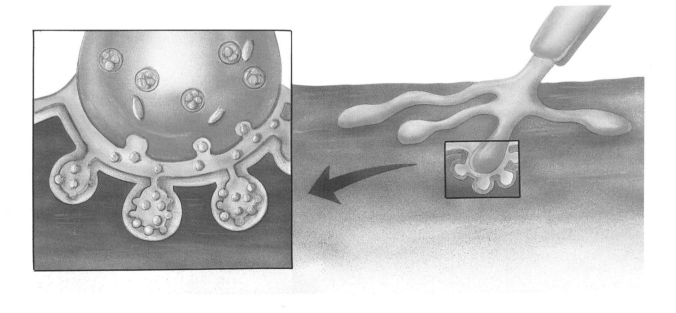

Figure 3.4   The neuromuscular junction.

Table 3.1   Classification of Neurotransmitters

Small-molecule, rapid-acting transmitters

Class I	Acetylcholine
Class II	Amines: norepinephrine, epinephrine, dopamine, serotonin, and histamine
Class III	Amino acids: GABA, glycine, glutamate, and aspartate

Neuropeptide, slow-acting transmitters

Hypothalamic-releasing hormones (e.g., thyrotropin-releasing hormone and somatostatin)

Pituitary peptides (e.g., β-endorphins, thyrotropin, and vasopressin)

Peptides that act on the gut and brain (e.g., cholecystokinin, neurotensin, and leucine enkephalin)

Peptides from other tissues (e.g., angiotensin II, bradykinin, and calcitonin)

KEY POINT

Acetylcholine and norepinephrine are the two major neurotransmitters—chemical substances that transmit nerve impulses across synapses and synaptic clefts.

Once the neurotransmitter binds to the postsynaptic receptor, the nerve impulse has been successfully transmitted. The neurotransmitter is then either destroyed by enzymes or actively transported back into the presynaptic terminals for reuse when the next impulse arrives.

The Postsynaptic Response

We have discussed generating an action potential, conducting the impulse the length of the neuron, and transmitting it to the next cell. We continue the story with what happens after the neurotransmitter binds with the postsynaptic receptors.

Once the neurotransmitter binds to the receptors, the chemical signal that traversed the synaptic cleft once again becomes an electrical signal. The binding causes a graded potential in the postsynaptic membrane. As mentioned earlier, an incoming impulse may be either excitatory or inhibitory. An excitatory impulse causes a depolarization, known as an excitatory postsynaptic potential (EPSP). An inhibitory impulse causes a hyperpolarization, known as an inhibitory postsynaptic potential (IPSP).

The discharge of a single presynaptic terminal generally changes the postsynaptic potential less than 1 mV. Clearly this is not sufficient to generate an action potential because reaching threshold requires a

---

IN REVIEW . . .

1. Neurons communicate with each other across synapses.
2. A synapse involves
   - the axon terminals of the presynaptic neuron,
   - the postsynaptic receptors on the dendrite or cell body of the next neuron, and
   - the space (the synaptic cleft) between the two neurons.
3. A nerve impulse causes chemicals called neurotransmitters to be released from the presynaptic axon terminals into the synaptic cleft.
4. Neurotransmitters diffuse across the cleft and are bound to the postsynaptic receptors.
5. Once neurotransmitters are bound, the impulse has been successfully transmitted and the neurotransmitter is then either destroyed by enzymes or actively returned to the presynaptic neuron for future use.
6. Neurotransmitter binding at the postsynaptic receptors opens ion gates in that membrane and can cause depolarization (excitation) or hyperpolarization (inhibition), depending on the specific neurotransmitter and the receptors to which it binds.
7. Neurons communicate with muscle cells at neuromuscular junctions. These involve presynaptic axon terminals (motor endplates), the synaptic cleft, and receptors on the sarcolemma of the muscle fiber. The neuromuscular junction functions much like a neural synapse.
8. The neurotransmitters most important to regulation of exercise are acetylcholine and norepinephrine.

---

change of at least 15 to 20 mV. But when a neuron transmits an impulse, several presynaptic terminals typically release their neurotransmitters so they can diffuse to the postsynaptic receptors. Also, presynaptic terminals from numerous axons can converge on the dendrites and cell body of a single neuron. When multiple presynaptic terminals discharge at the same time, or when only a few fire in rapid succession, more neurotransmitter is released. With an excitatory neurotransmitter, the more that is bound, the greater the EPSP will be.

Triggering an action potential at the postsynaptic neuron depends on the combined effects of all incoming impulses from these various presynaptic terminals. A number of impulses are needed to cause sufficient depolarization in order to generate an action potential. Specifically, the sum of all changes in the membrane potential must equal or exceed the threshold. This summing of their individual effects is called summation.

For summation, the postsynaptic cell must keep a running total of the neuron's responses, both EPSPs and IPSPs, to all incoming impulses. This task is done at the axon hillock, which lies on the axon just past the cell body. Only when the sum of all individual graded potentials meets or exceeds threshold can an action potential occur.

Now that we have carefully considered the function of the most basic units of the nervous system, the neurons, we are ready to examine how these cells work together. Individual neurons are grouped together into bundles. In the central nervous system (brain and spinal cord) these bundles are referred to as tracts, or pathways. Neuron bundles in the peripheral nervous system are referred to as nerves.

IN REVIEW . . .

1. EPSPs are depolarizations of the postsynaptic membrane. IPSPs are hyperpolarizations of that membrane.
2. A single presynaptic terminal cannot generate enough of a depolarization to fire an action potential. Multiple signals are needed. These may come from numerous neurons or from a single neuron when numerous axon terminals release neurotransmitters repeatedly and rapidly.
3. The axon hillock keeps a running total of all EPSPs and IPSPs. When their sum meets or exceeds the threshold for depolarization, an action potential occurs. This process of accumulating incoming signals is known as summation.

The Central Nervous System (CNS)

To comprehend how even the most basic stimulus can cause muscle activity, we must next consider the complexity of the nervous system. Let's turn our attention to the various components of the nervous system and how they effect movement. These components are listed in Figure 3.5. In this section we will consider an overview of the components of the central nervous system. We will briefly consider their functions.

The central nervous system houses more than 100 billion neurons.

The Brain

Your brain is composed of numerous parts. For our purposes, we will subdivide it into four regions:

1. The cerebrum
2. The diencephalon
3. The cerebellum
4. The brain stem

These parts of the brain are illustrated in Figure 3.6. Let's discuss them briefly.

The Cerebrum

The cerebrum is composed of the right and left cerebral hemispheres. These are connected to each other by fiber bundles (tracts) referred to as the corpus callosum, allowing the two hemispheres to communicate with each other. The cerebral cortex forms the outer portion of the cerebral hemispheres and has been referred to as the site of the mind and intellect. It is also called the gray matter, which simply reflects its distinctive

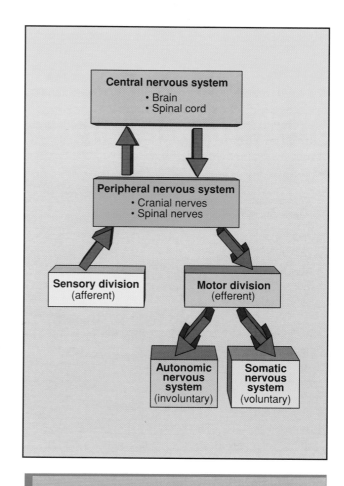

Figure 3.5   The functional organization of the nervous system.

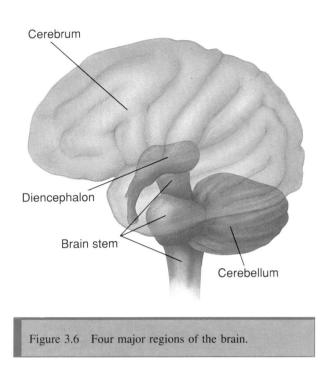

Cerebrum

Diencephalon

Brain stem

Cerebellum

Figure 3.6   Four major regions of the brain.

color resulting from lack of myelin on the cell bodies located in this area. The cerebral cortex is your conscious brain. It allows you to think, to be aware of sensory stimuli, and to voluntarily control your movements.

The cerebrum consists of five lobes—four outer lobes and the central insula, which we will not discuss.

Its four major lobes have the following general functions:

1. The frontal lobe: general intellect and motor control
2. The temporal lobe: auditory input and its interpretation
3. The parietal lobe: general sensory input and its interpretation
4. The occipital lobe: visual input and its interpretation

These lobes are shown in Figure 3.7.

The three areas in the cerebrum that are of primary concern to our discussion and which we will discuss later in this chapter are

1. the primary motor cortex, in the frontal lobe;
2. the basal ganglia, in the cerebral white matter; and
3. the primary sensory cortex, in the parietal lobe.

The Diencephalon

This region of the brain is mostly composed of the thalamus and the hypothalamus. The thalamus is an important sensory integration center. All sensory input (except smell) enters the thalamus and is relayed to the appropriate area of the cortex. The thalamus regulates what sensory input reaches your conscious brain, and thus is very important for motor control.

The hypothalamus, directly below the thalamus, is responsible for maintaining homeostasis by regulating

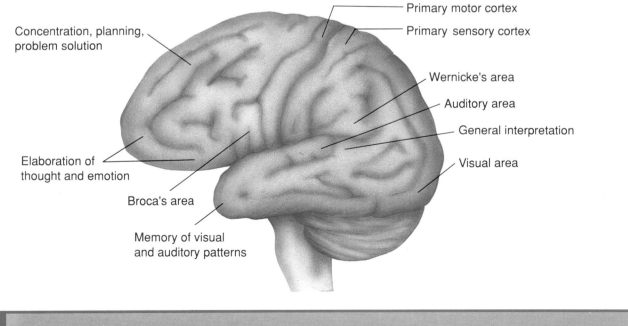

Concentration, planning, problem solution

Elaboration of thought and emotion

Broca's area

Memory of visual and auditory patterns

Primary motor cortex

Primary sensory cortex

Wernicke's area

Auditory area

General interpretation

Visual area

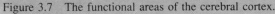

Figure 3.7   The functional areas of the cerebral cortex.

almost all processes that affect the body's internal environment. Neural centers here regulate

- the autonomic nervous system (and, through it, blood pressure, heart rate and contractility, respiration, digestion, etc.),
- body temperature,
- fluid balance,
- neuroendocrine control,
- emotions,
- thirst,
- food intake, and
- sleep-wake cycles.

The Cerebellum

The cerebellum is located behind the brain stem. It is connected to numerous parts of the brain and has a crucial role in controlling movement, as we shall see later in this chapter.

The Brain Stem

The brain stem, composed of the midbrain, the pons, and the medulla oblongata (Figure 3.8), is the stalk of your brain, connecting the brain and the spinal cord. All sensory and motor nerves pass through the brain stem as they relay information between the brain and the spinal cord. This is the site of origin for 10 of the 12 pairs of cranial nerves. The brain stem also contains the major autonomic regulatory centers that exert control over the respiratory and cardiovascular systems.

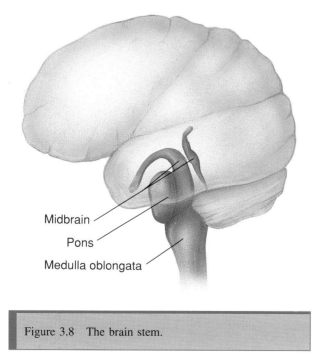

Midbrain

Pons

Medulla oblongata

Figure 3.8   The brain stem.

A specialized collection of neurons running the entire length of the brain stem, known as the reticular formation, are influenced by and have an influence on nearly all areas of the central nervous system. These neurons help

- coordinate skeletal muscle function,
- maintain muscle tone,
- control cardiovascular and respiratory functions, and
- determine our state of consciousness (both arousal and sleep).

The brain has a pain control system, called an analgesia system. The enkephalins and β-endorphin are important opiate substances that act on the opiate receptors in the analgesia system to help reduce pain. Exercise of long duration has been postulated to increase the natural levels of these opiate substances.

The Spinal Cord

The lowest part of the brain stem, the medulla oblongata, is continuous below with the spinal cord. The spinal cord is composed of tracts of nerve fibers that allow two-way conduction of nerve impulses. The sensory (afferent) fibers carry neural signals from sensory receptors, such as those in the muscles and joints, to the upper levels of the CNS. Motor (efferent) fibers from the brain and upper spinal cord travel down to end organs (muscles, glands).

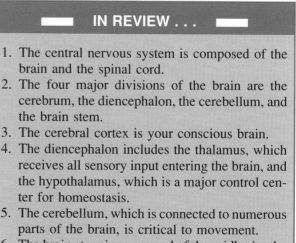

▬ IN REVIEW . . . ▬

1. The central nervous system is composed of the brain and the spinal cord.
2. The four major divisions of the brain are the cerebrum, the diencephalon, the cerebellum, and the brain stem.
3. The cerebral cortex is your conscious brain.
4. The diencephalon includes the thalamus, which receives all sensory input entering the brain, and the hypothalamus, which is a major control center for homeostasis.
5. The cerebellum, which is connected to numerous parts of the brain, is critical to movement.
6. The brain stem is composed of the midbrain, the pons, and the medulla oblongata.
7. The spinal cord carries both sensory and motor fibers between the brain and the periphery.

The Peripheral Nervous System (PNS)

The peripheral nervous system contains 43 pairs of nerves: 12 pairs of cranial nerves that connect with the brain and 31 pairs of spinal nerves that connect with the spinal cord. Spinal nerves directly supply the skeletal muscles. Recall the structure of a spinal nerve, as shown in Figure 3.9, from introductory anatomy. For each spinal nerve, sensory neurons enter the spinal cord through the dorsal root, and their cell bodies are located in the dorsal root ganglia. Motor neurons leave the cord through the ventral root; they are the final link in the chain of control for muscle activity, terminating at the neuromuscular junctions.

Functionally, the peripheral nervous system has two major divisions: the sensory division and the motor division. Let's examine each briefly.

The Sensory Division

The sensory division of your peripheral nervous system carries sensory information toward your central nervous system. Sensory (afferent) neurons originate in such areas as

- blood and lymph vessels,
- internal organs,
- organs of special sense (taste, touch, smell, hearing, vision),
- the skin, and
- muscles and tendons.

Sensory neurons in your PNS end either in your spinal cord or in your brain, and they continuously convey information to the CNS concerning the body's constantly changing status. By relaying this information, these neurons allow your brain to sense what is going on in all parts of your body and in your immediate environment. Sensory neurons within your CNS carry the sensory input to appropriate areas where the information can be processed and integrated with other incoming information.

The sensory division receives information from five primary types of receptors:

1. Mechanoreceptors that respond to mechanical forces such as pressure, touch, or stretch
2. Thermoreceptors that respond to changes in temperature
3. Nociceptors that respond to painful stimuli
4. Photoreceptors that respond to electromagnetic radiation (light) to allow vision
5. Chemoreceptors that respond to chemical stimuli, such as from foods, odors, or changes in blood concentrations of substances (oxygen, carbon dioxide, glucose, electrolytes, etc.)

Several of these receptors are important in exercise and sport. Let's consider just a few. Free nerve endings detect crude touch, pressure, pain, heat, and cold. Thus they function as mechanoreceptors, noci-

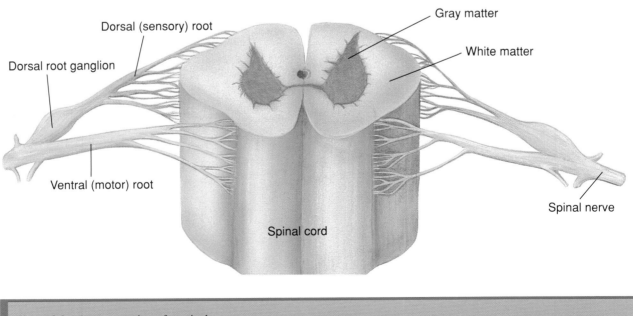

Figure 3.9 A cross section of a spinal nerve.

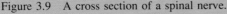

ceptors, and thermoreceptors. These nerve endings are important for the prevention of injury during athletic performance.

Special muscle and joint nerve endings are of many types and functions, and each type is sensitive to a specific stimulus. Here are some important examples:

- Joint kinesthetic receptors located in your joint capsules are sensitive to joint angles and rates of change in these angles. Thus they sense the position and any movement of your joints.
- Muscle spindles sense how much a muscle is stretched.
- Golgi tendon organs detect the tension applied by a muscle to its tendon, providing information about the strength of muscle contraction.

Muscle spindles and Golgi tendon organs are discussed later in this chapter.

The Motor Division

Your central nervous system transmits information out to various parts of your body through the motor, or efferent, division of your peripheral nervous system. Once your CNS has processed the information it receives from the sensory division, it decides how your body should respond to that input. From your brain and spinal cord, intricate networks of neurons go out to all parts of your body providing detailed instructions to the target areas—for our purposes, muscles.

The Autonomic Nervous System

The autonomic nervous system, often considered part of the motor division of the peripheral nervous system, controls your body's involuntary internal functions. Some of these functions that are important to the athlete include

- heart rate,
- blood pressure,
- blood distribution, and
- respiration.

The autonomic nervous system has two major divisions: the sympathetic nervous system and the parasympathetic nervous system. These originate from different sections of the spinal cord and from the base of the brain. The effects of the two systems are often antagonistic, but both systems always function together. Remember this as we examine each separately.

The Sympathetic Nervous System

The sympathetic nervous system is your fight-or-flight system—it prepares your body to face a crisis. When you're excited, your sympathetic nervous system produces a massive discharge throughout your body, preparing you for action. A sudden loud noise, a life-threatening situation, or those last few seconds before starting an athletic competition are examples of when you would experience this massive sympathetic discharge. The effects of sympathetic stimulation are important to the athlete:

- Heart rate and strength of cardiac contraction increase.
- Coronary vessels dilate, increasing the blood supply to the heart muscle to meet its increased demands.
- Vasodilation allows more blood to enter the active skeletal muscles.
- Vasoconstriction in most other tissues diverts blood away from them and to the active muscles.
- Blood pressure increases, allowing better perfusion of the muscles and improving the return of venous blood.
- Bronchodilation improves gas exchange.
- Metabolic rate increases, reflecting the body's increased effort to meet the increased demands of physical activity.
- Mental activity increases, allowing better perception of sensory stimuli and more concentration on performance.
- Glucose is released from the liver into the blood as an energy source.
- Functions not directly needed are slowed (renal function, digestion), conserving energy so it can be used for action.

These basic alterations in body function facilitate your motor response, demonstrating the importance of the autonomic nervous system in preparing you for acute stress or physical activity.

The Parasympathetic Nervous System

The parasympathetic nervous system is your body's housekeeping system. It has a major role in carrying out such processes as digestion, urination, glandular secretion, and conservation of energy. This system is more active when you are calm and at rest. Its effects tend to oppose those of the sympathetic system. It causes

- decreased heart rate,
- constriction of coronary vessels, and
- bronchoconstriction.

The various effects of the sympathetic and parasympathetic divisions of the autonomic nervous system are summarized in Table 3.2.

Table 3.2   Effects of the Sympathetic and Parasympathetic Nervous Systems on Various Organs

Target organ/system	Sympathetic effects	Parasympathetic effects
Heart muscle	Increases rate and force of contraction	Decreases rate of contraction
Heart: coronary blood vessels	Causes vasodilation	Causes vasoconstriction
Lungs	Causes bronchodilation; mildly constricts blood vessels	Causes bronchoconstriction
Blood vessels	Increases blood pressure; causes vasoconstriction in abdominal viscera and skin to divert blood when necessary; causes vasodilation in the skeletal muscles and heart during exercise	Little or no effect
Liver	Stimulates glucose release	No effect
Cellular metabolism	Increases metabolic rate	No effect
Adipose tissue	Stimulates lipolysis	No effect
Sweat glands	Increases sweating	No effect
Adrenal medulla	Stimulates secretion of epinephrine and norepinephrine	No effect
Digestive system	Decreases activity of glands and muscles; constricts sphincters	Increases peristalsis and glandular secretion; relaxes sphincters
Kidney	Causes vasoconstriction; decreases urine formation	No effect

IN REVIEW . . .

1. The peripheral nervous system contains 43 pairs of nerves: 12 cranial and 31 spinal.
2. The PNS can be subdivided into the sensory and motor divisions. The motor division also includes the autonomic nervous system.
3. The sensory division carries information from sensory receptors to the CNS so that the CNS is constantly aware of your current status and your environment.
4. The motor division carries motor impulses out from the CNS to the muscles.
5. The autonomic nervous system includes the sympathetic nervous system, which is your fight-or-flight system, and the parasympathetic system, which is your housekeeping system. Though these systems often oppose each other, they always function together.

Sensory-Motor Integration

Now that we have discussed the components and divisions of the nervous system, we are ready to discuss how a sensory stimulus gives rise to a motor response. How, for example, do the muscles in your hand know to pull your finger away from a hot stove? How, when you decide to run, do the muscles in your legs coordinate while supporting your weight and propelling you forward? To accomplish these tasks, the sensory and motor systems must communicate with each other.

This process is called sensory-motor integration, and it is depicted in Figure 3.10. For your body to respond to sensory stimuli, the sensory and motor divisions of your nervous system must function together in a specific sequence of events:

1. A sensory stimulus is received by sensory receptors (Figure 3.10a).
2. The sensory impulse is transmitted along sensory neurons to the CNS (Figure 3.10b).
3. The CNS interprets the incoming sensory information and determines which response is most appropriate (Figure 3.10c).
4. The signals for the response are transmitted from the CNS out along motor neurons (Figure 3.10d).
5. The motor impulse is transmitted to a muscle (Figure 3.10e) and the response occurs.

Sensory Input

Recall that sensations and physiological status are detected by sensory receptors throughout your body. The impulses resulting from sensory stimulation are transmitted via the sensory nerves to the spinal cord. When they reach the spinal cord, they can trigger a local reflex at that level or they can travel to the upper regions of the spinal cord or to the brain. Sensory pathways to the brain can terminate in sensory areas of the brain stem, the cerebellum, the thalamus, or the cerebral cortex. An area in which the sensory impulses terminate is referred to as an integration center. This is where the sensory input is interpreted and linked to the motor system. These integration centers vary in function:

- Sensory impulses that terminate in the spinal cord are integrated there. The response is typically a simple motor reflex, which is the simplest type of integration. We will discuss it later.

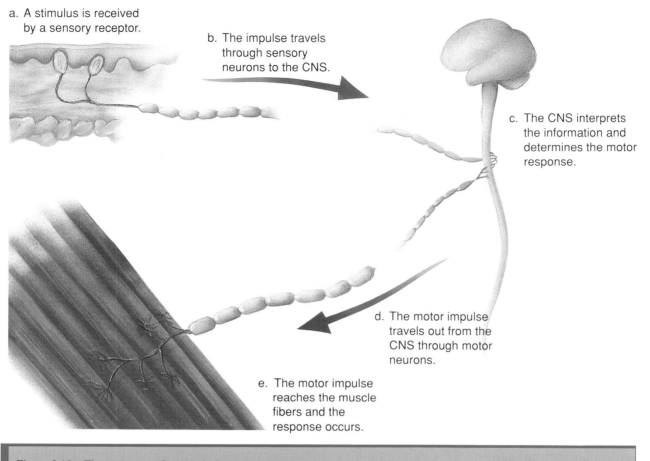

a. A stimulus is received by a sensory receptor.

b. The impulse travels through sensory neurons to the CNS.

c. The CNS interprets the information and determines the motor response.

d. The motor impulse travels out from the CNS through motor neurons.

e. The motor impulse reaches the muscle fibers and the response occurs.

Figure 3.10   The sequence of events in sensory-motor integration.

- Sensory signals that terminate in the lower brain stem result in subconscious motor reactions of a higher and more complex nature than simple spinal cord reflexes. Postural control when sitting, standing, or moving is an example of this level of sensory input.
- Sensory signals that terminate in the cerebellum also result in subconscious control of movement. This appears to be the center of coordination, smoothing out movements by coordinating the actions of the various contracting muscle groups to perform the desired movement. Both fine and gross motor movements appear to be coordinated by the cerebellum in concert with the basal ganglia. Without the control exerted by the cerebellum, all movement would be uncontrolled and uncoordinated.
- Sensory signals that terminate at the thalamus begin to enter the level of consciousness, and you begin to distinguish various sensations.
- Only when sensory signals enter the cerebral cortex can you discretely localize the signal. The primary sensory cortex, located in the postcentral gyrus (in the parietal lobe), receives general sensory input from receptors in the skin and from proprioceptors in the muscles, tendons, and joints. This area has a map of the body. Stimulation in a specific area of the body is recognized and its exact location is known instantly. Thus, this part of our conscious brain allows us to be constantly aware of our surroundings and our relationship to them.

Figure 3.11 illustrates various sensory receptors and their nerve pathways back to the spinal cord and up into various areas of the brain.

Motor Control

Once a sensory impulse is received, it typically evokes a response through a motor neuron, regardless of the level at which the sensory impulse stops. Skeletal muscles are controlled by impulses conducted by motor (efferent) neurons that originate from any of three levels:

1. The spinal cord
2. The lower regions of the brain
3. The motor area of the cerebral cortex

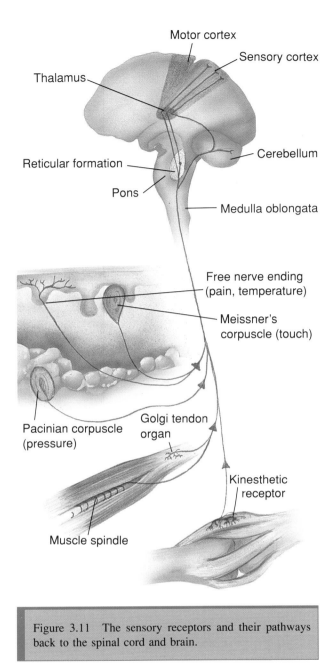

Figure 3.11   The sensory receptors and their pathways back to the spinal cord and brain.

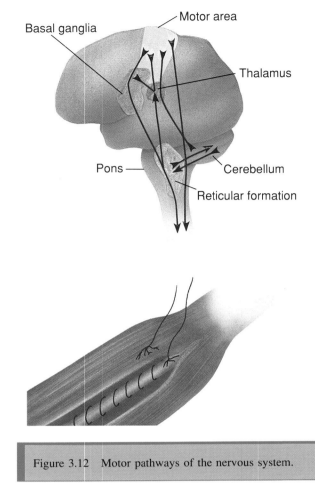

Figure 3.12   Motor pathways of the nervous system.

As the level of control moves from the spinal cord to the motor cortex, the degree of movement complexity increases from simple reflex control to complicated movements requiring basic thought processes. Motor responses for more complex movement patterns typically originate in the motor cortex of the brain. Some motor pathways are depicted in Figure 3.12.

At last, we are ready to tie the two systems together through sensory-motor integration. The simplest form of this is the reflex, so we will consider it first.

Reflex Activity

What happens when you unknowingly put your hand on a hot stove? First, the stimuli of heat and pain are received by the thermoreceptors and nociceptors in your hand, then travel to the spinal cord, terminating at the level of entry. Once in the spinal cord, these impulses are integrated instantly by interneurons that connect the sensory and motor neurons. The impulse moves to the motor neurons and travels to the effectors, the muscles controlling the withdrawal of your hand. The result is that you reflexively withdraw your hand from the hot stove without giving the action any thought.

A reflex is a preprogrammed response—any time your sensory nerves transmit specific impulses, your body responds instantly and identically. In our example, whether you touch something that is too hot or too cold, thermoreceptors will elicit a reflex for you to withdraw your hand. Whether the pain arises from heat or from a sharp object, the nociceptors will also cause a withdrawal reflex. By the time you are consciously aware of the specific stimulus, after sensory impulses have also been transmitted to your primary sensory cortex, the reflex activity is well under way, if not completed. All neural activity occurs extremely rapidly, but a reflex is the fastest mode of response because you don't need time to make a conscious decision. Only one response is possible—no options need to be considered.

Muscle Spindles

Now that you understand the basics of reflex activity, we can look more closely at two reflexes that help control muscle function. The first involves a special structure—the muscle spindle.

Muscle spindles, as seen in Figure 3.13, lie between regular skeletal muscle fibers, referred to as extrafusal (outside the spindle) fibers. A muscle spindle is composed of from 4 to 20 small specialized muscle fibers called intrafusal (inside the spindle) fi-

bers, and the nerve endings, sensory and motor, associated with these fibers. A connective tissue sheath surrounds the muscle spindle and attaches to the endomysium of the extrafusal fibers. The intrafusal fibers are controlled by specialized motor neurons, referred to as gamma motor neurons. In contrast, extrafusal fibers (the regular fibers) are controlled by alpha motor neurons.

The central region of an intrafusal fiber cannot contract because it contains no or only a few actin and myosin filaments. Thus, the central region can only stretch. Because the muscle spindle is attached to the extrafusal fibers, any time those fibers are stretched the central region of the muscle spindle will also be stretched.

Sensory nerve endings wrapped around this central region of the muscle spindle transmit information to the spinal cord when this region is stretched, informing the CNS of the muscle's length. In the spinal cord, the sensory neuron synapses with an alpha motor neuron, which triggers reflexive muscle contraction (in the extrafusal fibers) to resist further stretching.

Let's illustrate this action with an example. Your arm is bent at the elbow, and your hand is extended, palm up. Suddenly someone places a heavy weight in your palm. Your forearm starts to drop, which stretches the muscle fibers in your arm (biceps brachii), which, in turn, stretch the muscle spindle. In response to that stretch, the sensory neurons send impulses to the spinal cord, which then excites the alpha motor neurons. These cause the biceps to contract, overcoming the stretch.

Gamma motor neurons excite the intrafusal fibers, prestretching them slightly. Though the midsection of the intrafusal fibers cannot contract, the ends can. The gamma motor neurons cause slight contraction of the ends of these fibers, which stretches the central region slightly. This prestretch makes the muscle spindle highly sensitive to even small degrees of stretch.

The muscle spindle also assists normal muscle action. It appears that when the alpha motor neurons are stimulated to contract the extrafusal muscle fibers, the gamma motor neurons are also activated, contracting the ends of the intrafusal fibers. This stretches the central region of the muscle spindle, giving rise to sensory impulses that travel to the spinal cord and then to the motor neurons. In response, the muscle contracts. Thus neural muscle contraction is enhanced through this function of the muscle spindles.

Information brought into the spinal cord from the sensory neurons associated with muscle spindles does not merely end at that level. Impulses are also sent up to higher parts of the CNS, supplying the brain with information on the exact length and contractile state

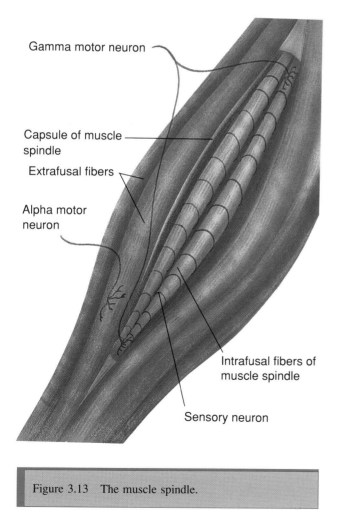

Gamma motor neuron

Capsule of muscle spindle

Extrafusal fibers

Alpha motor neuron

Intrafusal fibers of muscle spindle

Sensory neuron

Figure 3.13   The muscle spindle.

of the muscle, as well as the rate at which those are changing. This information is essential for maintaining muscle tone and posture, and for executing movements. Before the brain can tell a muscle what to do next, the brain must know what the muscle is currently doing.

Golgi Tendon Organs

Golgi tendon organs are encapsulated sensory receptors through which a small bundle of muscle tendon fibers pass. These organs are located just proximal to the tendon fibers' attachment to the muscle fibers, as shown in Figure 3.14. Approximately 5 to 25 muscle fibers are usually connected with each Golgi tendon organ. Whereas muscle spindles monitor the length of a muscle, these structures are sensitive to tension in the muscle-tendon complex and operate like a strain gauge, a device that senses changes in tension. Their sensitivity is so great that they can respond to the contraction of a single muscle fiber. These sensory receptors are inhibitory in nature, performing a protective function by reducing the potential for injury. When stimulated, these receptors inhibit the contracting (agonist) muscles and excite the antagonist muscles.

Some researchers speculate that reducing the influence of Golgi tendon organs results in disinhibition of the active muscles, allowing a more forceful muscle action. This mechanism may explain at least part of the gains in muscular strength that accompany strength training.

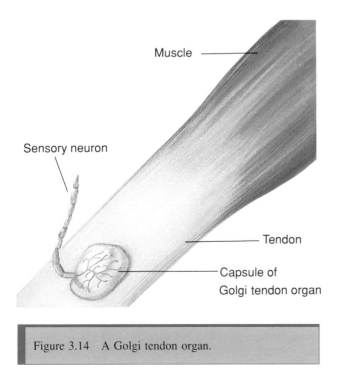

Muscle

Sensory neuron

Tendon

Capsule of Golgi tendon organ

Figure 3.14   A Golgi tendon organ.

The Higher Brain Centers

Reflexes involve the simplest form of neural integration. But most movements used in sport activities involve control and coordination through the higher brain centers, specifically

- the primary motor cortex,
- the basal ganglia, and
- the cerebellum.

Let's discuss some functions of each of these.

The Primary Motor Cortex

The primary motor cortex is responsible for the control of fine and discrete muscle movements. It is located in the frontal lobe, specifically within the precentral gyrus. Neurons here, known as pyramidal cells, let us consciously control movement of our skeletal muscles. Think of the primary motor cortex as the part of the brain that decides what movement you want to make. For example, if you are sitting in a chair and you want to stand up, the decision to do so is made in your primary motor cortex, where the entire body is carefully mapped out. The areas that require the finest motor control have a greater representation in the motor cortex, thus more neural control is provided to them.

The cell bodies of the pyramidal cells are housed in the primary motor cortex, and their axons form the extrapyramidal tracts. These are also known as the corticospinal tracts because the nerve processes extend from the cerebral cortex down to the spinal cord. These tracts provide the major voluntary control of our skeletal muscles.

The Basal Ganglia

The basal ganglia (nuclei) are not part of the cerebral cortex. Rather they are in the cerebral white matter, deep to the cortex. These ganglia are clusters of nerve cell bodies. The complex functions of the basal ganglia are not well understood, but the ganglia are known to be important in the initiation of movements of a sustained and repetitive nature (such as arm-swinging while walking), and thus they control complex semi-voluntary movements such as walking and running. These cells are also involved in maintaining posture and muscle tone.

The Cerebellum

The cerebellum is crucial to the control of all rapid and complex muscular activities. It helps coordinate the timing of motor activities and the rapid progression from one movement to the next by monitoring and making corrective adjustments in the motor activities that are elicited by other parts of the brain. The cerebellum assists the functions of both the primary motor cortex and the basal ganglia. It facilitates movement patterns by smoothing out the movement that would otherwise be jerky and uncontrolled.

The cerebellum acts as an integration system, comparing your programmed or intended activity with the actual changes occurring in your body, then initiating corrective adjustments through the motor system. It receives information from the cerebrum and other parts of your brain, and also from sensory receptors (proprioceptors) in your muscles and joints that keep your cerebellum informed about your body's current position. The cerebellum also receives visual and equilibrium input. Thus it notes all incoming information about the exact tension and position of all muscles, joints, and tendons and your body's current position relative to your surroundings, then determines the best plan of action to produce the desired movement.

Consider our previous example in which you were sitting but wanted to stand. Your primary motor cortex is the part of your brain that makes the decision to stand. This decision is relayed to the cerebellum. The cerebellum notes the desired action, then considers the current status of your body, based on all the sensory input it receives. Then the cerebellum decides, based on that input, what is the best plan of action to accomplish your desired movement, standing.

Engrams

When you learn a new motor skill, your initial periods of practice require intense concentration. As you become more familiar with the skill, you find that you don't need to concentrate as much. Finally, once you perfect the skill, it can be recalled with little or no conscious effort. How do you reach this point?

Specific learned motor patterns appear to be stored in the brain, to be replayed on request. These memorized motor patterns are referred to as motor programs, or engrams. Engrams are apparently stored in both the sensory and motor portions of the brain. Those in the sensory portion of the brain are for slower motor patterns, and those in the motor portion are for rapid movements. Little is known about engrams and the mechanisms of their action, so these are important areas for future research.

The Motor Response

Now that we have discussed how sensory input is integrated to determine the appropriate motor response, the last step in the process to consider is how muscles

---

━━ IN REVIEW . . . ━━

1. Sensory-motor integration is the process by which your PNS relays sensory input to your CNS, your CNS interprets this information, and then it sends out the appropriate motor signal to elicit the desired motor response.
2. Sensory input can terminate at various levels of the CNS. Not all of this information reaches the brain.
3. Reflexes are the simplest form of motor control. These are not conscious responses. For a given sensory stimulus, the motor response is always identical and instantaneous.
4. Muscle spindles trigger reflexive muscle action when the muscle spindle is stretched.
5. Golgi tendon organs trigger a reflex that inhibits contraction if the tendon fibers are overstretched.
6. The primary motor cortex, located in the frontal lobe, is the center of conscious motor control.
7. The basal ganglia, in the cerebral white matter, help initiate some movements (sustained and repetitive ones) and help control posture and muscle tone.
8. The cerebellum is involved in all rapid and complex movement processes and assists the primary motor cortex and the basal ganglia. It is an integration center that decides how to best execute the desired movement given your body's current position and your muscles' current status.
9. Though not well understood, engrams are memorized motor patterns, stored in both the sensory and motor areas of the brain, that are called upon as needed.

---

respond to motor impulses once they reach the muscle fibers.

The Motor Unit

Once an electrical impulse reaches a motor neuron, the impulse travels the length of the neuron to the neuromuscular junction. From there, the impulse spreads to all muscle fibers innervated by that particular motor neuron. Recall that the motor neuron and all muscle fibers it innervates form a single motor unit. Each muscle fiber is innervated by only one motor neuron, but each motor neuron innervates up to several thousand muscle fibers, depending on the function of the muscle. Muscles controlling fine movements, such as those controlling the eyes, have only a small number of muscle fibers per motor neuron. Muscles with more general functions have many fibers per motor neuron.

The muscles that control eye movements (the extraocular muscles) have an innervation ratio of 1:15, meaning that one motor neuron serves only 15 muscle fibers. In contrast, the gastrocnemius and tibialis anterior muscles have innervation ratios of almost 1:2,000.

The muscle fibers in a specific motor unit are homogeneous with respect to fiber type. Thus you won't find a motor unit that has both fast-twitch and slow-twitch fibers. In fact, as mentioned in chapter 2, it is generally believed that the characteristics of the motor neuron actually determine the fiber type in that motor unit.[1,3]

The Orderly Recruitment of Muscle Fibers

Most researchers agree that motor units are generally activated on the basis of a fixed order of recruitment. This is known as the principle of orderly recruitment, in which the motor units within a given muscle appear to be ranked. Let's use the biceps brachii as an example: Assuming a total of 200 motor units, they would be ranked on a scale of 1 to 200. For an extremely fine muscle action requiring very little force production, the motor unit ranked number 1 would be recruited. As the requirements for force production increased, numbers 2, 3, 4, and so on would be recruited, up to a maximal muscle action that would activate 50% to 70% of the motor units. For a given force production, the same motor units are recruited each time.

A mechanism that may partially explain the principle of orderly recruitment is the size principle, which states that the recruitment of a motor unit is directly related to the motor neuron size. Motor units with smaller motor neurons will be recruited first. Because the slow-twitch motor units have smaller motor neurons, they are the first units recruited in graded movement (going from very low to very high rates of force production). The fast-twitch motor units are then recruited as the force needed to perform the movement increases. Some questions remain about how the size principle relates to most athletic movements, because it has been examined only in graded movements that represent relative intensities of muscle action of less than 25%.

KEY POINT

Neuromuscular activity is graded on the basis of a fixed order of recruitment from the available pool of motor units. The more force that is needed to execute a certain movement, the more motor units are recruited.

IN REVIEW . . .

1. Each muscle fiber is innervated by only one neuron, but each neuron may innervate up to several thousand muscle fibers.
2. All muscle fibers within a single motor unit are of the same fiber type.
3. Motor units are recruited in an orderly manner, so that specific ones are called on each time a specific activity is performed.
4. Motor units with smaller neurons (slow-twitch units) are called on before those with larger neurons (fast-twitch).

In Closing . . .

What we have covered in this chapter is merely a tiny fragment of the complex role the nervous system plays in regulating movement. All divisions of the nervous system are involved:

- The sensory division of the PNS always keeps your CNS informed of what is happening in and around your body.
- The CNS interprets all incoming sensory information and decides how you should respond.
- The motor division of the PNS tells your muscles exactly when and how much to act.
- The autonomic division of the PNS adjusts physiological functions throughout your body to ensure that the needs of your active tissues are met.

We have seen how your muscles respond to neural stimulation, whether through reflexes or under complex control of the higher brain centers. We discussed how the individual motor units respond and how they are recruited in an orderly manner depending on the required force. Thus we have learned how your body functions to allow you to move. In the next chapter, we shall examine the effects that training has on this neuromuscular control.

Key Terms

action potential
axon terminal
depolarization
engram
excitatory postsynaptic
    potential (EPSP)
Golgi tendon organ
graded potential
hyperpolarization
inhibitory postsynaptic
    potential (IPSP)

motor reflex
muscle spindle
myelin sheath
nerve impulse
neuromuscular junction
neurotransmitter
principle of orderly re-
    cruitment
resting membrane poten-
    tial (RMP)
saltatory conduction

sensory-motor inte-
gration
summation

synapse
threshold

Study Questions

1. Name the different regions of a neuron.
2. Explain the resting membrane potential. What causes it? How is it maintained?
3. Describe an action potential. What is required before an action potential is fired? Once it is fired, what is the sequence of events?
4. Explain how an electrical impulse is transmitted from a presynaptic neuron to a postsynaptic neuron. Describe a synapse and a neuromuscular junction.
5. How is an action potential generated in a postsynaptic neuron?
6. What are the major divisions of the nervous system? What are their major functions?
7. What brain centers have major roles in controlling movement, and what are these roles?
8. How do the sympathetic and parasympathetic systems differ? What is their significance to performing physical activity?
9. Explain how movement occurs in response to touching a hot object.
10. Describe the role of the muscle spindle in controlling muscle action.
11. Describe the role of the Golgi tendon organ in controlling muscle action.
12. What is a motor unit, and how are motor units recruited?

References

1. Edström, L., & Grimby, L. (1986). Effect of exercise on the motor unit. *Muscle and Nerve*, **9**, 104-126.

2. Guyton, A.C. (1991). *Textbook of medical physiology* (8th ed.). Philadelphia: Saunders.

3. Pette, D., & Vrbová, G. (1985). Neural control of phenotypic expression in mammalian muscle fibers. *Muscle and Nerve*, **8**, 676-689.

Selected Readings

Åstrand, P.-O., & Rodahl, K. (1986). *Textbook of work physiology* (3rd ed.). New York: McGraw-Hill.
Brooks, G.A., & Fahey, T.D. (1984). *Exercise physiology: Human bioenergetics and its applications.* New York: Wiley.
Christensen, N.J., & Galbo, H. (1983). Sympathetic nervous activity during exercise. *Annual Review of Physiology*, **45**, 139-153.
Edington, D.W., & Edgerton, V.R. (1976). *The biology of physical activity*. Boston: Houghton Mifflin.
Emonet-Dénand, F., Hunt, C.C., & Laporte, Y. (1988). How muscle spindles signal changes of muscle length. *News in Physiological Sciences*, **3**, 105-109.
Enoka, R.M. (1988). *Neuromechanical basis of kinesiology*. Champaign, IL: Human Kinetics.
Enoka, R.M., & Stuart, D.G. (1984). Henneman's 'size principle': Current issues. *Trends in NeuroSciences*, **7**, 226-227.
Fox, E.L., Bowers, R.W., & Foss, M.L.. (1993). *The physiological basis for exercise and sport* (5th ed.). Dubuque, IA: Brown & Benchmark.
Gielen, C.C.A.M., & Denier van der Gon, J.J. (1990). The activation of motor units in coordinated arm movements in humans. *News in Physiological Sciences*, **5**, 159-163.
Ginzel, K.H. (1977). Interaction of somatic and autonomic functions in muscular exercise. *Exercise and Sport Sciences Reviews*, **4**, 35-86.
Goodwin, G.M. (1977). The sense of limb position and movement. *Exercise and Sport Sciences Reviews*, **4**, 87-124.
Hasan, Z., Enoka, R.M., & Stuart, D.G. (1985). The interface between biomechanics and neurophysiology in the study of movement: Some recent approaches. *Exercise and Sport Sciences Reviews*, **13**, 169-234.
Henneman, E., & Mendell, L.M. (1981). Functional organization of motoneuron pool and its inputs. In *Handbook of physiology. The nervous system: Motor control* (pp. 423-507). Bethesda, MD: American Physiological Society.
McArdle, W.D., Katch, F.I., & Katch, V.L. (1991). *Exercise physiology: Energy, nutrition, and human performance* (3rd ed.). Philadelphia: Lea & Febiger.
O'Donovan, M.J. (1985). Developmental regulation of motor function: an uncharted sea. *Medicine and Science in Sports and Exercise*, **17**, 35-43.
Roy, R.R., Baldwin, K.M., & Edgerton, V.R. (1991). The plasticity of skeletal muscle: Effects of neuromuscular activity. *Exercise and Sport Sciences Reviews*, **19**, 269-312.
Sale, D.G. (1987). Influence of exercise and training on motor unit activation. *Exercise and Sport Sciences Reviews*, **15**, 95-151.
Seals, D.R., & Victor, R.G. (1991). Regulation of muscle sympathetic nerve activity during exercise in humans. *Exercise and Sport Sciences Reviews*, **19**, 313-349.

Chapter 4

Neuromuscular Adaptations to Resistance Training

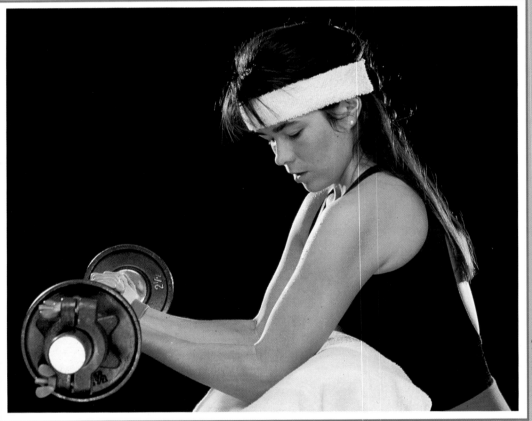

Chapter Overview

In the preceding chapters, we have discussed the functions of the muscular and nervous systems during exercise. But how do we account for the differences between the classic 90-lb weakling and an Olympic weight lifter? What enables a 9-year-old boy to lift a 2-ton car? Why do athletes engage in resistance training even in sports that don't require tremendous strength? Does no pain indeed equal no gain?

We cannot each be an Arnold Schwarzenegger, but nearly everyone can improve strength. In this chapter we will examine how strength is gained through resistance training, noting changes that occur in the muscles themselves and in the neural mechanisms controlling them. We will explore the phenomenon of muscle soreness and how to prevent it. Finally, we will discuss the major concerns in designing a resistance training program and the importance of tailoring it to the specific needs of the individual.

Chapter Outline

We know that athletes who use resistance training become much stronger. For a number of years, Dr. William Gonyea and his colleagues at the University of Texas Health Sciences Center Dallas have been trying to determine what changes that improve strength occur in the muscles of athletes. But Dr. Gonyea and his group have been working with a different type of athlete—cats! The cats receive food rewards for their daily workouts that entice them to work very hard "pumping iron." Like their human counterparts, these cats experience substantial increases in strength and in muscle size. Dogs beware—these are not cats that you want to mess around with!

With chronic exercise, many adaptations occur in the neuromuscular system. The extent of the adaptations depends on the type of training program followed: Aerobic training, such as jogging or swimming, results in little or no gain in muscular strength and power, but major neuromuscular adaptations occur with resistance training.

Resistance training was once considered inappropriate for athletes except for those in competitive weight lifting, weight events in track and field, and, on a limited basis, for those in football, wrestling, and boxing. But in the late 1960s and early 1970s, coaches and researchers discovered that strength and power training are beneficial for almost all sports and activities.

Most athletes now include strength and power training as important components of their overall training programs. This includes female athletes, who were traditionally excluded from such training. Much of this attitude change is attributable to research that has proven the performance benefits of resistance training and to innovations in training techniques and equipment. Resistance training is even now recognized as important for nonathletes who seek the health-related benefits of exercise.

Terminology

Before discussing the neuromuscular changes that result from resistance training, we'll first define the measurable components of muscular fitness.

Muscular Strength

The maximum force a muscle or muscle group can generate is termed strength. Someone with a maximum capacity to bench-press 300 lb has twice the strength of someone who can bench-press 150 lb. In this example, maximum capacity, or strength, is defined as the maximum weight the individual can lift just once. This is referred to as the one-repetition maximum, or the 1-RM.

Muscular Power

Power, the explosive aspect of strength, is the product of strength and speed of movement:

$$power = (force \times distance)/time.$$

Consider an example. Two individuals can each bench-press 250 lb, moving the weight the same distance. But the one who can do it in half the time has twice the power of the slower individual. This principle is illustrated in Figure 4.1.

KEY POINT
Power is the functional application of both strength and speed. It is the key component for most athletic performances.

Although absolute strength is an important component of performance, power is probably even more important for most activities. In football, for example, an offensive lineman with a bench-press 1-RM of 450 lb may be unable to control a defensive lineman with a bench-press 1-RM of only 350 lb if the defensive lineman can move his 1-RM at a much faster speed. The offensive lineman is 100 lb stronger, but the defensive lineman's faster speed coupled with good strength gives him the performance edge.

In this chapter, we primarily concern ourselves with issues of muscular strength, with only brief mention of muscular power. Recall that power has two components: strength and speed. Speed is more of an innate quality that changes little with training. Thus

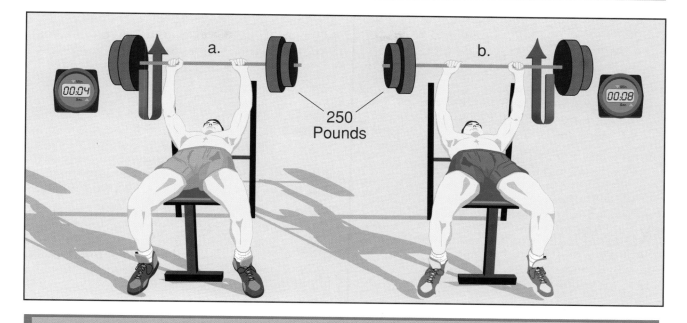

Figure 4.1   Athlete A has twice the power of Athlete B because he can bench press 250 lb in half as much time.

power is increased almost exclusively through gains in strength.

Muscular Endurance

Although this chapter focuses on maximal strength and power development, many sporting activities depend on your muscles' ability to repeatedly develop and sustain near-maximal or maximal forces. This capacity to sustain repeated muscle actions, such as when performing sit-ups or push-ups, or to sustain fixed or static muscle actions for an extended period of time, such as when attempting to pin an opponent in wrestling, is termed muscular endurance. It can be determined by assessing the maximum number of repetitions you can perform at a given percentage of your 1-RM. For example, if you can bench-press 200 lb, your muscular endurance could be evaluated independent of your muscular strength by noting how many repetitions you could perform at, say, 75% of that load (150 lb). Your muscular endurance is increased through gains in muscular strength and through changes in local metabolic and circulatory patterns. Metabolic adaptations that occur with training will be discussed in chapter 7, and circulatory adaptations are discussed in chapter 10.

Table 4.1 illustrates the functional differences between strength, power, and muscular endurance in three athletes. The actual values have been exaggerated for the purpose of illustration.

Table 4.1   Strength, Power, and Muscular Endurance While Performing the Bench-Press

Component	Athlete A—Bob	Athlete B—Ben	Athlete C—Bill
Strength[a]	200 lb	400 lb	400 lb
Power[b]	200 lb lifted 2 ft in 0.5 s, or 800 ft-lb · s⁻¹	400 lb lifted 2 ft in 2 s, or 400 ft-lb · s⁻¹	400 lb lifted 2 ft in 1 s, or 800 ft-lb · s⁻¹
Muscular endurance[c]	10 repetitions with 150 lb	10 repetitions with 300 lb	5 repetitions with 300 lb

[a]Strength was determined by the one-repetition maximum (1-RM).

[b]Power was determined by performing the 1-RM test as explosively as possible. Power was calculated as the product of force (weight lifted) times distance lifted divided by the time needed to complete the 1-RM.

[c]Muscular endurance was determined by the greatest number of repetitions that could be performed using 75% of the 1-RM.

Adapted from Wilmore, 1986.

Strength Gains From Resistance Training

Resistance training programs can produce substantial strength gains. Within three to six months, you can see from 25% to 100% improvement, sometimes even more. How do you become stronger? What physiological adaptations occur that allow you to exert greater levels of strength?

Muscle Size

For many years strength gains were assumed to result directly from increases in muscle size (hypertrophy). This assumption was logical because most who strength-trained regularly were men, and they often developed large, bulky muscles. Also, a limb immobilized in a cast for weeks or months starts to decrease in size (atrophy) and lose strength almost immediately. Gains in muscle size are generally paralleled by gains in strength, and losses in muscle size correlate highly with losses in strength. Thus, we are tempted to conclude that a cause-and-effect relationship exists between muscle size and muscle strength. However, muscle strength involves far more than mere muscle size. Let's consider some examples.

Superhuman Strength

Numerous media reports indicate that people can perform superhuman feats of strength during great psychological stress. Straightjackets were designed specifically to control patients in mental hospitals who suddenly go berserk and are impossible to restrain. Even the world of sport boasts isolated examples of superhuman athletic performances, such as Bob Beamon's long jump of 29 feet, 2-1/2 inches at the 1968 Olympic Games, a jump that exceeded the previous world record by nearly 2 feet! World records are usually broken by inches, or more often mere fractions of inches. Beamon's record stood unbroken until 1991.

Studies in Women

Women experience similar strength gains compared to men who participate in the same training program, but the women do not experience as much hypertrophy (see chapter 19). In fact, some women have doubled their strength without any observable change in their muscle size. Thus, strength gains don't require hypertrophy.

This doesn't mean that muscle size is unimportant in the ultimate strength potential of the muscle. Size is extremely important, as revealed by the existing men's and women's world records for competitive weight lifting, shown in Figure 4.2. As weight classification increases (implying increased muscle size), so does the record for the total weight lifted. However, examples of superhuman strength and studies on women indicate that the mechanisms associated with strength gains are very complex and are not completely understood at this time. How, then, can we explain strength gains with training?

Neural Control of Strength Gains

An important neural component explains at least some of the strength gains that result from resistance training. Enoka has made a convincing argument that strength gains can be achieved without structural changes in muscle, but not without neural adaptations.[10] Thus, strength is not solely a property of the muscle. Rather, it is a property of the motor system. Motor unit recruitment is quite important to strength gains. It may well explain most, if not all, strength gains that occur in the absence of hypertrophy, as well as episodic superhuman feats of strength.[26]

Recruitment of Additional Motor Units

Motor units are generally recruited asynchronously; they are not all called on at the same instant. They are controlled by a number of different neurons that can transmit either excitatory or inhibitory impulses (see chapter 3). Whether the muscle fibers contract or stay relaxed depends on the summation of the many impulses received by that motor unit at any one time. The motor unit is activated and its muscle fibers contract only when the incoming excitatory impulses exceed the inhibitory impulses and threshold is met.

Strength gains may result from recruitment of additional motor units to act synchronously, facilitating contraction and increasing the muscle's ability to generate force. Such improvement in recruitment pat-

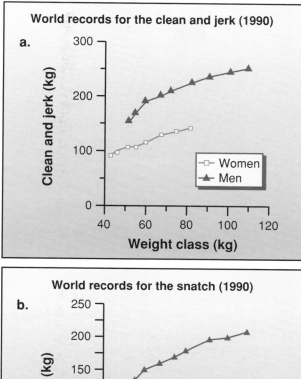

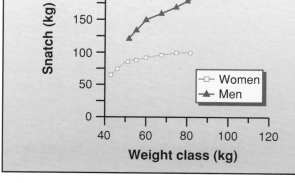

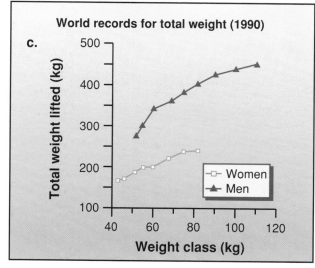

Figure 4.2   World records for (a) the clean and jerk, (b) the snatch, and (c) total weight for men and women through 1990.

terns could result from a blocking or reduction of inhibitory impulses, allowing more motor units to be activated simultaneously. But there is still controversy as to whether synchronization of motor unit activation will produce a more forceful contraction. An alternate possibility is simply that more motor units are recruited to perform the given task, independent of whether or not these motor units act in unison.

Autogenic Inhibition

Inhibitory mechanisms in the neuromuscular system, such as the Golgi tendon organs, might be necessary to prevent the muscles from exerting more force than the bones and connective tissues can tolerate. This control is referred to as autogenic inhibition. During superhuman feats of strength, major damage has often occurred to these structures, suggesting that the protective inhibitory mechanisms were overridden.

We discussed the function of Golgi tendon organs in chapter 3. When the tension on a muscle's tendons and internal connective tissue structures exceeds the threshold of the imbedded Golgi tendon organs, motor neurons to that muscle are inhibited. This reflex is called autogenic inhibition. Both the reticular formation in the brain stem and the cerebral cortex can also initiate and propagate inhibitory impulses.

Training may gradually reduce or counteract these inhibitory impulses, allowing the muscle to reach greater levels of strength. Thus strength gains may be achieved by reduced neurological inhibition. This theory is attractive because it can explain superhuman strength and strength gains in the absence of hypertrophy. Like any other theory, though, it must undergo the rigors of scientific testing before it can be accepted as fact.

Neural Activation and Hypertrophy

Research conducted thus far on resistance training indicates that early increases in voluntary strength are associated primarily with neural adaptations. These neural adaptations include

- improved coordination,
- improved learning, and
- increased activation of the prime mover muscles.

But long-term strength changes most likely result from hypertrophy of the trained muscle or muscle group.[30] This is illustrated in Figure 4.3. Notable exceptions to this generalization have been found. A 6-month study using strength-trained athletes found that neural activation explained most of the strength gains during the most intensive training months and that hypertrophy was not a major factor.[21]

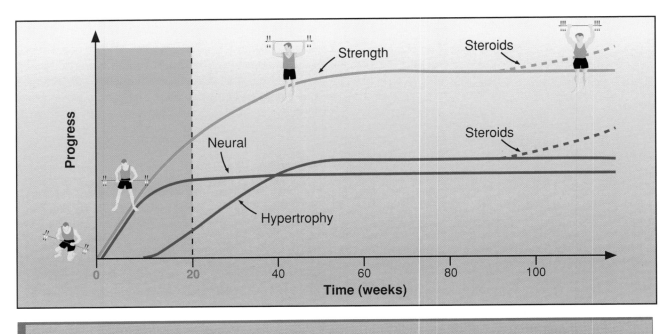

Figure 4.3   Neural and muscular adaptations during resistance training. Most training studies span only 8 to 20 weeks. However, long-term studies reveal that neural adaptations dominate early in training, whereas most changes that occur during later training phases are associated with muscle hypertrophy. Adapted from Sale (1988).

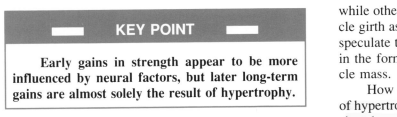

KEY POINT

Early gains in strength appear to be more influenced by neural factors, but later long-term gains are almost solely the result of hypertrophy.

Muscle Hypertrophy

When hypertrophy does occur with resistance training, what causes it? The hormone testosterone is thought to be at least partly responsible because one of its functions is the promotion of muscle growth (chapter 6). Males experience a significantly greater increase in muscle size than females for the same strength training program and even for the same relative increase in strength. Testosterone is an androgen—a substance that produces masculine characteristics. Anabolic steroids are also androgens, and it is well known that massive doses of anabolic steroids coupled with resistance training lead to marked increases in muscle mass (chapter 14).

Although testosterone plays a key role in hypertrophy, it alone does not determine the amount of hypertrophy resulting from resistance training. In fact, blood testosterone concentrations correlate poorly with the degree of training-induced muscle hypertrophy. Some women experience considerable hypertrophy while others experience essentially no change in muscle girth as a result of resistance training. Researchers speculate that the testosterone:estrogen ratio is higher in the former group, resulting in an increase in muscle mass.

How does a muscle's size increase? Two types of hypertrophy can occur: transient and chronic. Transient hypertrophy is that pumping up of the muscle that happens during a single exercise bout. This results mainly from fluid accumulation (edema) in the interstitial and intracellular spaces of the muscle. This fluid is lost from the blood plasma. Transient hypertrophy, as its name implies, lasts only for a short time. The fluid returns to the blood within hours after exercise.

Chronic hypertrophy refers to the increase in muscle size that occurs with long-term resistance training. This reflects actual structural changes in the muscle as a result of either an increased number of muscle fibers (hyperplasia) or an increased size of existing individual muscle fibers (hypertrophy). Controversy surrounds the theories that attempt to explain the underlying cause of this phenomenon.

Fiber Hypertrophy and Hyperplasia

Early research indicated that the number of muscle fibers in each of your muscles is established by birth or shortly thereafter, and that this number remains fixed throughout your life. If this is true, then chronic

The Moritani and deVries Model

Moritani and deVries proposed a model to explain strength gains based on both hypertrophy and neural activation of muscle.[27] This model allows us to estimate the relative contributions of hypertrophy and neural activation to strength gains. Refer to Figure 4.4, which illustrates how this model works.

In this model, force production and integrated electromyographic (IEMG) activation are measured simultaneously from low to maximal levels of force production. IEMG represents an integration of the electrical impulses picked up from the surface of the muscle and thus represents the muscle's level of neural activation. If strength gains result solely from neural factors, maximal IEMG activation must increase to explain the increase in force production or strength (Figure 4.4a). In this case, maximal IEMG activation is increased and more motor units are activated, but there is no change in the force exerted per individual muscle fiber or motor unit. If strength gains are due solely to muscular hypertrophy, then increases in force production capacity occur without increases in IEMG activation (Figure 4.4b). Figure 4.4c illustrates a more typical response to resistance training, in which the gains in force production or strength result from both increased neural activation and muscle hypertrophy.

From Figure 4.4c, we can calculate the relative contributions of both neural factors (N.F.) and muscle hypertrophy (M.H.). In this illustration, Point A represents the initial maximal force production of the muscle, Point C represents the maximal force production following resistance training, and Point B represents the force on the post-training curve where the pre-training maximal activation would have occurred. The relative contributions of M.H. and N.F. can be calculated as follows:

$$\% \text{ M.H.} = \frac{B - A}{C - A} \times 100, \text{ and}$$

$$\% \text{ N.F.} = \frac{C - B}{C - A} \times 100,$$

where C − A represents the total gain in force production capacity (strength), B − A represents the contribution from hypertrophy, and C − B represents the contribution from increased activation.

Using this model, Moritani and deVries demonstrated that 8 weeks of progressive resistance training in five young men (average 22 years old) and in five older men (average 70 years old) resulted in quite different adaptation patterns.[28] Neural activation explained most strength increases in the older

subjects throughout the 8-week training period. In the younger subjects, however, although neural activation was important over the first 4 weeks, hypertrophy became the dominant factor during the last 4 weeks. This suggests that the ability to increase muscle size may decrease with aging.

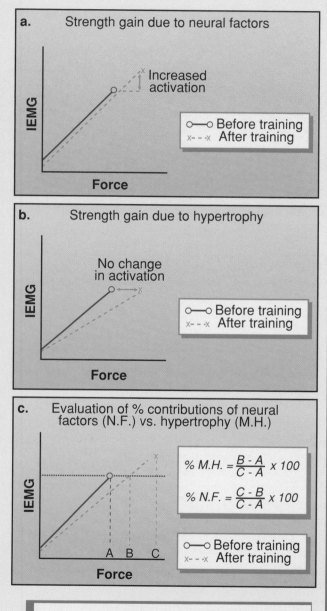

Figure 4.4   The Moritani and deVries model for estimating the training gains in muscular strength consequent to resistance training that result from (a) neural factors, (b) muscle hypertrophy, and (c) both. Adapted from Moritani and deVries (1980).

hypertrophy could result only from individual muscle fiber hypertrophy. This could be explained by

- more myofibrils,
- more actin and myosin filaments,
- more sarcoplasm,
- more connective tissue, or
- any combination of these.

As noted in the micrographs in Figure 4.5, intense resistance training can significantly increase the cross-sectional area of muscle fibers. In this example, fiber hypertrophy is probably caused by increased numbers of myofibrils and actin and myosin filaments, which would provide more cross-bridges for force production during maximal contraction. Such dramatic enlargement of muscle fibers does not occur, however, in all cases of muscle hypertrophy.

Direct Evidence for Hyperplasia

Recent research on animals suggests that hyperplasia may also be a factor in the hypertrophy of whole muscles. Studies on cats provide fairly clear evidence that fiber splitting occurs with extremely heavy weight training.[15] Cats were trained to move a heavy weight with a forepaw to get their food (Figure 4.6). They learned to generate considerable force. With this intense strength training, selected muscle fibers appeared to actually split in half, and each half then increased to the size of the parent fiber. This is seen in the cross-sectional cuts through the muscle fibers shown in Figure 4.7.

Subsequent studies, however, demonstrated that hypertrophy of selected muscles in chickens, rats, and mice that resulted from chronic exercise overload was due solely to hypertrophy of existing fibers, not hyperplasia.[13,14,38] In these studies, each fiber in the whole muscle was actually counted. These direct fiber counts revealed no change in fiber number.

This led the scientists who conducted the initial cat experiments to conduct an additional resistance training study with cats. This time they used actual fiber counts to determine if total muscle hypertrophy

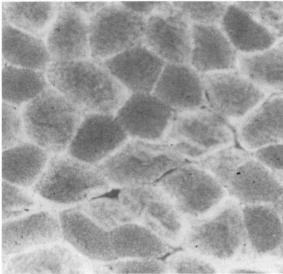

a.

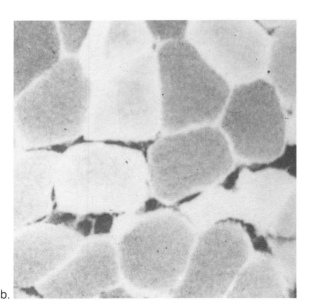

b.

Figure 4.5 Microscopic views of muscle cross-sections taken from the leg muscle of a man who had not trained during the previous two years (a) before he resumed training and (b) after he completed 6 months of dynamic strength training. Note the significantly larger fibers (hypertrophy) after training.

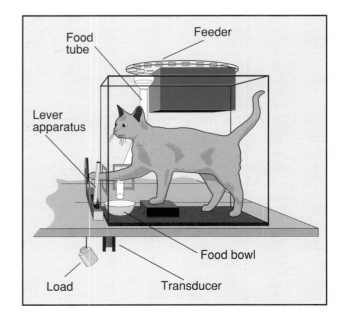

Figure 4.6 Heavy-resistance training in cats. Adapted from Gonyea (1980).

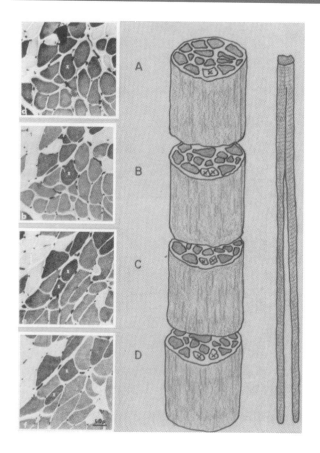

Figure 4.7   Muscle fiber splitting. The drawn models are assumed from the series of microscopic slides (a-d). Adapted from Gonyea, Ericson, and Bonde-Petersen (1977).

resulted from hyperplasia or fiber hypertrophy.[16] Following a resistance training program of 101 weeks, the cats were able to perform one-leg lifts with an average of 57% of their body weight, resulting in an 11% increase in muscle weight. Most importantly, the researchers found a 9% increase in the total number of muscle fibers, confirming that muscle fiber hyperplasia did occur.

The difference in results between the cat studies and those with other animals may be due to differences in the manner in which the animals were trained. The cats were trained with a pure form of resistance training—high resistance and low repetitions. The others were trained with more endurance-type activity—low resistance and high repetitions.

Indirect Evidence for Hyperplasia

Researchers are still uncertain about the roles played by hyperplasia and individual fiber hypertrophy in increasing human muscle size with resistance training. Most evidence indicates that individual fiber hypertro-

phy accounts for most whole-muscle hypertrophy. However, results of two studies on bodybuilders indicate that hyperplasia is possible in humans.

One study reported that the mean muscle fiber areas of the vastus lateralis and the deltoid muscles were smaller in a group of high-caliber bodybuilders than in a reference group of competitive power/weight lifters and were nearly identical to those in physical education students and non-strength-trained people. This suggested that individual fiber hypertrophy was not critical to the bodybuilders' gains in muscle mass.[37]

Similar results were found in a subsequent study comparing highly trained bodybuilders and active but untrained controls. Muscle fiber areas of the trained subjects were similar to those of the control subjects, despite the fact that the trained subjects had much greater limb circumferences.[25] The researchers also found more muscle fibers per motor unit in the trained bodybuilders than in the nonathlete control group. Because these men had substantially greater muscle girth but normal muscle fiber cross-sectional area, these findings suggest that the number of muscle fibers increased. An alternate explanation is that these athletes had more muscle fibers at birth.

In contrast, at least one study has found large differences in muscle fiber area when comparing bodybuilders to male and female physical education students.[31] Mean fiber areas of the vastus lateralis for each of the three groups were as follows:

- Bodybuilders, 8,400 μm^2
- Male physical education students, 6,200 μm^2
- Female physical education students, 4,400 μm^2

The differences between these studies might be explained by the nature of the training load or stimulus. Training at high intensities or high resistances is thought to cause greater fiber hypertrophy, particularly of the FT fibers, than training at lower intensities or resistances.[23]

Mechanisms for Fiber Hypertrophy

Individual muscle fiber hypertrophy from resistance training appears to result from a net increase in muscle protein synthesis. The muscle's protein content is in a continual state of flux. Protein is always being synthesized and degraded. But the rates of these processes vary with the demands placed on the body. During exercise, protein synthesis decreases while protein degradation apparently increases.[17] This pattern reverses during the post-exercise recovery period, even to the point of a net synthesis of protein.

In animals, research has established that exercise-induced muscular hypertrophy is accompanied by a long-term increase in protein synthesis and a decrease in protein degradation. This was illustrated by a study that used electrical stimulation in rats to produce a low repetition and high resistance training stimulus to a single hindlimb.[39] The opposite hindlimb acted as the untrained control. Following a 16-week training program, the investigators reported

- a 66% increase in work during a training bout,
- an 18% increase in the wet weight of the trained muscle,
- a 17% increase in the muscle's protein content, and
- a 26% increase in the muscle's RNA content.

Muscle Atrophy

When a trained muscle suddenly becomes inactive through immobilization, major changes are initiated within that muscle in a matter of hours (chapter 13). During the first 6 hr of immobilization, the rate of protein synthesis starts to decrease. This is likely related to the start of muscular atrophy, which is the wasting away or decrease in the size of muscle tissue. Atrophy occurs from lack of muscle use and results from the consequent loss of muscle protein that accompanies the inactivity. Strength decreases are most dramatic during the first week of immobilization, averaging 3% to 4% per day.[2] This is associated with the atrophy but is also associated with decreased neuromuscular activity of the immobilized muscle.

Atrophy appears to primarily affect the slow-twitch (ST) fibers. From various studies, researchers have observed disintegrated myofibrils, streaming Z disks (discontinuity of Z disks and fusion of the myofibrils), and mitochondrial damage in ST fibers. When muscle atrophies, both the cross-sectional fiber area and the percentage of ST fibers decrease. Whether ST fibers decrease from fiber necrosis (death) or conversion into fast-twitch (FT) fibers is unclear.[2]

Muscles can and often do recover from atrophy when activity is resumed. The recovery period is substantially longer than the period of immobilization, but it is more brief than the original training period.

Similarly, significant muscle alterations can occur when you stop training. In one study, women were resistance trained for 20 weeks, then their training was stopped for 30 to 32 weeks. Finally they were retrained for 6 weeks.[34]

The training program focused on the lower extremity, using a full squat, leg press, and leg extension. Strength increases were dramatic, as seen in Figure 4.8. Pre-20 and post-20 refer to the pre- and post-training results for the women before and after the 20-week training period. Pre-6 and post-6 refer to the pre- and post-training results following the final 6-week training period. Compare the women's strength after

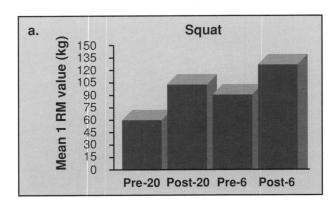

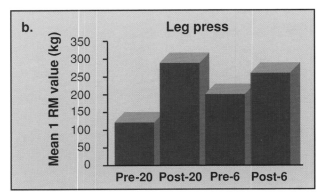

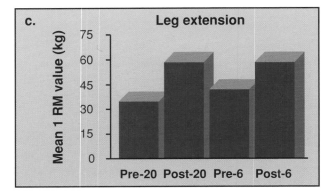

Figure 4.8   Changes in muscle strength with resistance training in women, assessed by (a) the full squat, (b) the leg press, and (c) leg extension. *Post-20* values indicate the changes following 20 weeks of training, *Pre-6* values indicate the changes following a period of detraining, and *Post-6* values indicate the changes following 6 weeks of retraining. Adapted from Staron et al. (1991).

their initial training period (post-20) to their strength after detraining (pre-6). This represents the strength loss they experienced with cessation of training.

During the two training periods, increases in strength were accompanied by increases in the cross-sectional area of all fiber types and a decrease in the percentage of FT_b fibers. Detraining had relatively little effect on fiber cross-sectional area, although the FT fiber areas tended to decrease (Figure 4.9).

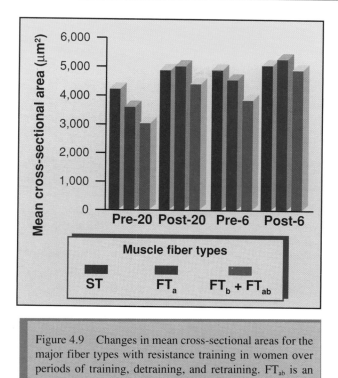

Figure 4.9 Changes in mean cross-sectional areas for the major fiber types with resistance training in women over periods of training, detraining, and retraining. FT$_{ab}$ is an intermediate fiber type. Adapted from Staron et al. (1991).

In another study, men and women resistance trained (with knee extensions) for either 10 or 18 weeks, then spent an additional 12 weeks with either no training or reduced training.[18] Knee extension strength increased 21.4% following the training period. Subjects who then stopped training lost 68% of their strength gains during the weeks they didn't train. But subjects who reduced their training by 1 day per week did not lose strength. Thus, it appears that strength can be maintained for at least up to 12 weeks with reduced training frequency.

To prevent losses in the strength gained through resistance training, basic maintenance programs must be established once the desired goals for strength development have been achieved. Maintenance programs are designed to provide sufficient stress to the muscles to maintain existing levels of strength while allowing a reduction in any of the following aspects of training:

- intensity,
- duration, or
- frequency.

Fiber-Type Alterations

Can muscle fibers change from one type to another through resistance training? The earliest research concluded that neither speed (anaerobic) nor endurance (aerobic) training could alter the basic fiber type.[7,12] These early studies did show, however, that fibers begin to take on certain characteristics of the opposite fiber type (for example, FT fibers might become more oxidative) if the training is of the opposite kind (aerobic).

More recent research with animals has shown that fiber-type conversion is indeed possible under conditions of cross-innervation, where a FT motor unit is innervated by a ST motor neuron, or vice versa. Also, chronic stimulation of FT motor units with low-frequency nerve stimulation transforms FT motor units into ST motor units within a matter of weeks.[29] Muscle fiber types in rats have changed in response to 15 weeks of high-intensity treadmill training, resulting in an increase in ST and FT$_a$ fibers and a decrease in FT$_b$ fibers.[19] The transition of fibers from FT$_b$ to FT$_a$ and from FT$_a$ to ST was confirmed by several different histochemical techniques.

Staron et al. found evidence of fiber-type transformation in women as a result of heavy resistance training.[35] Substantial increases in static strength and in the cross-sectional area of all fiber types were noted following a 20-week heavy resistance training program for the lower extremity. The mean percentage of FT$_b$ fibers decreased significantly, but the mean percentage of FT$_a$ fibers increased. In an extensive 1990 review of the research literature in this area, it was concluded that extreme and prolonged training may produce skeletal muscle fiber type conversion.[1]

Muscle Soreness

Muscle soreness can be present

- during the latter stages of an exercise bout and the immediate recovery period,
- between 12 and 48 hr after a strenuous bout of exercise, or
- at both times.

Let's examine soreness during both periods.

Acute Muscle Soreness

Pain felt during and immediately after exercise can result from accumulation of the end products of exercise, such as H$^+$ or lactate, and tissue edema, mentioned earlier, that is caused by fluid shifting from the blood plasma into the tissues. This is the pumped-up feeling that the athlete is conscious of following heavy endurance or strength training. This pain and soreness usually disappears within a few minutes to several hours after the exercise. Thus it is often referred to as acute muscle soreness

Delayed-Onset Muscle Soreness

Muscle soreness felt a day or two after a heavy bout of exercise is not clearly understood. Because this pain does not occur immediately, it is referred to as delayed-onset muscle soreness, or DOMS. In the following sections, we will discuss some theories that attempt to explain this form of muscle soreness. As we do so, realize that none of these theories yet has universal support. More research must be conducted before the exact mechanisms can be determined.

Almost all current theories acknowledge that eccentric action is the primary initiator of this muscle soreness. This was initially observed in a study that investigated the relationship of muscle soreness to eccentric, concentric, and static actions. It found that a group training solely with eccentric actions experienced extreme muscle soreness, while the static and concentric action groups experienced little.[36] This was further explored in studies where subjects were asked to run on a treadmill for 45 min on two separate days,

one day on a level grade and the other day on a 10% downhill grade.[32,33] No muscle soreness was associated with the level running. But the downhill running, which required extensive eccentric action, resulted in considerable soreness within 24 to 48 hours, even though the blood lactate levels, previously thought to cause muscle soreness, were much higher with level running.

Let's examine some of the proposed explanations for exercise-induced, delayed-onset muscle soreness.

Structural Damage

The presence of muscle enzymes in blood after intense exercise suggests that some structural damage may occur in the muscle membranes. It has been reported that these enzymes increase from 2 to 10 times their normal levels following bouts of heavy training. Recent studies support the idea that these changes might indicate various degrees of muscle tissue breakdown. Examination of tissue from the leg muscles of marathon runners has revealed remarkable damage to the muscle fibers after both training and marathon competition. The onset and timing of these muscle changes parallels the degree of muscle soreness experienced by the runners.

The electron micrograph in Figure 4.10 shows muscle fiber damage as a result of marathon running.[20] In this case, the sarcolemma (cell membrane) was totally ruptured, allowing the cell's contents to float freely between the other normal fibers. Fortunately, not all damage done to muscle cells is as severe.

Figure 4.11 shows changes in the contractile filaments and Z disks before and after a marathon race. Recall that Z disks are the points of contact for the contractile proteins. They provide structural support for the transmission of force when the muscle fibers are activated to shorten. Figure 4.11b, after the marathon, shows the Z disks pulled apart as a result of the force of eccentric actions or stretching of the tightened muscle fibers.

Although the effects of muscle damage on performance are not fully understood, experts generally agree that this damage is, in part, responsible for the localized muscle pain, tenderness, and swelling associated with delayed-onset muscle soreness. However, blood enzyme levels might rise and muscle fibers might be damaged frequently during daily exercise that produces no muscle soreness.

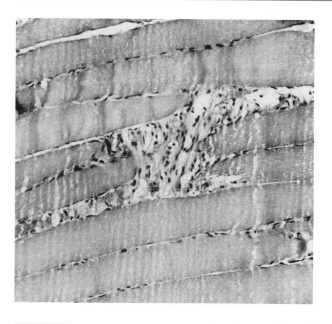

Figure 4.10   An electron micrograph of a muscle sample taken immediately after a marathon, showing the disruption of the cell membrane in one muscle fiber. Reprinted from Hagerman et al. (1984).

Inflammatory Reaction

White blood cells serve as a defense against foreign materials that enter your body or against conditions that threaten the normal function of its tissues. The white blood cell count tends to rise following activities that induce muscle soreness. This led some investigators to suggest that soreness results from inflammatory reactions in the muscle. But the link between these reactions and muscle soreness has been difficult to establish.

Researchers have tried to use drugs to block the inflammatory reaction, but these efforts have been unsuccessful in reducing either the amount of muscle soreness or the degree of inflammation.[24] Because both remain, conclusions about the role of inflammation in muscle soreness cannot be drawn from this research. More recent studies, however, are beginning to establish a link between muscle soreness and inflammation.

Sequence of Events in DOMS

In 1984, Armstrong conducted a review of possible mechanisms for exercise-induced, delayed-onset muscle

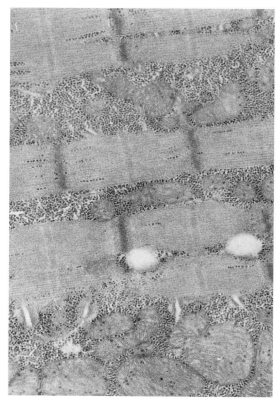

a.

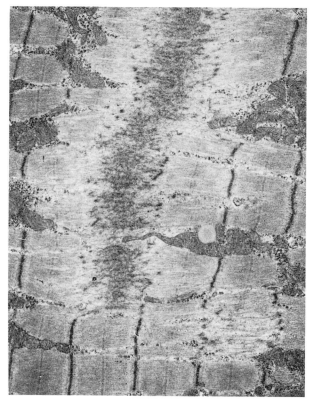

b.

Figure 4.11   (a) An electron micrograph showing the normal arrangement of the actin and myosin filaments and Z disk configuration in the muscle of a runner before a marathon race. (b) A muscle sample taken immediately after a marathon race shows Z disk streaming caused by the eccentric actions of running. Reprinted from Hagerman et al. (1984).

soreness.[3] He concluded that DOMS is associated with

- elevations in plasma enzymes,
- myoglobinemia (presence of myoglobin in the blood), and
- abnormal muscle histology and ultrastructure.

He developed a model of DOMS that proposed the following sequence of events:

1. High tension in the contractile-elastic system of muscle results in structural damage to the muscle and its cell membrane.
2. The cell membrane damage disturbs calcium homeostasis in the injured fiber, resulting in necrosis (cell death) that peaks about 48 hr after exercise.
3. The products of macrophage activity and intracellular contents (such as histamine, kinins, and K^+) accumulate outside the cells. These substances then stimulate the free nerve endings in the muscle. This process appears to be accentuated in eccentric exercise, in which large forces are distributed over relatively small cross-sectional areas of the muscle.

Recent comprehensive reviews have provided much greater insight into the cause of muscle soreness. We now are confident that muscle soreness results from injury or damage to the muscle itself, generally the muscle fiber, and possibly the sarcolemma.[4] This damage sets up a chain of events that includes the release of intracellular proteins and an increase in muscle protein turnover. The damage and repair process involves calcium ions, lysosomes, connective tissue, free radicals, energy sources, inflammatory reactions, and intracellular and myofibrillar proteins. But the precise cause of skeletal muscle damage and the mechanisms of repair are not well understood. Some evidence suggests that this process is an important step in muscle hypertrophy.

The Prevention of Muscle Soreness

The prevention of muscle soreness is important for maximizing training gains. The eccentric component of muscle action should be minimized during early training, but this is not possible for athletes in most sports. An alternative approach is to start training at a very low intensity and progress slowly through the first few weeks. Yet another approach is to initiate the training program with a high-intensity, exhaustive training bout. Muscle soreness would be great for the first few days, but some evidence suggests that subse-

---

IN REVIEW . . .

1. Acute muscle soreness occurs late in an exercise bout and during the immediate recovery period.
2. Delayed-onset muscle soreness (DOMS) occurs a day or two after the exercise bout. Eccentric action seems to be the primary instigator of this type of soreness.
3. Proposed causes of DOMS include structural damage to muscle cells and inflammatory reactions within the muscles.
4. Armstrong's proposed model of the sequence of events that cause DOMS includes
   - structural damage,
   - impaired calcium availability leading to necrosis,
   - accumulation of irritants, and
   - increased macrophage activity.
5. Muscle soreness can be prevented or minimized by
   - reducing the eccentric component of muscle action during early training,
   - starting training at a low intensity and gradually increasing it, or
   - beginning with a high-intensity, exhaustive bout, which will cause much soreness initially but will decrease future pain.

---

quent training bouts would cause considerably less muscle soreness.[9]

Designing Resistance Training Programs

Over the past 50 years, research has provided a substantial knowledge base concerning resistance training and its application to health and sport. The health aspects of resistance training are discussed in chapter 22. In this section, we will primarily concern ourselves with the use of resistance training for sport.

Resistance Training Actions

Resistance training actions are related to the types of muscle actions. Resistance training can use static actions (formerly referred to as isometric actions), dynamic actions, or both. Dynamic actions include the use of free weights, variable resistance, isokinetic actions, and plyometrics (see Figure 4.12).

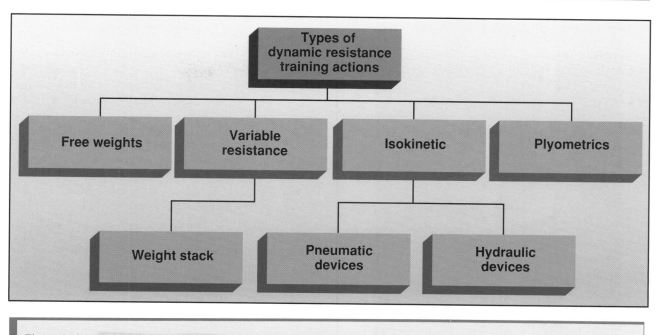

Figure 4.12 Examples of dynamic resistance training actions and devices.

With free weights, such as barbells and dumb-bells, the resistance or weight lifted remains constant throughout the dynamic range of movement. If you lift a 10-kg weight, it will always weigh 10 kg. In contrast, variable resistance action involves varying the resistance in an attempt to match it to your strength curve. Figure 4.13 illustrates how your strength varies throughout the range of motion in a two-arm curl. Maximal strength production by the elbow flexors occurs at approximately 100° in the range of movement. These muscles are weakest at 60° (elbows fully flexed) and at 180° (elbows fully extended).

With a variable resistance device, the resistance is decreased in the weakest points in the range of movement and increased in the strongest points. This is the basis for several popular resistance training devices. The underlying theory is that the muscle can be more fully trained if it is forced to act at higher constant percentages of its capacity throughout each point in its range of movement. Figure 4.14 illustrates a variable resistance device in which a cam alters the resistance through the range of motion.

In isokinetic action, movement speed is held constant by the device. Whether you apply very light force or an all-out maximal muscle action, the speed of movement does not vary. Using either electronics or hydraulics, the device can be preset to control the speed of movement (angular velocity) from $0° \cdot s^{-1}$ (static action) up to $300° \cdot s^{-1}$ or higher. An isokinetic device is illustrated in Figure 4.15. Theoretically, if properly motivated, the individual can contract the muscles at maximal force at all points in the range of motion.

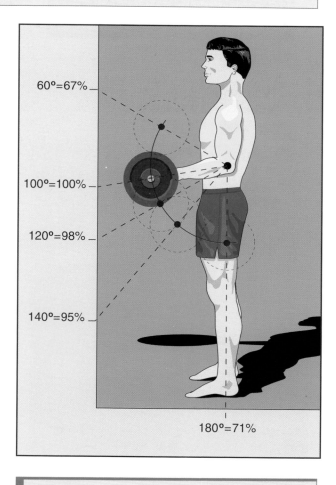

Figure 4.13 The variation in strength relative to the angle of the elbow flexors during the two-arm curl. Strength is optimized at an angle of 100°.

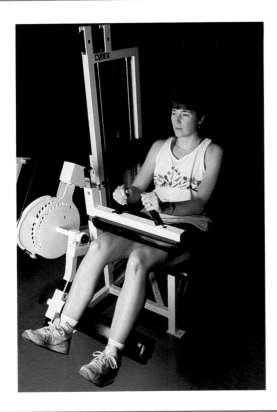

Figure 4.14   A variable resistance training device using a cam to alter the resistance through the range of motion.

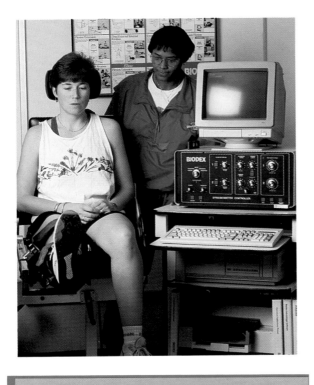

Figure 4.15   An isokinetic testing and training device.

A Training Needs Analysis

When you work with athletes, Fleck and Kraemer suggest a needs analysis should be the first step in designing and prescribing a resistance training program.[11] The needs analysis should include the following assessment:

- What major muscle groups need to be trained?
- What method of training should be used?
- What energy system should be stressed?
- What are the primary sites of concern for injury prevention?

Once this needs analysis has been completed, the resistance training program can be designed and prescribed. You can now logically select

- the exercises that will be performed,
- the order in which they will be performed,
- the number of sets for each exercise,
- the rest periods between sets and between exercises, and
- the load to be used (amount of resistance).

The last point is quite important. The role of load in training for strength, power, endurance, and muscle size has been an area of great confusion.

Selecting the Appropriate Resistance

The actual resistance (weight) to be lifted is generally expressed as a percentage of your maximal capacity. Recall that a 1-RM load is a maximum load—the highest resistance that can be moved only once. In contrast, a 25-RM load is very light. Strength development is optimized by low repetitions and high resistance, whereas muscular endurance is optimized by low resistance and high repetitions.

Less clear, at least from solid research, is how to best develop power and muscle size. Fleck and Kraemer feel that power training should be the same as strength training with respect to load. But when performing high-load (high-resistance) exercise, the speed of action is typically very slow. Because speed is an integral component of power, the principle of specificity of training would argue against this. Currently there is insufficient research to clarify this apparent inconsistency.

When the training objective is to increase muscle size, an important objective for bodybuilders, the load should be set within a range of 8-RM to 12-RM, but the number of sets should be increased to a minimum of 3 to 6 and up to as many as 10 to 15. Also, the rest interval should be very short, usually not more than 90 s.[11]

Periodization

Periodization refers to changes or variations in the resistance training program that are implemented over the course of a distinct period of time, such as a year. Periodization varies the exercise stimulus to keep the individual from overtraining or becoming stale.

According to Fleck and Kraemer, periodization consists of four phases in each training cycle. The first phase is characterized by high volume (repetitions and sets) and low intensity. During the next three phases, volume is decreased and intensity is increased. Generally, the four phases are followed by an active recovery phase where either light resistance training or some unrelated activity is used, allowing the body time to completely recover from the training cycle, both physically and mentally. Once the active recovery phase is completed, the entire periodization cycle is repeated.

Periodization cycles can vary in duration from one cycle per year to two or three per year. An example of a periodization program is illustrated in Table 4.2. The number of repetitions and sets can be varied to accommodate the sport. The main idea is to gradually decrease volume while gradually increasing intensity. Each of the four phases emphasizes a different component of muscular fitness:

- Phase I—muscular hypertrophy (muscle size)
- Phase II—strength
- Phase III—power
- Phase IV—peak strength

Forms of Resistance Training

Over the years, many claims have been made touting the advantages of specific forms of resistance training. Let's briefly evaluate some of these.

Static Action Training

Static action resistance training evolved in the early 20th century, but gained great popularity and support in the mid-1950s as a result of new research by several German scientists. These studies indicated that static resistance training causes tremendous strength gains, and that these gains exceed those from dynamic action procedures. Subsequent studies have not been able to reproduce the original studies' results, yet static actions remain an important form of training, particularly for postsurgical rehabilitation when the limb is immobilized and thus incapable of dynamic actions. Static actions facilitate recovery and reduce muscle atrophy and strength loss.

Plyometrics

A relatively new form of dynamic action resistance training is plyometrics, or jump training, which became popular during the late 1970s and early 1980s for improving jumping ability. Proposed to bridge the gap between speed and strength training, plyometrics uses the stretch reflex to facilitate recruitment of additional motor units. It also loads both the elastic and contractile components of muscle. As an example, to develop knee extensor muscle strength, you jump from an 18-in. box to the ground, land with your knees partly flexed, then rebound upward by a forceful maximal contraction of your knee extensor muscles. Figure 4.16 shows an example. The individual jumps down, landing in a semicrouched position, and immediately rebounds upward with an explosive movement. A number of variations can be performed, including repetitive jumping on and off a box and jumping while wearing weight belts.

Bobbert has conducted an extensive review of both the scientific and coaching literature on plyometrics and concludes that there is not a sufficient research base to establish the superiority of plyometrics over more traditional resistance training techniques.[6]

Eccentric Training

Another form of dynamic action resistance training emphasizes the eccentric phase. With eccentric actions, the muscle's ability to resist force is approximately 30% greater than with concentric actions. Subjecting

Table 4.2 Periodization Training for Strength/Power Sports Using Two Cycles Per Year

Variable	Phase I— hypertrophy	Phase II— strength	Phase III— power	Phase IV— peaking	Active rest
Sets	3 to 5	3 to 5	3 to 5	1 to 3	General activity
Repetitions	8 to 20	2 to 6	2 to 3	1 to 3	or light
Intensity	Low	High	High	Very high	resistance training
Duration	6 weeks	6 weeks	6 weeks	6 weeks	2 weeks

Reprinted from Fleck and Kraemer (1987).

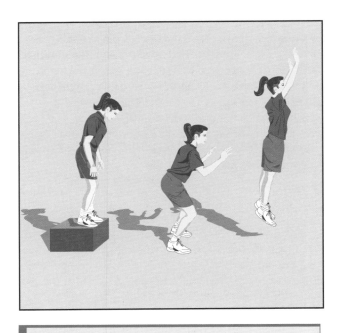

Figure 4.16 A plyometric depth jump.

the muscle to this greater stimulus theoretically would produce greater strength gains with training.

Although this is theoretically sound, the research to date has not shown a clear advantage of eccentric training over either concentric or static action training.[5,11] Most recently, however, several well-controlled studies showed the importance of including the eccentric phase of muscle action along with the concentric phase to maximize gains in strength and size.[8,22]

Free Weights

Many athletes are going back to free weights for resistance training instead of using the equipment that has flooded the market over the past 25 years. Athletes and strength training coaches alike feel that free weights offer advantages that resistance machines do not provide. The athlete must control the weight being lifted. To do this, an athlete must recruit more motor units, not only in the muscles being trained, but also in additional muscles to gain control of the bar and to maintain body balance. When training for a sport like football, the experience with free weights is more similar to that found in competition.

Electrical Stimulation Training

A muscle can be stimulated by passing an electric current directly across it or its motor nerve. This technique, called electrical stimulation training, has been proven effective in a clinical setting. It is used to reduce the loss of strength and muscle size during periods of immobilization and to restore strength and size during rehabilitation. It has also been used experimentally in training healthy subjects (including athletes) because it can increase muscular strength.

However, the gains reported are no greater than those achieved with more conventional training. Athletes have used this technique to supplement their regular training programs, but no evidence shows any additional gains in strength, power, or performance from this supplementation.

Specificity of Training Procedures

As discussed in chapter 1, training results are highly specific to the type of training program used. Long distance running does little, if anything, to improve a powerlifter's maximal weight lifting capacity. High-resistance weight training does little to improve a distance runner's marathon time. A resistance training program to develop strength and power should be carefully designed to match the requirements of the specific sport in which the athlete is involved.

Strength gains from resistance training are highly specific to the speed of training. If a person trains at high velocities, maximum strength gains are seen when testing is also done at high velocities. For this reason, most athletes should do at least part of their strength training at high velocities because that is the nature of most sport movements.

Evidence also indicates that strength gains are highly specific to movement patterns. This suggests that the closer the movement pattern mimics the actual sport performance, the greater the benefit from training.

At this time, it is unclear how specific training must be to provide maximal benefits from resistance training programs. Also, resistance training may not improve performance. Costill has found major increases in swimmers' strength following resistance training, but swimming performance did not improve any more than with swim training alone.

KEY POINT

Resistance training should be as sport-specific as possible. At least part of the training should involve movements that closely mimic those needed for the athlete's sport or activity, including movement patterns and speed.

IN REVIEW . . .

1. Resistance training actions can use static or dynamic actions. Dynamic actions include the use of free weights, variable resistance, isokinetic actions, and plyometrics.
2. A needs analysis should be completed before designing a training program to tailor the program to the athlete's specific needs.
3. Low-repetition, high-resistance training enhances strength development, whereas high-repetition, low-intensity training optimizes muscular endurance.
4. Periodization, through which various aspects of the training program are varied, is important to prevent overtraining or burnout. Typically the goal is to gradually decrease volume while increasing intensity. A typical cycle has four phases, each emphasizing a different muscle fitness component.
5. Strength gains are highly specific to the speed of training and the movement patterns used in training. For maximum benefit, a resistance training program must include activities quite similar to those experienced by the athlete in actual performance.

Analyzing the Importance of Resistance Training

Resistance training is widely regarded as appropriate only for young, healthy male athletes. This narrow concept has led many people to overlook the benefits of resistance training when planning their own activities. In this section, we will first consider gender and age stereotypes, then we will summarize the importance of this form of training to all athletes, regardless of gender, age, or sport.

Gender and Age Differences

In recent years, considerable interest has focused on the trainability of women, children, and the aging population. As mentioned in the introduction to this chapter, the use of resistance training by women, either for sport or for health-related benefits, is rather recent. Since the early 1970s, a substantial body of knowledge has developed in this area that reveals that women and men have the same ability to develop strength but women may not be able to achieve peak values as high

as those attained by men. This is primarily due to muscle size differences related to gender differences in anabolic hormones. Resistance training techniques developed for and applied to training men seem equally appropriate for training women. This is covered in more detail in chapter 19.

In 1984, the University of Arizona was the first Division I NCAA school to hire a woman as head strength coach for both the men's and women's athletic programs. The position went to Meg Ritchie, former Scottish discus thrower and shot-putter for Great Britain's Olympic team.

The wisdom of resistance training in children and adolescents has long been debated. The potential for injury, particularly growth plate injuries from the use of free weights, has sparked much concern. Many people also believed that children would not benefit from resistance training, based on the assumption that the hormonal changes associated with puberty are necessary for gaining muscle strength and mass. We now know that children and adolescents can train safely with minimal risk of injury if appropriate safeguards are followed. Furthermore, they can indeed gain both muscular strength and muscle mass (chapter 17).

Interest in the use of resistance training procedures for the elderly has increased. A substantial loss of the fat-free body mass accompanies aging. This mainly reflects the loss of muscle mass, occurring largely because most people become less active as they age. When a muscle isn't used regularly, it loses function, with predictable atrophy and loss of strength.

Can resistance training in the elderly reverse this process? The elderly can indeed gain strength and muscle mass in response to resistance training. This has important implications for both their health and the quality of their lives (chapter 18). With maintained or improved strength, falling is less likely. This is a significant benefit because falls are a major source of injury and debilitation for elderly people, and they often lead to death.

Resistance Training for Athletes

Gaining strength, power, or muscular endurance simply for the sake of being stronger, being more powerful, or possessing greater muscular endurance is of relatively little importance to athletes unless it also results in improvements in their athletic performance. The use of resistance training by field event athletes and competitive weight lifters makes intuitive sense. The need for its use by the gymnast, distance runner, base-ball player, high jumper, or ballerina is less obvious.

We do not have extensive research to document the specific benefits of resistance training for every sport or for every event within a sport. But clearly each has basic strength requirements that must be met to achieve optimal performance. Training beyond these requirements seems unnecessary.

Training is costly in terms of time, and athletes can't afford to waste time on activities that won't result in better athletic performances. Thus, in any resistance training program, it is imperative to have some performance measurement to evaluate the program's efficacy. To resistance train solely to become stronger, with no associated improvement in performance, is of questionable value.

IN REVIEW . . .

1. Resistance training can benefit almost everyone, regardless of a person's gender, age, or athletic involvement.
2. Most athletes in most sports can benefit from resistance training if an appropriate program is designed for them. But to ensure that the program is working, performance should be assessed periodically and adjustments made to the training regime as needed.

In Closing . . .

In this chapter we have carefully considered the role of resistance training in increasing muscular strength and improving performance. We have examined how muscle strength is gained, through both muscular and neural adaptations, what factors can lead to muscle soreness, and how to design an appropriate resistance training program that will meet the specific needs of the individual athlete. In the next chapter, we will turn our attention away from the neuromuscular aspects of physical activity as we begin exploring how this activity is fueled.

Key Terms

acute muscle soreness
atrophy
autogenic inhibition
chronic hypertrophy
delayed-onset muscle
    soreness (DOMS)
eccentric training
electrical stimulation
    training
hyperplasia
muscular endurance
needs analysis
periodization
plyometrics
power
static action resistance
    training
strength
transient hypertrophy

Study Questions

1. Define and differentiate the terms strength, power, and muscular endurance. How does each component relate to athletic performance?
2. Discuss possible mechanisms that might account for superhuman feats of strength.
3. Discuss the different theories that have attempted to explain how muscles gain strength with training.
4. What is autogenic inhibition? How might it be important to resistance training?
5. Differentiate transient and chronic muscle hypertrophy.
6. What is hyperplasia? How might it be related to gains in size and muscle strength with resistance training?
7. What is the definition of and the physiological basis for hypertrophy? For atrophy?
8. What is the physiological basis for muscle soreness?
9. Define and differentiate static, free weight, isokinetic, and variable resistance types of training.
10. Describe several important principles that need to be considered when designing resistance training programs.

References

1. Abernethy, P.J., Thayer, R., & Taylor, A.W. (1990). Acute and chronic responses of skeletal muscle to endurance and sprint exercise. *Sports Medicine*, **10**, 365-389.

2. Appell, H.-J. (1990). Muscular atrophy following immobilisation: A review. *Sports Medicine*, **10**, 42-58.

3. Armstrong, R.B. (1984). Mechanisms of exercise-induced delayed-onset muscular soreness: A brief review. *Medicine and Science in Sports and Exercise*, **16**, 529-538.

4. Armstrong, R.B., Warren, G.L., & Warren, J.A. (1991). Mechanisms of exercise-induced muscle fibre injury. *Sports Medicine*, **12**, 184-207.

5. Atha, J. (1982). Strengthening muscle. *Exercise and Sport Sciences Reviews*, **9**, 1-73.

6. Bobbert, M.F. (1990). Drop jumping as a training method for jumping ability. *Sports Medicine*, **9**, 7-22.

7. Costill, D.L., Coyle, E.F., Fink, W.F., Lesmes, G.R., & Witzmann, F.A. (1979). Adaptations in skeletal muscle following strength training. *Journal of Applied Physiology*, **46**, 96-99.

8. Dudley, G.A., Tesch, P.A., Miller, B.J., & Buchanan, P. (1991). Importance of eccentric actions in performance adaptations to resistance training. *Aviation, Space, and Environmental Medicine*, **62**, 543-550.

9. Ebbeling, C.B., & Clarkson, P.M. (1989). Exercise-induced muscle damage and adaptation. *Sports Medicine*, **7**, 207-234.

10. Enoka, R.M. (1988). Muscle strength and its development: New perspectives. *Sports Medicine*, **6**, 146-168.

11. Fleck, S.J., & Kraemer, W.J. (1987). *Designing resistance training programs.* Champaign, IL: Human Kinetics.

12. Gollnick, P.D., Armstrong, R.B., Saltin, B., Saubert IV, C.W., Sembrowich, W.L., & Shepherd, R.E. (1973). Effect of training on enzyme activity and fiber composition of human skeletal muscle. *Journal of Applied Physiology*, **34**, 107-111.

13. Gollnick, P.D., Parsons, D., Riedy, M., & Moore, R.L. (1983). Fiber number and size in overloaded chicken anterior latissimus dorsi muscle. *Journal of Applied Physiology*, **54**, 1292-1297.

14. Gollnick, P.D., Timson, B.F., Moore, R.L., & Riedy, M. (1981). Muscular enlargement and number of fibers in skeletal muscles of rats. *Journal of Applied Physiology*, **50**, 936-943.

15. Gonyea, W.J. (1980). Role of exercise in inducing increases in skeletal muscle fiber number. *Journal of Applied Physiology*, **48**, 421-426.

16. Gonyea, W.J., Sale, D.G., Gonyea, F.B., & Mikesky, A. (1986). Exercise induced increases in muscle fiber number. *European Journal of Applied Physiology*, **55**, 137-141.

17. Goodman, M.N. (1988). Amino acid and protein metabolism. In E.S. Horton & R.L. Terjung (Eds.), *Exercise, nutrition, and energy metabolism* (pp. 89-99). New York: Macmillan.

18. Graves, J.E., Pollock, M.L., Leggett, S.H., Braith, R.W., Carpenter, D.M., & Bishop, L.E. (1988). Effect of reduced training frequency on muscular strength. *International Journal of Sports Medicine*, **9**, 316-319.

19. Green, H.J., Klug, G.A., Reichmann, H., Seedorf, U., Wiehrer, W., & Pette, D. (1984). Exercise-induced fibre type transitions with regard to myosin, parvalbumin, and sarcoplasmic reticulum in muscles of the rat. *Pflugers Archive*, **400**, 432-438.

20. Hagerman, F.C., Hikida, R.S., Staron, R.S., Sherman, W.M., & Costill, D.L. (1984). Muscle damage in marathon runners. *Physician and Sportsmedicine*, **12**, 39-48.

21. Häkkinen, K., Alén, M. & Komi, P.V. (1985). Changes in isometric force and relaxation-time, electromyographic and muscle fibre characteristics of human skeletal muscle during strength training and detraining. *Acta Physiologica Scandinavica*, **125**, 573-585.

22. Hather, B.M., Tesch, P.A., Buchanan, P., & Dudley, G.A. (1991). Influence of eccentric actions on skeletal muscle adaptations to resistance training. *Acta Physiologica Scandinavica*, **143**, 177-185.

23. Kraemer, W.J., Deschenes, M.R., & Fleck, S.J. (1988). Physiological adaptations to resistance exercise: Implications for athletic conditioning. *Sports Medicine*, **6**, 246-256.

24. Kuipers, H., Keizer, H.A., Verstappen, F.T.J., & Costill, D.L. (1985). Influence of a prostaglandin-inhibiting drug on muscle soreness after eccentric work. *International Journal of Sports Medicine*, **6**, 336-339.

25. Larsson, L., & Tesch, P.A. (1986) Motor unit fibre density in extremely hypertrophied skeletal muscle in man: Electrophysiological signs of muscle fiber hyperplasia. *European Journal of Applied Physiology*, **55**, 130-136.

26. McDonagh, M.J.N., & Davies, C.T.M. (1984). Adaptive response of mammalian skeletal muscle to exercise with high loads. *European Journal of Applied Physiology*, **52**, 139-155.

27. Moritani, T., & deVries, H.A. (1979). Neural factors versus hypertrophy in the time course of muscle strength gain. *American Journal of Physical Medicine*, **58**, 115-130.

28. Moritani, T., and deVries, H.A. (1980). Potential for gross muscle hypertrophy in older men. *Journal of Gerontology*, **35**, 672-682.

29. Pette, D., & Vrbová, G. (1985). Neural control of phenotypic expression in mammalian muscle fibers. *Muscle and Nerve*, **8**, 676-689.

30. Sale, D.G. (1988). Neural adaptation to resistance training. *Medicine and Science in Sports and Exercise*, **20**, S135-S145.

31. Schantz, P., Randall-Fox, E., Hutchison, W., Tydén, A., & Åstrand, P.-O. (1983). Muscle fibre type distribution, muscle cross-sectional area and maximal voluntary strength in humans. *Acta Physiologica Scandinavica*, **117**, 219-226.

32. Schwane, J.A., Johnson, S.R., Vandenakker, C.B., & Armstrong, R.B. (1983). Delayed-onset muscular soreness and plasma CPK and LDH activities

after downhill running. *Medicine and Science in Sports and Exercise*, **15**, 51-56.

33. Schwane, J.A., Watrous, B.G., Johnson, S.R., & Armstrong, R.B. (1983). Is lactic acid related to delayed-onset muscle soreness? *Physician and Sportsmedicine*, **11**(3), 124-131.

34. Staron, R.S., Leonardi, M.J., Karapondo, D.L., Malicky, E.S., Falkel, J.E., Hagerman, F.C., & Hikida, R.S. (1991). Strength and skeletal muscle adaptations in heavy-resistance-trained women after detraining and retraining. *Journal of Applied Physiology*, **70**, 631-640.

35. Staron, R.S., Malicky, E.S., Leonardi, M.J., Falkel, J.E., Hagerman, F.C., & Dudley, G.A. (1990). Muscle hypertrophy and fast fiber type conversions in heavy resistance-trained women. *European Journal of Applied Physiology*, **60**, 71-79.

36. Talag, T.S. (1973). Residual muscular soreness as influenced by concentric, eccentric and static contractions. *Research Quarterly*, **44**, 458-469.

37. Tesch, P.A., & Karlsson, J. (1985). Muscle fiber types and size in trained and untrained muscles of elite athletes. *Journal of Applied Physiology*, **59**, 1716-1720.

38. Timson, B.F., Bowlin, B.K., Dudenhoeffer, G.A., & George, J.B. (1985). Fiber number, area, and composition of mouse soleus muscle following enlargement. *Journal of Applied Physiology*, **58**, 619-624.

39. Wong, T.S., & Booth, F.W. (1990). Protein metabolism in rat tibialis anterior muscle after stimulated chronic eccentric exercise. *Journal of Applied Physiology*, **69**, 1718-1724.

Selected Readings

Antonio, A., & Gonyea, W.J. (1993). Skeletal muscle fiber hyperplasia. *Medicine and Science in Sports and Exercise*, **25**(12), 1333-1345.

Armstrong, R.B. (1986). Muscle damage and endurance events. *Sports Medicine*, **3**, 370-381.

Behm, D.G., & Sale, D.G. (1993). Velocity specificity of resistance training. *Sports Medicine*, **15**(6), 374-388.

Booth, F.W. (1982). Effect of limb immobilization on skeletal muscle. *Journal of Applied Physiology*, **52**, 1113-1118.

Chesley, A., MacDougall, J.D., Tarnopolsky, M.A., Atkinson, S.A., & Smith, K. (1992). Changes in human muscle protein synthesis after resistance exercise. *Journal of Applied Physiology*, **73**, 1383-1388.

Chu, D.A. (1992). *Jumping into plyometrics*. Champaign, IL: Leisure Press.

Chu, D.A., & Plummer, L. (1984). The language of plyometrics. *National Strength Coaches Association Journal*, **1**, 30-31.

Clarke, D.H. (1973). Adaptations in strength and muscular endurance resulting from exercise. *Exercise and Sport Sciences Reviews*, **1**, 73-102.

Deschenes, M.R., Kraemer, W.J., Maresh, C.M., & Crivello, J.F. (1991). Exercise-induced hormonal changes and their effects upon skeletal muscle tissue. *Sports Medicine*, **12**, 80-93.

deVries, H.A. (1980). *Physiology of exercise for physical education and athletics* (3rd. ed.). Dubuque, IA: Brown.

Edgerton, V.R. (1976). Neuromuscular adaptations to power and endurance work. *Canadian Journal of Applied Sports Sciences*, **1**, 49-58.

Evans, W.J., & Cannon, J.G. (1991). The metabolic effects of exercise induced muscle damage. *Exercise and Sport Sciences Reviews*, **19**, 99-125.

Fleck, S.J., & Kraemer, W.J. (1988a). Resistance training: Basic principles. *Physician and Sportsmedicine*, **16**(3), 160-171.

Fleck, S.J., & Kraemer, W.J. (1988b). Resistance training: Physiological responses and adaptations. *Physician and Sportsmedicine*, **16**(4), 108-124.

Fleck, S.J., & Kraemer, W.J. (1988c). Resistance training: Physiological responses and adaptations. *Physician and Sportsmedicine*, **16**(5), 63-76.

Garfinkel, S., & Cafarelli, E. (1992). Relative changes in maximal force, EMG, and muscle cross-sectional area after isometric training. *Medicine and Science in Sports and Exercise*, **24**(11), 1220-1227.

Giddings, C.J., & Gonyea, W.J. (1992). Morphological observations supporting muscle fiber hyperplasia following weight-lifting exercise in cats. *The Anatomical Record*, **233**, 178-195.

Goldberg, A.L., Etlinger, J.D., Goldspink, D.F., & Jablecki, C. (1975). Mechanisms of work-induced hypertrophy of skeletal muscle. *Medicine and Science in Sports*, **7**, 248-261.

Gonyea, W.J., Ericson, G.C., & Bonde-Petersen, F. (1977). Skeletal muscle fiber splitting induced by weight-lifting exercise in cats. *Acta Physiologica Scandinavica*, **19**, 105-109.

Kannus, P., Jozsa, L., Renström, P., Järvinen, M., Kvist, M., Lehto, M., Oja, P., & Vuori, I. (1992). The effects of training, immobilization and remobilization on musculoskeletal tissue. 1. Training and immobilization. *Scandinavian Journal of Medicine and Science in Sports*, **2**, 100-118.

Knuttgen, H.G., & Kraemer, W.J. (1987). Terminology and measurement in exercise performance. *Journal of Applied Sport Science Research*, **1**, 1-10.

Komi, P.V., Viitasalo, J.H.T., Havu, M., Thorstensson, A., Sjödin, B., & Karlsson, J. (1977). Skeletal muscle fibres and muscle enzyme activities in monozygous and dizygous twins of both sexes. *Acta Physiologica Scandinavica*, **100**, 385-392.

Kraemer, W.J., & Fleck, S.J. (1988). Resistance training: Exercise prescription. *Physician and Sportsmedicine*, **16**(6), 69-81.

Larsson, L., & Ansved, T. (1985). Effects of long-term physical training and detraining on enzyme histochemical and functional skeletal muscle characteristics in man. *Muscle and Nerve*, **8**, 714-722.

MacDougall, J.D., Tuxen, D., Sale, D.G., Moroz, J.R., & Sutton, J.R. (1985). Arterial blood pressure response to heavy resistance exercise. *Journal of Applied Physiology*, **58**, 785-790.

Mikesky, A.E., Giddings, C.J., Matthews, W., & Gonyea, W.J. (1991). Changes in muscle fiber size and composition in response to heavy resistance exercise. *Medicine and Science in Sports and Exercise*, **23**, 1042-1049.

Sale, D., & MacDougall, D. (1981, March). Specificity in strength training: A review for the coach and athlete. *Science Periodical on Research and Technology in Sport*. Ottawa: The Coaching Association of Canada.

Salmons, S., & Henriksson, J. (1981). The adaptive response of skeletal muscle to increased use. *Muscle and Nerve*, **4**, 95-105.

Simoneau, J.A., Lortie, G., Boulay, M.R., Marcotte, M., Thibault, M.C., & Bouchard, C. (1985). Human skeletal muscle fiber type alteration with high-intensity intermittent training. *European Journal of Applied Physiology*, **54**, 250-253.

Smith, L.L. (1991). Acute inflammation: The underlying mechanism in delayed onset muscle soreness? *Medicine and Science in Sports and Exercise*, **23**, 542-551.

Stauber, W.T. (1989). Eccentric action of muscles: Physiology, injury and adaptation. *Exercise and Sport Sciences Reviews*, **17**, 157-185.

Stone, M.H., Fleck, S.J., Triplett, N.T., & Kraemer, W.J. (1991). Health and performance-related potential of resistance training. *Sports Medicine*, **11**, 210-231.

Tanaka, H., Costill, D.L., Thomas, R. Fink, W.J., & Widrick, J.J. (1993). Dry-land resistance training for competitive swimming. *Medicine and Science in Sports and Exercise*, **25**(8), 952-959.

Taylor, N.A.S., & Wilkinson, J.G. (1986). Exercise-induced skeletal muscle growth: Hypertrophy or hyperplasia? *Sports Medicine*, **3**, 190-200.

Tesch, P.A. (1988). Skeletal muscle adaptations consequent to long-term heavy resistance exercise. *Medicine and Science in Sports and Exercise*, **20** (Suppl.), S132-S134.

Tesch, P.A., & Larsson, L. (1982). Muscle hypertrophy in bodybuilders. *European Journal of Applied Physiology*, **49**, 301-306.

Timson, B.F. (1990). Evaluation of animal models for the study of exercise-induced muscle enlargement. *Journal of Applied Physiology*, **69**, 1935-1945.

Walker, J.A., Cerny, F.J., Cotter, J.R., & Burton, H.W. (1992). Attenuation of contraction-induced skeletal muscle injury by bromelain. *Medicine and Science in Sports and Exercise*, **24**, 20-25.

Energy for Movement

In the previous part, we studied the structure and function of the skeletal muscles, how muscles are controlled by the nervous system, and muscle and neural adaptations that occur in response to resistance training. We understand the basic mechanical aspects of muscles and how the muscles are controlled, but for them to produce movement they must use energy. In Part B, we turn our attention to how the body meets the energy needs of our skeletal muscles. In chapter 5, Basic Energy Systems, we examine our primary source of energy—ATP—and how it is provided through three energy systems. We will discuss the body's energy expenditure, how it varies from when we are at rest to when we are engaged in maximal levels of exercise, and how fatigue can result if energy demands exceed energy supply. In chapter 6, Hormonal Regulation of Exercise, we will see how endocrine glands and their hormones assist in the control of energy metabolism and fluid and electrolyte balance. Finally, in chapter 7, Metabolic Adaptations to Training, we will study adaptations in the skeletal muscles and the energy systems that occur in response to aerobic and anaerobic training and that can improve performance.

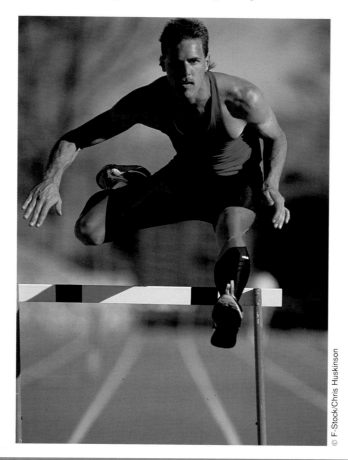

© F-Stock/Chris Huskinson

Chapter 5

Basic Energy Systems

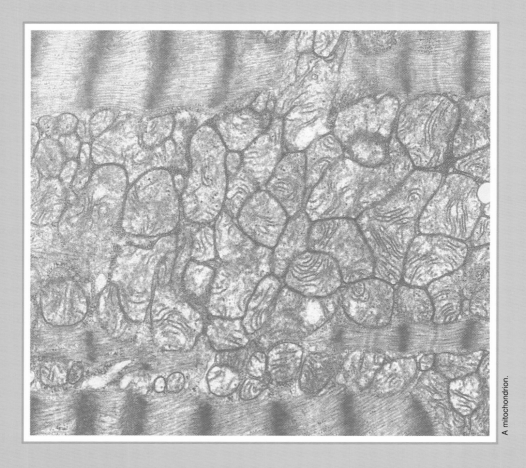

A mitochondrion.

Chapter Overview

All plants and animals depend on energy to sustain life. As humans, we derive this energy from food. Whether we eat the freshest fruits and vegetables or indulge in greasy french fries and burgers, each bite provides us with energy that our bodies require.

You cannot understand exercise physiology without understanding some key concepts about energy. In the previous chapters, we saw that movement does not occur without cost. We pay this cost with ATP, a form of chemical energy stored within our cells. We produce ATP by processes that are known collectively as metabolism, our focus for this chapter. We will review the biochemical processes that are basic to understanding how our muscles use food to create energy for movement. Then we will discuss how measurement of energy production and consumption helps us understand the effects of acute and chronic exercise on performance and conditioning.

Chapter Outline

In 1978, Tom Osler, a world-ranked marathon and ultramarathon runner, came to the Ball State University Human Performance Laboratory to be studied during his attempt to run and walk continuously for 72 hr. Laboratory measurements indicated that his muscles were using mostly carbohydrate for energy during the first hours of exercise. As the hours passed, more and more of the energy needed to continue this ordeal was obtained from fat. Ultimately, during the final 24 hr of effort, nearly all of his energy was provided by his body's fat stores, in spite of his continued intake of milk saturated with sugar and his consumption of an 18 in. × 21 in. birthday cake. Despite the intake of more than 9,000 kcal during the first 24 hr, Tom was forced to end his effort at 70 hr, exhausted and out of energy, having completed 200 miles.

Many dictionaries define the term energy as the capacity to perform work. Unfortunately this says nothing about the many biological functions that depend on the production and liberation of energy.

Energy can take a number of forms, such as

- chemical,
- electrical,
- electromagnetic,
- thermal,
- mechanical, and
- nuclear.

According to the laws of thermodynamics, all forms of energy are interchangeable. Chemical energy, for example, can be used to create the electrical energy stored in a battery, which can then be used to accomplish mechanical work by powering a motor. Energy is never lost or newly created. Instead, it undergoes a steady degradation from one form to another, ultimately becoming heat. Typically 60% to 70% of the total energy in the human body is degraded to heat. How do our bodies use energy before it reaches this final stage?

Energy for Cellular Activity

All energy originates from the sun as light energy. Chemical reactions in plants (photosynthesis) convert light into stored chemical energy. In turn, we obtain energy by eating plants, or animals that feed on plants. Energy is stored in food in the forms of carbohydrates, fats, and proteins. These basic food components can be broken down in our cells to release the stored energy.

Because all energy is eventually degraded to heat, the amount of energy released in a biological reaction is calculated from the amount of heat produced. Energy in biological systems is measured in kilocalories (kcal). By definition, 1 kcal equals the amount of heat energy needed to raise 1 kg of water 1 °C at 15 °C. The burning of a match, for example, liberates approximately 0.5 kcal, whereas the complete combustion of a gram of carbohydrate generates about 4.0 kcal.

Some free energy in the cells is used for growth and repair throughout the body. Such processes, as we saw earlier, build muscle mass during training and repair muscle damage after exercise or injury. Energy is also needed for active transport of many substances, such as glucose and Ca^{++}, across cell membranes. Active transport is critical to the survival of cells and the maintenance of homeostasis. Some of the energy released in our bodies is also used by the myofibrils to cause sliding of the actin and myosin filaments, resulting in muscle action and force generation, as we saw in chapter 2. This use is our main concern.

Energy Sources

Foods are composed primarily of carbon, hydrogen, oxygen, and, in the case of protein, nitrogen. Molecular bonds in foods are relatively weak and provide little energy when broken. Consequently, food is not used directly for cellular operations. Rather, the energy in food molecules' bonds is chemically released within our cells, then stored in the form of a high-energy compound called adenosine triphosphate (ATP).

**　KEY POINT　**

The formation of ATP provides the cells with a means of storing and conserving energy in a high-energy compound.

At rest, the energy your body needs is derived almost equally from the breakdown of carbohydrates (CHO) and fats. Proteins are your body's building blocks, usually providing little energy for cellular function. During mild to severe muscular effort, more carbohydrate is used, with less reliance on fat. In maximal short-duration exercise, ATP is generated almost exclusively from carbohydrate.

Carbohydrate

Your muscle's dependence on carbohydrate during exercise is related to carbohydrate availability and your muscle's well developed system for its metabolism. Carbohydrates are ultimately converted to glucose, a monosaccharide (one-unit sugar) that is transported via your blood to all body tissues. Under resting conditions, ingested carbohydrate is taken up by your muscles and liver, then converted into a more complex sugar molecule—glycogen. Glycogen is then stored in the cytoplasm until your cells use it to form ATP. The glycogen stored in your liver is converted back to glucose as needed, then transported by your blood to active tissues, where it is metabolized.

Liver and muscle glycogen reserves are limited and can be depleted unless the diet contains a reasonable amount of carbohydrate. Thus, we rely heavily on dietary sources of starches and sugars to replenish our carbohydrate reserves. Without adequate carbohydrate intake, the muscles and liver can be deprived of their primary energy source.

Fat

Fat and protein are also used as energy sources. Your body stores much more fat than it does carbohydrate. As noted in Table 5.1, the body's energy reserve from fat is far greater than from carbohydrate. But fat is less accessible for cellular metabolism because it must first be reduced from its complex form—triglyceride—

to its basic components: glycerol and free fatty acids (FFA). Only free fatty acids are used to form ATP.

KEY POINT

Carbohydrate stores in the liver and skeletal muscle are limited to less than 2,000 kcal of energy, or the equivalent of the energy needed for about 32 km (20 mi) of running. Fat stores, however, generally exceed 70,000 kcal of stored energy.

As seen in Figure 5.1, substantially more energy is derived from a given quantity of fat (9 kcal · g^{-1}) than from the same amount of carbohydrate (4 kcal · g^{-1}). Nonetheless, the rate of energy release from these compounds is too slow to meet all of the energy demands of intense muscular activity.

Protein

The process by which protein or fat is converted into glucose is called gluconeogenesis. Alternatively, protein can be converted through a series of reactions into fatty acids. This is called lipogenesis.

Protein can supply up to 5% to 10% of the energy needed to sustain prolonged exercise. Only the most basic units of protein—the amino acids—can be used for energy.

Table 5.1 Body Stores of Fuels and Energy

		g	kcal
Carbohydrates			
Liver glycogen		110	451
Muscle glycogen		250	1,025
Glucose in body fluids		15	62
	Total	375	1,538
Fat			
Subcutaneous		7,800	70,980
Intramuscular		161	1,465
	Total	7,961	72,445

Note. These estimates are based on an average body weight of 65 kg with 12% body fat.

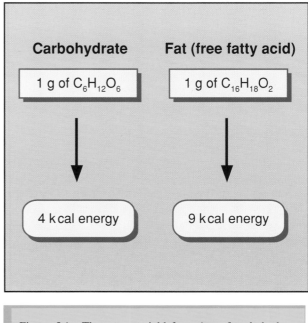

Figure 5.1 The energy yield from 1 g of carbohydrate and from 1 g of fat.

Rate of Energy Release

To be useful, free energy must be released from chemical compounds at a controlled rate. This rate is partially determined by the choice of the primary fuel source. Large amounts of one particular fuel can cause cells to rely more on that source than on alternatives. This influence of energy availability is termed the mass action effect.

Specific enzymes provide more structured control of the free-energy release rate. Many of these special proteins facilitate the breakdown (catabolism) of chemical compounds (Figure 5.2). Although the enzyme names are quite complex, all end with the suffix -ase. For example, an important enzyme that acts on ATP is termed adenosine triphosphatase (ATPase).

Now that we have the energy sources, we can look at how that energy is stored. In the next section, we will examine the production of the energy-storing compound ATP.

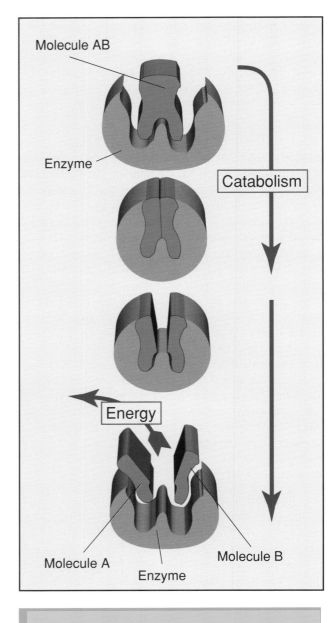

Figure 5.2   The action of enzymes in the catabolism (breakdown) of compounds.

▬▬ IN REVIEW . . . ▬▬

1. About 60% to 70% of the energy in the human body is degraded to heat. The remainder is used for mechanical work and cellular activities.
2. We derive our energy from food sources—carbohydrates, fats, and proteins.
3. The energy we derive from food is stored in a high-energy compound—ATP.
4. Carbohydrate provides about 4 kcal of energy per gram, compared to about 9 kcal · g⁻¹ for fat. But CHO energy is more accessible. Protein can also provide energy.

Bioenergetics: ATP Production

An ATP molecule (Figure 5.3a) consists of adenosine (a molecule of adenine joined to a molecule of ribose) combined with three inorganic phosphate (P_i) groups. When acted on by the enzyme ATPase, the last phosphate group splits away from the ATP molecule, rapidly releasing a large amount of energy (7.6 kcal · mole⁻¹ of ATP). This reduces the ATP to ADP (adenosine diphosphate) and P_i (Figure 5.3b). But how was that energy originally stored?

The process of storing energy by forming ATP from other chemical sources is called phosphorylation. Through various chemical reactions, a phosphate group is added to a relatively low-energy compound, adeno-sine diphosphate (ADP), converting it to adenosine triphosphate (ATP). When these reactions occur without oxygen, the process is called anaerobic metabolism. When these reactions occur with the aid of oxygen, the overall process is called aerobic metabolism, and the aerobic conversion of ADP to ATP is oxidative phosphorylation.

Cells generate ATP by three methods:

1. The ATP-PCr system
2. The glycolytic system
3. The oxidative system

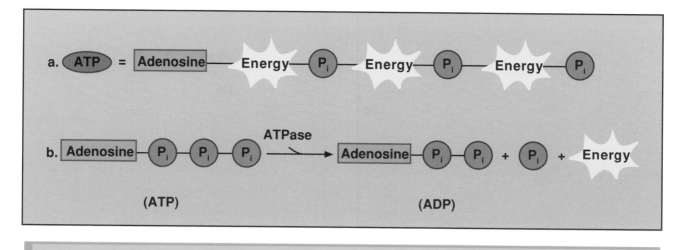

Figure 5.3   (a) The structural make-up of an ATP molecule, showing the high-energy phosphate bonds, and (b) energy release.

ATP-PCr System

The simplest of the energy systems is the ATP-PCr system. In addition to ATP, your cells have another high-energy phosphate molecule that stores energy. This molecule is called phosphocreatine, or PCr (also called creatine phosphate). Unlike with ATP, energy released by the breakdown of PCr is not used directly to accomplish cellular work. Instead, it rebuilds ATP to maintain a relatively constant supply.

The release of energy from PCr is facilitated by the enzyme creatine kinase (CK), which acts on PCr to separate P_i from creatine. The energy released can then be used to couple P_i to an ADP molecule, forming ATP. This process is depicted in Figure 5.4. With this system, as energy is released from ATP by the splitting of a phosphate group, your cells can prevent ATP depletion by reducing PCr, providing energy to form more ATP.

This process is rapid and can be accomplished without any special structures within the cell. Although it can occur in the presence of oxygen, this process does not require oxygen, so the ATP-PCr system is said to be anaerobic.

During the first few seconds of intense muscular activity, such as sprinting, ATP is maintained at a relatively constant level, but the PCr level declines steadily as the compound is used to replenish the depleted ATP (see Figure 5.5). At exhaustion, however, both ATP and PCr levels are quite low, and are unable to provide the energy for further contractions and relaxations.

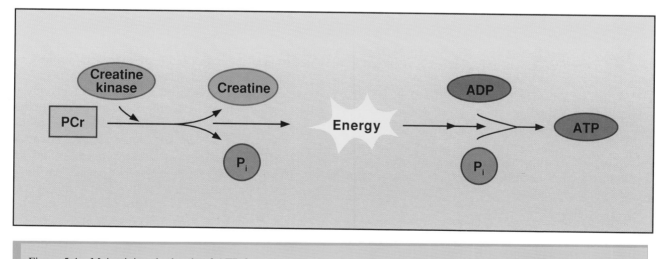

Figure 5.4   Maintaining the levels of ATP from the energy stored in PCr.

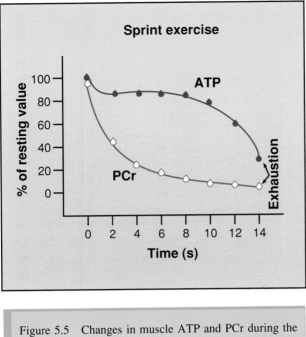

Figure 5.5 Changes in muscle ATP and PCr during the first seconds of maximal muscular effort.

Thus your capacity to maintain ATP levels with the energy from PCr is limited. Your ATP and PCr stores can sustain your muscles' energy needs for only 3 to 15 s during an all-out sprint. Beyond that point the muscles must rely on other processes for ATP formation: the glycolytic and oxidative combustion of fuels.

The Glycolytic System

Another method of ATP production involves the liberation of energy through the breakdown (lysis) of glucose. This system is called the glycolytic system because it involves the process of glycolysis, which is the breakdown of glucose via special glycolytic enzymes. An overview of this process is depicted in Figure 5.6.

Glucose accounts for about 99% of all sugars circulating in the blood. Blood glucose comes from the digestion of carbohydrate and the breakdown of liver glycogen. Glycogen is synthesized from glucose by a process called glycogenesis. It is stored in the liver or in muscle until needed. At that time, the glycogen is broken down to glucose-1-phosphate through the process of glycogenolysis.

Before either glucose or glycogen can be used to generate energy, they must be converted to a compound called glucose-6-phosphate. Conversion of a molecule of glucose requires one molecule of ATP.

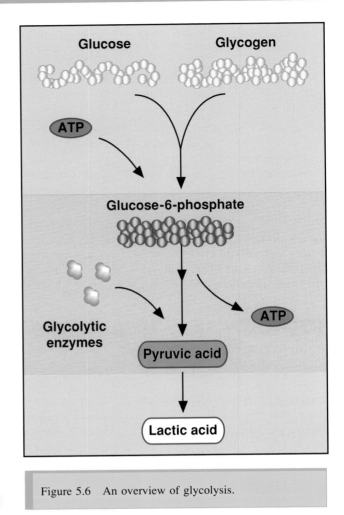

Figure 5.6 An overview of glycolysis.

In the conversion of glycogen, glucose-6-phosphate is formed from glucose-1-phosphate without this energy expenditure. Glycolysis begins once the glucose-6-phosphate is formed.

Glycolysis ultimately produces pyruvic acid. This process doesn't require oxygen, but the use of oxygen determines the fate of the pyruvic acid formed by glycolysis. In this text, when we refer to the glycolytic system we are referring to the process of glycolysis as it occurs without the involvement of oxygen. In this case, the pyruvic acid is converted to lactic acid.

Glycolysis, which is far more complex than the ATP-PCr system, requires 12 enzymatic reactions for the breakdown of glycogen to lactic acid. All these enzymes operate within the cells' cytoplasm. The net gain from this process is 3 moles of ATP formed for each mole of glycogen broken down. If glucose is used instead of glycogen, the gain is only 2 moles of ATP because 1 mole is used for the conversion of glucose to glucose-6-phosphate.

This energy system does not produce large amounts of ATP. Despite this limitation, the combined actions of the ATP-PCr and glycolytic systems allow the muscles to generate force even when the oxygen supply is limited. These two systems predominate during the early minutes of high-intensity exercise.

Another major limitation of anaerobic glycolysis is that it causes an accumulation of lactic acid in the muscles and body fluids. In all-out sprint events lasting 1 or 2 min, the demands on the glycolytic system are high, and muscle lactic acid levels can increase from a resting value of about 1 mmol · kg^{-1} of muscle to more than 25 mmol · kg^{-1}. This acidification of muscle fibers inhibits further glycogen breakdown because it impairs glycolytic enzyme function. In addition, the acid decreases the fibers' calcium-binding capacity and thus may impede muscle contraction.

KEY POINT

Lactic acid and lactate are not the same compound. Lactic acid is an acid with the chemical formula $C_3H_6O_8$. Lactate is any salt of lactic acid. When lactic acid releases H^+, the remaining compound joins with Na^+ or K^+ to form a salt. Anaerobic glycolysis produces lactic acid, but it quickly dissociates and the salt—lactate—is formed. For this reason, the terms are often used interchangeably.

A muscle fiber's rate of energy use during exercise can be 200 times greater than at rest. The ATP-PCr and glycolytic systems alone cannot supply all the needed energy. Without another energy system, our exercise capacity might be limited to only a few minutes. Let's turn our attention to the third energy system.

The Oxidative System

The final system of cellular energy production is the oxidative system. This is the most complex of the three energy systems, but we will avoid cumbersome details. The process by which the body disassembles fuels with the aid of oxygen to generate energy is called cellular respiration. Because oxygen is used, this is an aerobic process. This oxidative production of ATP occurs within special cell organelles—the mitochondria. In muscles, these are adjacent to the myofibrils and are also scattered throughout the sarcoplasm.

Muscles need a steady supply of energy to continuously produce the force needed during long-term ac-

---

IN REVIEW . . .

1. ATP is generated through three energy systems:
   - The ATP-PCr system
   - The glycolytic system
   - The oxidative system
2. In the ATP-PCr system, P_i is separated from phosphocreatine through the action of creatine kinase. The P_i can then combine with ADP to form ATP. This system is anaerobic, and its main function is to maintain ATP levels. The energy yield is 1 mole of ATP per 1 mole of PCr.
3. The glycolytic system involves the process of glycolysis, through which glucose or glycogen is broken down to pyruvic acid via glycolytic enzymes. When conducted without oxygen, the pyruvic acid is converted to lactic acid. One mole of glucose yields 2 moles of ATP, but 1 mole of glycogen yields 3 moles of ATP.
4. The ATP-PCr and glycolytic systems are major contributors of energy during the early minutes of high-intensity exercise.

---

tivity. Unlike anaerobic ATP production, the oxidative system has a tremendous energy yield, so aerobic metabolism is the primary method of energy production during endurance events. This places considerable demands on the body's ability to deliver oxygen to the active muscles.

Oxidation of Carbohydrate

To follow this discussion, please refer to the schematic diagram in Figure 5.7. Oxidative production of ATP involves three processes:

1. Glycolysis
2. Krebs cycle
3. Electron transport chain

Glycolysis. In carbohydrate metabolism, glycolysis plays a role in both anaerobic and aerobic ATP production. The process of glycolysis is the same whether or not oxygen is present. Presence of oxygen determines only the fate of the end product—pyruvic acid. Recall that anaerobic glycolysis produces lactic acid and only 3 moles of ATP per mole of glycogen. In the presence of oxygen, however, the pyruvic acid is converted into a compound called acetyl coenzyme A (acetyl CoA).

The Krebs Cycle. Once formed, acetyl CoA enters the Krebs cycle (citric acid cycle), a complex series of

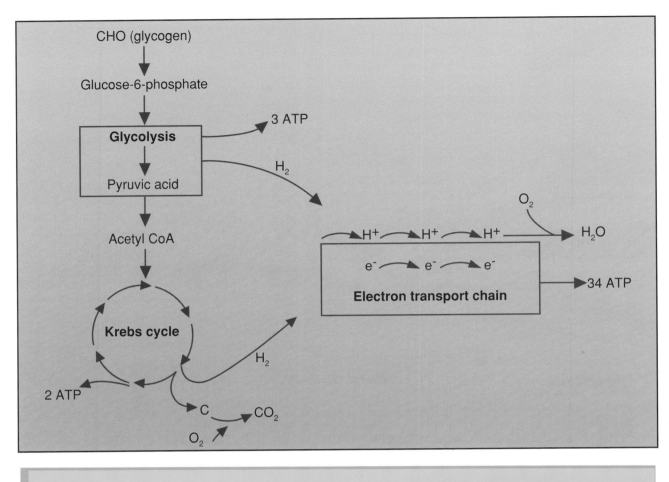

Figure 5.7   The oxidation of carbohydrate.

chemical reactions that permits the complete oxidation of acetyl CoA. At the end of the Krebs cycle, 2 moles of ATP have been formed and the substrate (the compound upon which the enzymes act—in this case the original carbohydrate) has been broken down into carbon and hydrogen. The remaining carbon then combines with oxygen to form carbon dioxide. This CO_2 easily diffuses out of the cells and is transported by the blood to the lungs to be expired.

The Electron Transport Chain.   During glycolysis, hydrogen is released as glucose is metabolized to pyruvic acid. More hydrogen is released during the Krebs cycle. If it remains in the system, the inside of the cell becomes too acidic. What happens to this hydrogen?

The Krebs cycle is coupled to a series of reactions known as the electron transport chain. The hydrogen released during glycolysis and during the Krebs cycle combines with two coenzymes: NAD (nicotinamide adenine dinucleotide) and FAD (flavin adenine dinucleotide). These carry the hydrogen atoms to the electron transport chain, where they are split into protons and electrons. At the end of the chain, the H^+ combines with oxygen to form water, thus preventing acidification.

The electrons that were split from the hydrogen pass through a series of reactions, hence the name electron transport chain, and ultimately provide energy for the phosphorylation of ADP, thus forming ATP. Because this process relies on oxygen, it is referred to as oxidative phosphorylation.

Energy Yield From Carbohydrate.   The oxidative system of energy production can generate up to 39 molecules of ATP from one molecule of glycogen. If the process begins with glucose, the net gain is 38 ATP molecules (recall that one ATP molecule is used for conversion to glucose-6-phosphate before glycolysis begins). The energy gained is summarized in Table 5.2.

Oxidation of Fat

As noted earlier, fat also contributes to muscles' energy needs. Muscle and liver glycogen stores may be able to provide only 1,200 to 2,000 kcal of energy, but the

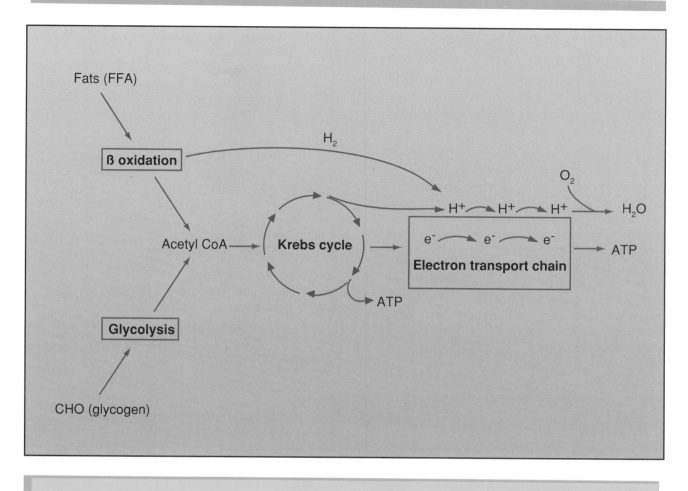

Figure 5.8   The metabolism of fat and carbohydrate share some common pathways.

Table 5.2   Energy Production From the Oxidation of Liver Glycogen

| | ATP produced from 1 mole of liver glycogen | |
Stage of process	Direct	By oxidative phosphorylation[a]
Glycolysis (glucose to pyruvic acid)	3	6
Pyruvic acid to acetyl CoA	0	6
Krebs cycle	2	22
Subtotal	5	34
Total		39

[a]Refers to ATP produced by transferring H^+ and electrons to the electron transport chain.

fat stored inside your muscle fibers and in your fat cells can supply about 70,000 to 75,000 kcal.

Although many chemical compounds (such as triglycerides, phospholipids, and cholesterol) are classified as fats, only triglycerides are major energy sources. Triglycerides are stored in fat cells and in skeletal muscle fibers. To be used for energy, a triglyceride must be broken down to its basic units: one molecule of glycerol and three molecules of free fatty acids. This process is called lipolysis, and it is carried out by enzymes known as lipases. The FFA are the primary energy source, so they will be our focus.

Once freed from glycerol, FFA can enter the blood and be transported throughout the body, entering muscle fibers by diffusion. Their rate of entry into the muscle fibers depends on the concentration gradient. Increasing the FFA concentration in the blood drives them into the muscle fibers.

β Oxidation.   Although the various free fatty acids in the body differ structurally, their metabolism is essentially the same, as shown in Figure 5.8. Upon entering the muscle fiber, free fatty acids are enzymatically activated with energy from ATP, preparing them for catabolism (breakdown) within the mitochondria. This enzymatic catabolism of fat by the mitochondria is termed beta oxidation (β oxidation).

In this process, the carbon chain of a free fatty acid is cleaved into separate 2-carbon units of acetic acid. For example, if a free fatty acid originally has a 16-carbon chain, β oxidation yields 8 molecules of acetic acid. Each acetic acid is then converted to acetyl CoA.

The Krebs Cycle and the Electron Transport Chain. From this point on, fat metabolism follows the same path as carbohydrate metabolism. Acetyl CoA formed by β oxidation enters the Krebs cycle. The Krebs cycle generates hydrogen that is transported to the electron transport chain, along with the hydrogen generated during β oxidation, to undergo oxidative phosphorylation. As in glucose metabolism, the by-products of FFA oxidation are ATP, H_2O, and CO_2. However, the complete combustion of a free fatty acid molecule requires more oxygen because that molecule contains considerably more carbon than a glucose molecule.

KEY POINT

Although fat provides more kcal of energy per gram than carbohydrate, fat oxidation requires more oxygen than carbohydrate oxidation. The energy yield from fat is 5.6 ATP molecules per O_2 molecule used, compared to carbohydrate's yield of 6.3 ATP per O_2. Oxygen delivery is limited by the oxygen transport system, so carbohydrate is the preferred fuel during high-intensity exercise.

The advantage of having more carbon in free fatty acids than in glucose is that more acetyl CoA is formed from the metabolism of a given amount of fat, so more enters the Krebs cycle and more electrons are sent to the electron transport chain. This is why fat metabolism can generate so much more energy than glucose metabolism.

Consider the example of palmitic acid, a rather abundant 16-carbon free fatty acid. The combined reactions of oxidation, the Krebs cycle, and the electron transport chain produce 129 molecules of ATP from one molecule of palmitic acid (as seen in Table 5.3), compared to only 38 molecules of ATP from glucose or 39 from glycogen. Although this yield seems quite high, only about 40% of the energy released by the metabolism of either glucose or free fatty acid mole-

Table 5.3   Energy Production From the Oxidation of Palmitic Acid ($C_{16}H_{32}O_2$)

Stage of process	ATP produced from 1 molecule of palmitic acid	
	Direct	By oxidative phosphorylation
Fatty acid activation		−2
β oxidation		35
Krebs cycle	8	88
Subtotal	8	121
Total	129	

cules is captured to form ATP. The remaining 60% is given off as heat.

Protein Metabolism

As noted earlier, carbohydrates and fatty acids are our bodies' preferred fuels. But proteins, or rather the amino acids that form them, are also used. Some amino acids can be converted into glucose (by gluconeogenesis). Alternatively, some can be converted into various intermediates of oxidative metabolism (such as pyruvate or acetyl CoA) to enter the oxidative process.

Protein's energy yield is not as easily determined as that of carbohydrate or fat, because protein also contains nitrogen. When amino acids are catabolized, some of the released nitrogen is used to form new amino acids, but the remaining nitrogen cannot be oxidized by the body. Instead it is converted into urea and then excreted, primarily in the urine. This conversion requires the use of ATP, so some energy is spent in this process.

When protein is broken down through combustion in the laboratory, the energy yield is 5.65 kcal per gram. However, when metabolized in the body, because of the energy expended in converting nitrogen to urea, the energy yield is only about 5.20 kcal per gram, 8% less than the laboratory value.

To accurately assess the rate of protein metabolism, the amount of nitrogen being eliminated from the body must be determined. These measurements require urine collection for 12- to 24-hr periods, clearly a time-consuming process. Because the healthy body utilizes little protein during rest and exercise (usually far less than 5% to 10% of total energy expended), estimates of energy expenditure generally ignore protein metabolism.

The Oxidative Capacity of Muscle

We have seen that the processes of oxidative metabolism have the highest energy yields. It would be ideal if these processes always functioned at peak capacity. But, as with all physiological systems, they operate within certain constraints. The oxidative capacity, termed the $\dot{Q}_{O_2}$, of a muscle is a measure of its maximal capacity to use oxygen. In this section, we'll look at the limitations of your muscles' oxidative capacity.

Enzyme Activity

Muscle fibers' capacity to oxidize carbohydrate and fat is difficult to determine. Numerous studies have shown a close relationship between a muscle's ability to perform prolonged aerobic exercise and the activity of its oxidative enzymes. Because many enzymes are required for oxidation, the enzyme activity of your muscle fibers provides a reasonable indication of their oxidative potential.

Measuring all of the enzymes in muscles is impractical, so a few representatives have been selected to reflect the aerobic capacity of the fibers. The enzymes most frequently measured include succinate dehydrogenase (SDH) and citrate synthase (CS), mitochondrial enzymes involved in the Krebs cycle. Figure 5.9 illustrates the relationship between SDH activity in the vastus lateralis muscle and the muscle's oxidative capacity. Endurance athletes' muscles have oxidative enzyme activities nearly two to four times greater than those of untrained men and women.[2,3,5]

Fiber-Type Composition and Endurance Training

A muscle's fiber-type composition determines, in part, its oxidative capacity. As noted in chapter 3, slow-twitch (ST) fibers have a greater capacity for aerobic activity than the fast-twitch (FT) fibers because ST fibers have more mitochondria and higher concentrations of oxidative enzymes. FT fibers are better suited for glycolytic energy production. Thus, in general, the more ST fibers in your muscles, the greater your muscles' oxidative capacity. Elite distance runners, for example, have been reported to possess more ST fibers, more mitochondria, and higher muscle oxidative enzyme activities than untrained individuals.[5,6]

Endurance training enhances the oxidative capacity of all fibers, especially FT fibers. Training that places demands on oxidative phosphorylation stimulates the muscle fibers to develop more mitochondria that are also larger and contain more oxidative enzymes. By increasing the fiber's enzymes for β oxida-

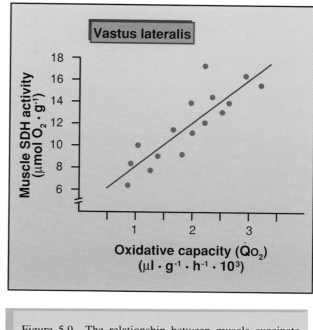

Figure 5.9 The relationship between muscle succinate dehydrogenase (SDH) activity and oxidative capacity ($\dot{Q}_{O_2}$).

tion, this training also enables the muscle to rely more heavily on fat for ATP production.

Thus, with endurance training, even people with large percentages of FT fibers can increase their muscles' aerobic capacities. But it is generally agreed that an endurance-trained FT fiber will not develop the same high-endurance capacity as a similarly trained ST fiber.

Oxygen Needs

Although your muscles' oxidative capacity is determined by the number of mitochondria and the amount of oxidative enzymes present, oxidative metabolism ultimately depends on an adequate supply of oxygen. When at rest, your body's need for ATP is relatively small, requiring minimal oxygen delivery. As your exercise intensity increases, so do your energy demands. To meet them, your rate of oxidative ATP production also increases. In an effort to satisfy your muscles' need for oxygen, the rate and depth of your respiration increase, improving gas exchange in the lungs, and your heart beats faster, pumping more oxygenated blood to your muscles.

The human body stores little oxygen. Because of this, the amount of oxygen entering your blood as it passes through your lungs is directly proportional to the amount used by your tissues for oxidative metabolism. Consequently, a reasonably accurate estimate of aerobic energy production can be made by measuring the amount of oxygen consumed at the lungs.

IN REVIEW . . .

1. The oxidative system involves breakdown of fuels with the aid of oxygen. This system yields more energy than the ATP-PCr or glycolytic system.
2. Oxidation of carbohydrate involves glycolysis, the Krebs cycle, and the electron transport chain. The end result is H_2O, CO_2, and 38 or 39 ATP molecules per carbohydrate molecule.
3. Fat oxidation begins with β oxidation of free fatty acids, then follows the same path as carbohydrate oxidation: the Krebs cycle and the electron transport chain. The energy yield for fat oxidation is much higher than for carbohydrate oxidation, and it varies with the free fatty acid being oxidized.
4. Protein oxidation is more complex because protein (amino acids) contains nitrogen, which cannot be oxidized. Protein contributes relatively little to energy production, so its metabolism is often overlooked.
5. Your muscles' oxidative capacity depends on their oxidative enzyme levels, their fiber-type composition, and oxygen availability.

Measuring Energy Use During Exercise

The energy turnover in muscle fibers cannot be directly measured. But numerous indirect laboratory methods can be used to calculate the rate and quantity of energy expenditure when your body is at rest and during exercise. Several of these methods have been in use since the early 1900s. Others are new and only recently have been used in exercise physiology. In the following sections we will review some of these methods of measurement.

Direct Calorimetry

As noted earlier, only about 40% of the energy liberated during the metabolism of glucose and fats is used to produce ATP. The remaining 60% is converted to heat, so one way to gauge the rate and quantity of energy production is to measure your body's heat production. This technique is called direct calorimetry.

This approach was first described by Zuntz and Hagemann in the late 1800s. They developed the calorimeter (illustrated in Figure 5.10), which is an insulated airtight chamber. The walls of the chamber contain copper tubing through which water is passed. When you're placed inside the chamber, the heat produced by your body radiates to the walls and warms the water. The water's temperature change is recorded, as are temperature changes in the air entering and leaving the chamber as you breathe. These changes are due to the heat your body generates. By using the resulting values, it is possible to calculate your metabolism.

Calorimeters are expensive to construct and to use and are slow to generate results. Their only real advantage is that they measure heat directly. Although a calorimeter can provide an accurate measure of total body energy expenditure, it cannot follow rapid changes in energy release. For that reason, energy metabolism during intense exercise cannot be studied with a calorimeter. Consequently, this method is seldom used today because it is easier and less expensive to measure energy expenditure by assessing the exchange of oxygen and carbon dioxide that occurs during oxidative phosphorylation.

Indirect Calorimetry

As noted earlier, glucose and fat metabolism depend on O_2 availability and produce CO_2 and water. The amount of O_2 and CO_2 exchanged in the lungs normally equals that used and released by body tissues. Knowing this, your caloric expenditure can be estimated by measuring your respiratory gases. This method of estimating energy expenditure is called indirect calorimetry because heat production is not measured directly. Rather, it is calculated from the respiratory exchange of CO_2 and O_2.

Figure 5.11 shows some of the equipment used to measure CO_2 production and O_2 consumption. Though this equipment is cumbersome and limits movement, it has been adapted for use under a variety of conditions in the laboratory, on the playing field, and elsewhere.

The Respiratory Exchange Ratio

To estimate the amount of energy used by the body, it is necessary to know the type of food (carbohydrate, fat, or protein) being oxidized. The carbon and oxygen contents of glucose, free fatty acids, and amino acids differ dramatically. As a result, the amount of oxygen used during metabolism depends on the type of fuel being oxidized. Indirect calorimetry measures the amount of CO_2 released ($\dot{V}_{CO_2}$) and oxygen consumed

Calorimeter

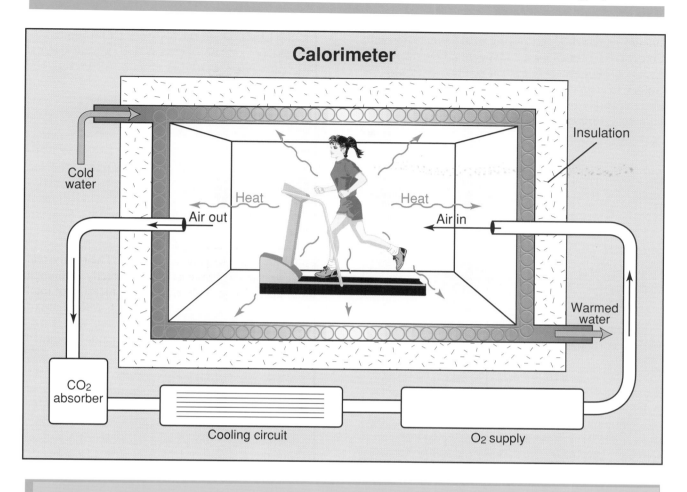

Figure 5.10   A calorimetric chamber.

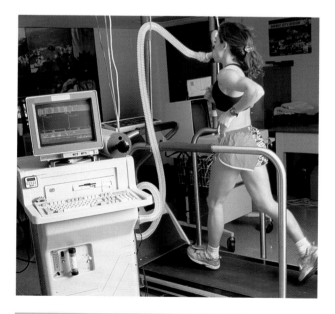

Figure 5.11   The equipment used to measure the respiratory exchange of oxygen and carbon dioxide.

($\dot{V}O_2$). The ratio between these two values is termed the respiratory exchange ratio, or RER.

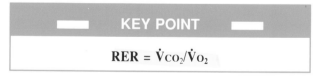

KEY POINT

$$RER = \dot{V}CO_2/\dot{V}O_2$$

In general, the amount of oxygen needed to completely oxidize a molecule of carbohydrate or fat is proportional to the amount of carbon in that fuel. For example, glucose ($C_6H_{12}O_6$) contains six carbon atoms. During glucose combustion, six molecules of oxygen are used to produce 6 CO_2 molecules, 6 H_2O molecules, and 38 ATP molecules:

$$6O_2 + C_6H_{12}O_6 \rightarrow 6CO_2 + 6H_2O + 38ATP$$

By evaluating how much CO_2 is released compared to the amount of O_2 consumed, we find that the respiratory exchange ratio is 1.0:

$$RER = \dot{V}CO_2/\dot{V}O_2, \; 6CO_2/6O_2 = 1.0$$

As shown in Table 5.4, the RER value varies with the type of fuels being used for energy. Free fatty acids have considerably more carbon and hydrogen but less oxygen than glucose. Consider palmitic acid, $C_{16}H_{32}O_2$. To completely oxidize this molecule to CO_2 and H_2O requires 23 molecules of oxygen:

$$16C + 16O_2 \rightarrow 16CO_2$$
$$\underline{32H + 8O_2 \rightarrow 16H_2O}$$

$$\begin{aligned} \text{Total} &= 24\ O_2 \text{ needed} \\ &\underline{-\ 1\ O_2 \text{ provided by the palmitic acid}} \\ &23\ O_2 \text{ must be added} \end{aligned}$$

Ultimately this oxidation results in 16 molecules of CO_2, 16 molecules of H_2O, and 129 molecules of ATP:

$$C_{16}H_{32}O_2 + 23O_2 \rightarrow 16CO_2 + 16H_2O + 129ATP$$

Combustion of this fat molecule requires significantly more oxygen than combustion of a carbohydrate molecule. During carbohydrate oxidation, approximately 6.3 molecules of ATP are produced for each molecule of O_2 used (38 ATP per 6 O_2), compared to 5.6 molecules of ATP per molecule of oxygen during palmitic acid metabolism (129 ATP per 23 O_2).

Although fat provides more energy than carbohydrate, more oxygen is needed to oxidize fat than carbohydrate. This means that the RER value for fat is substantially lower than for carbohydrate. Using palmitic acid, the RER value is 0.70:

$$RER = \dot{V}_{CO_2}/\dot{V}_{O_2} = 16/23 = 0.70.$$

Once the RER value is determined from measurement of the respiratory gases, the value can be compared to a table (Table 5.4) to determine the food mixture being oxidized. If, for example, the RER value is 1.0, the cells are using only glucose or glycogen, and each liter of oxygen consumed would generate 5.05 kcal. The oxidation of only fat would yield 4.69 kcal $\cdot$ L^{-1} O_2, and the oxidation of protein would yield 4.46 kcal $\cdot$ L^{-1} O_2 consumed. Thus, if the muscles were using only glucose and the body were consuming 2 L of oxygen per minute, then the rate of heat energy production would be 10.1 kcal $\cdot$ min^{-1} (2 L $\cdot$ min^{-1} $\times$ 5.05 kcal).

Limitations

Even indirect calorimetry is far from perfect. Calculations of gas exchange assume that the body's O_2 content remains constant, and that CO_2 exchange in the lung is proportional to its release from the cells. Arterial blood remains almost completely oxygen-saturated (about 98%) even during intense effort. We can accurately assume that the oxygen being removed from the air we breathe is in proportion to its cellular uptake. Carbon dioxide exchange, however, is less constant. Body CO_2 pools are quite large and can be altered simply by deep breathing or by performing highly intense exercise. Under these conditions, the amount of CO_2 released in the lung may not represent that being produced in the tissues. So calculations of carbohydrate and fat used based on gas measurements appear to be valid only during rest or steady state exercise.

Use of the respiratory exchange ratio can also lead to inaccuracies. Recall that protein is not completely oxidized in the body because nitrogen is not oxidizable. This makes it impossible to calculate the body's protein use from the respiratory exchange ratio. As a result, the RER is sometimes referred to as a nonprotein RER and it simply ignores protein oxidation.

Traditionally, protein was thought to contribute little to the energy used during exercise, so exercise physiologists felt justified in using the nonprotein RER when making calculations. But more recent evidence suggests that in exercise lasting for several hours, protein may contribute up to 10% of the total energy.

The body normally uses a combination of fuels. RER values vary depending on the specific mixture being oxidized. At rest, the RER value is typically in the range of 0.78 to 0.80. During exercise, though, muscles rely increasingly on carbohydrate for energy, resulting in a higher RER. As exercise intensity increases, the muscles' carbohydrate demand also increases. As more carbohydrate is used, the RER value approaches 1.0.

This rise in the RER value to 1.0 reflects the demands on blood glucose and muscle glycogen, but it may also indicate that more CO_2 is being unloaded from the blood than is being produced by the muscles. At or near exhaustion, lactate accumulates in the blood. Your body tries to reverse this acidification by releasing more CO_2. Lactate accumulation increases CO_2 production because excess acid causes carbonic acid in the blood to be converted to CO_2. As a consequence, the excess CO_2 diffuses out of the blood and into the

Table 5.4   Caloric Equivalence of the Respiratory Exchange Ratio and % kcal From CHO and Fats

Respiratory exchange ratio	Energy kcal · L⁻¹ O₂	% kcal Carbohydrates	Fats
0.71	4.69	0	100
0.75	4.74	15.6	84.4
0.80	4.80	33.4	66.6
0.85	4.86	50.7	49.3
0.90	4.92	67.5	32.5
0.95	4.99	84.0	16.0
1.00	5.05	100.0	0

lung for exhalation, increasing the amount of CO_2 released. For this reason, RER values approaching 1.0 may not accurately estimate the type of fuel being used by the muscles.

As another complication, glucose production from the catabolism of amino acids and fats in the liver produces a respiratory exchange ratio below 0.70. Thus calculations of carbohydrate oxidation from the RER value will be underestimated if energy is derived from this process.

Despite shortcomings of indirect calorimetry, it still provides our best estimate of energy expenditure during rest and at submaximal exercise.

Isotopic Measurements of Energy Metabolism

In the past, determining an individual's total daily energy expenditure depended on recording food intake over several days and measuring body composition changes during that period. This method, although widely used, is limited by the individual's ability to keep accurate records and by the ability to match the individual's activities to accurate energy costs.

Fortunately, the use of isotopes has expanded our ability to investigate energy metabolism. Isotopes are elements with an atypical atomic weight. They can be either radioactive (radioisotopes) or nonradioactive (stable isotopes). As an example, carbon-12 (^{12}C) has a molecular weight of 12, is the most common natural form of carbon, and is nonradioactive. In contrast, carbon-14 (^{14}C) has 2 more neutrons than carbon-12, giving it an atomic weight of 14. Carbon-14 is created in the laboratory and is radioactive.

Carbon-13 (^{13}C) constitutes about 1% of the carbon in nature and is used frequently for studying energy metabolism. Because carbon-13 is nonradioactive, it is less easily traced within the body than carbon-14. But although radioactive isotopes are easily detected in the body, they pose a hazard to body tissues and thus are infrequently used in human research.

Carbon-13 and other isotopes such as hydrogen-2 (deuterium, or ^2H) are used as tracers, meaning that they can be selectively followed in the body. Tracer techniques involve infusing isotopes into an individual, then following their distribution and movement.

Although the method was described more than 30 years ago, studies with doubly labeled water have only recently been introduced for monitoring energy expenditure during normal daily living. The subject ingests a known amount of water labeled with two isotopes ($^2H_2{}^{18}O$), hence the term doubly labeled water. The deuterium (^2H) diffuses throughout the body's water, and the oxygen-18 (^{18}O) diffuses throughout both the water and the bicarbonate stores (where much of the carbon dioxide derived from metabolism is stored). The rate at which the two isotopes leave the body can be determined by analyzing their presence in a series of urine, saliva, or blood samples. These turnover rates can then be used to calculate how much carbon dioxide is produced, and that value can be converted to energy expenditure using calorimetric equations.

Because isotope turnover is relatively slow, measurement of energy metabolism must be conducted for several weeks. Thus this method is not well suited for measurements of acute exercise metabolism. However, its accuracy (more than 98%) and low risk make it well suited for determining day-to-day energy expenditure. Nutritionists have hailed the doubly labeled water method as the most significant technical advance of the past century in the field of energy metabolism.

IN REVIEW . . .

1. Direct calorimetry involves using a calorimeter to directly measure heat produced by the body.
2. Indirect calorimetry involves measuring O_2 consumption and CO_2 release, calculating the RER value (the ratio of these two gas measurements), comparing it to standard values to determine the foods being oxidized, then calculating the energy expended per liter of oxygen consumed.
3. The RER value at rest is usually 0.78 to 0.80.
4. Isotopes can be used to determine metabolic rate. They are injected into the body or ingested then traced as they move through it. The rates at which they are cleared can be used to calculate CO_2 production and then caloric expenditure.

Estimates of Anaerobic Effort

We have discussed how your aerobic metabolism can be measured. But these methods ignore the anaerobic processes. How can the interaction of the aerobic (oxidative) processes and the anaerobic processes be evaluated? The most common methods for estimating anaerobic effort involve the examination of either the excess post-exercise oxygen consumption or the lactate threshold. Let's consider both.

Post-Exercise Oxygen Consumption

Your body's ability to gauge your muscles' need for oxygen is not perfect. When you begin exercise, your oxygen transport system (respiration and circulation) does not immediately supply the needed quantity of oxygen to the active muscles. Your oxygen consumption requires several minutes to reach the required (steady state) level at which the aerobic processes are fully functional, but your body's oxygen requirements increase markedly the moment exercise begins.

Because oxygen needs and oxygen supply differ during the transition from rest to exercise, your body incurs an oxygen deficit, as shown in Figure 5.12, even with low levels of exercise. The oxygen deficit is calculated simply as the difference between the oxygen required for a given rate of work (steady state), and the oxygen actually consumed. In spite of insufficient oxygen, your muscles still generate the ATP needed through the anaerobic pathways.

During the initial minutes of recovery, even though your muscles are no longer actively working, oxygen demand does not immediately decrease. Instead, oxygen consumption remains elevated temporarily (Figure 5.12). This consumption exceeding that usually required when at rest has traditionally been referred to as the oxygen debt. A more common term today is excess post-exercise oxygen consumption (EPOC). The EPOC is in addition to the oxygen normally consumed at rest. Think of what happens when you finish an exercise bout: A quick run down the block to catch a departing bus or a fast climb up several flights of stairs leaves you with a rapid pulse and feeling out of breath. After several minutes of recovery, your pulse and breathing return to resting rates.

For many years, the EPOC curve was described as having two distinct components: an initial fast com-

ponent and a secondary slow component. By classical theory, the fast component of the curve represented the oxygen required to rebuild the ATP and PCr used during exercise, especially its initial stages. Without sufficient oxygen, the high-energy phosphate bonds in these compounds were broken to supply the required energy. During recovery, these bonds would need to be reformed, via oxidative processes, to replenish the energy stores, or repay the debt. The slow component of the curve was thought to result from removal of accumulated lactate from the tissues, by either conversion to glycogen or oxidization to CO_2 and H_2O, thus providing the energy needed to restore glycogen stores.

With this theory, both the fast and the slow components of the curve were thought to reflect the anaerobic activity that had occurred during exercise. The belief was that by examining the post-exercise oxygen consumption, one could estimate the amount of anaerobic activity that had occurred.

However, more recent studies concluded that the classical explanation of EPOC is too simplistic. For example, during the initial phase of exercise, some oxygen is borrowed from the oxygen stores (hemoglobin and myoglobin). That oxygen must be replenished during recovery. Also, respiration remains elevated temporarily following exercise, partly in an effort to clear CO_2 that has accumulated in the tissues as a by-product of metabolism. Body temperature is also elevated, which keeps the metabolic and respiratory rates high, thus requiring more oxygen, and elevated levels of norepinephrine and epinephrine during exercise have similar effects.

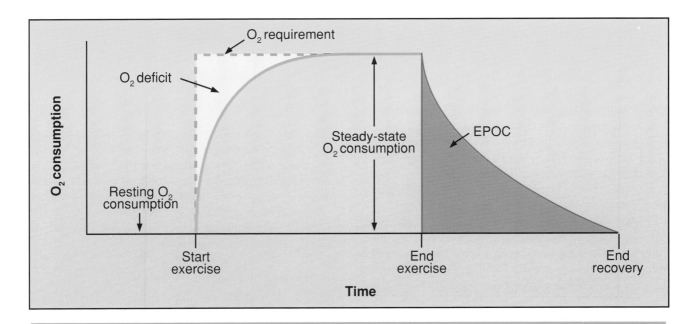

Figure 5.12 Oxygen need during exercise and recovery. Illustration of the oxygen deficit and excess post-exercise oxygen consumption (EPOC).

Thus more is involved than what the classical theory allows. The oxygen debt depends on many factors other than merely rebuilding ATP and PCr and clearing the lactate produced by anaerobic metabolism. The physiological mechanisms responsible for the EPOC need to be clearly defined.

The Lactate Threshold

Many investigators consider the lactate threshold to be a good indicator of an athlete's potential for endurance exercise. The lactate threshold (LT) is defined as the point at which blood lactate begins to accumulate above resting levels during exercise of increasing intensity. During light to moderate activity, blood lactate remains only slightly above the resting level. With more intense effort, lactate accumulates more rapidly. Look at Figure 5.13. At low swimming velocities, blood lactate levels remain at or near resting levels. But as swimming velocity increases above about 1.4 m · s^{-1}, the blood lactate levels increase rapidly. This breakpoint in the curve represents the lactate threshold.

By definition, the lactate threshold has been thought to reflect the interaction of the aerobic and anaerobic energy systems. Some researchers have suggested that the lactate threshold represents a significant shift toward anaerobic glycolysis, which forms lactate. Consequently, the sudden increase in blood lactate with increasing effort has also been referred to as the anaerobic threshold.

However, considerable controversy surrounds the relationship of the lactate threshold to anaerobic metabolism in muscle. Muscles are likely producing lactate well before the lactate threshold is reached, but it is being removed by other tissues. In addition, a clear breakpoint is not always apparent. Because of this, researchers often set an arbitrary value of either 2.0 or 4.0 mmol lactate per liter of oxygen consumed to represent the point at which blood lactate accumulation begins. This allows a standard point of reference, known as the onset of blood lactate accumulation, or OBLA, from which to work.

The lactate threshold is usually expressed in terms of the %$\dot{V}O_2$ max at which it occurs. The ability to exercise at a high intensity without accumulating lactate is beneficial to the athlete because lactate formation contributes to fatigue. Consequently, a lactate threshold at 80% $\dot{V}O_2$ max suggests a greater exercise tolerance than a threshold at 60% $\dot{V}O_2$ max. Generally, in two individuals with the same maximal oxygen uptake, the person with the highest lactate threshold or OBLA exhibits the best endurance performance.

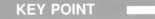

> **KEY POINT**
>
> **Lactate threshold, when expressed as a percentage of $\dot{V}O_2$ max, is one of the best determinants of an athlete's pace in endurance events such as distance running and cycling.**

In untrained people, the lactate threshold typically occurs at around 50% to 60% of their $\dot{V}O_2$ max. Elite endurance athletes may not reach lactate threshold until around 70% or 80% of $\dot{V}O_2$ max.

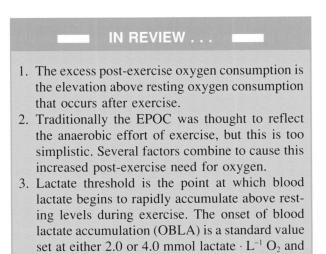

> **IN REVIEW . . .**
>
> 1. The excess post-exercise oxygen consumption is the elevation above resting oxygen consumption that occurs after exercise.
> 2. Traditionally the EPOC was thought to reflect the anaerobic effort of exercise, but this is too simplistic. Several factors combine to cause this increased post-exercise need for oxygen.
> 3. Lactate threshold is the point at which blood lactate begins to rapidly accumulate above resting levels during exercise. The onset of blood lactate accumulation (OBLA) is a standard value set at either 2.0 or 4.0 mmol lactate · L^{-1} O$_2$ and is used as a common reference point.
> 4. Generally, individuals with higher lactate thresholds or OBLA values, expressed as a percent of their $\dot{V}O_2$ max, are capable of the best endurance performance.

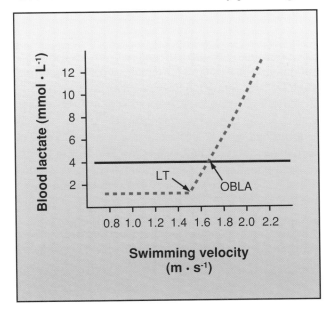

Figure 5.13   The relationship between exercise intensity (swimming velocity) and blood lactate accumulation.

Energy Expenditure at Rest and During Exercise

Now that we have discussed the energy-producing systems in our bodies, we can turn our attention to how this energy is used.

The Metabolic Rate

The rate at which your body uses energy is your metabolic rate. As noted earlier, estimates of energy expenditure during rest and exercise are based on measurement of whole-body oxygen consumption and its caloric equivalent. At rest, an average person consumes about 0.3 L $O_2 \cdot min^{-1}$. This equals 18 L $\cdot$ hr^{-1} or 432 L $\cdot$ day^{-1}.

Now let's calculate this person's daily caloric expenditure. At rest, recall that the body usually burns a mixture of carbohydrate and fat. An RER value of 0.80 when at rest is fairly common for most individuals on a mixed diet. The caloric equivalence of an RER value of 0.80 is 4.80 kcal $\cdot$ L^{-1} O_2 consumed (from Table 5.4). Using these common values, we can calculate this individual's caloric expenditure as follows:

kcal per day
$= $ L O_2 consumed per day $\times$ kcal used per L O_2
$= 432$ L $O_2 \cdot day^{-1} \times 4.80$ kcal $\cdot L^{-1}$ O_2
$= 2,074$ kcal $\cdot day^{-1}$

This value is in close agreement with the average resting energy expenditure expected for a 70-kg (154-lb) man. Of course, it does not include the energy needed for normal daily activity.

One standardized measure of energy expenditure when at rest is the basal metabolic rate (BMR). The BMR is the rate of energy expenditure for an individual at rest in a supine position, measured immediately after at least 8 hr of sleep and at least 12 hr of fasting. This value reflects the minimum amount of energy required to carry on your body's essential physiological functions.

Your basal metabolic rate is directly related to your fat-free mass and is generally reported in kcal per kg of fat-free mass per minute. The more fat-free mass, the more total calories expended in a day. Recall that women tend to have a greater fat mass than men. Because of this, women tend to have lower BMRs than men of similar weight.

Your body's surface area is equally important. The more surface area you have, the more heat loss occurs across your skin, which raises your basal metabolic rate because more energy is needed to maintain your body temperature. For this reason the BMR is also often reported in kcal per m^2 of body surface area per hour. Because we are discussing daily energy expenditure, we've opted for a simpler unit, kcal per day.

Many other factors affect your BMR. Among them are the following:

- Age: BMR gradually decreases with increasing age.
- Body temperature: BMR increases with increasing temperature.
- Stress: Stress increases activity of the sympathetic nervous system, which increases the BMR.
- Hormones: Thyroxine from the thyroid gland and epinephrine from the adrenal medulla both increase the BMR.

Instead of basal metabolic rate, most researchers now use the term resting metabolic rate, because most measurements follow the same conditions required for measuring BMR but don't require the individual to sleep over in the facility. The BMR may vary between $1,200$ and $2,400$ kcal $\cdot day^{-1}$. But the average total metabolic rate of an individual engaged in normal daily activity ranges from 1,800 to 3,000 kcal.

The energy expenditure for very large athletes engaged in intense daily training can exceed 10,000 kcal per day!

Maximal Capacity for Exercise

As your body shifts from rest to exercise, your energy needs increase. Your metabolism increases in direct proportion to the increase in your rate of work. But when faced with increasing energy demands, your body eventually reaches a limit for oxygen consumption. At this point, as illustrated in Figure 5.14, oxygen consumption ($\dot{V}O_2$) peaks and remains constant or drops slightly, even though your work intensity continues to increase. This peak value is referred to as your aerobic capacity, maximal oxygen uptake, or $\dot{V}O_{2\,max}$. $\dot{V}O_{2\,max}$ is regarded by some as the best single measurement of cardiorespiratory endurance and aerobic fitness.

Although some sport scientists have suggested $\dot{V}O_{2\,max}$ as a good predictor of success in endurance events, the winner of a marathon race cannot be predicted from the runner's laboratory-measured $\dot{V}O_{2\,max}$.[4] Likewise, an endurance-running performance test is only a modest predictor of one's $\dot{V}O_{2\,max}$. This suggests that a good performance entails more than a high $\dot{V}O_{2\,max}$.[1]

Also, research has documented that $\dot{V}O_{2\,max}$ increases with physical training only for 8 to 12 weeks, then this value plateaus, despite continued, higher intensity training. Although $\dot{V}O_{2\,max}$ doesn't continue

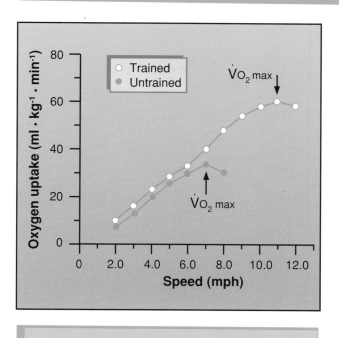

Figure 5.14   The relationship between exercise intensity (speed) and oxygen uptake, illustrating $\dot{V}O_2$ max in trained and untrained men.

to increase, the participants continue to improve their endurance performance. People may develop a greater ability to perform at a higher percentage of their $\dot{V}O_2$ max. Most runners, for example, can complete a 42-km (26.2-mi) race at an average pace that requires them to use approximately 75% to 80% of their $\dot{V}O_2$ max.[1]

Consider the case of Alberto Salazar, the former world record holder in the marathon. His measured $\dot{V}O_2$ max was 70 ml · kg⁻¹ · min⁻¹. That is below the $\dot{V}O_2$ max expected based on his record performance of 2 hr 8 min. He was, however, able to run at 86% of his $\dot{V}O_2$ max when performing at his racing pace, a percentage considerably higher than that of other runners. This may partly explain his world-class running ability.

The major determinants of successful endurance performance discussed thus far are both $\dot{V}O_2$ max and the percentage of $\dot{V}O_2$ max that an athlete can maintain for a prolonged period. The latter is probably related to the lactate threshold, because the lactate threshold is likely the major determinant of the pace that can be tolerated during a long-term endurance event. So the ability to perform at a higher percentage of $\dot{V}O_2$ max likely reflects a higher lactate threshold.

Because individual needs for energy vary with body size, $\dot{V}O_2$ max is generally expressed relative to body weight, in milliliters of oxygen consumed per kilogram of body weight per minute (ml · kg⁻¹ · min⁻¹). This allows a more accurate comparison of different-

sized individuals who exercise in weight-bearing events, such as running. In non-weight-bearing activities, such as swimming and cycling, endurance performance is more closely related to $\dot{V}O_2$ max measured in liters per minute.

Normally active 18- to 22-year-old college students have average $\dot{V}O_2$ max values of 38 to 42 ml · kg⁻¹ · min⁻¹ for women and 44 to 50 ml · kg⁻¹ · min⁻¹ for men. After the age of 25 to 30 years, inactive people's $\dot{V}O_2$ max values decrease about 1% per year. This is probably due to a combination of biological aging and sedentary lifestyle. In addition, adult females generally have $\dot{V}O_2$ max values considerably below those of their male counterparts. Two reasons for these gender differences are body composition differences (women generally have less fat-free mass) and blood hemoglobin content (women have less, thus they have less oxygen-carrying capacity). But it's unclear how much of the gender difference in $\dot{V}O_2$ max is due to actual physiological differences and how much might be due to a culture that may impose a sedentary lifestyle on women after sexual maturity. This will be discussed further in chapter 19.

Aerobic capacities of 80 to 84 ml · kg⁻¹ · min⁻¹ have been observed among elite male long-distance runners and cross-country skiers. The highest $\dot{V}O_2$ max value recorded for a male is from a champion Norwegian cross-country skier who had a $\dot{V}O_2$ max of 94 ml · kg⁻¹ · min⁻¹. The highest value recorded for a female is 74 ml · kg⁻¹ · min⁻¹ in a Russian cross-country skier. In contrast, poorly conditioned adults may have values below 20 ml · kg⁻¹ · min⁻¹.

Economy of Effort

As you become more skillful at performing an exercise, your energy demands during that exercise are reduced. You become more efficient. This is illustrated in Figure 5.15 by the data from two distance runners. At all running speeds faster than 200 m · min⁻¹ (7.5 mph), runner A used significantly less oxygen than runner B. These men had similar $\dot{V}O_2$ max values (64 to 65 ml · kg⁻¹ · min⁻¹), so runner A's lower energy use would be a decided advantage during competition.

These two runners competed on numerous occasions. During marathon races, they ran at paces requiring them to use 85% of their $\dot{V}O_2$ max. On the average, runner A's running efficiency gave him a 13-min advantage in these competitions. Because their $\dot{V}O_2$ max values are so similar but their energy needs so different during these events, much of runner A's competitive advantage can be attributed to his greater running efficiency. Unfortunately, we have no explanation for the underlying causes of these efficiency differences.

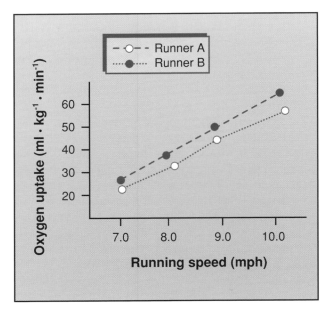

Figure 5.15 The oxygen requirements for two distance runners while they ran at various speeds. Although they had similar $\dot{V}O_2$ max values (64 to 65 ml · kg⁻¹ · min⁻¹), Runner A was more efficient and therefore faster.

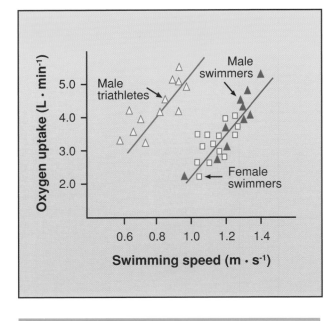

Figure 5.16 The oxygen requirements in trained swimmers and in highly trained triathletes.

Various studies with sprint, middle-distance, and marathon runners have shown that marathon runners are generally the most efficient. In general, these ultra-long-distance runners use 5% to 10% less energy than middle-distance and sprint runners. However, this economy of effort has been studied at only relatively slow speeds (10 to 19 kph [6 to 12 mph] paces). We can reasonably assume that distance runners are less efficient at sprinting than runners who train specifically for short, faster races.

Variations in running form and the specificity of training for sprint and distance running may account for these differences in running economy. Film analyses reveal that middle-distance and sprint runners have significantly more vertical movement when running at 11 to 19 kph (7 to 12 mph) than marathoners do. But such speeds are well below those required during middle-distance races and probably don't accurately reflect the running efficiency of competitors in shorter events of 1,500 m or less.

Performance in other athletic events might be even more affected by efficiency of movement than in running. Part of the energy expended during swimming, for example, is used to support the body on the surface of the water and to generate enough force to overcome the water's resistance to motion. Although the energy needed for swimming depends on body size

and buoyancy, the efficient application of force against the water is the major determinant of swimming economy.

Figure 5.16 illustrates the oxygen requirements of trained competitive male and female swimmers, and a group of highly trained male triathletes. Oxygen uptake is plotted at various swimming speeds. Although the triathletes trained daily for swimming, none had a background in competitive swimming. Interestingly, though many triathletes had markedly higher aerobic capacities than the competitive swimmers, few could perform as well as even the poorest competitive swimmer. Several female competitive swimmers with $\dot{V}O_2$ max values of 2.1 to 2.3 L · min⁻¹ swam 400 m as fast as male triathletes with values above 5.0 L · min⁻¹. The competitive swimmers were notably more efficient than the triathletes.

Performance in many activities may be limited more by athletes' skill than by their energy production capacity. Training time and effort spent on the mechanical aspects (skill) of the sport may be as important as the time dedicated to improving strength and endurance. But, for endurance activities, success appears to be dictated by at least the following factors:

• High $\dot{V}O_2$ max value
• High lactate threshold or OBLA
• High economy of effort, or low $\dot{V}O_2$ value for the same rate of work
• High percentage of ST muscle fibers

Table 5.5 Energy Expenditure During Various Physical Activities

Activity	Male (kcal · min^{-1})	Female (kcal · min^{-1})	Relative to body mass (kcal · kg^{-1} · min^{-1})
Basketball	8.6	6.8	0.123
Cycling			
7.0 mph	5.0	3.9	0.071
10.0 mph	7.5	5.9	0.107
Handball	11.0	8.6	0.157
Running			
7.5 mph	14.0	11.0	0.200
10.0 mph	18.2	14.3	0.260
Sitting	1.7	1.3	0.024
Sleeping	1.2	0.9	0.017
Standing	1.8	1.4	0.026
Swimming (crawl), 3.0 mph	20.0	15.7	0.285
Tennis	7.1	5.5	0.101
Walking, 3.5 mph	5.0	3.9	0.071
Weight lifting	8.2	6.4	0.117
Wrestling	13.1	10.3	0.187

Note. Values presented are for a 154-lb (70-kg) man and a 121-lb (55-kg) woman. These values will vary depending on individual differences.

━━━ KEY POINT ━━━

Success in endurance activities depends largely on the following:

- **High $\dot{V}_{O_2 \text{ max}}$ value**
- **High lactate threshold or OBLA**
- **High economy of effort, or low $\dot{V}_{O_2}$ value for the same rate of work**
- **High percentage of ST muscle fibers**

Energy Cost of Various Activities

The amount of energy expended for different activities varies with the intensity and type of exercise. The energy cost of many activities has been determined, usually by monitoring the oxygen consumption during the activity to determine an average oxygen uptake per unit of time. Kilocalories of energy used per minute (kcal · min^{-1}) can then be calculated from this value.

These values typically ignore the anaerobic aspects of exercise and the excess post-exercise oxygen consumption. This is important because an activity that costs a total of 300 kcal during the actual exercise period may cost an additional 100 kcal during the recovery period. Thus, the total cost of that activity would be 400, not 300, kcal.

An average body requires 0.20 to 0.35 L of oxygen per minute to satisfy its resting energy requirements. This would amount to 1.0 to 1.8 kcal · min^{-1}, 60 to 108 kcal · hr^{-1}, or 1,440 to 2,592 kcal · day^{-1}. Obviously, any activity above resting levels will add to the projected daily expenditure. The range for total daily caloric expenditure is highly variable. It depends on many factors, including

- activity level,
- age,
- gender,
- size,
- weight, and
- body composition.

The energy costs of sport activities also differ. Some, such as archery or bowling, require only slightly more energy than when at rest. Others, such as sprinting, require so much energy that they can be maintained for only seconds. In addition to exercise intensity, the duration of the activity must be considered. For example, approximately 29 kcal · min^{-1} are expended while running at 25 kph (15.5 mph), but this pace can be endured only for brief periods. Jogging at an 11 kph (7 mph) pace, on the other hand, expends only 14.5 kcal · min^{-1}, half that of running at 25 kph (15.5 mph). But jogging can be maintained for considerably longer, resulting in a greater total energy expenditure.

Table 5.5 provides an estimate of energy expenditure for various activities for average mature men and women. These values are mere averages. Most activities involve moving the body mass, so these figures may vary considerably with individual differences such as those previously listed and with individual skill (efficiency of movement).

Causes of Fatigue

What exactly is the meaning of the term fatigue during exercise? Sensations of fatigue are markedly different when exercising to exhaustion in events lasting 45 to 60 s, such as the 400-m run, than those experienced during prolonged exhaustive muscular effort (such as marathon running). We typically use the term fatigue to describe general sensations of tiredness and accompanying decrements in muscular performance.

Most efforts to describe underlying causes and sites of fatigue focus on

- the energy systems (ATP-PCr, glycolysis, and oxidation),
- the accumulation of metabolic by-products,
- the nervous system, and
- the failure of the fiber's contractile mechanism.

None of these alone can explain all aspects of fatigue. For example, although the lack of available energy can reduce the muscles' capacity to generate force, the energy systems are not wholly responsible for all forms of fatigue. The sensations of tiredness we often experience at the end of a workday have little to do with

ATP availability. Fatigue may also result from environmental stress altering homeostasis. Many questions about fatigue remain unanswered.

The Energy Systems and Fatigue

The energy systems are an obvious area to explore when considering possible causes of fatigue. When we feel fatigued, we often express it by saying "I have no energy." But this use of the term energy is far removed from its physiological meaning. What role does energy, in this narrower sense, play in fatigue during exercise?

Phosphocreatine Depletion

Recall that phosphocreatine (PCr) is used under anaerobic conditions to rebuild the high-energy ATP as it is used, and thus maintain your body's ATP stores. Biopsy studies of human thigh muscles have shown that, during repeated maximal contractions, fatigue coincides with PCr depletion. Although ATP is directly responsible for the energy used during such activities, it is depleted less rapidly than PCr during muscular effort because ATP is being produced by other systems. But as PCr is depleted, your body's ability to quickly replace the spent ATP is seriously hindered. ATP use continues, but the ATP-PCr system is less able to replace it. Thus ATP levels also drop. At exhaustion, both ATP and PCr may be depleted.

To delay fatigue, the athlete must control the rate of effort through proper pacing to insure that PCr and ATP are not prematurely exhausted. If the beginning pace is too rapid, the ATP and PCr available will quickly decrease, leading to early fatigue and inability to maintain the pace in the event's final stages. Training and experience allow the athlete to judge the optimal pace that permits the most efficient use of ATP and PCr for the entire event.

Glycogen Depletion

Muscle ATP levels are also maintained by the aerobic and anaerobic breakdown of muscle glycogen. In events lasting longer than a few seconds, muscle glycogen becomes the primary energy source for ATP synthesis. Unfortunately, glycogen reserves are limited and are depleted quickly.

As with PCr use, the rate of muscle glycogen depletion is controlled by the intensity of the activity. Increasing the rate of work results in a disproportionate decrease in muscle glycogen. During sprint running, for example, muscle glycogen may be used 35 to 40 times faster than during walking. Muscle glycogen can be a limiting factor even during mild effort. The muscle depends on a constant supply of glycogen to meet the high energy demands of exercise.

Muscle glycogen is used more rapidly during the first few minutes of exercise than in the later stages, as seen in Figure 5.17. The illustration shows the change in muscle glycogen content in the subject's gastrocnemius (calf) muscle during the test. Although the test was run at a steady pace, the rate of muscle glycogen metabolized from the gastrocnemius was greatest during the first 90 min.

The subject reported his perceived exertion (how difficult his effort seemed to be) at various times during the test. He felt only moderately stressed early in the run, when his glycogen stores were still high, even though he was using glycogen at a high rate. He didn't perceive severe fatigue until his muscle glycogen levels were nearly depleted. Thus, sensation of fatigue in long-term exercise coincides with the decrease of muscle glycogen. Marathon runners commonly refer to the sudden onset of fatigue that they experience at

29 to 35 km (18 to 22 mi) as "hitting the wall." At least part of this sensation can be attributed to muscle glycogen depletion.

Glycogen Depletion in Different Fiber Types.
Muscle fibers are recruited and deplete their energy reserves in selected patterns. The individual fibers most frequently recruited during exercise may become depleted of glycogen. This would reduce the number of fibers capable of producing the muscular force needed for exercise.

This is illustrated in Figure 5.18, which shows a micrograph of muscle fibers taken from a runner before and after a 30-km run. Figure 5.18a has been stained to differentiate slow-twitch (ST) and fast-twitch (FT) fibers. One of the FT fibers is circled. Figure 5.18b shows a second sample from the same muscle, stained to show glycogen. The more red (darker) the stain, the more glycogen is present. Before the run, all fibers are full of glycogen and appear red (not depicted). In Figure 5.18b (after the run) the circled FT fiber still has plenty of glycogen. But the ST fibers on either side of it are almost completely depleted of glycogen. This suggests that ST fibers are used more heavily during endurance exercise that requires only moderate force development, such as the 30-km run.

The pattern of glycogen depletion from ST and FT fibers depends on the exercise intensity. Recall that ST fibers are the first fibers to be recruited during light exercise. As muscle tension requirements increase, FT_a fibers are added to the workforce. In exercise approaching maximum intensities, the FT_b fibers are added to the pool of recruited fibers. Glycogen depletion should follow a similar pattern.

Figure 5.19 illustrates the amount of the total glycogen being used by the ST, FT_a, and FT_b fibers in the vastus lateralis muscle during cycling at various percentages of a typical subject's $\dot{V}O_2$ max. During relatively low-intensity exercise (40% to 60% $\dot{V}O_2$ max), ST fibers are the most active, and FT_a and FT_b fibers are relatively inactive. At higher intensities of effort (75% to 90% $\dot{V}O_2$ max), FT fibers are recruited more frequently and are depleted of their glycogen at a greater rate than the ST fibers.

This does not mean that ST fibers are used less than FT fibers during maximal contractions. It simply reflects the FT fibers' greater reliance on glycogen. All fiber types are recruited during highly intense muscular actions.

When glycogen stores in the ST fibers are depleted, it appears that FT fibers either are unable to generate enough tension or cannot be sufficiently recruited to compensate for the loss in muscle tension. For that reason, it has been theorized that the sensations of muscle fatigue and heaviness during long-term exercise may reflect some muscle fibers' inability to respond to exercise demands.

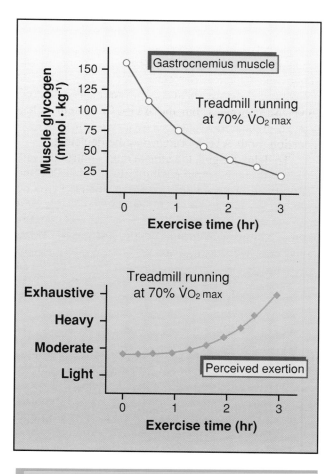

Figure 5.17 Glycogen use and relative perception of effort during 3 hr of treadmill running at 70% of $\dot{V}O_2$ max. Adapted from Costill (1986).

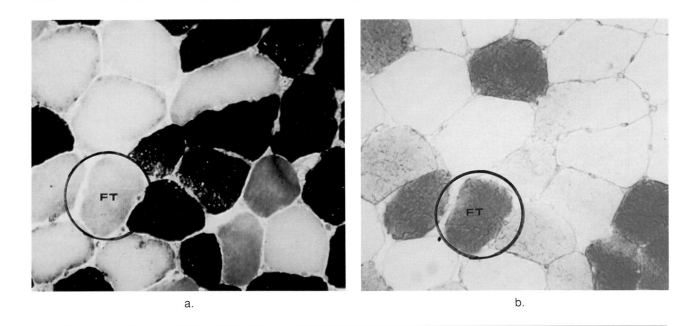

a.   b.

Figure 5.18   Histochemical staining for muscle glycogen (a) before and (b) after a 30-km run.

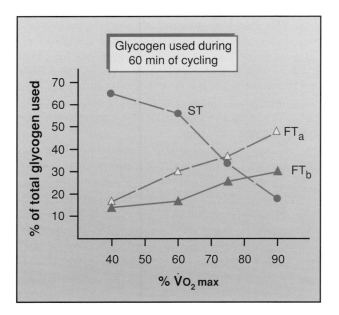

Figure 5.19   Glycogen use in ST, FT_a and FT_b fibers during cycling at 40%, 60%, 75%, and 90% $\dot{V}O_2$ max. Data from Wilmore and Costill (1988).

Glycogen Depletion in Different Muscle Groups.   In addition to selectively depleting glycogen from ST or FT fibers, exercise may place unusually heavy demands on select muscle groups. In one study, subjects ran on a treadmill positioned for uphill, downhill, and level run-ning for 2 hr at 70% $\dot{V}O_2$ max. Figure 5.20 compares the resultant glycogen depletion in three muscles of the lower extremity:

- Vastus lateralis (knee extensor)
- Gastrocnemius (ankle extensor)
- Soleus (also an ankle extensor)

The results show that whether you run uphill, downhill, or level, the gastrocnemius uses more glyco-gen than the vastus lateralis or the soleus. This suggests that the ankle extensor muscles, which are worked more during distance running, are more likely to be-come depleted during distance running than are the thigh muscles, isolating the site of fatigue to the lower leg muscles.

Glycogen Depletion and Blood Glucose

Muscle glycogen alone can't provide enough carbohy-drate for exercise lasting several hours. Glucose deliv-ered by the blood to the muscles contributes a lot of energy during endurance exercise. The liver breaks down its stored glycogen to provide a constant supply of blood glucose. In the early stages of exercise, energy production requires relatively little blood glucose, but in the later stages of an endurance event, blood glucose may make a large contribution. To keep pace with the muscles' glucose uptake, the liver must break down increasingly more glycogen as exercise duration in-creases.

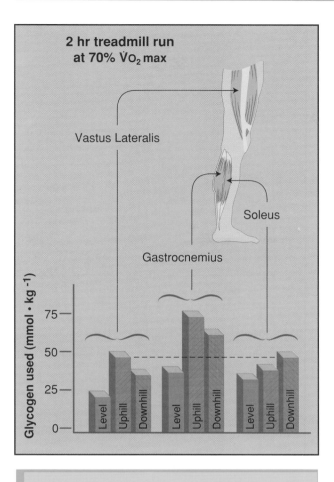

Figure 5.20   Muscle glycogen use from the gastrocnemius, soleus, and vastus lateralis muscles during uphill, level, and downhill running.

The liver's glycogen stores are limited, and it can't produce glucose rapidly from other substrates. Consequently, blood glucose levels can drop when muscle uptake exceeds the liver's glucose output. Unable to obtain sufficient glucose from the blood, the muscles must rely more heavily on their glycogen reserves, accelerating muscle glycogen depletion and leading to earlier exhaustion.

Effects on Performance

Not surprisingly, endurance performances improve when the muscle glycogen supply is elevated at the start of activity. The importance of muscle glycogen storage for endurance performance will be discussed in chapter 15. For now, note that glycogen depletion and hypoglycemia (low blood sugar) limit performance in activities lasting 30 min or longer. Fatigue in shorter events more likely results from accumulation of metabolic by-products, such as lactate and H⁺, within the muscles.

Metabolic By-Products and Fatigue

Recall that lactic acid is a by-product of glycolysis. Although most people believe that it is responsible for fatigue and exhaustion in all types of exercise, lactic acid only accumulates within the muscle fiber during relatively brief, highly intense muscular effort. Marathon runners, for example, may have near-resting lactic acid levels at the end of the race, despite their exhaustion. As noted in the previous section, their fatigue is caused by inadequate energy supply, not excess lactic acid.

Sprints in running, cycling, and swimming all lead to large accumulations of lactic acid. But the presence per se of lactic acid should not be blamed for the feeling of fatigue. When not cleared, the lactic acid dissociates, converting to lactate and causing an accumulation of hydrogen ions. This H^+ accumulation causes muscle acidification, resulting in a condition known as acidosis.

Activities of short duration and high intensity, such as sprint running and sprint swimming, depend heavily on glycolysis and produce large amounts of lactate and H^+ within the muscles. Fortunately, the cells and body fluids possess buffers, such as bicarbonate (HCO_3), that minimize the disrupting influence of the H^+. Without these buffers H^+ would lower the pH to about 1.5, killing the cells. Because of the body's buffering capacity, the H^+ concentration remains low even during the most severe exercise, allowing muscle pH to fall from a resting value of 7.1 to no lower than 6.6 to 6.4 at exhaustion.

However, pH changes of this magnitude adversely affect energy production and muscle contraction. An intracellular pH below 6.9 inhibits the action of phosphofructokinase (PFK), an important glycolytic enzyme, slowing the rate of glycolysis and ATP production. At a pH of 6.4, the influence of H^+ stops any further glycogen breakdown, causing a rapid decrease in ATP and ultimately exhaustion. In addition, H^+ may displace calcium within the fiber, interfering with the coupling of the actin-myosin cross-bridges and decreasing the muscle's contractile force. Most researchers agree that low muscle pH is the major limiter of performance and the primary cause of fatigue during maximal short-term exercise.

As seen in Figure 5.21, reestablishing the pre-exercise muscle pH after an exhaustive sprint bout requires about 30 to 35 min of recovery. Even when normal pH is restored, blood and muscle lactate levels can remain quite elevated. However, experience has shown that an athlete can continue to exercise at relatively high intensities even with a muscle pH below 7.0 and a blood lactate level above 6 or 7 mmol · L⁻¹, four to five times the resting value.

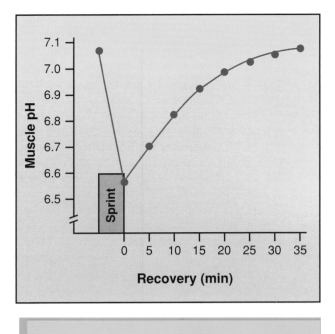

Figure 5.21 Changes in muscle pH during sprint exercise and recovery.

Currently, some coaches and sport physiologists are attempting to use blood lactate measurements to gauge the intensity and volume of training needed to produce an optimal training stimulus. Such measurements provide an index of training intensity, but they might not be related to the anaerobic processes or the state of acidosis in the muscles. As lactate and H$^+$ are generated in the muscles, both diffuse out of the cells. They are then diluted in the body fluids and transported to other areas of the body to be metabolized. Consequently, blood lactate values are dependent on the rates of production, diffusion, and oxidation. A variety of factors can influence these processes, so lactate values are of questionable use when prescribing training.

Neuromuscular Fatigue

Thus far we have considered only factors within the muscle that might be responsible for fatigue. Evidence also suggests that under some circumstances fatigue may result from an inability to activate the muscle fibers, a function of the nervous system. As noted in chapter 3, the nerve impulse is transmitted across the motor end plate to activate the fiber's membrane and causes the fiber's sarcoplasmic reticulum to release calcium. The calcium, in turn, binds with troponin to initiate muscle contraction. Let's examine two possible neural mechanisms that could disrupt this process and possibly contribute to fatigue.

Neural Transmission

Fatigue may occur at the motor end plate, preventing nerve impulse transmission to the muscle fiber membrane. Studies early in this century clearly established such a failure of nerve impulse transmission in fatigued muscle. This failure may involve one or more of the following processes:

- The release or synthesis of acetylcholine (ACh), the neurotransmitter that relays the nerve impulse from the motor nerve to the muscle membrane, might be reduced.
- Cholinesterase, the enzyme that breaks down ACh once it has relayed the impulse, might become hyperactive, preventing sufficient concentration of ACh to initiate an action potential.
- Cholinesterase activity might become hypoactive (inhibitive), allowing ACh to accumulate excessively, paralyzing the fiber.
- The muscle fiber membrane might develop a higher threshold.
- Some substance might compete with ACh for the receptors on the muscle membrane without activating the membrane.
- Potassium might leave the intracellular space of the contracting muscle, decreasing the membrane potential to half of its resting value.

Although most of these causes for a neuromuscular block have been associated with neuromuscular diseases (such as myasthenia gravis), they may also cause some forms of neuromuscular fatigue. Some evidence also suggests that fatigue may be due to calcium retention within the T tubules, which would decrease the calcium available for muscle contraction. In fact, depletion of PCr and lactate buildup might simply increase the rate of calcium accumulation within the T tubules. However, these theories of fatigue remain speculative.

The Central Nervous System

The central nervous system (CNS) might also be a site of fatigue, although there is evidence both for and against this theory. Early studies showed that when a subject's muscles appeared to be nearly exhausted, verbal encouragement, shouting, or even direct electrical stimulation of the muscle could increase the strength of muscle contraction. These studies suggest that the limits of performance in exhaustive exercise may, to a great extent, be psychological. The precise mechanisms underlying such CNS fatigue are not fully understood. Whether this form of fatigue is isolated to the CNS or linked to peripheral nerve transmission is also difficult to determine.

The recruitment of muscle depends, in part, on conscious control. The psychological trauma of exhaustive exercise may consciously or subconsciously inhibit the athlete's willingness to tolerate further pain. The CNS may slow the exercise pace to a tolerable level to protect the athlete. Indeed, researchers generally agree that the perceived discomfort of fatigue precedes the onset of a physiological limitation within the muscles. Unless they are highly motivated, most individuals terminate exercise before their muscles are physiologically exhausted. To achieve peak performance, athletes train to learn proper pacing and tolerance for fatigue.

IN REVIEW . . .

1. Fatigue may result from depletion of PCr or glycogen. Either of these situations impairs ATP production.
2. Lactic acid has often been blamed for fatigue, but it is actually the H^+ generated by lactic acid that leads to fatigue. The accumulation of H^+ decreases muscle pH, which impairs the cellular processes that produce energy and muscle contraction.
3. Failure of neural transmission may be a cause of some fatigue. Many mechanisms can lead to such failure, and all need further research.
4. The CNS may also cause fatigue, perhaps as a protective mechanism. Perceived fatigue usually precedes physiological fatigue, and athletes who feel exhausted can often be psychologically encouraged to continue.

In Closing . . .

In previous chapters, we discussed how muscles and the nervous system function together to produce movement. Now in this chapter we have focused on metabolism. We considered the energy needed for movement. We saw how energy is stored in the form of ATP, examined the three systems that generate energy, and explored how its production and availability can limit your performance. We also learned that your metabolic needs vary considerably. In the next chapter, we turn

our attention to the regulation of metabolism as we focus on the endocrine system and hormonal regulation.

Key Terms

acetyl coenzyme A
    (acetyl CoA)
adenosine diphosphate
    (ADP)
adenosine triphosphate
    (ATP)
adenosine triphosphatase
    (ATPase)
aerobic metabolism
ATP-PCr system
basal metabolic rate
    (BMR)
beta oxidation
    (β oxidation)
direct calorimetry
electron transport chain
excess post-exercise
    oxygen consumption
    (EPOC)

fatigue
glycolysis
glycolytic system
indirect calorimetry
Krebs cycle
lactate threshold (LT)
maximal oxygen uptake
    ($\dot{V}O_{2\ max}$)
onset of blood lactate
    accumulation (OBLA)
oxidative capacity ($\dot{Q}O_2$)
oxidative system
phosphocreatine (PCr)
respiratory exchange
    ratio (RER)

Study Questions

1. What is the role of PCr?
2. Describe the relationship between muscle ATP and PCr during sprint exercise.
3. Why are the ATP-PCr and glycolytic energy systems considered anaerobic?
4. What role does oxygen play in the process of aerobic metabolism?
5. Describe the by-products of energy production from ATP-PCr, glycolysis, and oxidation.
6. What is the respiratory exchange ratio (RER)? Explain how it is used to determine the oxidation of carbohydrate and fat.
7. What is the relationship between oxygen consumption and energy production?
8. What is the lactate threshold?
9. How can we use measurements of oxygen consumption to estimate one's exercise efficiency?
10. Why do athletes with high $\dot{V}O_{2\ max}$ values perform better in endurance events than those with lower values?
11. Why is oxygen consumption often expressed as milliliters of oxygen per kilogram of body weight per minute ($ml \cdot kg^{-1} \cdot min^{-1}$)?
12. Describe the possible causes of fatigue during exercise bouts lasting 15 to 30 s and 2 to 4 hr.

References

1. Costill, D.L. (1970). Metabolic responses during distance running. *Journal of Applied Physiology*, **28**, 251-255.

2. Costill, D.L., Daniels, J., Evans, W., Fink, W., Krahenbuhl, G., & Saltin, B. (1976). Skeletal muscle enzymes and fiber composition in male and female track athletes. *Journal of Applied Physiology*, **40**, 149-154.

3. Costill, D.L., Fink, W.J., Flynn, M., & Kirwan, J. (1987). Muscle fiber composition and enzyme activities in elite female distance runners. *International Journal of Sports Medicine*, **8**, 103-106.

4. Costill, D.L., & Fox, E.L. (1969). Energetics of marathon running. *Medicine and Science in Sports*, **1**(2), 81-86.

5. Gollnick, P.D., Armstrong, R., Saubert, C., Piehl, K., & Saltin, B. (1972). Enzyme activity and fiber composition in skeletal muscle of untrained and trained men. *Journal of Applied Physiology*, **33**, 312-319.

6. Ivy, J.L., Withers, R.T., Van Handel, P.J., Elger, D.H., & Costill, D.L. (1980). Muscle respiratory capacity and fiber type as determinants of the lactate threshold. *Journal of Applied Physiology*, **48**, 523-527.

Selected Readings

Armstrong, R.B. (1979). Biochemistry: Energy liberation and use. In R.H. Strauss (Ed.), *Sports medicine and physiology*. Philadelphia, PA: W.B. Saunders.

Bergstrom, J. (1967). Local changes of ATP and phosphocreatine in human muscle tissue in connection with exercise. In *Physiology of muscular exercise* (Monograph No. 15), pp. 191-196. New York: American Heart Association.

Blom, P., Vollestad, N.K., & Costill, D.L. Factors affecting changes in muscle glycogen concentration during and after prolonged exercise. *Acta Physiologica Scandinavica*, **128**:(Suppl. 556).

Brooks, G.A. (1987). Amino acid and protein metabolism during exercise and recovery. *Medicine and Science in Sports and Exercise*, **19**(5), S150-S156.

Brooks, G.A., Brauner, K.E. & Cassens, R.G. (1973). Glycogen synthesis and metabolism of lactic acid after exercise. *American Journal of Physiology*, **224**, 1162-1166.

Coggan, A.R., & Coyle, E.F. (1991) Carbohydrate ingestion during prolonged exercise: Effects on metabolism and performance, *Exercise and Sports Sciences Reviews*, **19**, 1-40.

Costill, D.L., Coyle, E., Dalsky, G., Evans, W., Fink, W., & Hoopes, D. (1977). Effects of elevated plasma FFA and insulin on muscle glycogen usage during exercise. *Journal of Applied Physiology*, **43**, 695-699.

Costill, D.L., Gollnick, P.D., Jansson, E.D., Saltin, B., & Stein, E.M. (1973). Glycogen depletion pattern in human muscle fibers during distance running. *Acta Physiologica Scandinavica*, **89**, 374-383.

Costill, D.L., Jansson, E., Gollnick, P.D. & Saltin, B. (1974). Glycogen utilization in leg muscles of men during level and uphill running. *Acta Physiologica Scandinavica*, **91**, 475-481.

Farrell, P.A., Wilmore, J.H., Coyle, E.F., Billing, J.E., & Costill, D.L. (1979). Plasma lactate accumulation and distance running performance. *Medicine and Science in Sports*, **11**, 338-344.

Henriksson, J., & Reitman, J. (1976). Quantitative measures of enzyme activities in type I and type II muscle fibers of man after training. *Acta Physiologica Scandinavica*, **97**, 392-397.

Ingjer, F. (1991). Maximal oxygen uptake as a predictor of performance ability in women and men elite cross-country skiers. *Scandinavian Journal of Medicine & Science in Sports*, **1**, 25-30.

Ivy, J.L., Costill, D.L., & Maxwell, B.D. (1980). Skeletal muscle determinants of maximum aerobic power in man. *European Journal of Applied Physiology*, **44**(1), 1-8.

Katz, A. & Sahlin, K. (1990). Role of oxygen in regulation of glycolysis and lactate production in human skeletal muscle. *Exercise and Sport Science Reviews*, **18**, 1-28.

Medbø, J.I., Mohn, A.-C., Tabata, I., Bahr, R., Vaage, O., & Sejersted, O.M. (1988). Anaerobic capacity determined by maximal accumulated O_2 deficit. *Journal of Applied Physiology*, **64**(1), 50-60.

Needham, D.M. (1971). *The biochemistry of muscular contraction in its historical development*. Cambridge, MA: University Press.

Pernow, B., & Saltin, B. (1986). *Muscle metabolism during exercise* (pp. 67-74). New York: Plenum Press 1971.

Scott, C.B., Roby, F.B., Lohman, T.B., & Bunt, J.C. (1991). The maximally accumulated oxygen deficit as an indicator of anaerobic capacity. *Medicine and Science in Sports and Exercise*, **23**(5), 618-624.

Simonson, E. (1971). *Physiology of work capacity and fatigue*. C.C Thomas: Springfield, IL.

Sjøgaard, G. (1991). Role of exercise-induced potassium fluxes underlying muscle fatigue: A brief review. *Canadian Journal of Physiology and Pharmacology*, **69**, 238-245.

Vandewalle, G.P., & Monod, H. (1987). Standard anaerobic exercise tests. *Sports Medicine*, **4**, 268-289.

Vollestäd, N.K., & Blom, P.C.S. (1988). Effect of varying exercise intensity on glycogen depletion in human muscle fibers. *Acta Physiologica Scandinavica*, **125**, 395-405.

Zuntz, N. & Hagemann, O. (1898). *Untersuchungen über den Stroffwechsel des Pferdes bei Ruhe und Arbeit* (p. 438). Parey: Berlin.

Chapter 6

Hormonal Regulation of Exercise

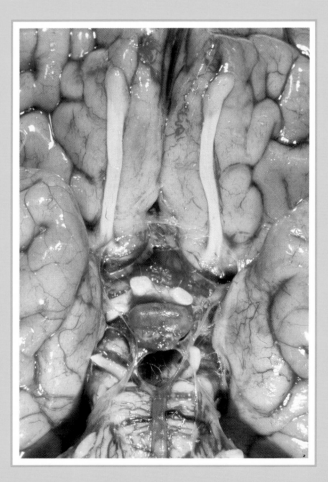

Chapter Overview

During exercise, your body is faced with tremendous demands, which lead to many physiological changes. The rate of energy use increases. Metabolic by-products that must be cleared often begin to accumulate. Water shifts between the fluid compartments and is lost through sweating. Even at rest, your body's internal environment is in a constant state of flux. But during exercise, it can become quite chaotic.

Yet we know that homeostasis must be maintained for you to survive. The more rigorous the exercise, the more difficult this maintenance becomes. Much of the regulation required during exercise is accomplished by the nervous system. But another system is in contact with virtually every cell in your body. It constantly monitors your body's internal milieu, noting all changes that occur and responding quickly to ensure that homeostasis is not drastically disrupted. It is your endocrine system, which exerts its control through the hormones it releases. In this chapter, we will focus on the importance of your endocrine system, both in allowing physical activity and in ensuring that homeostasis is reasonably maintained even amidst all the internal chaos.

In 1972, I [DLC] convinced my coauthor [JHW] to run 16 km (10 mi) per day for 5 successive days. To add to the physical stress, these runs were performed in the bright summer sun and heat (approximately 30 to 35 °C, or 86 to 95 °F) of Davis, California. We each lost 3 to 4 kg (6.6 to 8.8 lb) of sweat daily, leaving us somewhat dehydrated and overheated. Nevertheless, blood samples taken each day during this period revealed that our hemoglobin levels and hematocrits (percentage of blood composed of red blood cells) were declining. Isotope studies of our blood revealed that we were not losing hemoglobin or blood cells. Rather, our plasma, the fluid part of our blood, was increasing day by day. Thus it appeared that our bodies were trying to offset the detrimental effects of daily dehydration by retaining water to minimize the loss of plasma volume that accompanied such heavy sweating. But how did our bodies know that we needed to expand our plasma? What was responsible for the water retention? We now know that at least three hormones—aldosterone, renin, and antidiuretic hormone—all function to maintain appropriate plasma volume and minimize the risk of dehydration.

Muscular activity requires coordinated integration of many physiological and biochemical systems. Such integration is possible only if your body's various tissues and systems can communicate with each other. Although your nervous system is responsible for much of this communication, fine-tuning your body's physiological responses to any disturbance of its equilibrium is primarily the responsibility of your endocrine system. The endocrine and nervous systems work in concert to initiate and control movement and all physiological processes it involves. The nervous system functions quickly, having short-lived localized effects, whereas the endocrine system functions much more slowly, having longer lasting and more general effects.

The endocrine system includes all tissues or glands that secrete hormones. The major endocrine glands are illustrated in Figure 6.1. Endocrine glands secrete their hormones directly into the blood. Hormones act as chemical signals throughout the body. When secreted by the specialized endocrine cells, they are transported via the blood to specific target cells. Upon reaching their destinations, they can control the activity of the target tissue. A unique feature of hormones is that they travel away from the cells that secrete them and specifically affect the activities of other cells and organs. Some affect many body tissues, whereas others affect only specific target cells.

The Nature of Hormones

Hormones are involved in most physiological processes, so their actions are relevant to many aspects of exercise and sport performance. Before examining specific roles played by hormones, we need a better understanding of the nature of these substances. In the following sections, we will examine the chemical nature of hormones and their general mechanisms of action.

Chemical Classification of Hormones

Hormones can be categorized as two basic types: steroid hormones and nonsteroid hormones. Steroid hormones have a chemical structure similar to cholesterol, and most are derived from it. For this reason, they are lipid soluble and diffuse rather easily through cell membranes. This group includes the hormones secreted by

- the adrenal cortex (such as cortisol and aldosterone),
- the ovaries (estrogen and progesterone),
- the testes (testosterone), and
- the placenta (estrogen and progesterone).

Nonsteroid hormones are not lipid soluble, so they cannot easily cross cell membranes. The nonsteroid hormone group can be subdivided into two groups: protein or peptide hormones and amino acid derivative hormones. The two hormones from the thyroid gland (thyroxine and triiodothyronine) and the two from the adrenal medulla (epinephrine and norepinephrine) are amino acid hormones. All other nonsteroid hormones are protein or peptide hormones.

Hormone Actions

Because hormones travel in the blood, they contact virtually all body tissues. How, then, can they limit their effects to specific targets? This ability is due to the specific hormone receptors possessed by the target

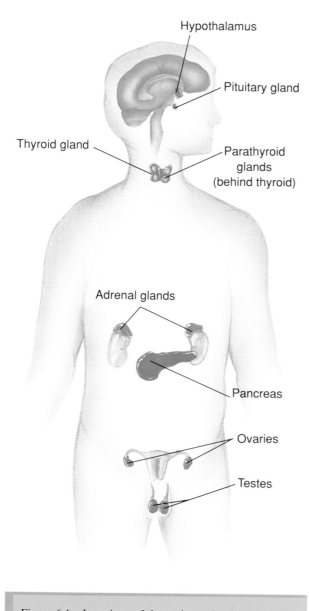

Hypothalamus

Pituitary gland

Thyroid gland

Parathyroid glands (behind thyroid)

Adrenal glands

Pancreas

Ovaries

Testes

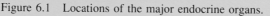

Figure 6.1   Locations of the major endocrine organs.

tissues. The interaction between the hormone and its specific receptor has been compared to a lock (receptor) and key (hormone) arrangement, in which only the correct key can unlock a given action within the cells. The combination of a hormone bound to its receptor is referred to as a hormone-receptor complex.

Each cell typically has from 2,000 to 10,000 receptors. Receptors for nonsteroid hormones are located on the cell membrane, whereas those for steroid hormones are found either in the cell's cytoplasm or in its nucleus. Each hormone is usually highly specific for a single type of receptor and binds only with receptors that are specific to it, thus affecting only tissues that contain those specific receptors.

Numerous mechanisms allow hormones to control the actions of cells. Let's examine the primary modes of action for both the steroid and the nonsteroid hormones.

Steroid Hormones

As mentioned earlier, steroid hormones are lipid soluble and thus pass easily through the cell membrane. Their mechanism of action is illustrated in Figure 6.2. Once inside the cell, a steroid hormone binds to its specific receptors. The hormone-receptor complex then enters the nucleus, binds to part of the cell's DNA, and activates certain genes. This process is referred to as direct gene activation. In response to this activation, mRNA is synthesized within the nucleus. The mRNA then enters the cytoplasm and promotes protein synthesis. These proteins may be

- enzymes that can have numerous effects on cellular processes,
- structural proteins to be used for tissue growth and repair, or
- regulatory proteins that can alter enzyme function.

Nonsteroid Hormones

Because nonsteroid hormones cannot easily cross the cell membrane, they react with specific receptors outside the cell, on the cell membrane. A nonsteroid hormone molecule binding to its receptor triggers a series of enzymatic reactions that lead to the formation of an intracellular second messenger. The most studied and most widely distributed second messenger is cyclic adenosine monophosphate (cyclic AMP, or cAMP). This mechanism of action is depicted in Figure 6.3. In this case, attachment of the hormone to the appropriate membrane receptor activates an enzyme termed adenylate cyclase, situated within the cell membrane. This enzyme catalyzes the formation of cyclic AMP from cellular ATP. Cyclic AMP can then produce specific physiological responses, which may include

- activation of cellular enzymes,
- change in membrane permeability,
- promotion of protein synthesis,
- change in cellular metabolism, or
- stimulation of cellular secretions.

Thus, nonsteroid hormones typically activate the cAMP system of the cell, which then leads to changes in intracellular functions.

Control of Hormone Release

Hormones appear to be released in relatively brief bursts, so plasma levels of specific hormones fluctuate

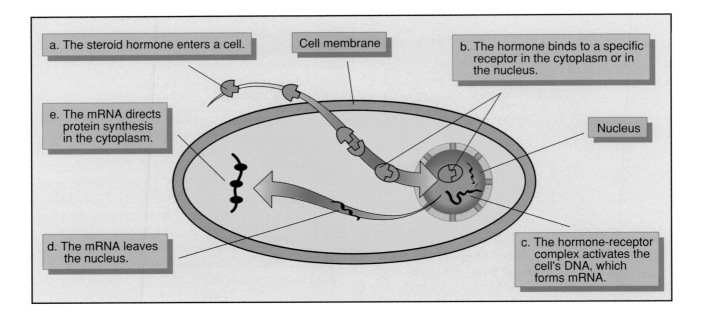

Figure 6.2   The mechanism of action of a steroid hormone, leading to direct gene activation.

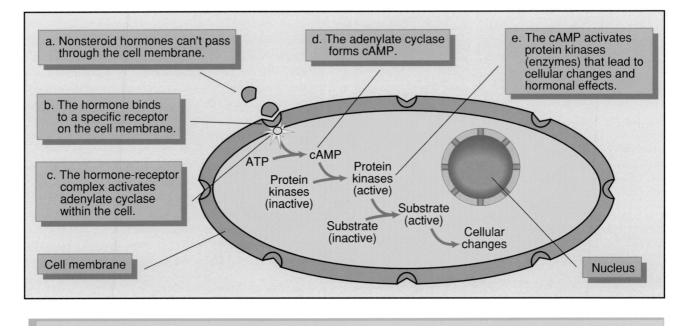

Figure 6.3   The mechanism of action of a nonsteroid hormone, utilizing a second messenger (cAMP) within the cell.

over short periods such as an hour or less. But these levels also fluctuate over longer periods of time, showing daily or even monthly cycles (such as monthly menstrual cycles). How do endocrine glands know when to release their hormones?

Negative Feedback

Most hormone secretion is regulated by a negative feedback system. Secretion of a hormone causes some change in the body, and this change in turn inhibits further hormone secretion. Consider how a home thermostat works. When the room temperature falls below some preset level, the thermostat signals the furnace to produce heat. When the room temperature rises to the preset level, the thermostat's signal ends, and the furnace stops producing heat. When the temperature again falls below the preset level, the cycle begins anew. Thus, in the body, secretion of a specific hormone is turned on or off by specific physiological changes.

Negative feedback is the primary mechanism through which your endocrine system maintains homeostasis. Let's consider the case of plasma glucose levels and the hormone insulin. When the plasma glucose concentration is high, the pancreas releases insulin. Insulin increases cellular uptake of glucose, lowering plasma concentration of glucose. When plasma glucose concentration returns to normal, insulin release is inhibited until the plasma glucose level rises again.

Number of Receptors

The plasma levels of specific hormones are not always the best indicators of actual hormone activity because the number of receptors on a cell can be altered to increase or decrease that cell's sensitivity to a certain hormone. Most commonly, an increased amount of a specific hormone causes a decrease in the number of cell receptors available to it. When this happens, the cell becomes less sensitive to that hormone because with fewer receptors, less hormone can bind. This is referred to as down-regulation or desensitization. In

Prostaglandins

Prostaglandins, though technically not hormones, are often considered to be a third class of hormones. These substances are derived from a fatty acid, arachidonic acid, and they are associated with the plasma membranes of almost all body cells. Prostaglandins typically act as local hormones, exerting their effects in the immediate area where they are produced. But some also survive long enough to circulate through the blood to exert their effects on distant tissues. Prostaglandin release can be triggered by many stimuli, such as other hormones and local injury. Their functions are quite numerous because there are several different types of prostaglandins. They often mediate the effects of other hormones. They are also known to act directly on blood vessels, causing increased vascular permeability (which promotes swelling) and vasodilation. In this capacity, they are important mediators of the inflammatory response. They also sensitize nerve endings of pain fibers; thus they promote both inflammation and pain.

some people with obesity, for example, the number of insulin receptors on their cells appears to be reduced. Their bodies respond by increasing insulin secretion from the pancreas, so their plasma insulin levels rise. To obtain the same degree of plasma glucose control as normal, healthy people, these individuals must release much more insulin.

Conversely, a cell may respond to the prolonged presence of large amounts of a hormone by increasing its number of available receptors. When this happens, the cell becomes more sensitive to that hormone because more can be bound at one time. This is referred to as up-regulation. In addition, one hormone can occasionally regulate the receptors for another hormone.

The Endocrine Glands and Their Hormones

Now that we have discussed the general nature of hormones, we are prepared to look at specific hormones and their functions. The endocrine glands and their respective hormones are listed in Table 6.1. This table also lists each hormone's stimulus for release, its target, and its actions. Please keep in mind that the endocrine system is extremely complex. The presentation here has been greatly simplified to focus on those hormones of greatest importance to sport and physical activity. Also, as you read this, please realize that research on hormone actions during exercise is limited

and available information is often conflicting. Much remains to be learned in this area.

The Pituitary Gland

The pituitary gland, also referred to as the hypophysis, is a marble-sized gland at the base of the brain. This gland was at one time considered the human body's master gland because it secretes a number of hormones that affect a wide variety of other glands and organs. However, the secretory action of the pituitary is itself controlled by either neural mechanisms or other hormones secreted by the hypothalamus. Therefore, the pituitary gland is perhaps more appropriately thought of as the relay between central nervous system control centers and peripheral endocrine glands.

KEY POINT

The pituitary gland was once thought to be the master endocrine gland controlling many other glands and organs. It is now recognized that the pituitary gland is largely controlled by the hypothalamus.

The pituitary gland is composed of three lobes—anterior, intermediate, and posterior (Figure 6.4). The intermediate lobe is very small and is thought to play

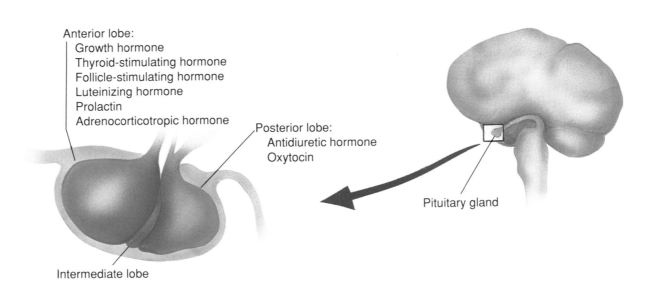

Anterior lobe:
  Growth hormone
  Thyroid-stimulating hormone
  Follicle-stimulating hormone
  Luteinizing hormone
  Prolactin
  Adrenocorticotropic hormone

Posterior lobe:
  Antidiuretic hormone
  Oxytocin

Pituitary gland

Intermediate lobe

Figure 6.4   The location and make-up of the pituitary gland.

Table 6.1 The Endocrine Glands, Their Hormones, Their Target Organs, and Major Functions of the Hormones

Endocrine gland	Hormone	Target organ	Major functions
Pituitary			
Anterior lobe	Growth hormone (GH)	All cells in the body	Promotes development and enlargement of all body tissues up through maturation; increases rate of protein synthesis; increases mobilization of fats and uses fat as an energy source; decreases rate of carbohydrate utilization
	Thyrotropin or thyroid-stimulating hormone (TSH)	Thyroid gland	Controls the amount of thyroxin and triiodothyronine produced and released by the thyroid gland
	Adrenocorticotropin (ACTH)	Adrenal cortex	Controls the secretion of hormones from the adrenal cortex
	Prolactin	Breasts	Stimulates breast development and milk secretion
	Follicle-stimulating hormone (FSH)	Ovaries, testes	Initiates growth of follicles in the ovaries and promotes secretion of estrogen from the ovaries; promotes development of sperm in testes
	Luteinizing hormone (LH)	Ovaries, testes	Promotes secretion of estrogen and progesterone, and causes the follicle to rupture, releasing the ovum; causes testes to secrete testosterone
Posterior lobe (from hypothalamus)	Antidiuretic hormone (ADH or vasopressin)	Kidneys	Assists in controlling water excretion by the kidneys; elevates blood pressure by constricting blood vessels
	Oxytocin	Uterus, breasts	Stimulates contraction of uterine muscles; milk secretion
Thyroid	Thyroxine and triiodothyronine	All cells in the body	Increases the rate of cellular metabolism; increases rate and contractility of the heart
	Calcitonin	Bones	Controls calcium-ion concentration in the blood
Parathyroid	Parathormone or parathyroid hormone	Bones, intestine, and kidneys	Controls calcium-ion concentration in extracellular fluid through its influence on bone, intestine, and kidneys
Adrenal			
Medulla	Epinephrine	Most cells in the body	Mobilizes glycogen; increases skeletal muscle blood flow; increases heart rate and contractility; oxygen consumption
	Norepinephrine	Most cells in the body	Constricts arterioles and venules thereby elevating blood pressure
Cortex	Minerocorticoids (aldosterone)	Kidneys	Increases sodium retention and potassium excretion through the kidneys
	Glucocorticoids (cortisol)	Most cells in the body	Controls metabolism of carbohydrates, fats, and proteins; anti-inflammatory action
	Androgens and estrogens	Ovaries, breasts, and testes	Assists in the development of the female and male sex characteristics
Pancreas	Insulin	All cells in the body	Controls blood glucose levels by lowering glucose levels; increases the utilization of glucose and the synthesis of fat
	Glucagon	All cells in the body	Increases blood glucose; stimulates the breakdown of protein and fat
	Somatostatin	Islets of Langerhans and gastro-intestinal tract	Depresses the secretion of both insulin and glucagon
Gonads			
Testes	Testosterone	Sex organs, muscle	Promotes development of male sex characteristics, including growth of testes, scrotum, and penis; facial hair and change in voice; promotes muscle growth
Ovaries	Estrogen	Sex organs, adipose tissue	Promotes development of female sex organs and characteristics; provides increased storage of fat; assists in regulating the menstrual cycle
Kidneys	Renin	Adrenal cortex	Assists in blood pressure control
	Erythropoietin	Bone marrow	Erythrocyte production

Note. These represent the major endocrine glands and hormones. Others of lesser importance to sport and physical activity have not been included.

little or no role in humans, but both the posterior and anterior lobes have major endocrine functions.

The Posterior Lobe of the Pituitary Gland

The pituitary's posterior lobe is an outgrowth of neural tissue from the hypothalamus. For this reason, it is also referred to as the neurohypophysis. It secretes two hormones—antidiuretic hormone (ADH or vasopressin) and oxytocin. But these hormones are actually produced in the hypothalamus. They travel down through the neural tissue and are stored in vesicles within nerve endings in the posterior pituitary. These hormones are released into capillaries as needed in response to neural impulses from the hypothalamus.

Of the two posterior pituitary hormones, only ADH is known to play an important role in exercise. ADH promotes water conservation by increasing the water permeability of the kidneys' collecting ducts. As a result, less water is excreted in the urine.

Little is known about the effects of exercise on the secretions from the posterior lobe of the pituitary gland. We do know, however, that injecting a concentrated electrolyte solution into the blood causes the release of large quantities of ADH from this gland. This hormone's role in conserving body water minimizes the risk of dehydration during periods of heavy sweating and hard exercise.

Figure 6.5 shows this mechanism at work. Muscular activity and sweating cause concentration of the electrolytes in the blood plasma. This is called hemoconcentration, and it increases the plasma osmolality. This is the primary physiological stimulus for ADH release. The increased osmolality is sensed by osmoreceptors located in the hypothalamus. In response, the hypothalamus sends neural impulses to the posterior pituitary, stimulating ADH release. The ADH enters the blood, travels to the kidneys, and promotes water retention in an effort to dilute the plasma electrolyte concentration back to normal levels.

The Anterior Lobe of the Pituitary Gland

The anterior pituitary, also called the adenohypophysis, secretes six hormones in response to releasing or inhibiting factors (hormones) secreted by the hypothalamus. Communication between the hypothalamus and the anterior lobe of the pituitary occurs through a specialized circulatory system that transports the releasing and inhibiting hormones from the hypothalamus to the anterior pituitary. The major functions of each of the anterior pituitary hormones, along with their releasing and inhibiting factors, are listed in Table 6.2. Exercise appears to be a strong stimulant to the hypothalamus, because exercise increases the release rate of all anterior pituitary hormones.

Of the six anterior pituitary hormones, four are tropic hormones, meaning they affect the functioning of other endocrine glands. The exceptions to this are growth hormone (GH) and prolactin (PRL). Growth hormone is a potent anabolic agent. It promotes muscle growth and hypertrophy by facilitating amino acid transport into the cells. In addition, GH directly stimulates fat metabolism (lipolysis) by increasing the synthesis of enzymes involved in this process. Growth hormone levels are elevated during aerobic exercise, apparently in proportion to the exercise intensity, and typically remain elevated for some time after exercise.

The Thyroid Gland

The thyroid gland is located along the midline of the neck, immediately below the larynx. It secretes two important hormones that regulate metabolism in general, triiodothyronine (T_3) and thyroxine (T_4), and an additional hormone, calcitonin, which assists in regulating calcium metabolism.

Triiodothyronine and Thyroxine

The two metabolic thyroid hormones share similar functions. Triiodothyronine and thyroxine increase the metabolic rate of almost all tissues and can increase the body's basal metabolic rate by as much as 60% to 100%. These hormones also

- increase protein synthesis (thus also enzyme synthesis),
- increase the size and number of mitochondria in most cells,
- promote rapid cellular uptake of glucose,
- enhance glycolysis and gluconeogenesis, and
- enhance lipid mobilization, increasing free fatty acid availability for oxidation.

Release of thyroid stimulating hormone (TSH) from the anterior pituitary increases during exercise. TSH controls the release of triiodothyronine and thyroxine so the exercise-induced increase in TSH would be expected to stimulate the thyroid gland. Exercise indeed produces an increase in plasma thyroxine levels, but a delay occurs between the rise in TSH levels during exercise and the increase in plasma thyroxine levels. Furthermore, during prolonged submaximal exercise, thyroxine levels remain relatively constant after a sharp initial increase as exercise begins, and triiodothyronine levels tend to decrease.

Calcitonin

Calcitonin decreases the plasma calcium concentration. It acts primarily on two targets: the bones and the kidneys. In bone, calcitonin inhibits the activity of

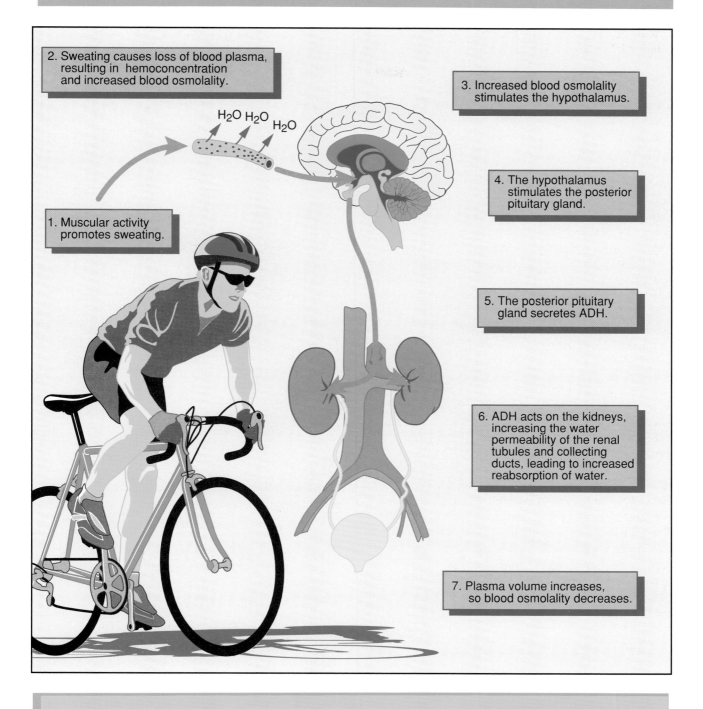

1. Muscular activity promotes sweating.

2. Sweating causes loss of blood plasma, resulting in hemoconcentration and increased blood osmolality.

H_2O H_2O H_2O

3. Increased blood osmolality stimulates the hypothalamus.

4. The hypothalamus stimulates the posterior pituitary gland.

5. The posterior pituitary gland secretes ADH.

6. ADH acts on the kidneys, increasing the water permeability of the renal tubules and collecting ducts, leading to increased reabsorption of water.

7. Plasma volume increases, so blood osmolality decreases.

Figure 6.5   The mechanism by which antidiuretic hormone (ADH) conserves body water.

the osteoclasts (the bone-resorbing cells), thus inhibiting bone resorption. The osteoclasts may be calcitonin's only target in the bone. In the kidney, calcitonin increases urinary excretion of calcium by decreasing calcium reabsorption from the renal tubules.

Calcitonin is primarily important in children, while their bones are rapidly growing and developing strength. This hormone is not a major regulator of calcium homeostasis in adults. But it does appear to offer some protection against excessive bone reabsorption.

The Parathyroid Glands

The parathyroid glands are located on the back of the thyroid gland. They secrete parathyroid hormone

Table 6.2 The Hormones of the Anterior Lobe of the Pituitary Gland

Hormone	Controlling factors	Major functions
Adrenocorticotropic hormone (ACTH)	Stimulated by cortioctropic-releasing hormone (CRH)	Promotes release of hormones from adrenal cortex
Growth hormone (GH)	Stimulated by growth hormone-releasing hormone (GHRH) Inhibited by somatostatin, also called growth hormone-inhibiting hormone (GHIH)	Promotes growth of bone and muscle; promotes use of fat for energy, sparing glucose
Thyroid-stimulating hormone (TSH)	Stimulated by thyroid-releasing hormone (TRH)	Promotes release of thyroid hormones
Follicle-stimulating hormone (FSH)	Stimulated by gonadotropin-releasing hormone (GnRH)	Females: promotes maturation of follicles in ovary and production of estrogen Males: stimulates production of sperm
Luteinizing hormone (LH)	Stimulated by GnRH	Females: stimulates production of estrogen and progesterone Males: promotes production of testosterone
Prolactin (PRL)	Stimulated by prolactin-releasing hormone (PRH) Inhibited by prolactin-inhibiting hormone (PIH)	Promotes lactation

(PTH, or parathormone). This hormone is the principal regulator of plasma calcium concentration, and it also regulates plasma phosphate. Its release is stimulated by a decrease in plasma calcium levels.

Parathyroid hormone exerts its effects on three targets: the bones, the intestines, and the kidneys. In the bone, PTH stimulates osteoclast activity. This increases bone resorption, which releases both calcium and phosphate into the blood. In the intestines, PTH increases calcium absorption indirectly by stimulating an enzyme that is required for the process. Increased intestinal absorption of calcium is accompanied by increased absorption of phosphate. Because PTH raises plasma levels of phosphate ions, the excess phosphate must be removed. This is accomplished by PTH's action in the kidneys, where it increases calcium reabsorption but decreases phosphate reabsorption, which promotes urinary excretion of phosphate.

Over an extended period, exercise increases bone formation. This results primarily from increased intestinal absorption of Ca^{++}, decreased urinary excretion of Ca^{++}, and increased PTH levels. Conversely, immobilization or complete bedrest promotes bone resorption. During such a period, PTH levels decrease.

The Adrenal Glands

The adrenal glands are situated directly atop each kidney and are composed of the inner adrenal medulla and the outer adrenal cortex. The hormones secreted by these parts are quite different, so we will consider them separately.

The Adrenal Medulla

The adrenal medulla produces and releases two hormones—epinephrine and norepinephrine—which are referred to as catecholamines. When the adrenal medulla is stimulated by the sympathetic nervous system, approximately 80% of the secretion is epinephrine and 20% is norepinephrine, although these percentages vary with different physiological conditions. The catecholamines have powerful effects similar to those of the sympathetic nervous system, but the hormones' effects last longer because these substances are removed from the blood relatively slowly. These two hormones prepare you for immediate action, eliciting the fight-or-flight response.

Epinephrine and norepinephrine help you face a real or perceived crisis. Although some of the specific actions of these two hormones differ, the two work together. Their combined effects include

- increased rate and force of heart contraction,
- increased metabolic rate,
- increased glycogenolysis (breakdown of glycogen to glucose) in the liver and muscle,
- increased release of glucose and free fatty acids into the blood,
- redistribution of blood to the skeletal muscles (through vasodilation of vessels supplying skeletal muscles, and vasoconstriction in vessels to the skin and viscera),

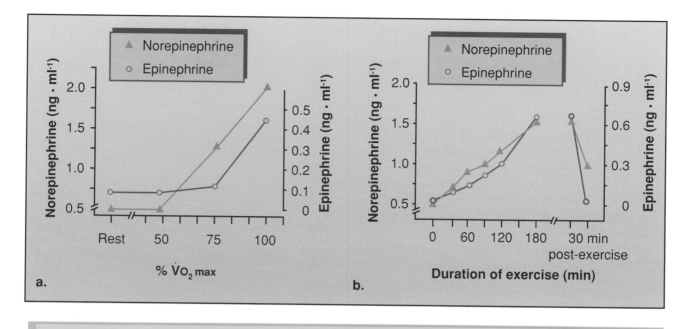

Figure 6.6   Changes in blood concentrations of epinephrine and norepinephrine (a) at rest and at various intensities (% $\dot{V}O_2$ max) of treadmill running and (b) during prolonged treadmill running at 60% $\dot{V}O_2$ max and during recovery.

- increased blood pressure, and
- increased respiration.

Release of epinephrine and norepinephrine is affected by a wide variety of factors, including changes in body position, psychological stress, and exercise. Figure 6.6a shows the changes in plasma levels of these hormones when individuals gradually increase their exercise intensity. Plasma norepinephrine levels increase markedly at work rates above 50% of $\dot{V}O_2$ max. But the epinephrine level doesn't increase significantly until the exercise intensity exceeds 60% to 70% of $\dot{V}O_2$ max. Figure 6.6b shows that during steady-state activity lasting more than 3 hr at 60% of $\dot{V}O_2$ max, blood levels of both hormones rise. When the exercise bout ends, epinephrine levels return to resting levels within only a few minutes of recovery, but norepinephrine can remain elevated for several hours.

The Adrenal Cortex

The adrenal cortex secretes over 30 different steroid hormones, referred to as corticosteroids. These are generally classified into three major types:

1. mineralocorticoids,
2. glucocorticoids, or
3. gonadocorticoids (sex hormones).

Mineralocorticoids.   The mineralocorticoids maintain electrolyte balance in the extracellular fluids, especially that of sodium and potassium. Aldosterone is the major mineralocorticoid, responsible for at least 95% of all mineralocorticoid activity. It works primarily by promoting renal reabsorption of sodium (Na$^+$), thus causing the body to retain sodium. When sodium is retained, so is water; thus, aldosterone fights dehydration. Sodium retention also leads to enhanced K$^+$ excretion, so aldosterone plays a role in potassium balance as well. For these reasons, aldosterone secretion is stimulated by many factors, including decreased plasma sodium, decreased blood volume, decreased blood pressure, and increased plasma potassium concentration. We'll further discuss the actions of aldosterone later in this chapter.

Glucocorticoids.   The glucocorticoids are essential to life. They enable us to adapt to external changes and stress. They also maintain fairly consistent plasma glucose levels even when we go for long periods without ingesting food. Cortisol, also known as hydrocortisone, is the major corticosteroid. It is responsible for about 95% of all glucocorticoid activity in the body. Cortisol is known to

- stimulate gluconeogenesis to ensure an adequate fuel supply;
- increase mobilization of free fatty acids, making them a more available energy source;
- decrease glucose utilization, sparing it for the brain;
- stimulate protein catabolism to release amino acids for use in repair, enzyme synthesis, and energy production;
- act as an anti-inflammatory agent;

- depress immune reactions; and
- increase the vasoconstriction caused by epinephrine.

We will discuss cortisol's important role in exercise later in this chapter, when we discuss the regulation of glucose and fat metabolism.

Gonadocorticoids. The adrenal cortex also synthesizes and releases the gonadocorticoids. These hormones are mostly androgens, although estrogens and progesterones are released in small amounts. These hormones are the same as those produced by the reproductive organs. Apparently these cortical secretions have little effect in adults—the amounts secreted are insignificant compared to the amounts released from the reproductive glands. Thus the exact role played by gonadocorticoids is unclear.

The Pancreas

The pancreas is located behind and slightly below the stomach. Its two major hormones are insulin and glucagon. These provide the major control of plasma glucose levels. When plasma glucose levels are elevated (hyperglycemia), such as after a meal, the pancreas receives signals to release insulin into the blood.

Among its actions, insulin

- facilitates glucose transport into the cells, especially those in muscle and connective tissue;
- promotes glycogenesis; and
- inhibits gluconeogenesis.

Insulin's main function is to reduce the amount of glucose circulating in the blood. But it is also involved in protein and fat metabolism, promoting cellular uptake of amino acids and enhancing synthesis of protein and fat.

The pancreas secretes glucagon when the plasma glucose concentration falls below normal levels (hypoglycemia). Its effects generally oppose those of insulin. Glucagon promotes increased breakdown of liver glycogen to glucose (glycogenolysis) and increased gluconeogenesis. Both processes increase plasma glucose levels.

During exercise lasting 30 min or longer, insulin levels tend to decline, as shown in Figure 6.7, although the plasma glucose concentration may remain relatively constant. Research has shown that the number or availability of insulin receptors increases during exercise, increasing the body's sensitivity to insulin. This reduces the need to maintain high plasma insulin levels for transporting glucose into the muscle cells. Plasma glucagon, on the other hand, shows a gradual rise throughout the period of exercise. Glucagon primarily maintains plasma glucose concentrations by

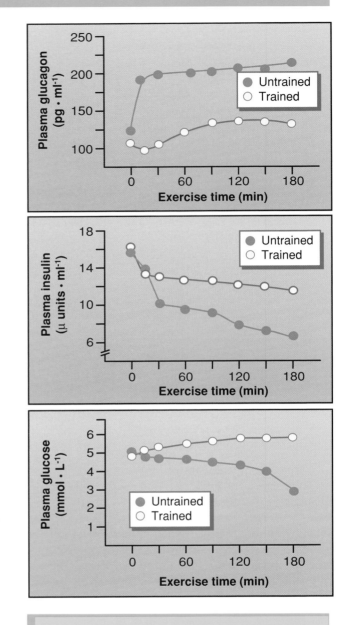

Figure 6.7   Changes in plasma levels of glucagon, insulin, and glucose during prolonged exercise.

stimulating liver glycogenolysis. This increases glucose availability to the cells, maintaining adequate plasma glucose levels to meet increased metabolic demands. As can be seen by Figure 6.7, the hormone response is usually blunted in trained people.

The Gonads

The gonads are the reproductive glands: the testes and the ovaries. The hormones they secrete are generally anabolic, meaning they promote anabolism, the constructive phase of metabolism. The testes secrete androgens, of which testosterone is the most important. Testosterone is responsible for the development of male secondary sex characteristics and spermatogenesis. It is also essential for normal growth, development, and maturation of the male skeletal system. Another critical role of the androgens is the promotion of skeletal muscle growth, which is particularly important to our understanding of strength training and gender differences in muscle growth. The androgenic effects of testosterone are responsible, in part, for muscle protein retention and muscle hypertrophy observed during strength training. This has led to some athletes' use of it and other anabolic steroids to artificially promote muscle building beyond natural levels. We will discuss this illegal and dangerous use of testosterone and other anabolic steroids in more detail in chapter 14.

The ovaries secrete two types of hormones: estrogens and progesterone. Estrogens promote development of the female secondary sex characteristics, the proliferative phase of the menstrual cycle, oogenesis, ovulation, and many changes during pregnancy. Progesterone promotes the secretory (luteal) phase of the menstrual cycle, prepares the uterus for pregnancy, and prepares the breasts for lactation.

The Kidneys

Although not typically considered major endocrine organs, we will discuss the kidneys here because they release a hormone called erythropoietin. Erythropoietin regulates red blood cell (erythrocyte) production by stimulating bone marrow cells. The red blood cells are essential for transporting oxygen to the tissues and removing carbon dioxide, so this hormone is extremely important in our adaptation to training and altitude. Research has shown that part of the adaptation when training at high elevations is an increased release of erythropoietin, which in turn stimulates more red blood cell production, increasing the blood's oxygen-carrying capacity. Because of this, some athletes have used injections of this hormone to build up their red blood cell count, hoping to gain an edge over their competitors. This will be discussed further in chapter 14.

The Endocrine Response to Exercise

Endocrine responses to an acute bout of exercise are summarized in Table 6.3. This table focuses on the hormones suspected of playing major roles in sport and physical activity.

Hormonal Effects on Metabolism and Energy

As noted in chapters 5 and 15, carbohydrate and fat metabolism are responsible for maintaining muscle ATP levels during prolonged exercise. Various hormones work to ensure glucose and free fatty acid (FFA) availability for muscle energy metabolism. In this section, we will examine how the metabolism of glucose and fat are affected by these hormones during exercise. Because carbohydrate is the primary fuel used during both brief and prolonged exhaustive exercise, we shall first consider the hormones that regulate its availability.

Regulation of Glucose Metabolism During Exercise

As we saw in the previous two chapters, for your body to meet the heightened energy demands of exercise, more glucose must be available to the muscles. Recall that glucose is stored in the body as glycogen located primarily in the muscles and the liver. Glucose must be freed from storage, so glycogenolysis must increase. Glucose freed from the liver enters the blood to circulate throughout the body, allowing it access to the active tissues. Plasma glucose levels can also be increased through gluconeogenesis. Let's examine the hormones involved in both glycogenolysis and gluconeogenesis.

Plasma Glucose Levels

Four hormones work to increase the amount of circulating plasma glucose:

1. glucagon,
2. epinephrine,
3. norepinephrine, and
4. cortisol.

The plasma glucose concentration during exercise depends on a balance between glucose uptake by the muscles and its release by the liver. At rest, glucose release from the liver is facilitated by glucagon which promotes liver glycogen breakdown and glucose formation from amino acids. During exercise, glucagon secretion increases. Muscular activity also increases the rate of catecholamine release from the adrenal medulla, and these hormones (epinephrine and norepinephrine) work with glucagon to further increase glycogenolysis. Evidence suggests that cortisol levels also increase during exercise. Cortisol increases protein catabolism, freeing amino acids to be used within the

Table 6.3 A Summary of Hormonal Changes During Exercise

Hormone	Exercise response	Special relationships	Probable significance
Catecholamines	Increases	Greater increase with intense exercise, norepinephrine > epinephrine, increase less after training	Increased blood glucose
GH	Increases	Increases more in unfit person; declines faster in fit person	Unknown
ACTH-cortisol	Increases	Greater increase with intense exercise; increase less after training with submaximal exercise	Increased gluconeogenesis in liver (kidney)
TSH-thyroxine	Increases	Increased thyroxine turnover with training but no toxic effects evident	Unknown
LH	No change	None	None
Testosterone	Increases	None	Unknown
Estradiol-progesterone	Increases	Increases during luteal phase of cycle	Unknown
Insulin	Decreases	Decreases less after training	Decreased stimulus to utilize blood glucose
Glucagon	Increases	Increases less after training	Increased blood glucose via glycogenolysis and gluconeogenesis
Renin-angiotensin-aldosterone	Increases	Same increase after training in rats	Sodium retention to maintain plasma volume
ADH	Expected increase	None	Water retention to maintain plasma volume
PTH-calcitonin	Unknown	None	Needed to establish proper bone development
Erythropoietin	Unknown	None	Would be important to increase erythropoiesis
Prostaglandins	May increase	May increase in response to sustained isometric contractions— may need ischemic stress	May be local vasodilators

liver for gluconeogenesis. Thus all four of these hormones can increase the amount of plasma glucose by enhancing the processes of glycogenolysis and gluconeogenesis. In addition, growth hormone increases mobilization of free fatty acids and decreases cellular uptake of glucose, so less glucose is used by the cells (more remains in circulation), and the thyroid hormones promote glucose catabolism and fat metabolism.

The amount of glucose released by the liver depends on your exercise intensity and the duration. As intensity increases, so does your rate of catecholamine release. This can cause the liver to release more glucose than is being taken up by the active muscles. Figure 6.8 shows the glucose level following an explosive, short-term bout of sprinting. By the end of the 60-s sprint cycling bout, the plasma glucose level exceeds the resting level, indicating that glucose release exceeds glucose uptake. Why is the excess glucose not being used?

The greater your exercise intensity, the greater your catecholamine release. So your glycogenolysis rate is significantly increased. This process occurs not only in the liver, but also in the muscle. The glucose released from the liver enters the blood to become available to the muscle. But the muscle has a more readily available source of glucose: its own glycogen. The muscle will use its own glycogen stores before using the plasma glucose during explosive, short-term exercise. Glucose released from the liver is not used as readily, so it remains in circulation, elevating the plasma glucose. Following exercise, plasma glucose levels decrease as the glucose enters the muscle to replenish the depleted muscle glycogen stores.

During exercise bouts that last for several hours, however, the rate of liver glucose release more closely matches the muscle's needs, keeping plasma glucose at or only slightly above the resting levels. As muscle uptake of glucose increases, the liver's rate of glucose release also increases. In most cases, plasma glucose

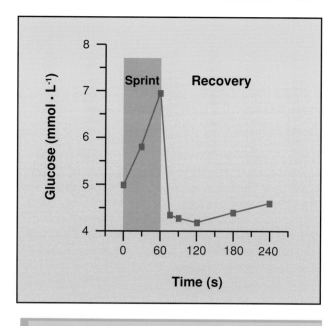

Figure 6.8 Changes in blood glucose during 1 min of sprint cycling.

glucose during 3 hr of cycling. Although the hormonal regulation of glucose remains intact throughout such long-term activities, the liver's glycogen supply may fall critically low. As a result, the liver's rate of glucose release may be unable to keep pace with the muscle's rate of glucose uptake. Under this condition, the plasma glucose level may decline, despite strong hormonal stimulation. At this point, glucose ingested during the activity can play a major role in maintaining plasma glucose levels.

Glucose Uptake by the Muscles

Merely releasing sufficient amounts of glucose into the blood does not ensure that the muscle cells will have enough glucose to meet their energy demands. The glucose must not only be delivered to these cells, it must also be taken up by them. That job relies on insulin. Once glucose is delivered to the muscle, insulin facilitates its transport into the fibers.

Surprisingly, as seen in Figure 6.10, plasma insulin levels tend to decrease during prolonged submaximal exercise despite an increase in plasma glucose concentration and glucose uptake by muscle. This apparent contradiction between the plasma insulin concentrations and the muscle's need for glucose reminds us that a hormone's activity is not always determined by its concentration in blood. In this case, the cell's sensitivity to insulin may be as important as the amount of circulating hormone. Exercise may enhance insulin binding to receptors on the muscle fiber.[5,6] Muscle

levels don't begin to decline until late in the activity as liver glycogen stores become depleted, at which time glucagon levels rise significantly. Glucagon and cortisol together enhance gluconeogenesis, providing more fuel.

Figure 6.9 illustrates the changes in plasma levels of epinephrine, norepinephrine, glucagon, cortisol, and

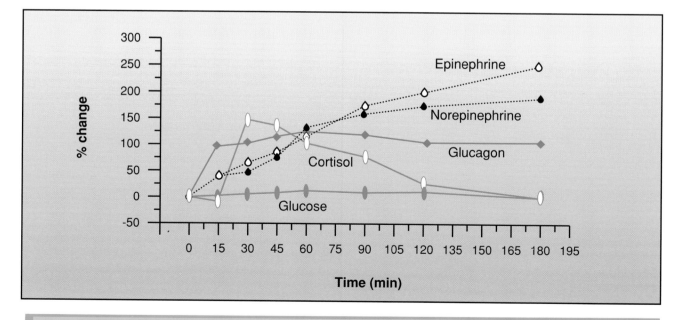

Figure 6.9 Changes in plasma levels of epinephrine, norepinephrine, glucagon, cortisol, and glucose during 3 hr of cycling at 65% $\dot{V}O_2$ max.

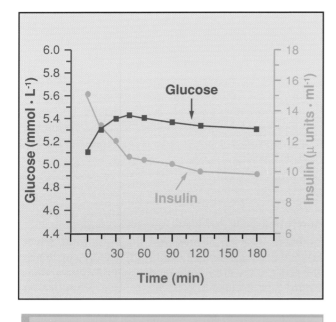

Figure 6.10 · Changes in plasma levels of glucose and insulin during prolonged cycling at 65% to 70% $\dot{V}O_2$ max.

to release glucose from its storage sites and creating new glucose. High insulin levels would oppose their action, preventing this needed increase in plasma glucose supply.

Regulation of Fat Metabolism During Exercise

Although fat generally contributes less than carbohydrate to muscles' energy needs during exercise, mobilization and oxidation of free fatty acids (FFA) are critical to performance in endurance exercise bouts. During such activity, carbohydrate reserves become depleted and your body must rely more heavily on the oxidation of fat for energy production. When carbohydrate reserves are low (low plasma glucose and low muscle glycogen), the endocrine system can accelerate the oxidation of fats (lipolysis), thus ensuring that your muscles' energy needs can be met. Lipolysis is also enhanced through the elevation of epinephrine and norepinephrine.

Recall that FFA are stored as triglycerides in fat cells and inside muscle fibers. Triglycerides must be broken down to release the FFA, which are then transported to the muscle fibers. The rate of FFA uptake by active muscle is highly correlated to the plasma FFA concentration. Increasing this concentration would increase cellular uptake of the FFA. We can assume that increased plasma FFA concentration causes increased FFA oxidation because increased cellular uptake of FFA provides more for oxidation.[1] Thus, the rate of triglyceride breakdown may, in part,

action, for reasons not completely understood, appears to have an insulinlike effect in recruiting receptors—more receptors appear on the cells, and their activity may be increased, thereby reducing the need for high levels of plasma insulin to transport glucose across the muscle cell membranes into the cell. This is important, because during exercise you have four hormones trying

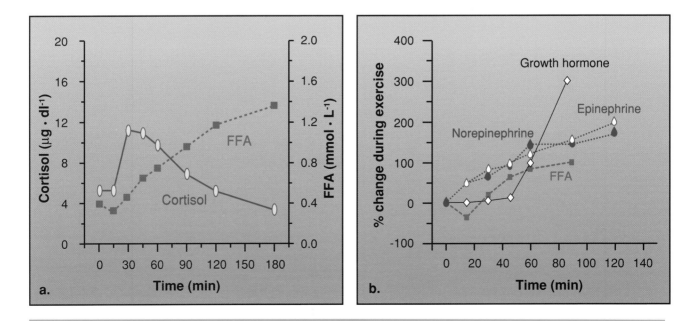

Figure 6.11   Changes (a) in plasma levels of FFA and cortisol and (b) in plasma levels of epinephrine, norepinephrine, growth hormone, and FFA during prolonged exericse.

determine the rate at which muscles use fat as a fuel source during exercise.

Triglycerides are reduced to FFA and glycerol by a special enzyme called lipase, which is activated by at least four hormones:

1. Cortisol
2. Epinephrine
3. Norepinephrine
4. Growth hormone

In addition to cortisol's role in gluconeogenesis, it also accelerates the mobilization and use of FFA for energy during exercise. Figure 6.11a illustrates the changes in the plasma concentrations of FFA and cortisol during prolonged exercise. Plasma cortisol levels peak after 30 to 45 min of exercise, then decrease to near normal levels. But the plasma FFA concentration continues to rise throughout the activity, meaning that lipase must continue to be activated by other hormones. The hormones that continue this process are the catecholamines and growth hormone. As shown in Figure 6.11b, the plasma levels of these hormones continue to rise throughout exercise, progressively increasing FFA release and fat oxidation. The thyroid hormones have similar effects.

Thus, the endocrine system plays a critical role in the regulation of ATP production during exercise and may be responsible for controlling the balance between carbohydrate and fat metabolism.

IN REVIEW . . .

1. Plasma glucose is increased by the combined actions of glucagon, epinephrine, norepinephrine, and cortisol. These hormones promote glycogenolysis and gluconeogenesis, thus increasing the amount of glucose available for use as a fuel source. Growth hormone and the thyroid hormones share these functions.
2. Insulin helps the released glucose enter the cells where it can be used for energy production. But insulin levels decline during prolonged exercise, indicating that exercise facilitates the action of insulin so that less of the hormone is required during exercise than when at rest.
3. When carbohydrate reserves are low, the body turns more to fat oxidation for energy, and this process is facilitated by cortisol, epinephrine, norepinephrine, and growth hormone.
4. Cortisol accelerates lipolysis, releasing free fatty acids into the blood so they can be taken up by the cells and used for energy production. But cortisol levels peak and then return to near normal levels during prolonged exercise. When this happens, the catecholamines and growth hormone take over cortisol's role.

Hormonal Effects on Fluid and Electrolyte Balance During Exercise

Fluid balance during exercise is critical for optimal cardiovascular and thermoregulatory function. At the onset of exercise, water is shifted from the plasma volume to the interstitial and intracellular spaces.[2,3] This water shift is related to the muscle mass that is active and the intensity of effort. Metabolic by-products begin to accumulate in and around the muscle fibers, increasing the osmotic pressure there. Water is drawn into these areas. Also, increased muscle activity increases your blood pressure, which, in turn, drives water out of your blood. In addition, sweating increases during exercise. The combined effect of these actions is that your muscles gain water at the expense of your plasma volume. For example, running at approximately 75% $\dot{V}O_2$ max results in a 5% to 10% decrease in plasma volume. Reduced plasma volume decreases your blood pressure and the amount of blood flow to your skin and muscles. Both of these can seriously impede athletic performance.

The endocrine system plays a major role in monitoring fluid levels and correcting imbalances. This is accomplished along with regulation of the electrolyte balance, especially that of sodium. The two major hormones involved in this regulation are aldosterone and antidiuretic hormone (ADH), and the kidneys are their primary targets. Let's examine these hormones' effects.

Aldosterone and the Renin-Angiotensin Mechanism

The kidneys have a strong regulatory influence on blood pressure. This influence also allows them to regulate fluid balance. Plasma volume is a major determinant of blood pressure: When plasma volume decreases, so does blood pressure. Your blood pressure is constantly monitored by specialized cells within your kidneys. During exercise, these cells can be stimulated by decreased blood pressure, decreased blood flow to the kidneys through increased sympathetic nervous activity accompanying exercise, or by direct stimulation from the sympathetic nerves.

The mechanism involved in renal control of blood pressure is depicted in Figure 6.12. This is the renin-angiotensin mechanism. The kidneys respond to decreased blood pressure or blood flow by forming an enzyme called renin. Renin, in turn, converts a plasma protein called angiotensinogen into an active form called angiotensin I, which is finally converted to angiotensin II. Angiotensin II acts in two ways. First, it is a potent arteriole constrictor. Through this action,

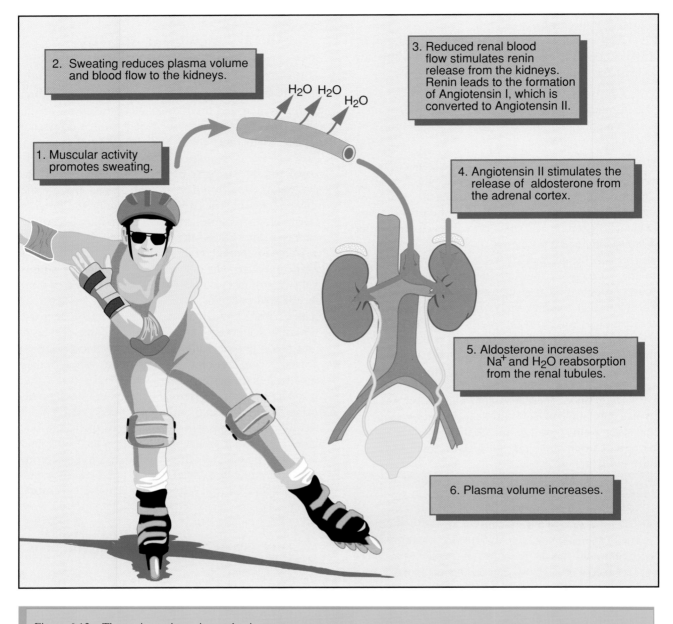

1. Muscular activity promotes sweating.

2. Sweating reduces plasma volume and blood flow to the kidneys.

3. Reduced renal blood flow stimulates renin release from the kidneys. Renin leads to the formation of Angiotensin I, which is converted to Angiotensin II.

4. Angiotensin II stimulates the release of aldosterone from the adrenal cortex.

5. Aldosterone increases Na^+ and H_2O reabsorption from the renal tubules.

6. Plasma volume increases.

H_2O H_2O H_2O

Figure 6.12   The renin-angiotensin mechanism.

your peripheral resistance increases, which raises your blood pressure. The second job of angiotensin II is to trigger aldosterone release from the adrenal cortex.

Recall that aldosterone's primary action is to promote sodium reabsorption in the kidneys. Because water follows sodium, this renal conservation of sodium requires that your kidneys also retain water. The net effect is to increase your body's fluid content, thus replenishing your plasma volume and raising your blood pressure toward normal. Figure 6.13 illustrates the changes in plasma volume and aldosterone concentrations during 2 hr of exercise.

Antidiuretic Hormone (ADH)

The other major hormone involved in fluid balance is antidiuretic hormone (ADH). ADH is released in response to increasing solute concentration of the blood. During exercise, the shifting of water out of the plasma leaves the blood more concentrated, and sweating promotes dehydration, which also causes plasma concentration. This elevates the blood osmolality. The concentrated plasma circulates and reaches the hypothalamus, which houses osmoreceptors that constantly monitor blood osmolality. When the osmo-

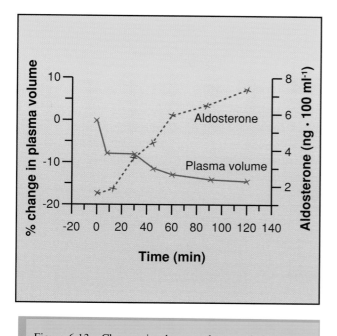

Figure 6.13   Changes in plasma volume and aldosterone concentrations during 2 hr of exericse.

lality increases, the hypothalamus triggers ADH release from the posterior pituitary. Recall that ADH promotes water reabsorption in the kidneys, leading to water conservation. As with aldosterone, although the stimuli and mechanisms of action are different, the net effect of ADH secretion is also to increase the body's fluid content, restoring normal plasma volume and blood pressure.

Following the initial drop in plasma volume, it remains relatively constant throughout the exercise. In addition to the actions of aldosterone and ADH, some evidence suggests that, despite continued sweat losses during the exercise, plasma volume is protected from a further reduction by water returning from the exercising muscles back into the blood. Also, as exercise progresses, the amount of metabolic water production via oxidation increases.

Post-Exercise Hormone Activity and Fluid Balance

The hormonal influences of aldosterone and ADH persist for 12 to 48 hr after exercise, reducing urine production and protecting the body from further dehydration.[3,4] In fact, aldosterone's prolonged enhancement of Na+ reabsorption causes the body's Na+ concentration to increase above normal following an exercise bout. In an effort to compensate for this eleva-

tion in Na+ levels, more of the water you ingest shifts into the extracellular compartment.

As shown in Figure 6.14, individuals who are subjected to repeated days of exercise and dehydration show a significant increase in plasma volume that continues to rise throughout the period of activity. When the daily bouts of activity are terminated, the excess Na+ and water are excreted in urine.

KEY POINT

Loss of fluid (plasma) from the blood results in a concentration of the constituents of the blood, a phenomenon referred to as hemoconcentration. Conversely, a gain of fluid into the blood results in a dilution of the constituents of the blood, which is referred to as hemodilution.

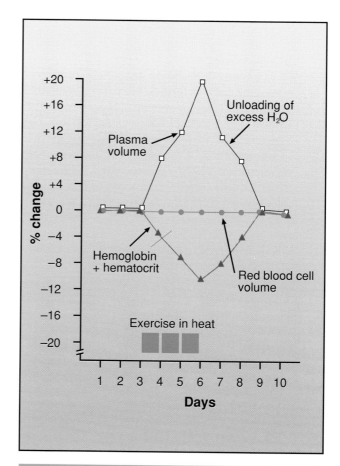
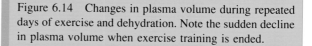

Figure 6.14   Changes in plasma volume during repeated days of exercise and dehydration. Note the sudden decline in plasma volume when exercise training is ended.

Most athletes involved in heavy training have an expanded plasma volume, which dilutes various blood constituents. The actual amount of substances within the blood remains unaltered, but they are dispersed throughout a greater volume of water (plasma), so they are diluted. This phenomenon is called hemodilution.

Hemoglobin is one of the substances diluted by plasma expansion. For this reason, some athletes who actually have normal hemoglobin levels may appear to be anemic as a consequence of this Na^+-induced hemodilution. This condition, not to be confused with true anemia, can be remedied with a few days of rest, allowing time for aldosterone levels to return to normal and for the kidneys to unload the extra Na^+ and water.

IN REVIEW . . .

1. The two primary hormones involved in the regulation of fluid balance are aldosterone and antidiuretic hormone (ADH).
2. When plasma volume or blood pressure decreases, the kidneys form an enzyme called renin that, in turn, converts angiotensinogen into angiotensin I, which later becomes angiotensin II. Angiotensin II increases peripheral resistance, raising the blood pressure.
3. Angiotensin II also triggers the release of aldosterone from the adrenal cortex. Aldosterone promotes sodium reabsorption in the kidneys, which in turn causes water retention, thus increasing the plasma volume.
4. ADH is released in response to increased plasma osmolality. When osmoreceptors in the hypothalamus sense this increase, the hypothalamus triggers ADH release from the posterior pituitary.
5. ADH acts on the kidneys, promoting water conservation. Through this mechanism, the plasma volume is increased, which results in dilution of the plasma solutes. Blood osmolality decreases.

In Closing . . .

In this chapter, we have focused on the role of the endocrine system in regulating physiological processes accompanying exercise. We concentrated on the role of hormones in the metabolism of glucose and fat, and also in maintaining fluid balance. Our primary interest in this chapter has been what happens during acute exercise. In the next chapter, we will examine adaptations in the body's metabolic processes that occur as a result of training.

Key Terms

catecholamines
direct gene activation
down-regulation
hemoconcentration
hemodilution
hormones
inhibiting factors
negative feedback
   system

nonsteroid hormones
releasing factors
renin-angiotensin
   mechanism
second messenger
steroid hormones
target cells
up-regulation

Study Questions

1. What is an endocrine gland, and what are the functions of hormones?
2. Explain the difference between steroid hormones and nonsteroid hormones.
3. How can hormones have very specific functions when they reach nearly all parts of the body through the blood?
4. How are plasma levels of specific hormones controlled?
5. Explain the rather complex relationship between the hypothalamus and the pituitary gland.
6. Briefly outline the major endocrine glands, their hormones, and the specific action of these hormones.
7. Which of the hormones outlined in the previous question would be of major significance during exercise?
8. What is hemoconcentration, and how does the endocrine system relate to it?
9. Describe the hormonal regulation of metabolism during exercise. What hormones are involved, and how do they influence the availability of carbohydrates and fats for energy during exercise lasting for several hours?
10. Describe the hormonal regulation of fluid balance during exercise.
11. What is hemodilution and how does the endocrine system relate to it?

References

1. Costill, D.L., Coyle, E., Dalsky, G., Evans, W., Fink, W., & Hoopes, D. (1977). Effects of elevated plasma FFA and insulin on muscle glycogen usage during exercise. *Journal of Applied Physiology*, **43**, 695-699.

2. Costill, D.L., & Fink, W.J. (1974). Plasma volume

changes following exercise and thermal dehydration. *Journal of Applied Physiology*, **37**, 521-525.

3. Dill, D.B., & Costill, D.L. (1974). Calculation of percentage changes in volumes of blood, plasma, and red cells in dehydration. *Journal of Applied Physiology*, **37**, 247-248.

4. Edington, D.W., & Edgerton, V.R. (1976). *The biology of physical activity*. Boston: Houghton Mifflin.

5. Krotkiewski, M., & Gorski, J. (1986). Effect of muscular exercise on plasma C-peptide and insulin in obese non-diabetics and diabetics, Type II. *Clinical Physiology*, **6**, 499-506.

6. Sutton, J.R., & Farrell, P.A. (1988). Endocrine responses to prolonged exercise. In D. Lamb and R. Murray (Eds.), *Perspectives in exercise science and sports medicine: Prolonged exercise* (Vol. 1). Indianapolis, IN: Benchmark Press.

Selected Readings

Costill, D.L., Branam, G., Fink, W., & Nelson, R. (1976). Exercise induced sodium conservation: Changes in plasma renin and aldosterone. *Medicine and Science in Sports*, **8**, 209-213.

Costill, D.L., Cote, R., Miller, E., Miller, T., & Wynder, S. (1975). Water and electrolyte replacement during repeated days of work in heat. *Aviation, Space, and Environmental Medicine*, **46**, 795-800.

Farrell, P.A., Gates, W.K., Morgan, W.P., & Pert, C.B. (1983). Plasma leucine enkephalin-like radioreceptor activity and tension-anxiety before and after competitive running. In H.G. Knuttgen, J.A. Vogel, & J. Poortmans (Eds.), *Biochemistry of exercise* (pp. 637-644). Champaign, IL: Human Kinetics.

Galbo, H. (1983). *Hormonal and metabolic adaptation to exercise*. New York: Thieme-Stratton.

Ginzel, K.H. (1977). Interaction of somatic and autonomic functions in muscular exercise. *Exercise and Sport Sciences Reviews*, **4**, 35-86.

Grossman, A., Bouloux, P., Price, P., Drury, P.L., Lam, K.S.L., Turner, T., Thomas, J., Besser, G.M., & Sutton, J. (1984). The role of opioid peptides in the hormonal responses to acute exercise in man. *Clinical Science*, **67**, 483-491.

Shangold, M.M. (1984). Exercise and the adult female: hormonal and endocrine effects. *Exercise and Sport Sciences Reviews*, **12**, 53-79.

Shephard, R.J., & Sidney, K.H. (1975). Effects of physical exercise on plasma growth hormone and cortisol levels in human subjects. *Exercise and Sport Sciences Reviews*, **3**, 1-30.

Sutton, J.R., Farrell, P.A., & Harber, V.J. (1990). Hormonal adaptations to physical activity. In C. Bouchard, R. Shephard, T. Stephens, J. Sutton, & B. McPherson (Eds.), *Exercise fitness and health*. Champaign, IL: Human Kinetics Publishers.

Terjung, R. (1979). Endocrine response to exercise. *Exercise and Sport Sciences Reviews*, **7**, 153-180.

Vander, A.J., Sherman, J.H., & Luciano, D.S. (1980). *Human physiology: The mechanisms of body function* (3rd ed.). New York: McGraw-Hill.

Wade, C.E. (1984). Response, regulation, and actions of vasopressin during exercise: A review. *Medicine and Science in Sports and Exercise*, **16**, 506-511.

Winder, W.W. (1985). Regulation of hepatic glucose production during exercise. *Exercise and Sport Sciences Reviews*, **13**, 1-31.

Chapter 7

Metabolic Adaptations to Training

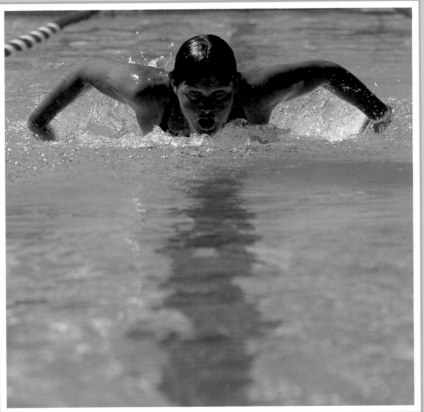

© F-Stock/Chris Huskinson

Chapter Overview

We have discussed how our bodies utilize the foods we eat and the nutrients we store to produce the energy needed for physical activity, and we've examined the endocrine system's role in regulating the various metabolic processes that occur during exercise. But how can we maximize our potential to perform? How can we maximize our energy?

The answer is we train. In this chapter, we turn our attention to the ways in which our bodies adapt to the repeated stimulus of training. Our focus will be on the metabolic adaptations that enhance our capacity for physical activity. We will discuss adaptations occurring within the muscles and in the energy systems that allow us to more efficiently use our energy. We will examine the effects of both aerobic and anaerobic training and consider how we can maximize the improvements we gain from these types of training.

Chapter Outline

Jim's wife thought he was crazy when he began jogging, at age 37, a few times per week with some friends. After all, he had never been interested in sports and had always shied away from any form of exercise. Despite his muscle soreness and inability to keep pace with the other runners, Jim increased his training sessions to six times per week. After eight weeks of this new exercise regimen, he suddenly realized that it was relatively easy to keep pace with the other runners. In fact, he had become the leader of the group and often felt as if he had to slow down to stay with the others. When the other runners decided to increase their training in preparation to run the Boston marathon, Jim considered it a challenge and joined the group in running 60 to 70 miles per week. During the race, he was able to run well ahead of his training partners, finishing more than an hour before them in a time of 2 hr 45 min—a time that placed him in the top 3% of the 9,540 runners in the race. Suddenly, it was apparent that Jim was gifted with an unusual capacity for endurance running, a talent that could only be realized after his body had been stimulated to adapt to the stresses of hard training.

Not all of the mechanisms that are responsible for improving muscular strength and endurance are fully understood. Nevertheless, we have been able to identify many of the metabolic and morphological changes that accompany days and weeks of daily activity. Aerobic training, for example, leads to improved central and peripheral blood flow and an enhanced capacity of the muscle fibers to generate greater amounts of ATP. Anaerobic training, on the other hand, leads to increased muscular strength and a greater tolerance for acid-base imbalances during highly intense effort. In the following pages we discuss the importance of various metabolic changes that accompany physical training, and we discover how these changes can benefit physical performance.

Adaptations to Aerobic Training

Improvements in endurance that accompany daily aerobic training, such as jogging or swimming, result from many adaptations to the training stimulus. Some adaptations occur within the muscles, and many involve changes in the energy systems. Still other changes occur in the cardiovascular system, improving circulation to and within the muscles. In the following discussion, we will focus on the muscular adaptations that occur with endurance training. (Cardiorespiratory adaptations to endurance training will be discussed in detail in chapter 10).

Adaptations in Muscle

Repeated use of muscle fibers stimulates changes in their structure and function. Many of these were dis-

cussed in chapter 4 with reference to resistance training but our main interest here will be on endurance training and the changes it produces in

- muscle fiber type,
- capillary supply,
- myoglobin content,
- mitochondrial function, and
- oxidative enzymes.

Muscle Fiber Type

Aerobic activities such as jogging and low- to moderate-intensity cycling rely extensively on the slow-twitch (ST) fibers. In response to the training stimulus, these fibers become 7% to 22% larger than the corresponding fast-twitch (FT) fibers.[5] But fiber size varies considerably in different athletes. Some individuals have unusually large ST fibers, but others have large FT fibers. This observation may be of only academic importance though, because muscle fiber sizes in endurance athletes seem to have little relationship to the athletes' aerobic capacity or performance. Fiber size may be more critical in events that demand great power and strength, such as sprinting and weight lifting, in which larger FT fibers would be beneficial.

Most studies have shown that endurance training doesn't change the percentage of ST and FT fibers. Current evidence tends to support this concept, but some subtle changes have been noted among FT fiber subtypes. FT_b fibers are apparently used less often than FT_a fibers, and for that reason they have a lower aerobic capacity. Long-duration exercise may eventually recruit these fibers into action, demanding them to perform in a manner normally expected of the FT_a fibers. Recent evidence indicates that many years of endurance training can cause some FT$_b$ fibers to take on some characteristics of the more oxidative FT$_a$ fibers. Neither the cause nor the consequences of this change are known. This subtle conversion of FT$_b$ to FT$_a$ fibers may simply reflect the greater use of the fast-twitch fibers during long, exhaustive training.

Capillary Supply

One of the most important adaptations to endurance training is an increase in the number of capillaries surrounding each muscle fiber. The micrographs shown in Figure 7.1 illustrate that endurance-trained men can have 5% to 10% more capillaries in their leg muscles than sedentary individuals.[9,11] With longer periods of endurance training, the number of capillaries has been shown to increase by as much as 15%.[9] Having more capillaries allows greater exchange of gases, heat, wastes, and nutrients between the blood and the working muscle fibers. This maintains an environment well suited to energy production and repeated muscle contractions. Substantial increases in muscle capillary number occur within the first few weeks or months

of training. But little research has been performed to determine what capillary changes occur with longer training periods.

KEY POINT

Aerobic training increases both the number of capillaries per muscle fiber and the number of capillaries for a given cross-sectional area of muscle. Both of these changes improve blood perfusion in the muscles.

Myoglobin Content

When oxygen enters the muscle fiber, it binds to myoglobin, a compound similar to hemoglobin. This iron-containing compound shuttles the oxygen molecules from the cell membrane to the mitochondria. The ST fibers contain large quantities, which give these fibers their red appearance (myoglobin is a pigment that turns red when bound to oxygen). The FT fibers, on the

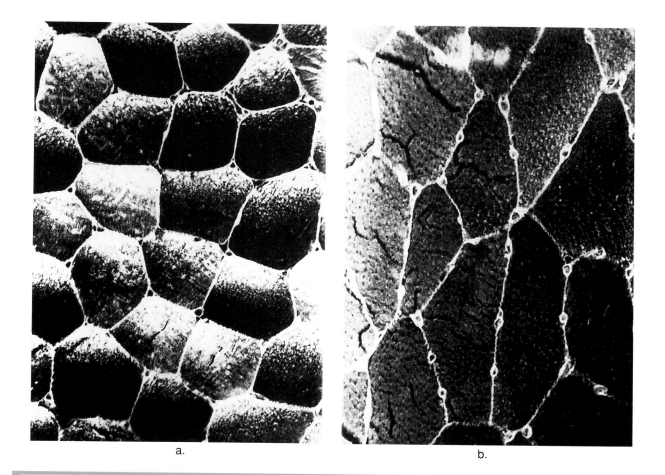

a.   b.

Figure 7.1   Micrographs of the capillaries around the muscle fibers of (a) an untrained man and (b) a trained distance runner.

other hand, are highly glycolytic, so they require (and have) little myoglobin, giving them a whiter appearance. More importantly, their limited myoglobin supply limits their oxygen capacity, resulting in poor aerobic endurance.

Myoglobin stores oxygen and releases it to the mitochondria when oxygen becomes limited during muscle action. This oxygen reserve is used during the transition from rest to exercise, providing oxygen to the mitochondria during the lag between the beginning of exercise and the increased cardiovascular delivery of oxygen.

Myoglobin's precise contributions to oxygen delivery are not yet fully understood. But endurance training has been shown to increase muscle myoglobin content by 75% to 80%. This adaptation would be expected only if it furthers a muscle's capacity for oxidative metabolism.

Mitochondrial Function

As noted in chapter 5, aerobic energy production is conducted in the mitochondria. Not surprisingly then, endurance training also induces changes in mitochondrial function that improve the muscle fibers' capacity to produce ATP. The ability to use oxygen and produce ATP via oxidation depends on the number, size, and efficiency of the muscle's mitochondria. All three of these qualities improve with endurance training.

During one study that involved endurance training in rats, the actual number of mitochondria increased approximately 15% during 27 weeks of exercise.[10] At the same time, the average mitochondrial size also increased, by about 35%, over the entire period. We now know that as the volume of aerobic training is increased, so are the number and the size of the mitochondria.

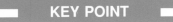

KEY POINT

Skeletal muscle mitochondria increase both in size and number with aerobic training, providing the muscle with much more efficient oxidative metabolism.

Oxidative Enzymes

Increasing the number and size of the mitochondria alone increases our muscles' aerobic capacity, but these changes are further enhanced by an increase in mitochondrial efficiency. Recall from chapter 5 that the oxidative breakdown of fuels and the ultimate production of ATP depends on the action of mitochondrial enzymes. Endurance training increases these enzymes' activities.

Figure 7.2 illustrates the changes in the activity of succinate dehydrogenase (SDH), one of the muscles' key oxidative enzymes, during 7 months of gradually increased swimming training. Interestingly, although these enzyme activities continued to rise throughout the period of training, little change in the body's maximal oxygen uptake ($\dot{V}O_2$ max) occurred during the final 6 weeks of training. This suggests that $\dot{V}O_2$ max might be more influenced by the circulatory system's limitations for transporting oxygen than by the muscles' oxidative potential.

The activities of muscle enzymes such as succinate dehydrogenase and citrate synthase are dramatically influenced by endurance training. This is seen in Figure 7.3, which compares the activities of these enzymes in untrained (UT), moderately trained (MT), and highly trained (HT) people. Even moderate amounts of daily exercise increase these enzyme activities and thus the muscles' aerobic capacity. For example, jogging or cycling for as little as 20 min per

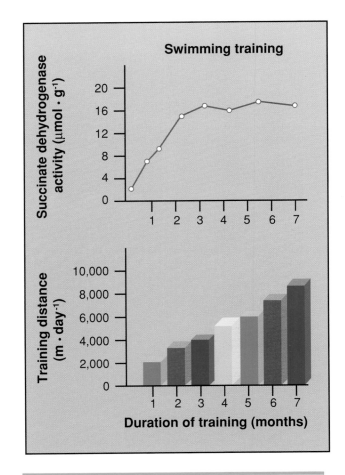

Figure 7.2 Changes in succinate dehydrogenase activity (deltoid muscle) during gradually increased swimming training.

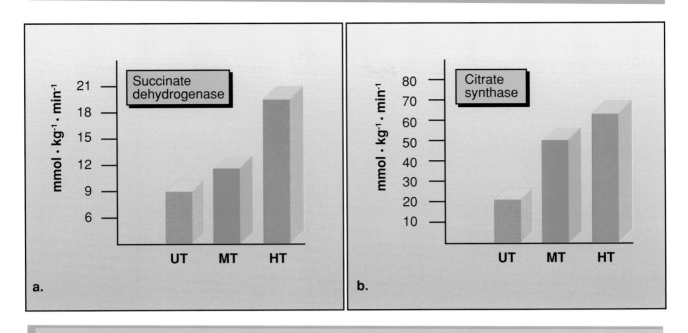

Figure 7.3   Leg muscle (gastrocnemius) enzyme activities of untrained (UT) subjects, moderately trained (MT) joggers, and highly trained (HT) marathon runners. Enzyme levels shown are for (a) succinate dehydrogenase and (b) citrate synthase, two of many enzymes that participate in the oxidative production of ATP. Adapted from Costill et al., (1979).

day has been shown to increase the leg muscles' SDH activity by more than 25% above that in sedentary individuals. Training more vigorously, such as 60 to 90 min per day, produces a 2.6-fold increase in this activity.

The training-induced increase in the activities of these oxidative enzymes reflects both the increase in the number and size of a muscle's mitochondria and an improved capacity for ATP production. Initially, the enzyme activity increase coincides with improvements in the individual's $\dot{V}O_2$ max. But we are uncertain whether there is a cause and effect relationship. Little is known about why training enhances oxidative enzyme activities within skeletal muscles. Moreover, the role of this increased activity is not well understood. These changes can be regarded as important either for the tissue's utilization of oxygen during exercise or to induce a glycogen-saving effect. Either can enhance endurance performance. But at best, only a weak relationship exists between muscle oxidative enzyme activities and enhancement of $\dot{V}O_2$ max.[8,14]

Some researchers argue that $\dot{V}O_2$ max is controlled by the oxygen transport system (circulation), but others believe that a muscle's oxidative capacity dictates its aerobic capacity. The debate over which system is most important for physiological endurance might be purely academic, however, because adaptations in both systems are essential to enhance the functioning of the oxidative system and endurance performance.

IN REVIEW . . .

1. Endurance training stresses ST muscle fibers more than FT fibers. Consequently, the ST fibers tend to enlarge with training. Although the percentages of ST and FT fibers do not appear to change, endurance training may cause FT_b fibers to take on more FT_a fiber characteristics.
2. The number of capillaries supplying each muscle fiber increases with training.
3. Endurance training increases muscle myoglobin content by about 75% to 80%. Myoglobin stores oxygen.
4. Endurance training increases both the number and the size of the mitochondria.
5. Activities of many oxidative enzymes are increased with training.
6. All of these changes occurring in the muscles, combined with adaptations in the oxygen transport system, lead to enhanced functioning of the oxidative system and improved endurance.

Adaptations Affecting Energy Sources

Aerobic training places repeated demands on muscles' stores of both glycogen and fat. Not surprisingly, our bodies will adapt to this repeated stimulus to make energy production more efficient and to reduce our risk of fatigue. Let's examine the adaptations in the way a trained body metabolizes both carbohydrate and fat for energy.

Carbohydrate for Energy

Muscle glycogen is used extensively during each training bout, so the mechanisms responsible for its resynthesis are stimulated after each session while the depleted glycogen stores are being replenished. With adequate rest and sufficient dietary carbohydrate, trained muscle stores considerably more glycogen than untrained muscle does. When distance runners, for example, stop training for several days and eat a diet rich in carbohydrates (400 to 550 g · day⁻¹), their muscle glycogen levels increase to nearly twice the levels of sedentary people who follow the same dietary regimen. More glycogen storage allows the athlete to better tolerate the subsequent demands of training because more fuel is available for use. Additional information regarding the dietary needs for training will be provided in chapter 15.

Fat for Energy

In addition to its greater glycogen content, endurance-trained muscle contains substantially more fat, stored as triglyceride, than is found in untrained fibers. Although information is limited about the mechanisms responsible for this improvement in fuel storage with endurance training, a 1.8-fold increase in muscle triglyceride content has been reported after only 8 weeks of endurance running.[7] In general, as shown in Figure 7.4, the vacuoles that contain triglyceride are distributed throughout the muscle fiber but are generally close to the mitochondria. Thus they can be easily accessed for use as fuel during exercise.

In addition, activities of many muscle enzymes responsible for the β oxidation of fat are increased with endurance training. This adaptation enables endurance-trained muscle to burn fat more efficiently, lessening the demands placed on a muscle's glycogen supply. Muscle samples taken from men's thighs before and after cycle training have shown a 30% increase in the ability to oxidize free fatty acids. Endurance training also increases the rate at which free fatty acids

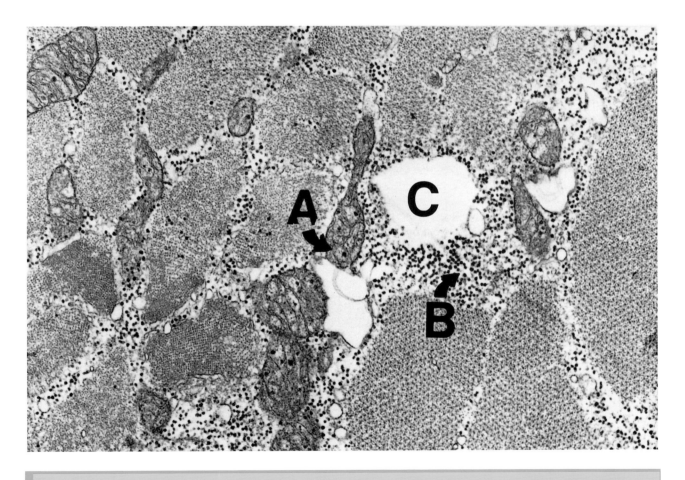

Figure 7.4   An electron micrograph showing (A) mitochondria, (B) muscle glycogen granules, and (C) triglyceride vacuoles.

are released from storage during prolonged exercise, making them readily available for the muscles' use.

Issekutz et al. observed that this elevation of blood levels of FFA enables the muscle to burn more fat and less carbohydrate.[12] Subsequent studies have shown that by elevating blood FFA levels, muscle glycogen can be spared, postponing exhaustion.[3,13] For any given rate of work, trained individuals tend to use more fat than carbohydrate for energy than untrained people do.

KEY POINT

With aerobic training, you become much more efficient at using fat as an energy source for exercise. This allows muscle and liver glycogen to be used at a slower rate.

IN REVIEW . . .

1. Endurance-trained muscle stores considerably more glycogen than does untrained muscle.
2. Endurance-trained muscle also stores more fat (triglyceride) than does untrained muscle.
3. The activities of many enzymes involved in β oxidation of fat increase with training, thus free fatty acid levels increase. This leads to increased use of fat as an energy source, sparing glycogen.

To summarize, improvements in muscle's aerobic energy system result in a greater capacity to produce energy, with a shift toward more reliance on fat for ATP production. Endurance-trained muscle's improved capacity to utilize fat is due to the enhanced ability to mobilize FFA and the improved capacity to oxidize fat. In activities lasting several hours, these adaptations prevent early muscle glycogen depletion and thus insure a continued supply of ATP. Thus endurance performance is enhanced.

Training the Aerobic System

In the laboratory, researchers can measure the aerobic capacity of a specimen of muscle obtained by a needle biopsy. By grinding the muscle sample in a solution containing other essential items, the mitochondria are stimulated to use oxygen and to produce ATP. As a result, the maximal rate at which the muscle's mitochondria use oxygen to generate ATP can be measured. This procedure, therefore, measures the muscle's maximal respiratory capacity, or $\dot{Q}_{O_2}$. In effect, $\dot{Q}_{O_2}$ is a measure of the muscle's maximal oxygen uptake (in contrast to $\dot{V}_{O_2 max}$, which is a measure of the body's maximal oxygen uptake).

For Figure 7.5, samples from the gastrocnemius muscles of three groups of people showed that untrained muscles have $\dot{Q}_{O_2}$ values of about 1.5 L of oxygen per hour for each gram of muscle ($L \cdot hr^{-1} \cdot g^{-1}$). In contrast, muscles from individuals who expend

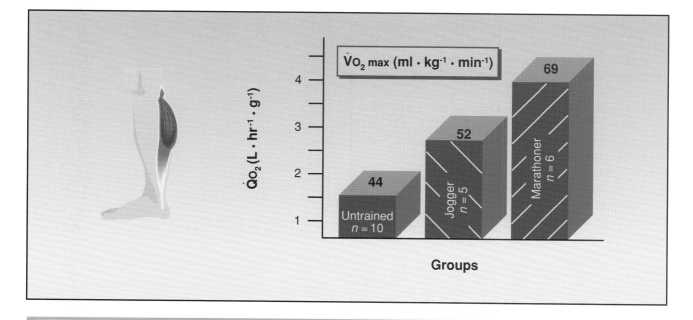

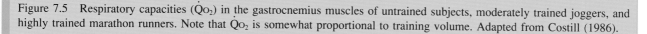

Figure 7.5   Respiratory capacities ($\dot{Q}_{O_2}$) in the gastrocnemius muscles of untrained subjects, moderately trained joggers, and highly trained marathon runners. Note that $\dot{Q}_{O_2}$ is somewhat proportional to training volume. Adapted from Costill (1986).

1,500 to 2,500 kcal · week⁻¹ during training (such as jogging 25 to 40 km · week⁻¹) have $\dot{Q}_{O_2}$ values around 2.7 L · hr⁻¹ · g⁻¹, which is 1.8 times greater than that of untrained people. Highly trained marathon runners, such as those who expend over 5,000 kcal · week⁻¹ (about 80 km · week⁻¹) in training, have displayed $\dot{Q}_{O_2}$ values in excess of 4.0 L · hr⁻¹ · g⁻¹, nearly 2.7 times greater than people with untrained muscle.

As you increase your total body's aerobic capacity, there is also an increase in the maximal oxidative or respiratory capacity ($\dot{Q}_{O_2}$) of your muscle. The highest average $\dot{Q}_{O_2}$ values reported in human muscle (5.2 L · hr⁻¹ · g⁻¹) are those in the deltoid muscles of swimmers who had expended more than 10,000 kcal · week⁻¹ during training.[1]

Clearly, endurance-trained individuals have an advantage over those who are less trained. But how do they gain this advantage? In the following sections, we will examine various aspects of endurance training in an effort to understand how we can maximize aerobic benefits from training.

Volume of Training

Training adaptations are best achieved when an optimal amount of work is performed in each training session and over a given period of time. Although this optimal load may differ from one individual to another, observations with distance runners suggest that, on the average, the ideal training regimen may be equivalent to an energy expenditure of between 5,000 and 6,000 kcal · week⁻¹ (approximately 715 to 860 kcal · day⁻¹). This translates to between 80 and 95 km of running per week.[2] To achieve the same aerobic benefits, swimmers would need to swim roughly 4,000 to 6,000 m · day⁻¹.[6] Of course, these are only estimates of the stimulus required for muscular conditioning. Some individuals may show greater improvement with less training, but others may require more.

How much your aerobic capacity improves is determined, in part, by how many calories you expend during each training bout and how much work you accomplish over a period of weeks. Many athletes and coaches believe this means that gains in aerobic endurance will be proportional to the volume of training. If training volume were the most important stimulus for muscular adaptations, individuals who expend the most energy during training should have the highest $\dot{V}_{O_2\,max}$ values. But this is not the case.

The amount of improvement attainable with endurance training seems to have an upper limit. Athletes who train with progressively greater work loads will eventually reach a maximal level of improvement beyond which additional increases in training volume won't improve endurance or $\dot{V}_{O_2\,max}$. This is illustrated in Figure 7.6, which shows the changes in $\dot{V}_{O_2\,max}$ for two distance runners prior to and at various levels of training. The runners' $\dot{V}_{O_2\,max}$ increased dramatically with the initiation of training (40 km · week⁻¹), and continued to improve when they increased their training to 80 km · week⁻¹. Beyond that level of training, however, these individuals had no additional gains in endurance. During a 1-month period, they increased their training to over 350 km (217 mi) per week, and still showed no further improvement in endurance.[2]

Some athletes try to perform more physical work by training twice each day, doubling their normal training volume. If an athlete is already expending 1,000 kcal · day⁻¹ in training, a second training session is unlikely to produce additional benefits. (This is discussed further in chapter 13.)

Intensity of Training

The degree of adaptation to endurance training depends not only on training volume, but also on training intensity. Let's briefly consider the importance of training intensity for performance in prolonged events (this topic will be examined more closely in chapter 13).

Muscular adaptations are specific to both the speed and duration of effort performed during training.

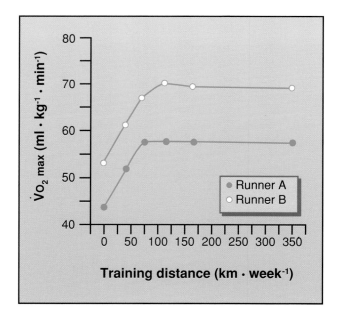

Figure 7.6   Changes in $\dot{V}_{O_2}$ max for two distance runners while they trained at various distances. Training 40 to 80 km per week resulted in improvement in aerobic capacity, whereas greater training distances produced no additional increase. Adapted from Costill (1986).

Runners, cyclists, and swimmers who incorporate intermittent, high-intensity bouts of exercise into their training regimen show more improvement in performance than those who perform only long, slow, low-intensity training bouts. Long-distance, low-intensity training doesn't develop the neurological patterns of muscle fiber recruitment and the high rate of energy production required for maximal endurance performance.

High-intensity speed training can include either intermittent exercise (intervals) or continuous exercise at near-competition pace. Let's look at the benefits from each type of training.

Interval Training

Although it has been used for many years, most athletes use interval training mainly to improve their anaerobic capacity. Consequently, most repeated exercise bouts are performed at speeds that produce large amounts of lactate. But this training format can also be used to develop the aerobic system. Repeated fast-paced and brief exercise bouts that allow short rest intervals between bouts achieve the same aerobic benefits as long, high-intensity continuous exercise.

This form of aerobic interval training has become the framework for aerobic conditioning, particularly in competitive swimming. It involves repeated short efforts lasting from 30 s to 5 min (50 to 400 m of swimming) performed slightly slower than race pace, but with very brief rest intervals (5 to 15 s). Such short rest intervals force the participant to exercise at an aerobic level, placing little reliance on the glycolytic lactate-producing system.

Table 7.1 offers an example of an aerobic interval training program for runners. Because volume is the key to successful aerobic training, the runner must perform a large number of these repeated runs. In this example, 20 repetitions of 400 m are performed, resulting in a total run of 8,000 m (approximately 5 mi). The pace maintained is slightly slower than that used during the 10-km race, in this case slower by 8 to 10 s per 400 m. Yet this pace is generally faster than could be sustained easily during a continuous 8,000-m run. The difficulty of this interval set is that

the prescribed rest between repetitions must be relatively brief— only about 10 to 15 s. Such short rest intervals allow little time for muscles to recover, yet they provide a brief respite from the muscular stress.

Continuous Training

It can be argued that a single, continuous bout of high-intensity exercise can give the same aerobic benefits as a set of aerobic intervals. But some athletes find continuous endurance exercise to be boring. For the aerobic aspects of training, personal preference may be the deciding factor. At present, no direct evidence shows that aerobic interval training produces greater muscular adaptations than continuous training bouts. Whether the training is performed as one long bout of continuous exercise or in a series of shorter intervals, the aerobic muscular benefits seem to be about the same.

IN REVIEW . . .

1. The ideal training regimen should have a caloric expenditure of about 5,000 to 6,000 kcal · week^{-1}. There seems to be little benefit beyond this level.
2. Intensity is also a critical factor in improving performance. Adaptations are specific to the speed and duration of training bouts, so those who perform at higher intensities must train at higher intensities.
3. Aerobic interval training involves repeated bouts of high-intensity performance separated by brief rest periods. This training, although traditionally considered only anaerobic, generates aerobic benefits because the rest period is so brief that full recovery can't occur, thus the aerobic system is stressed.
4. Continuous training is done as one prolonged bout of exercise, but many athletes find it boring.
5. The aerobic benefits from both interval training and continuous high-intensity training seem to be about the same.

Table 7.1 Example of Aerobic Intervals for Runners Training to Run a 10-km Race

Best 10 km (min:s)	Reps	Interval distance (m)	Rest (s)	Pace (min:s)
46:00	20	400	10-15	2:00
43:00	20	400	10-15	1:52
40:00	20	400	10-15	1:45
37:00	20	400	10-15	1:37
34:00	20	400	10-15	1:30

Adaptations to Anaerobic Training

In muscular activities that require near-maximal force production, such as sprint running and swimming, much of the energy needs are met by the ATP-PCr system and the anaerobic breakdown of muscle glycogen (glycolysis). In the following discussion, we'll focus on the trainability of these two systems.

Adaptations in the ATP-PCr System

Activities that emphasize maximal muscle force production, such as sprinting and weight lifting events, rely most heavily on the ATP-PCr system for energy. Maximal efforts lasting less than about 6 s place the greatest demands on the breakdown and resynthesis of ATP and PCr. Few studies have examined the training adaptations to short, maximal exercise bouts that are aimed specifically at developing the ATP-PCr system. In 1979, however, Costill et al. reported their findings from one such study.[4] The participants performed maximal knee extensions for training. One leg was trained using 6-s maximal work bouts that were repeated 10 times. This type of training preferentially stresses the ATP-PCr energy system. The other leg was trained with repeated 30-s maximal bouts, which, instead, preferentially stresses the glycolytic system.

Both forms of training produced the same muscular strength gains (about 14%) and the same resistance to fatigue. As seen in Figure 7.7, the activities of the muscle enzymes creatine phosphokinase (CPK) and myokinase (MK) increased as a result of the 30-s training bouts, but were unchanged in the leg trained with repeated 6-s maximal efforts. These findings lead us to conclude that maximal sprint bouts (6-s) might improve muscular strength, but contribute little to the mechanisms responsible for ATP breakdown. Such training will enhance performance by improving strength, but will result in little or no improvement in the energy release from ATP and PCr.

Another study, however, showed improvements in these ATP-PCr enzyme activities with training bouts lasting only 5 s.[16] Regardless of the conflicting results, these studies suggest that the major value for training bouts that last only a few seconds (sprints) is the development of muscular strength. Such strength gains enable the individual to perform a given task with less effort, which reduces the risk of fatigue. Whether or not these changes allow the muscle to perform more anaerobic work remains unanswered, although a 60-s sprint-fatigue test suggests that short sprint-type anaerobic training does not enhance anaerobic endurance.[4]

Adaptations in the Glycolytic System

Anaerobic training (30-s bouts) increases the activities of several key glycolytic and oxidative enzymes. The most frequently studied glycolytic enzymes are phosphorylase, phosphofructokinase (PFK), and lactate dehydrogenase (LDH). The activities of these three enzymes increase 10% to 25% with repeated 30-s training bouts, but change little with short (6-s) bouts that stress primarily the ATP-PCr system.[4] Because both PFK and phosphorylase are essential to the anaerobic yield of ATP, such training might be thought to en-

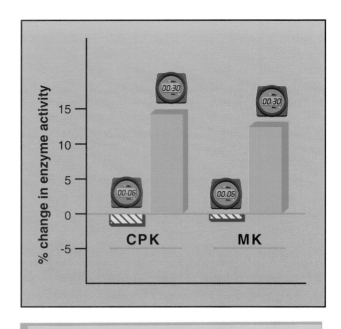

Figure 7.7   Changes in creatine phosphokinase (CPK) and muscle myokinase (MK) activities as a result of 6-s and 30-s bouts of maximal anaerobic training.

hance glycolytic capacity and to allow the muscle to develop greater tension for a longer period of time.

However, as seen in Figure 7.8, this conclusion is not supported by results of the 60-s sprint performance test, in which the subjects performed maximal knee extensions and flexions. Power output and the rate of fatigue (shown by a decrease in power production) were affected to the same degree after sprint training with both 6- and 30-s training bouts. Thus we must conclude that performance gains with these forms of training result from improvements in strength rather than improvements in the anaerobic yield of ATP.

> ### ■ KEY POINT ■
>
> **Anaerobic training increases the ATP-PCr and glycolytic enzymes but has no effect on the oxidative enzymes. Conversely, aerobic training leads to increases in the oxidative enzymes, but has no effect on the ATP-PCr or glycolytic enzymes. This reinforces a recurring theme — physiological alterations resulting from training are highly specific to the type of training pursued.**

Other Adaptations to Anaerobic Training

How else might anaerobic (sprint) training improve performance? In addition to strength gains, at least

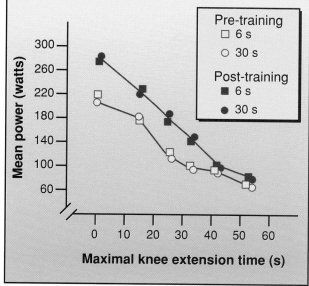

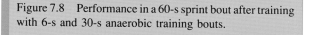

Figure 7.8   Performance in a 60-s sprint bout after training with 6-s and 30-s anaerobic training bouts.

three other changes may enhance performance and delay fatigue in highly anaerobic events. These three changes are improvements in

- efficiency of movement,
- aerobic energetics, and
- buffering capacity.

Efficiency of Movement

Training at high speeds improves your skill and your coordination for performing at higher intensities. From our discussion of selective muscle fiber recruitment in chapter 2, we can assume that anaerobic training optimizes fiber recruitment to allow more efficient movement. Training at fast speeds and with heavy loads improves your efficiency, economizing your use of the muscles' energy supply.

Aerobic Energetics

Anaerobic training doesn't stress only the anaerobic energy systems. Part of the energy needed for sprints that last at least 30 s is derived from oxidative metabolism. Consequently, repeated bouts of sprint-type exercise (such as with 30-s maximal effort bouts) also increase the muscles' aerobic capacity.[4,14] Although this change is often small, we can reasonably expect that this enhancement of the muscles' oxidative potential will assist the anaerobic energy systems' efforts

to meet muscle energy needs during highly anaerobic effort.

Buffering Capacity

Anaerobic training improves the muscles' capacity to tolerate the acid that accumulates within them during anaerobic glycolysis. As discussed in chapter 5, lactic acid accumulation is considered a major cause of fatigue during sprint-type exercise because the H^+ that dissociates from it is thought to interfere with both metabolism and the contractile process. Buffers (such as bicarbonate and muscle phosphates) combine with hydrogen to reduce the fiber's acidity; thus they can delay the onset of fatigue during anaerobic exercise.

Eight weeks of anaerobic training has been shown to increase muscle buffering capacity by 12% to 50%.[15] Aerobic training, on the other hand, has no effect on buffer potential. As with other training adaptations, changes in muscle buffering capacity are specific to the intensity of exercise performed during training.

KEY POINT

Although anaerobic training improves muscle buffering capacity, aerobic training does little to enhance the muscles' capacity to tolerate sprint-type activities.

With this increased buffering capacity, sprint-trained subjects can accumulate more lactate in their blood and muscles during and following an all-out sprint to exhaustion than untrained individuals can. This is because the H^+ that dissociates from the lactic acid, not the lactate that accumulates, leads to fatigue. With enhanced buffering capacity, muscles can generate energy for longer periods before a critically high concentration of H^+ inhibits the contractile process.

Interestingly, under similar circumstances (such as sprinting to exhaustion), endurance-trained subjects neither accumulate as much muscle lactate as nor experience the unusually low pH values seen in sprint-trained men. This difference is difficult to explain, but muscle pH doesn't appear to limit sprint performance for endurance-trained people. Table 7.2 shows the activities of selected muscle enzymes from the three energy systems. These enzyme activities are shown for untrained, anaerobically trained, and aerobically trained individuals. This table shows that aerobically trained muscles have significantly lower glycolytic enzyme activities. Thus they might have less capacity for anaerobic metabolism or they might rely less on energy from glycolysis. More research is needed to

Table 7.2 Selected Muscle Enzyme Activities (mmol • g^{-1} • min^{-1}) for Untrained, Anaerobically Trained, and Aerobically Trained Men

	Untrained	Anaerobically trained	Aerobically trained
Aerobic enzymes			
Oxidative system			
Succinate dehydrogenase	8.1	8.0	20.8[a]
Malate dehydrogenase	45.5	46.0	65.5[a]
Carnitine palmityl transferase	1.5	1.5	2.3[a]
Anaerobic enzymes			
ATP-PCr system			
Creatine phosphokinase	609.0	702.0[a]	589.0
Myokinase	309.0	350.0[a]	297.0
Glycolytic system			
Phosphorylase	5.3	5.8	3.7[a]
Phosphofructokinase	19.9	29.2[a]	18.9
Lactate dehydrogenase	766.0	811.0	621.0

[a]Denotes a significant difference from the untrained value.

explain the implications of the muscular changes accompanying both anaerobic and aerobic training.

■ IN REVIEW . . . ■

1. Anaerobic training bouts improve anaerobic performance, but the improvement appears to result more from strength gains than from improvements in the functioning of the anaerobic energy systems.
2. Anaerobic training also improves the efficiency of movement, and more efficient movement requires less energy expenditure.
3. Although sprint-type exercise is anaerobic by nature, part of the energy used during longer sprint bouts comes from oxidation, so muscle aerobic capacity can also be increased with this type of training.
4. Muscle buffering capacity is increased by anaerobic training, allowing the achievement of higher muscle and blood lactate levels. This allows the H^+ that dissociates from lactic acid to be neutralized, thus delaying fatigue.

Monitoring Training Changes

The goal of any training program is simple: Improve performance. Muscular adaptations are not instantaneous and maximal improvements in the muscles' energy systems can require months of training. To be sure that a particular program is meeting the athlete's expectations, the results must be monitored throughout the training period. Unfortunately, judging improvements gained from training is not easy. In this section we will examine how assessing some physiological changes can be used to monitor an individual's progress.

Some investigators feel that the best way to judge cardiorespiratory and muscular adaptations that accompany training is to evaluate the athlete's aerobic capacity—$\dot{V}O_{2\ max}$. This requires the sophisticated equipment found in an exercise physiology laboratory. Because the ability to employ this test is limited by access to a properly equipped laboratory, the test is unavailable to most coaches and athletes. Additionally, it doesn't measure muscular adaptations associated with anaerobic and aerobic training.

In recent years, sports physiologists have proposed that the blood lactate level during training might provide a gauge of training stress and a means to monitor muscle adaptations. Blood lactate accumulates suddenly during incremental exercise. This sudden change might provide a means by which to judge the exercise intensity (the training stimulus). As illustrated in Figure 7.9, endurance training raises the lactate threshold (the point at which blood lactate begins to accumulate). Endurance-trained individuals can exercise at a higher percentage of their $\dot{V}O_{2\ max}$ before blood lactate begins to accumulate. Although this phenomenon has been interpreted in different ways, most view it as a good predictor of endurance performance, and it is more sensitive than $\dot{V}O_{2\ max}$ for detecting training-induced changes.

Blood lactate measurement has been adapted for use with various sports, such as running and swimming. Athletes are asked to perform a series of standard fixed-pace exercise bouts at varied intensities, with 30 to 60 min of rest between efforts. Blood drawn from a forearm vein or fingertip is used to measure lactate after each exercise bout. These values are then graphed against the athlete's running or swimming velocity.

Although these tests offer sensitive methods for monitoring both exercise intensity and training adaptations, they require far too much time and technology to be routinely used in most sports. The need for repeated blood samples and the time required for these measurements do not justify the value of such testing. This has led to use of a simpler protocol to monitor training: measurement of blood lactate accumulation after a single standard fixed-pace exercise bout. The slope of the blood lactate–swimming velocity curve remains relatively unchanged with training. Thus we can judge the training effect on muscle metabolism by having the swimmer perform a single exercise trial at a controlled speed. For example, a 200-m swim in which the swimmer's pace is regulated has been used to study adaptations during a training season. The swimmer performs this swim at the same pace at various points during training.

The results of a study using this technique are shown in Figure 7.10. Blood lactate accumulation following such a standardized swim declined steadily in these swimmers over a 7-month training period. This suggests that they were developing either a greater aerobic capacity or a reduced reliance on the glycolytic system for energy, and perhaps both.

Other attempts to monitor training appear to be less sensitive and less reliable, as well as more expen-

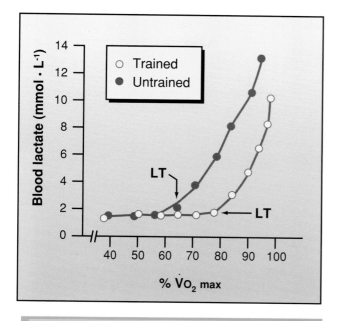

Figure 7.9   Effects of endurance training on blood lactate threshold (LT).

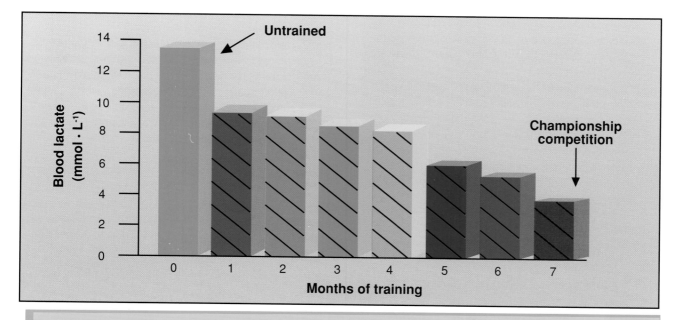

Figure 7.10   Effects of training on blood lactate concentration after a 200-m swim at a predetermined speed. The lowest lactate values were recorded during the period when the swimmers produced their best performances.

KEY POINT

The concentration of lactate in the blood following a fixed-pace swim or run provides an excellent means of monitoring the physiological changes that occur with training. As you become better trained, the blood lactate concentration is lower for the same rate of work.

sive and too time-consuming for use with athletes. But even this single measurement of blood lactate requires expensive equipment and trained personnel. In addition, controversy surrounds the use and interpretation of the findings from such testing. Should the results be used to vary the intensity of training? What physiological adaptations underlie these changes in lactate threshold? These and other questions remain unanswered, but such information is vital to the proper use and interpretation of tests to monitor athletes' muscular adaptations to training.

IN REVIEW . . .

1. Many have considered $\dot{V}O_2$ max to be the best means for evaluating training adaptations. But the test is too impractical for widespread use, and it cannot measure muscle adaptations to training.
2. Multiple measurements of blood lactate levels during an exercise bout of increasing intensity have been proposed as a good means for monitoring progress of training, but these tests are also impractical.
3. Various methods for monitoring training adaptations have been tried, but the easiest seems to be comparing single blood lactate values taken at various times during a training period, after a fixed-pace activity is performed. Even with this method, many questions remain unanswered about what actually happens within the body in response to the training stimulus.

In Closing . . .

In this section, we have focused on the energy needed for physical performance. In chapter 5, we reviewed the systems responsible for the production of energy. In chapter 6, we discussed the regulatory role of the endocrine system. And finally, in this chapter, keeping our focus on energy, we have looked at the adaptations occurring within the muscles and in the energy systems

themselves that accompany aerobic and anaerobic training, and have seen how these types of training can improve performance.

In the next section, we turn our attention to the oxygen transport system. We will begin in chapter 8 with a discussion of the cardiovascular system and its role in transporting oxygen, fuels, nutrients, and hormones throughout our bodies.

Key Terms

aerobic interval training
aerobic training
anaerobic training
buffers

continuous training
interval training
muscle buffering capacity
sprint training

Study Questions

1. What are the effects of aerobic and anaerobic training on muscle fibers?
2. How does aerobic training improve oxygen delivery to the muscle fibers?
3. What effect does aerobic training have on the type of fuels used during exercise?
4. Describe the factors responsible for the improvements in muscle respiratory capacity ($\dot{Q}O_2$) that occur with aerobic training.
5. Give examples of interval training sessions that might be used to develop the ATP-PCr, glycolytic, and oxidative systems for a runner.
6. What changes occur in muscle during anaerobic training that might reduce its fatiguability during highly glycolytic exercise?
7. Describe the changes in muscle buffering capacity resulting from aerobic and anaerobic training. How might this improve performance?
8. What changes might be expected in the lactate threshold as a result of aerobic training? Illustrate the relationship between running speed and blood lactate accumulation.

References

1. Costill, D.L. (1985). Practical problems in exercise physiology research. *Research Quarterly*, **56**, 379-384.

2. Costill, D.L. (1986). *Inside running: Basics of sports physiology* (p. 178). Indianapolis: Benchmark Press.

3. Costill, D.L., Coyle, E., Dalsky, G., Evans, W., Fink, W.W., & Hoopes, D. (1977). Effects of elevated plasma FFA and insulin on muscle glycogen usage during exercise. *Journal of Applied Physiology*, **43**, 695-699.

4. Costill, D.L., Coyle, E.F., Fink, W.F., Lesmes, G.R., & Witzmann, F.A. (1979). Adaptations in skeletal muscle following strength training. *Journal of Applied Physiology: Respiratory Environmental Exercise Physiology*, **46**, 96-99.

5. Costill, D.L., Daniels, J., Evans, W., Fink, W., Krahenbuhl, G., & Saltin, B. (1976). Skeletal muscle enzymes and fiber composition in male and female track athletes. *Journal of Applied Physiology*, **40**, 149-154.

6. Costill, D.L., Thomas, R., Robergs, R.A., Pascoe, D.D., Lambert, C.P., Barr, S.I., & Fink, W.J. (1991). Adaptations to swimming training: Influence of training volume. *Medicine & Science in Sport & Exercise*, **23**, 371-377.

7. Essén, B., Hagenfeldt, L., & Kaijser, L. (1977). Utilization of blood-borne and intramuscular substrates during continuous and intermittent exercise in man. *Journal of Physiology*, **265**, 480-506.

8. Gollnick, P.D., Armstrong, R.B., Saubert IV, C.W., Piehl, K., & Saltin, B. (1972). Enzyme activity and fiber composition in skeletal muscle of untrained and trained men. *Journal of Applied Physiology*, **33**, 312-319.

9. Hermansen, L., & Wachtlova, M. (1971). Capillary density of skeletal muscle in well-trained and untrained men. *Journal of Applied Physiology*, **30**, 860-863.

10. Holloszy, J.O., Oscai, L.B., Mole, P.A., & Don, I.J. (1971). Biochemical adaptations to endurance exercise in skeletal muscle. In B. Pernow and B. Saltin (Eds.), *Muscle metabolism during exercise*. New York: Plenum.

11. Ingjer, F. (1979). Capillary supply and mitochondrial content of different skeletal muscle fiber types in untrained and endurance trained men: A histochemical and ultra structural study. *European Journal of Applied Physiology*, **40**, 197-209.

12. Issekutz, B., Miller, H.I., Paul, P., & Rodahl, K. (1965). Aerobic work capacity and plasma FFA turnover. *Journal of Applied Physiology*, **20**, 293-296.

13. Rennie, M.J., Winder, W.W., & Holloszy, J.O. (1976). A sparing effect of increased plasma fatty acids on muscle and liver glycogen content in exercising rat. *Biochemistry Journal*, **156**, 647-655.

14. Saltin, B., Nazar, K., Costill, D.L., Stein, E., Jansson, E., Essen, B., & Gollnick, P.D. (1976). The nature of the training response: Peripheral and central adaptations to one-legged exercise. *Acta Physiologica Scandinavica*, **96**, 289-305.

15. Sharp, R.L., Costill, D.L., Fink, W.J., & King, D.S. (1986). Effects of eight weeks of bicycle ergometer sprint training on human muscle buffer capacity. *International Journal of Sports Medicine*, **7**, 13-17.

16. Thorstensson, A. (1975). Enzyme activities and muscle strength after sprint training in man. *Acta Physiologica Scandinavica*, **94**, 313-318.

Selected Readings

Åstrand, P.-O., & Rodahl, K. (1986). *Textbook of work physiology* (3rd ed.). New York: McGraw-Hill.

Beltz, J.D., Costill, D.L., Thomas, R., Fink, W.J., & Kirwan, J.P. (1988). Energy demands of interval training for competitive swimming. *Journal of Swimming Research*, **4**(3), 5-9.

Brooks, G.A. (1985). Response to Davis' manuscript. *Medicine and Science in Sports and Exercise*, **17**, 19-21.

Costill, D.L., Fink, W.J., Hargreaves, M., King, D.S., Thomas, R., & Fielding, R. (1985). Metabolic characteristics of skeletal muscle during detraining from competitive swimming. *Medicine and Science in Sports and Exercise*, **17**, 339-343.

Costill, D.L., Fink, W.J., Ivy, J.L., Getchell, L.H., & Witzmann, F.A. (1979). Lipid metabolism in skeletal muscle of endurance-trained males and females. *Journal of Applied Physiology*, **28**, 251-255.

Davis, J.A. (1985). Anaerobic threshold: Review of the concept and directions for future research. *Medicine and Science in Sports and Exercise*, **17**, 6-18.

Davis, J.A., Frank, M.H., Whipp, B.J., & Wasserman, K. (1979). Anaerobic threshold alterations caused by endurance training in middle-aged men. *Journal of Applied Physiology*, **46**, 1039-1046.

Henriksson, J., & Reitman, J.S. (1977). Time course of changes in human skeletal muscle succinate dehydrogenase and cytochrome oxidase activities and maximal oxygen uptake with physical activity and inactivity. *Acta Physiologica Scandinavica*, **99**, 91-97.

Hickson, R.C. (1980). Interference of strength development by simultaneously training for strength and endurance. *European Journal of Applied Physiology*, **45**, 255-263.

Houmard, J.A., Costill, D.L., Mitchell, J.B., Park, S.H., & Chenier, T.C. (1991). The role of anaerobic ability in middle distance running performance. *European Journal of Applied Physiology*, **62**, 40-43.

Lesmes, G.R., Costill, D.L., Coyle, E.F., & Fink, W.J. (1978). Muscle strength and power changes during maximal isokinetic training. *Medicine and Science in Sports*, **10**, 266-269.

Prud'Homme, D., Bouchard, G., Leblanc, C., Landry, F., & Fontaine, E. (1984). Sensitivity of maximal aerobic power to training is genotype-dependent. *Medicine and Science in Sports and Exercise*, **16**, 489-493.

Saltin, B., Blomqvist, G., Mitchell, J.H., Johnson, Jr., R.L., Wildenthal, K., & Chapman, C.B. (1968). Response to submaximal and maximal exercise after bed rest and training. *Circulation*, **38**(Suppl. 7).

Saltin, B., & Karlsson, J. (1971). Muscle ATP, CP, and lactate during exercise after physical conditioning. In B. Pernow and B. Saltin (Eds.), *Muscle metabolism during exercise*. New York: Plenum.

Saltin, B., & Rowell, L.B. (1980). Functional adaptations to physical activity and inactivity. *Federation Proceedings*, **39**, 1506-1513.

Wasserman, K. (1984). The anaerobic threshold measurement to evaluate exercise performance. *American Review of Respiratory Diseases*, **129**(Suppl.), S35-S40.

Cardiorespiratory Function and Performance

In the previous part, we learned how the body produces energy through metabolism to fuel its movement. But merely producing energy is useless if the energy does not reach the active muscles. In Part C, we will focus on how the cardiovascular and respiratory systems provide oxygen and fuel to the active muscles, how they rid the body of carbon dioxide and metabolic wastes, and how these systems adapt to aerobic training. In chapter 8, Cardiovascular Control During Exercise, we will look at the structure and function of the cardiovascular system—the heart, the blood vessels, and the blood. Our primary focus will be how this system provides active muscles with an adequate blood supply to meet their demands during increasing rates of work. In chapter 9, Respiratory Regulation During Exercise, we will examine the mechanics and regulation of breathing, the process of gas exchange in the lungs and at the muscles, and the transportation of oxygen and carbon dioxide in the blood. We will also see how this system regulates the body's pH within a very narrow range. In chapter 10, Cardiorespiratory Adaptations to Training, we will study the concept of endurance capacity. We will consider how it is evaluated in the laboratory and how it is improved with aerobic training, concentrating on cardiorespiratory adaptations that occur in response to aerobic training and that can improve performance.

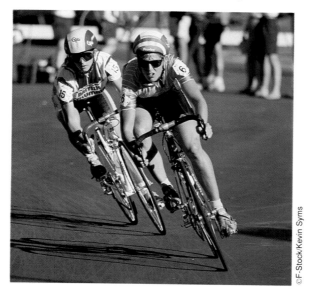

©F-Stock/Kevin Syms

Chapter 8

Cardiovascular Control During Exercise

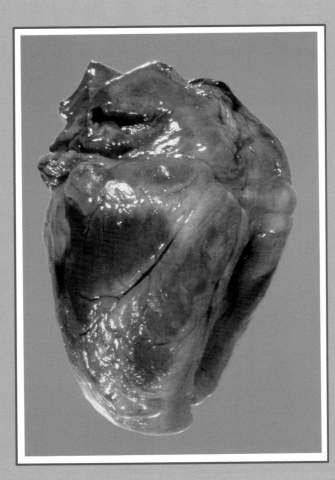

Chapter Overview

Your cardiovascular system, which includes your heart, blood vessels, and blood, has many roles, including nurturer, protector, and even garbage hauler. This system must reach every cell in your body, and it must be able to immediately respond to any change in your internal environment to keep all body systems functioning at peak efficiency. Even when you are at rest, your cardiovascular system constantly works to meet the demands of your body tissues. But during exercise you place numerous and far more urgent demands on this system.

In this chapter, we will explore the amazing role the cardiovascular system plays in physical activity. In the first part of the chapter we will review the structure and function of the cardiovascular system, emphasizing its complexities. In the second part, we will focus on how the cardiovascular system responds to increased demands during exercise. We will learn how each component of this system adapts to changes in the body's internal environment that result from increased rates of physical activity and how the system controls our ability to perform.

Chapter Outline

On January 5, 1988, the sports world lost one of its greatest athletes. "Pistol Pete" Maravich, former National Basketball Association star, collapsed and died of cardiac arrest at 40 years of age during a pickup basketball game. His death came as a shock, and the cause of his death surprised the medical experts. Maravich's heart was abnormally enlarged due primarily to the fact that he was born with only a single coronary artery on the right side of his heart—he was missing the two coronary arteries that supply the left side of the heart! The medical community was amazed that this single right coronary artery had taken over supplying the left side of Maravich's heart, and that this adaptation had allowed him to compete for many years as one of the top players in the history of basketball.

The cardiovascular system serves a number of important functions in the body. Most of these support other physiological systems. The major cardiovascular functions fall into five categories:

1. Delivery
2. Removal
3. Transport
4. Maintenance
5. Prevention

Consider some examples. The cardiovascular system delivers oxygen and nutrients to, and removes carbon dioxide and metabolic waste products from, every cell in the body. It transports hormones from endocrine glands to their target receptors. The system maintains body temperature, and the blood's buffering capabilities help control the body's pH. The cardiovascular system maintains appropriate fluid levels to prevent dehydration and helps prevent infection by invading organisms.

Although this is an abbreviated list, the cardiovascular functions listed here are important for understanding the physiological bases of physical activity. But before examining specific cardiovascular responses to activity, we need to review the components of the cardiovascular system and how they work together.

Structure and Function of the Cardiovascular System

The cardiovascular system is impressive in its ability to respond immediately to your body's many and ever-changing needs. All bodily functions and virtually every cell in your body depend in some way on this system.

Any system of circulation requires three components:

1. A pump (the heart)
2. A system of channels (the blood vessels)
3. A fluid medium (the blood)

Let's examine each of these separately.

The Heart

The heart, shown in Figure 8.1, has two atria acting as receiving chambers and two ventricles acting as sending units. The heart is the primary pump that circulates blood through the entire vascular system. Let's review the path of the blood as it moves through the heart.

Blood Flow Through the Heart

Blood that has coursed its way between the cells of the body, delivering oxygen and nutrients and picking up waste products, returns through the great veins—the superior vena cava and inferior vena cava—to the right atrium. This chamber receives all the body's deoxygenated blood.

From the right atrium, blood passes through the tricuspid valve into the right ventricle. This chamber pumps the blood through the pulmonary semilunar valve into the pulmonary artery, which carries the blood to the right and left lungs. Thus the right side of the heart is known as the pulmonary side, sending the blood that has circulated throughout the body into the lungs for reoxygenation.

After receiving a fresh supply of oxygen, the blood exits the lungs through the pulmonary veins, which carry it back to the heart and into the left atrium. All freshly oxygenated blood is received by this chamber. From the left atrium, the blood passes through the bicuspid (mitral) valve into the left ventricle. Blood leaves the left ventricle by passing through the aortic semilunar valve into the aorta, which ultimately sends it out to all body parts and systems. The left side of

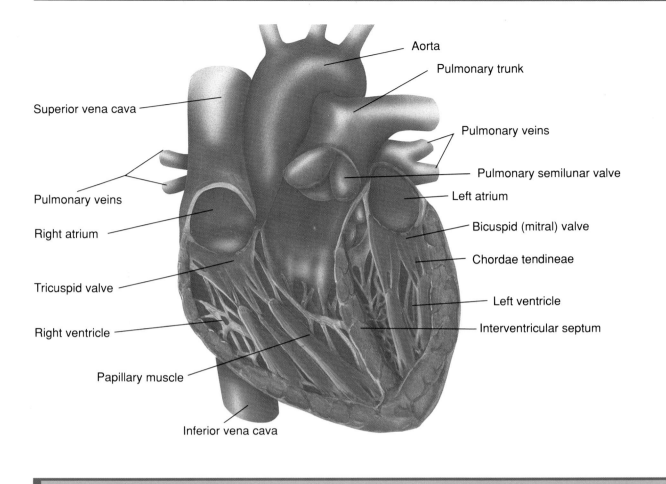

Figure 8.1   The anatomy of the human heart.

Heart Murmur

The four heart valves prevent backflow of blood, ensuring one-way flow through the heart. These valves maximize the amount of blood pumped out of the heart during contraction. A heart murmur is a condition in which abnormal heart sounds are detected with the aid of a stethoscope. Normally a heart valve makes a distinct clicking sound when it snaps shut. With a murmur, the click is replaced by a sound similar to blowing. This abnormal sound can indicate the turbulent flow of blood through a narrowed or leaky valve. It could also indicate errant blood flow through a hole in the wall separating the right and left sides of the heart (septal defect).

Heart murmurs are quite common in growing children and adolescents. During growth periods, valve development doesn't always keep up with enlargement of the heart openings. Valves can leak even in an adult. With mitral valve prolapse, the mitral (bicuspid) valve allows some blood to flow back into the left atrium during ventricular contraction. This disorder, common in adults (6% to 17% of the population), including athletes, usually has little clinical significance unless there is significant backflow.

Most murmurs in athletes are benign, affecting neither the heart's pumping nor the athlete's performance. But heart murmurs can indicate diseased valves, such as those with stenosis, in which the valve is narrowed and often thickened and rigid. This condition can require surgical replacement of the valve.

the heart is known as the systemic side. It receives the oxygenated blood from the lungs then sends it out to supply all body tissues.

The Myocardium

Cardiac muscle is collectively called the myocardium. Myocardial thickness varies directly with the stress placed on the heart chambers' walls. The left ventricle is the most powerful of the four heart chambers. Through its contractions, this chamber must pump blood out through the entire systemic route. When the body is sitting or standing, the left ventricle must contract with enough force to overcome the effect of gravity, which tends to pool blood in the lower extremities.

The left ventricle's tremendous power is reflected by the greater size (hypertrophy) of its muscular wall compared to the other heart chambers. This hypertrophy is simply the result of the demands placed on it at rest or under normal conditions of moderate activity. With more vigorous exercise—particularly intense aerobic activity, during which the working muscles' need for blood increases considerably—the demands on the left ventricle are high. Over time it responds by increasing its size, like skeletal muscle.

Although striated in appearance, the myocardium differs from skeletal muscle in one important way. Cardiac muscle fibers are anatomically interconnected end-to-end by dark-staining regions called intercalated disks, seen in Figure 8.2. These disks have desmosomes, which are structures that anchor the individual cells together so they don't pull apart during contraction, and gap junctions, which allow rapid transmission of the impulse signaling contraction. These features allow the myocardium in all four chambers to act as one large muscle fiber: All fibers contract together.

To understand how cardiac contractions are coordinated, we must understand how the signal for contraction originates and travels through the heart. These functions are accomplished by the cardiac conduction system.

The Cardiac Conduction System

Cardiac muscle has the unique ability to generate its own electrical signal, called autoconduction, that allows it to contract rhythmically without neural stimulation. With neither neural nor hormonal stimulation, the intrinsic heart rate averages 70 to 80 beats (contractions) per minute, but can drop below this rate in endurance-trained people.

Figure 8.3 illustrates the four components of the cardiac conduction system:

1. Sinoatrial (SA) node
2. Atrioventricular (AV) node

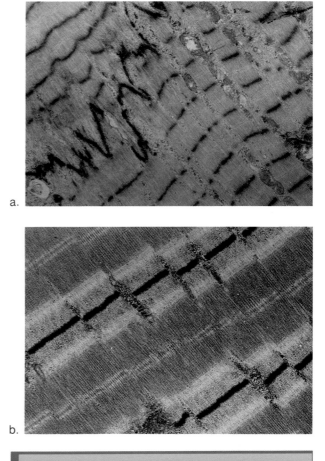

a.

b.

Figure 8.2 Micrographs of (a) cardiac muscle and (b) skeletal muscle. Both muscle types appear striated, but only the cardiac muscle fibers are connected by dark-staining intercalated disks.

3. Atrioventricular (AV) bundle (bundle of His)
4. Purkinje fibers

The impulse for heart contraction is initiated in the sinoatrial (SA) node, a group of specialized cardiac muscle fibers located in the posterior wall of the right atrium. Because this tissue generates the impulse, typically at a frequency of about 60 to 80 beats per minute, the SA node is known as the heart's pacemaker, and the beating rate it establishes is called the sinus rhythm. The electrical impulse generated by the SA node spreads through both atria and reaches the atrioventricular (AV) node, located in the right atrial wall near the center of the heart. As the impulse spreads through the atria, they are signalled to contract, which they do almost immediately.

The AV node conducts the impulse from the atria into the ventricles. The impulse is delayed by about 0.13 s as it passes through the AV node, then it enters the AV bundle. This delay allows the atria to fully

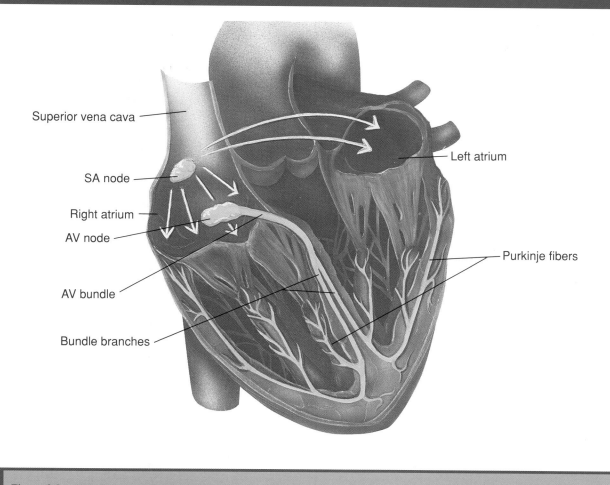

Superior vena cava

SA node

Right atrium

AV node

AV bundle

Bundle branches

Left atrium

Purkinje fibers

Figure 8.3   The cardiac conduction system.

contract before the ventricles do, maximizing ventricular filling. The AV bundle travels along the ventricular septum and then sends right and left bundle branches into both ventricles. These branches send the impulse toward the apex of the heart, then outward. Each bundle branch subdivides into many smaller ones that spread throughout the entire ventricular wall. These terminal branches of the AV bundle are the Purkinje fibers. They transmit the impulse through the ventricles approximately six times faster than through the rest of the cardiac conduction system. This rapid conduction allows all parts of the ventricle to contract at about the same time.

Extrinsic Control of Heart Activity

Although the heart initiates its own electrical impulses (intrinsic control), their timing and effects can be altered. Under normal conditions, this is accomplished primarily through three extrinsic systems:

1. The parasympathetic nervous system
2. The sympathetic nervous system
3. The endocrine system (hormones)

Occasionally, chronic problems develop within the cardiac conduction system, hampering its ability to maintain appropriate sinus rhythm throughout the heart. In such cases, an artificial pacemaker can be surgically installed. This is a small battery-operated electrical stimulator, usually implanted under the skin, with electrodes attached to the right ventricle. An example of when this is useful is a condition called AV block. With this disorder, the SA node fires its impulse, but the impulse is blocked at the AV node and can't reach the ventricles. The artificial pacemaker takes over the role of the disabled AV node, supplying the needed electrical impulse and thus controlling ventricular contraction.

Though an overview of their effects is offered here, these are discussed in more detail in chapters 3 and 6.

The parasympathetic system, a branch of the autonomic nervous system, acts on the heart through the vagus nerve (cranial nerve X). At rest, parasympathetic system activity predominates in a state referred to as vagal tone. The vagus nerve has a depressant effect on the heart—it slows impulse conduction and thus decreases the heart rate. Maximal vagal stimulation can lower the heart rate to between 20 and 30 beats per minute. The vagus nerve also decreases the force of cardiac contraction.

The sympathetic nervous system, the other branch of the autonomic system, has opposite effects. Sympathetic stimulation increases impulse conduction speed and thus heart rate. Maximal sympathetic stimulation will allow the heart rate to soar up to 250 beats per minute. Sympathetic input also increases the contraction force. The sympathetic system predominates during times of physical or emotional stress, when the body's demands are higher. After the stress subsides the parasympathetic system again predominates.

The endocrine system exerts its effect through the hormones released by the adrenal medulla: norepinephrine and epinephrine. These hormones are also known as catecholamines. Like the sympathetic nervous system, these hormones stimulate the heart, increasing its rate. In fact, release of these hormones is triggered by sympathetic stimulation during times of stress and their actions prolong the sympathetic response.

Normal resting heart rate typically varies between 60 and 85 beats per minute. With extended periods of endurance training (months to years), the resting heart rate can decrease to 35 beats per minute or less. We have observed a resting heart rate of 28 beats per minute in a world-class long-distance runner. These lower resting rates are postulated to result from increased parasympathetic stimulation (vagal tone), with a reduced sympathetic activity probably playing a lesser role.

Cardiac Arrhythmias

Occasionally disturbances in the normal sequence of cardiac events can lead to an irregular heart rhythm, called an arrhythmia. These disturbances vary in degree of seriousness. Bradycardia and tachycardia are two types of arrhythmias. Bradycardia means ''slow heart'' and indicates a resting heart rate lower than 60 beats per minute, whereas tachycardia means ''fast heart'' and indicates a resting rate greater than 100 beats per minute. With these arrhythmias, the sinus rhythm itself is usually altered. The heart's function may be normal, but its timing is abnormal, which can affect circulation. Symptoms of both arrhythmias include fatigue, dizziness, lightheadedness, and fainting. Tachycardia also can cause palpitations.

Other arrhythmias also occur. For example, premature ventricular contractions, which result in the feeling of skipped or extra beats, are relatively common and result from impulses orignating outside the SA node. Atrial flutter, in which the atria contract at

rates of 200 to 400 beats per minute, and atrial fibrillation, in which the atria contract in a rapid and uncoordinated manner, are more serious arrythmias which cause the atria to pump little or no blood. Ventricular tachycardia, defined as three or more consecutive premature ventricular contractions, is a very serious arrhythmia that can lead to ventricular fibrillation, in which contraction of the ventricular tissue is uncoordinated. When this happens, the heart cannot pump blood. Most cardiac deaths result from ventricular fibrillation. Use of a defibrillator to shock the heart back into a normal sinus rhythm must occur within minutes if the victim is to survive. Cardiopulmonary resuscitation imposes a normal rhythm on the heart and can maintain life for several hours, but chances of survival are greater if emergency treatment, including defibrillation, is provided quickly.

Interestingly, highly trained endurance athletes often develop low resting heart rates, an advantageous adaptation, as a result of training. Also, your heart rate naturally accelerates during physical activity to meet the increased demands of exertion. These adaptations should not be confused with bradycardia or tachycardia, which are abnormal alterations in the resting heart rate that usually indicate a pathological disturbance.

The ECG

The electrical activity of the heart can be recorded to diagnose potential cardiac problems or to monitor cardiac changes. The principle involved is simple—body fluids are good electrical conductors. Electrical impulses generated in the heart are conducted through body fluids to the skin, where they can be detected and printed out by a sensitive machine called an electrocardiograph. This printout is called an electrocardiogram, or ECG (see Figure 8.4). Three components of the ECG represent aspects of cardiac function:

1. The P wave
2. The QRS complex
3. The T wave

The P wave represents atrial depolarization and occurs when the electrical impulse travels from the SA node through the atria to the AV node. The QRS complex represents ventricular depolarization and occurs as the impulse spreads from the AV bundle to the Purkinje fibers and through the ventricles. The T wave represents ventricular repolarization. Atrial repolarization cannot be seen as it occurs during ventricular depolarization (QRS complex).

Often electrocardiograms are obtained during exercise. These are valuable diagnostic tests. As exercise intensity increases, the heart must beat faster and work harder to deliver more blood to active muscles. If the heart is diseased, an indication may show up on the electrocardiogram as the heart increases its rate of work. Exercise ECGs have also been invaluable tools for research in exercise physiology because they provide a convenient method for tracking cardiac changes during acute and chronic exercise.

Terminology of Cardiac Function

The following terms are essential to an understanding of the work done by the heart and to our future discussions of cardiac response during activity:

- Cardiac cycle
- Stroke volume
- Ejection fraction
- Cardiac output ($\dot{Q}$)

The Cardiac Cycle. The cardiac cycle includes all events occurring between two consecutive heartbeats. In mechanical terms, it consists of all heart chambers under-

a. Resting electrocardiogram   Heart rate: 75 beats/min

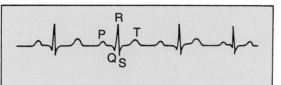

b. Exercise electrocardiogram   Heart rate: 150 beats/min

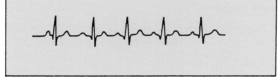

c. Ischemic response during exercise

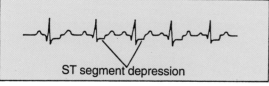

ST segment depression

d. Premature ventricular contraction

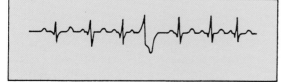

Figure 8.4   (a) A normal resting ECG, (b) a normal exercise ECG, (c) an exercise ECG showing an ischemic response (ST segment depression) that could indicate coronary artery disease, and (d) an ECG showing a premature ventricular contraction.

going a relaxation phase (diastole) and a contraction phase (systole). During diastole, the chambers fill with blood. During systole, the chambers contract and expel their contents. The diastolic phase is longer than the systolic phase. Consider an individual with a heart rate of 74 beats per minute. At this heart rate, the entire cardiac cycle takes 0.81 s to complete (60 s / 74 beats). Of the total cardiac cycle at this rate, diastole accounts for 0.50 s, or 62% of the cycle, and systole accounts for 0.31 s, or 38%. As the heart rate increases, these absolute time intervals shorten proportionately.

Refer back to the normal ECG in Figure 8.4a. One cardiac cycle spans the time between one systole and the next. Ventricular contraction (systole) begins during the QRS complex and ends in the T wave. Ventricular relaxation (diastole) occurs during the T wave and continues until the next contraction. You can see from this illustration that although the heart seems to always be at work, it actually spends slightly more time in the resting phase than in the working phase.

Stroke Volume. During systole, a certain volume of blood is ejected from the left ventricle. This amount is the stroke volume (SV) of the heart, or the volume of blood pumped per stroke (contraction). This is depicted in Figure 8.5a. To understand stroke volume, consider the amount of blood in the ventricle before and after contraction. At the end of diastole, just before contraction, the ventricle has completed filling. The volume of blood it now contains is called the end-diastolic volume, or EDV. At the end of systole, just after contraction, the ventricle has completed its ejection phase. The volume of blood remaining in the ventricle is called the end-systolic volume, or ESV. Stroke volume is the volume

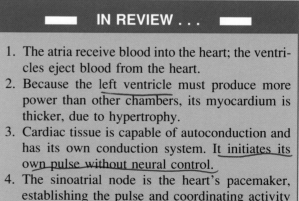

IN REVIEW . . .

1. The atria receive blood into the heart; the ventricles eject blood from the heart.
2. Because the left ventricle must produce more power than other chambers, its myocardium is thicker, due to hypertrophy.
3. Cardiac tissue is capable of autoconduction and has its own conduction system. It initiates its own pulse without neural control.
4. The sinoatrial node is the heart's pacemaker, establishing the pulse and coordinating activity throughout the heart.
5. Heart rate and contraction strength can be altered by the autonomic nervous system or the endocrine system.
6. The ECG is a recording of the heart's electrical functioning. An exercise ECG may reveal underlying cardiac disorders.

of blood that was ejected, and is merely the difference between the amount originally there and the amount remaining in the ventricle after contraction. So stroke volume is simply the difference between the EDV and the ESV.

Ejection Fraction. The proportion of the blood pumped out of the left ventricle at each beat is the ejection fraction (EF). This value, as seen in Figure 8.5b, is determined by dividing the stroke volume by the end-diastolic volume. It reveals how much of the blood entering the ventricle is actually ejected during contraction. The ejection fraction, generally expressed as a percentage, averages 60% at rest. Thus 60% of the blood in the ventricle at the end of diastole is ejected with the next contraction and 40% remains.

Cardiac Output. Cardiac output ($\dot{Q}$), as shown in Figure 8.5c, is the total volume of blood pumped by the ventricle per minute, or simply the product of heart rate (HR) and stroke volume (SV). The stroke volume at rest in the standing position averages between 60 and 80 ml of blood in most adults. Thus at a resting heart rate of 80 beats per minute the resting cardiac output will vary between 4.8 and 6.4 L · min⁻¹. The average adult body contains about 5 L of blood, so this means all of our blood is pumped through our hearts about once every minute.

Understanding the mechanical activity of the heart provides a basis for understanding the work of the cardiovascular system, but the heart is only one part of this system. Let's next turn our attention to the vast system of vessels that carries the blood to all body tissues.

The Vascular System

The vascular system is composed of a series of vessels that transport blood from the heart to the tissues and back:

- Arteries
- Arterioles
- Capillaries
- Venules
- Veins

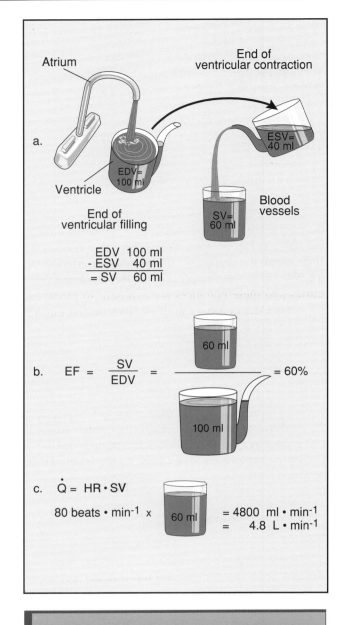

Figure 8.5 Calculations of (a) stroke volume (SV), which is the difference between end-diastolic volume (EDV) and end-systolic volume (ESV), (b) ejection fraction (EF), and (c) cardiac output ($\dot{Q}$).

KEY POINT

$$SV = EDV - ESV$$

$$EF = (SV \, / \, EDV) \times 100$$

$$\dot{Q} = HR \times SV$$

Recall that arteries are typically the largest, most muscular, and most elastic vessels, and they always carry blood away from the heart to the arterioles. From the arterioles, blood enters the capillaries. These are the narrowest vessels, often with walls only one cell thick. Virtually all exchange between the blood and the tissues occurs at the capillaries. Blood leaves the capillaries to begin the return trip to the heart in the venules, and the venules form larger vessels— the veins—that complete the circuit.

In addition to the pulmonary and systemic divisions of the vascular system, the heart, as an active muscle, requires its own vascular system to supply necessary nutrients and to clear waste products. The coronary arteries, which originate from the base of the aorta as it leaves the heart, supply the myocardium. These arteries are very susceptible to atherosclerosis, or narrowing, which can lead to coronary artery disease. This disease will be discussed in much greater detail in chapter 20.

During contraction, when blood is forced out of the left ventricle under high pressure, the aortic semilunar valve is forced open. When this valve is open, its flaps block the entrances to the coronary arteries. As the pressure in the aorta decreases, the semilunar valve closes and these entrances are exposed, so blood can then enter the coronary arteries. This design ensures that the coronary arteries are spared the very high blood pressure created by contraction of the left ventricle, thus protecting these vessels from damage.

Return of Blood to the Heart

Because we spend so much time in an upright position, the cardiovascular system requires assistance to overcome the force of gravity when returning blood from the lower parts of the body back to the heart. Three basic mechanisms assist in this process:

1. Breathing
2. The muscle pump
3. Valves

Each time you inhale and exhale, pressure changes in the abdominal and thoracic cavities assist blood return to the heart. As they contract, the skeletal muscles in the legs or abdomen share this function. During breathing and skeletal muscle contraction, the veins in the immediate vicinity are compressed and blood is pushed upwards toward the heart. These actions are aided by a series of valves in the veins that allow blood to flow in only one direction, thus preventing backflow and pooling of the blood in the lower body.

Distribution of Blood

Distribution of blood to the various body tissues varies tremendously depending on the immediate needs of a specific tissue and of the whole body. At rest under normal conditions, the most metabolically active tissues receive the greatest blood supply. The liver and kidneys combined receive almost half the blood being circulated (27% and 22%, respectively), and resting skeletal muscles receive only about 15%.

During exercise, blood is redirected to the areas where it is needed most. During heavy endurance exercise, for example, this redistribution is rather remarkable—muscles receive up to 80% or more of the available blood. This, along with increases in cardiac output (to be discussed later), allows up to 25 times more blood flow to active muscles. Figure 8.6 illustrates a typical distribution of blood throughout the body at rest and during heavy exercise. The values are expressed both as relative percentages of the total blood available and as absolute volumes.

Similarly, after you eat a big meal, your digestive system receives more blood than when you are at rest. During increasing environmental heat stress, the skin's blood supply increases as the body attempts to maintain normal temperature. Considering that the needs of the various body tissues are constantly changing, it is indeed amazing that the cardiovascular system can respond so efficiently, guaranteeing an adequate blood supply to the areas where it is most needed.

Distribution of blood to various areas is controlled primarily by the arterioles. These vessels have two important characteristics. They have a strong muscular wall that can significantly alter vessel diameter. They also respond to the mechanisms that control blood flow: autoregulation and extrinsic neural control. Let's examine these mechanisms.

Autoregulation. Local control of blood distribution is called autoregulation because the arterioles in specific areas control themselves. Autoregulation refers to the vessels' ability to self-regulate their own blood flow depending on the immediate needs of the tissues they supply. The arterioles undergo vasodilation, opening up to allow more blood to enter an area in need.

This increased blood flow is a direct response to changes in the tissue's local chemical environment. Oxygen demand appears to be the strongest stimulus. As the tissue's oxygen use increases, available oxygen is diminished. Local arterioles dilate to allow more blood, and thus more oxygen, to perfuse that area. Other chemical changes that can provide stimuli are decreases in other nutrients and increases in by-products (CO_2, K^+, H^+, lactic acid) or inflammatory chemicals. Increased blood supply can either bring in needed substances or clear out harmful ones.

Extrinsic Neural Control. Although the concept of autoregulation explains local redistribution of blood within an organ or tissue mass, it can't explain how the cardiovascular system as a whole knows to send less blood to one part of the body when more is needed

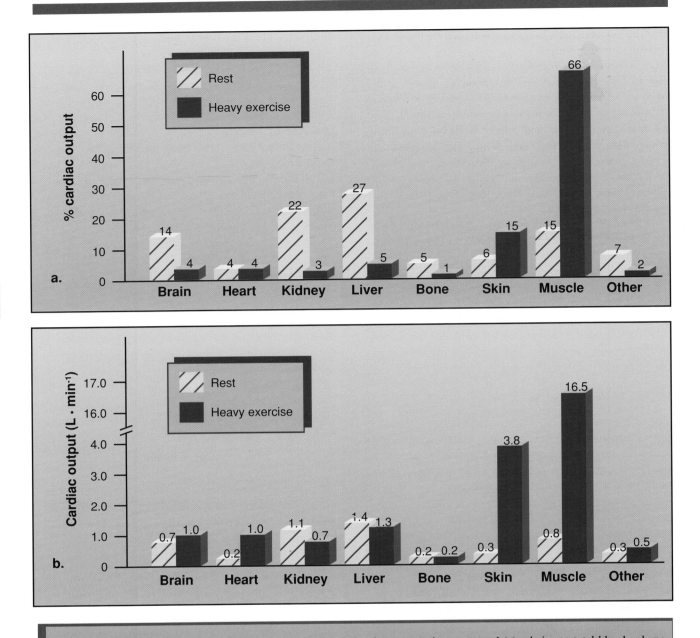

Figure 8.6   The distribution of cardiac output at rest and during heavy exercise, expressed (a) relative to total blood volume and (b) in absolute values.

elsewhere. Redistribution at the system or body level is controlled by neural mechanisms. This is known as extrinsic neural control of blood flow because the control comes from outside the specific area (extrinsic) instead of from inside the tissues (intrinsic) as in autoregulation.

Blood flow to all body parts is regulated largely by the sympathetic nervous system. The muscle within the walls of all vessels of systemic circulation is supplied by sympathetic nerves. In most vessels, stimulation by these nerves causes the muscle cells to contract, constricting that vessel so that less blood can pass through it.

Under normal conditions, the sympathetic nerves transmit impulses continuously to the blood vessels, keep-ing the vessels in a state of moderate constriction to maintain adequate blood pressure. This state of partial constriction is referred to as vasomotor tone. When sympathetic stimulation increases, further constriction of the blood vessels in a specific area decreases blood flow into that area and allows more blood to shift elsewhere. But if sympathetic stimulation decreases below that needed to maintain tone, constriction of vessels in that area is lessened, so the vessels dilate, increasing blood flow into that area. Therefore, sympathetic stimulation will cause vasoconstriction in most vessels, but blood flow is altered by either increasing or decreasing the amount of vasoconstriction relative to normal vasomotor tone.

The sympathetic system can also directly cause vasodilation through some of its fibers. A different type of sympathetic fiber supplies some blood vessels in skeletal muscles and in the heart. Stimulation of these fibers causes vasodilation, increasing blood flow into the muscles and heart. This system functions during the classic fight-or-flight response and increases blood flow into skeletal muscles and the heart in times of crisis. This response is also active during exercise, when the skeletal muscles and the heart are working harder, requiring much more blood than when at rest.

Redistribution of Venous Blood.   We have now discussed the mechanisms that control the redistribution of blood from one area of the body to another. But the distribution of blood throughout the body varies not only with the tissues being supplied, but also by the blood's location in the vascular system. At rest, the blood volume is distributed amongst the vasculature as shown in Figure 8.7. The majority of blood is located in the venous return channels (veins, venules, venous sinuses). Thus the venous system provides a large reservoir of blood readily available to meet increased need. When this need arises, sympathetic stimulation of the venules and veins constricts these vessels. This causes rapid redistribution of blood from peripheral venous circulation back to the heart, and then out to those areas that have greater needs. Not only is blood diverted away from other tissues, but more blood is sent into arterial circulation from the venous system, thereby ensuring a substantial increase of blood flow to a needy area.

Blood Pressure

Blood pressure is the pressure exerted by the blood on the vessel walls, and the term usually refers to arterial blood pressure. It is expressed by two numbers: the systolic pressure and the diastolic pressure. The higher number is the systolic blood pressure. It represents the highest pressure in the artery and corresponds to ventricular systole of the heart. Ventricular contraction pushes the blood through the arteries with tremendous force, which exerts high pressure on the arterial wall. The lower number is the diastolic blood pressure and represents the lowest pressure in the artery, corresponding to ventricular diastole when the heart is at rest. Blood moving through the arteries during that phase isn't pushed along by a forceful contraction.

Mean arterial pressure represents the average pressure exerted by the blood as it travels through the arteries. An approximation of mean arterial pressure is as follows (b.p. = blood pressure):

Mean arterial pressure
= diastolic b.p.
+ [0.333 (systolic b.p. − diastolic b.p.)].

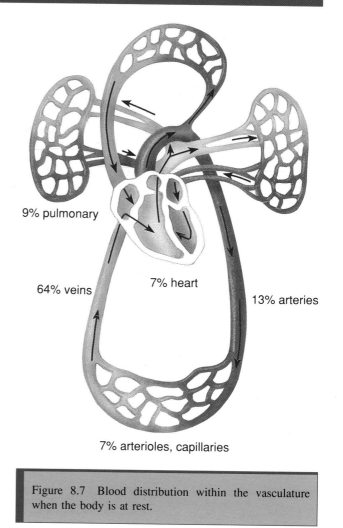

Figure 8.7   Blood distribution within the vasculature when the body is at rest.

9% pulmonary

64% veins

7% heart

13% arteries

7% arterioles, capillaries

To illustrate, with a systolic pressure of 120 mmHg and a diastolic pressure of 80 mmHg, the mean arterial pressure = 80 + [0.333 × (120-80)] = 93 mmHg. Note that this relationship is not a simple average of the systolic and diastolic values. Recall that the heart is in diastole longer than in systole, so the arteries experience diastolic pressure longer than systolic; that is factored into the equation.

Alterations in blood pressure are largely controlled by the specific changes in the arteries, arterioles, and veins previously described. Generalized constriction of blood vessels increases blood pressure, and generalized dilation reduces it. Hypertension is the clinical term describing the condition in which blood pressure is chronically elevated above normal, healthy values. The cause of hypertension is generally unknown in approximately 90% of cases, but it can usually be controlled effectively by weight loss, proper diet, and exercise, although appropriate medication may also be required. This is discussed in more detail in chapter 20.

The Blood

The third component of any system of circulation is a circulating substance. In the human body, this is the blood and lymph. These fluids are responsible for the actual transportation of various materials between the different cells or tissues of the body.

Recall from basic physiology the relationship between blood and lymph: Some blood plasma filters out of the capillaries into the tissues, becoming interstitial (tissue) fluid. Much of the interstitial fluid returns to the capillaries after exchange occurs, but less is returned than was originally filtered out. The excess fluid enters the lymph capillaries, and it is then referred to as lymph, which ultimately returns to the blood.

Clearly the lymphatic system plays a crucial role in maintaining appropriate fluid levels in the tissues as well as maintaining proper blood volume by ensuring that interstitial fluid is returned. This function becomes more important during exercise when increased blood flow to the active muscles and increased blood pressure lead to the formation of more interstitial fluid. The lymphatic system prevents swelling in the active areas and keeps the cardiovascular system working efficiently. This system is extremely important to coordinated physiological function and general health. But at the present time, beyond its role in fluid return, the lymphatic system is not a major area of concern for

exercise and sport physiology. We will instead focus on the blood.

Blood serves many useful purposes in the regulation of normal body function. The three functions of primary importance to exercise and sport are

1. transportation,
2. temperature regulation, and
3. acid-base (pH) balance.

We are most familiar with blood's transportation functions. In addition, blood is critical in temperature regulation during physical activity, picking up heat from the body core or from areas of increased metabolic activity and dissipating it throughout the body during normal conditions and to the skin when the body is overheated (see chapter 11). Blood can buffer the acids produced by anaerobic metabolism, maintaining the proper pH for efficient activity of metabolic processes (see chapter 9).

Blood Volume and Composition

The total volume of blood in the body varies considerably with the individual's size and the state of training. Larger blood volumes are associated with larger body size and high levels of endurance training. The blood volumes of people of average body size and normal physical activity (not training aerobically) generally range from 5 to 6 L in men and 4 to 5 L in women.

Blood is composed of plasma (primarily water) and formed elements (see Figure 8.8). Plasma normally constitutes about 55% to 60% of total blood volume, but can decrease by 10% or more with intense exercise in heat or increase by 10% or more with endurance training or acclimatization to heat and humidity. Approximately 90% of the plasma volume is water, 7% is plasma proteins, and the remaining 3% is cellular nutrients, electrolytes, enzymes, hormones, antibodies, and wastes.

The formed elements, which normally constitute about 40% to 45% of total blood volume, are the red blood cells (erythrocytes), white blood cells (leukocytes), and platelets (thrombocytes). Red blood cells constitute more than 99% of the formed element volume; white blood cells and platelets together account for less than 1%. The percentage of the total blood volume composed of red blood cells is referred to as the hematocrit. It typically varies between 40% and 45%.

White blood cells protect the body from disease organism invasion by either directly destroying invading agents through phagocytosis (ingestion) or forming antibodies to destroy them. Adults have about 7,000 white blood cells per cubic millimeter of blood.

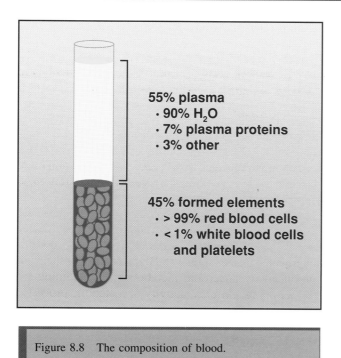

55% plasma
- 90% H₂O
- 7% plasma proteins
- 3% other

45% formed elements
- > 99% red blood cells
- < 1% white blood cells and platelets

Figure 8.8   The composition of blood.

The remaining formed element is the blood platelet. These are not really cells at all, but rather are cell fragments. These small discs are required for blood coagulation (clotting), which prevents excessive blood loss. We are most concerned with red blood cells, however, so our discussion will focus on them.

Red Blood Cells

Mature red blood cells (erythrocytes) have no nucleus, so they can't reproduce. They must be replaced with new cells. The normal life span of a red blood cell is only about 4 months. Thus these cells are continuously produced and destroyed at about equal rates. This balance is very important, because adequate oxygen delivery to body tissues depends on having a sufficient number of carriers—the red blood cells. Decreases in their count or function can hinder oxygen delivery and thus affect performance.

Red blood cells can be destroyed during exercise. The cell membrane appears to be disrupted by the wear and tear associated with increased circulation rate as well as by increased body temperature. Studies have even demonstrated that the constant pounding of the sole of the foot in the shoe during distance running can increase fragility and destruction of red blood cells.

Red blood cells transport oxygen primarily bound to their hemoglobin. Hemoglobin is composed of a protein (globin) and a pigment (heme). Heme contains iron, which binds oxygen. Each red blood cell contains approximately 250 million hemoglobin molecules, each able to bind 4 oxygen molecules, so each red blood cell can bind up to a billion molecules of oxygen! There are an average of 15 g of hemoglobin per 100 ml of whole blood. Each gram of hemoglobin can combine with 1.33 ml of oxygen, so as much as 20 ml of oxygen can be bound for each 100 ml of blood.

Blood Viscosity

Viscosity refers to the thickness or stickiness of the blood. The more viscous a fluid, the more resistant it is to flow. The viscosity of blood is normally about twice that of water. Blood viscosity, and thus resistance to flow, are increased with higher hematocrits.

Because of oxygen transport by the red blood cells, an increase in their number would be expected to maximize oxygen transport. But if an increase in red blood cell count is not accompanied by a similar increase in plasma volume, blood viscosity will increase, which could restrict blood flow. Generally this is not a problem unless the hematocrit reaches 60% or more.

Conversely, the combination of a low hematocrit with a high plasma volume, decreasing the blood's viscosity, appears to have certain benefits for the blood's transport function because the blood can flow more easily. Unfortunately, a low hematocrit frequently results from a reduced red blood cell count, as in diseases such as anemias. Under these circumstances the blood can flow easily, but it contains fewer carriers, so oxygen transport is impeded. For physical activity, a low hematocrit with a normal or slightly elevated number of red blood cells is desirable. This combination should facilitate oxygen transport. Many endurance athletes achieve this condition as part of their cardiovascular system's normal adaptation to training. This will be discussed in chapter 10.

When donating blood, the removal of one unit, or nearly 500 ml, represents approximately an 8% to 10% reduction in both the total blood volume and in the number of circulating red blood cells. Donors are advised to drink plenty of fluids. Because plasma is primarily water, simple fluid replacement returns plasma volume to normal within 24 to 48 hr. However, it will take at least six weeks to reconstitute the red blood cells, as they must go through full development before they are functional. This greatly compromises the performance of endurance athletes by reducing oxygen delivery capacity.

Cardiovascular Response to Exercise

Now that we have reviewed the basic anatomy and physiology of the cardiovascular system, we can look specifically at how this system responds to the increased demands placed on the body during exercise. During exercise, oxygen demand in the active muscles increases sharply. More nutrients are utilized. Metabolic processes speed up, so more waste is created. During prolonged exercise or exercise in a hot environ-ment, body temperature increases. In intense exercise, hydrogen ion concentration increases in the muscle and blood, lowering their pH.

Numerous cardiovascular changes occur during exercise. All share a common goal: to allow the system to meet the increased demands placed upon it by carrying out its functions with maximum efficiency. To better understand the changes that occur, we must look more closely at specific cardiovascular functions. We will examine changes in all components of the cardiovascular system, looking specifically at the following:

- Heart rate
- Stroke volume
- Cardiac output
- Blood flow
- Blood pressure
- The blood

Heart Rate

The heart rate (HR) is one of the simplest and most informative of the cardiovascular parameters. Measuring it involves simply taking the subject's pulse, usually at the radial or carotid site, as shown in Figure 8.9. Heart rate reflects the amount of work the heart must do to meet the increased demands of the body when engaged in activity. To understand this, we must compare the heart rate at rest and during exercise.

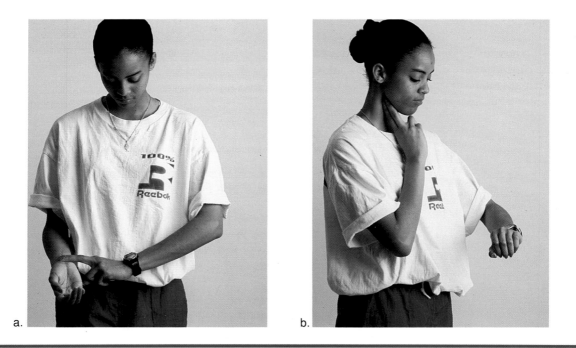

a.　　　　　　　　　　　　　　　b.

Figure 8.9　The procedure for taking (a) the radial pulse and (b) the carotid pulse.

Resting Heart Rate

Resting heart rate averages 60 to 80 beats per minute. In middle-aged, unconditioned, sedentary individuals the resting rate can exceed 100 beats per minute. In highly conditioned endurance-trained athletes, resting rates in the range of 28 to 40 beats per minute have been reported. Your resting heart rate typically decreases with age. It is also affected by environmental factors; for example, it increases with extremes in temperature and altitude.

Before the start of exercise, your pre-exercise heart rate usually increases well above normal resting values. This is called an anticipatory response. This response is mediated through release of the neurotransmitter norepinephrine from your sympathetic nervous system, and the hormone epinephrine from your adrenal gland. Vagal tone probably also decreases. Because the pre-exercise heart rate is elevated, reliable estimates of actual resting heart rate should be made only under conditions of total relaxation, such as early in the morning before arising from a restful night's sleep. Pre-exercise heart rates should not be used as estimates of resting heart rate.

Heart Rate During Exercise

When you begin to exercise, your heart rate increases rapidly in proportion to your exercise intensity. This is illustrated in Figure 8.10. In this figure, exercise intensity is represented by oxygen uptake because the two are directly related. When the rate of work (intensity) is accurately controlled and measured (for example, on a cycle ergometer), the oxygen uptake can be predicted. Thus, expressing the rate of work or exercise intensity in terms of oxygen uptake is not only accurate but is appropriate for comparing either different people or an individual under different circumstances.

Maximum Heart Rate. Your heart rate increases directly as you increase your exercise intensity (see Figure 8.10), until you are near the point of exhaustion. As that point is approached, your heart rate begins to level off. This indicates that you are approaching your maximum value. The maximum heart rate (HR max) is the highest heart rate value you achieve in an all-out effort to the point of exhaustion. This is a highly reliable value that remains constant from day to day and changes only slightly from year to year.

Estimates of maximum heart rate can be made based on your age because maximum heart rate shows a slight but steady decrease of about 1 beat per year beginning at 10 to 15 years of age. Subtracting your age from 220 provides an approximation of your average maximum heart rate. However, this is only an estima-

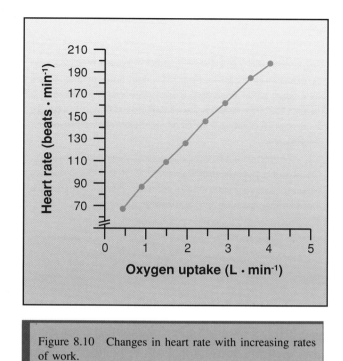

Figure 8.10   Changes in heart rate with increasing rates of work.

tion—individual values vary considerably from this average value. To illustrate, for a 40 year old, maximum heart rate would be estimated at 180 beats per minute (HR max = 220 − 40). For all 40 year olds, however, 68% will have actual maximum heart rate values between 168 and 192 beats per minute (mean ± 1 standard deviation), and 95% will fall between 156 and 204 beats per minute (mean ± 2 standard deviations). This demonstrates the potential for error in estimating a person's maximum heart rate.

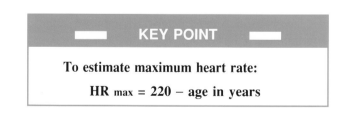

KEY POINT

To estimate maximum heart rate:

HR max = 220 − age in years

Steady State Heart Rate.   When the rate of work is held constant at submaximal levels of exercise, heart rate increases fairly rapidly until it reaches a plateau. This plateau is the steady state heart rate, and it is the optimal heart rate for meeting the circulatory demands at that specific rate of work. For each subsequent increase in intensity, heart rate will reach a new steady-state value within 1 to 2 min. However, the more intense the exercise, the longer it takes to achieve this steady-state value.

The concept of steady state heart rate forms the basis for several tests that have been developed to estimate physical fitness. In one such test, individuals are placed on an exercise device, such as a cycle ergometer, and are exercised at two or three standardized rates of work. Those in better physical condition, based on their cardio-respiratory endurance capacity, will have lower steady state heart rates at a given rate of work than those who are less fit. Thus steady state heart rate is a valid predictor of heart efficiency—a lower rate reflects a more efficient heart.

When exercise is performed at a constant rate over a prolonged period, particularly under conditions of heat stress, the heart rate tends to drift upward instead of maintaining its steady-state value. This response is part of a phenomenon called cardiovascular drift (discussed later in this chapter).

Stroke Volume

Stroke volume also changes during exercise to allow the heart to work more efficiently. It has become increasingly clear that with near-maximal and maximal rates of work, stroke volume is a major determinant of cardiorespiratory endurance capacity. Let's examine the basis for this.

Stroke volume is determined by four factors:

1. The volume of venous blood returned to the heart
2. Ventricular distensibility, or the capacity to enlarge the ventricle
3. Ventricular contractility
4. Aortic or pulmonary artery pressure (the pressure against which the ventricles must contract)

The first two factors influence the filling capacity of the ventricle, determining how much blood is available for filling the ventricle and the ease with which the ventricle is filled at the available pressure. The last two factors influence the ventricle's ability to empty, determining the force with which blood is ejected and the pressure against which it must flow in the arteries. These four factors directly control the alterations in stroke volume in response to increasing exercise intensity.

Stroke Volume Increase With Exercise

Researchers agree that stroke volume increases above resting values during exercise. But there are conflicting reports about stroke volume changes as you go from very low rates of work to maximal work or exhaustion. Most researchers agree that stroke volume increases with increasing rates of work, but only up to exercise intensities between 40% and 60% of maximal capacity. At that point, stroke volume is thought to plateau, as shown in Figure 8.11, remaining essentially unchanged up to and including the point of exhaustion.

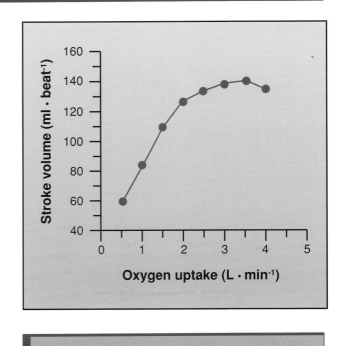

Figure 8.11 Changes in stroke volume with increasing rates of work.

When the body is in an upright position, stroke volume almost doubles from resting to maximal values. For example, in active but untrained individuals, it increases from about 50 to 60 ml at rest to 100 to 120 ml at maximal exercise. In highly trained endurance athletes, stroke volume can increase from 80 to 110 ml at rest to 160 to 200 ml at maximal exercise. During supine exercise, such as swimming, stroke volume also increases, but usually by only about 20% to 40%, not nearly as much as in an upright position. Why is there such a difference depending on body position?

When the body is in the supine position, blood does not pool in the lower extremities. Because of this, blood returns more easily to the heart, which means that resting stroke volume values are much higher in the supine position than in the upright position. Thus the increase in stroke volume with maximal exercise is not as great in the supine position as in the upright position. Interestingly, the highest stroke volume attainable in upright exercise is only slightly greater than the resting value in the reclining position. The majority of the stroke volume increase during low to moderate levels of work appears to be compensating for the force of gravity.

Explanations of Stroke Volume Increase

Although there is agreement that stroke volume increases from rest to exercise, until recently just how this increase occurs was not well documented. One

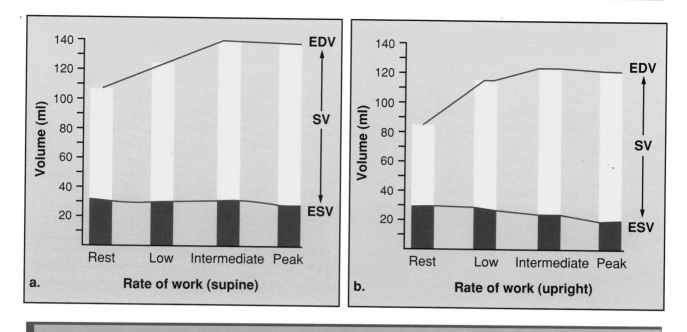

Figure 8.12   Changes in left ventricular end-diastolic volume, end-systolic volume, and stroke volume at rest and during a low rate of work, an intermediate rate of work, and a peak rate of work when the subject is (a) in the supine position and (b) in the upright position. Adapted from Poliner et al. (1980).

explanation is the Frank-Starling law, which states that the primary factor in controlling stroke volume is the extent that the ventricle stretches. When the ventricle stretches more, it will contract with more force. For example, if a larger volume of blood enters the chamber when your ventricle fills during diastole, the ventricle's walls will be stretched more than when a smaller volume enters. In order to eject the greater amount of blood, your ventricle must react to this increased stretching by contracting more strongly. This is referred to as the Frank-Starling mechanism. Conversely, stroke volume could also increase if the ventricle's contractility was greater, even without an increased end diastolic volume. Which of these mechanisms is responsible for increased stroke volume?

Several newer cardiovascular diagnostic techniques have made it possible to determine exactly how stroke volume changes with exercise. Echocardiography (using sound waves) and radionuclide (using electromagnetic radiation) techniques have been used successfully to determine how the heart chambers respond to increasing oxygen demands during exercise. With both techniques, continuous pictures can be taken of the heart at rest and up to near-maximal rates of exercise.

Figure 8.12 illustrates the results of one study of normal, active, but untrained subjects. In this study, participants were tested during both supine and upright cycle ergometry under four conditions:

1. Rest
2. A low work rate
3. An intermediate work rate
4. A peak work rate[13]

An increase in left ventricular end-diastolic volume (greater filling) would indicate that the Frank-Starling mechanism is operating, and a decrease in the left ventricular end-systolic volume (greater emptying) would indicate an increased degree of contractility.

These results indicate that both the Frank-Starling mechanism and increased contractility are important in increasing stroke volume. The Frank-Starling mechanism appears to have its greatest influence at the lower rates of work, and contractility has its greatest effects at the higher rates of work. Several other studies have supported this interpretation.

Recall that heart rate increases with exercise intensity. The plateau or small decrease in left ventricular end-diastolic volume could be caused by reduced ventricular filling time. One study observed that ventricular filling time was reduced from about 500 to 700 ms at rest to about 150 ms at higher heart rates (about 150 to 200 beats per minute).[17] So with increasing work rates approaching maximum heart rates, the diastolic filling time could be shortened enough to limit filling. As a result, end-diastolic volume might plateau or start to decrease.

For the Frank-Starling mechanism to work, the amount of blood entering the ventricle must increase.

Conflicting Research on Stroke Volume Increase

Although researchers agree that stroke volume increases as work rates increase up to around 40% to 60% of maximum, reports about what happens after that point differ widely. A review of studies conducted between the mid-1960s and the early 1990s reveals no clear pattern of stroke volume increases beyond the 40% to 60% work rate range. Examining both early and recent research reveals that the conflict continues. Several studies have found a plateau in stroke volume at approximately 50% of $\dot{V}O_2$ max, with little or no change occurring with further increases.[1,3,8,12,16] However, several other studies have shown that stroke volume continues to increase beyond that rate.[3,5,7,14]

This apparent disagreement might be the result of the mode of exercise testing or the participant's training level. Studies that show plateaus in the 40% to 60% $\dot{V}O_2$ max range have typically used cycle ergometers. Previous studies have shown that blood is trapped in the legs during cycle ergometer exercise. Thus the plateau in stroke volume might be unique to exercise on cycle ergometers, resulting from decreased venous return of blood from the legs.

In studies where stroke volume continued to increase up to maximal rates of exercise, subjects were generally highly trained athletes. Many highly trained athletes can continue to increase their stroke volumes after exceeding the 40% to 60% $\dot{V}O_2$ max level, perhaps because of adaptations to training. Finally, stroke volume is difficult to assess, particularly at higher work rates, so differences between studies could result from differences in the techniques used to measure cardiac output or stroke volume, and the accuracy of these techniques at different exercise intensities. Definitive research has yet to be done.

For this to occur, venous blood return to the heart must increase. This can happen rapidly with redistribution of blood by sympathetic activation of arteries and arterioles in inactive areas of the body and general sympathetic activation of the venous system. Also, the muscles are more active during exercise, so their pumping action increases. In addition, respiration increases, so intrathoracic and intra-abdominal pressure changes are increased. All of these changes enhance venous return.

Cardiac Output

Now that we have discussed both of the components of cardiac output, we can put this information together to understand what happens to cardiac output during exercise. Changes in cardiac output, because it is the product of both heart rate and stroke volume, are predictable with increasing work levels, as seen in Figure 8.13. The resting value for cardiac output is approximately 5.0 L · min⁻¹. Cardiac output increases directly with increasing exercise intensity to at least 20 to 40 L · min⁻¹. The absolute value varies with body size and endurance conditioning. The linear relationship between cardiac output and work rate should not be surprising, though, because the major purpose of the increase in cardiac output is to meet the muscles' increased demand for oxygen.

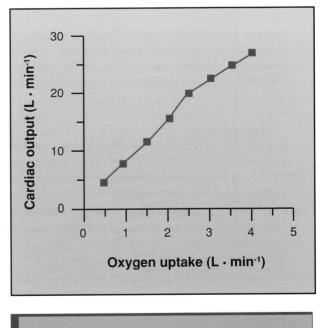

Figure 8.13 Changes in cardiac output with increasing rates of work.

Overall Changes in Cardiac Function

Because $\dot{Q} = HR \times SV$, changes in either heart rate or stroke volume will have an impact on the other component. Having viewed them each separately, we now need to put them together.

Consider the following example. You rise from a reclining position to a sitting position and then stand. You start walking. Your walk gives way to a jog, and finally you are running. How does your heart respond? As you progress from the reclined position to a full run, your cardiovascular system continuously makes adjustments that allow you to progressively increase your work rate.

If your heart rate when reclining was 50 beats per minute, it will increase to about 55 beats per minute when sitting and to about 60 beats per minute when standing. Why does your heart rate increase? When your body shifts from a reclining to a standing position, stroke volume immediately drops. This is due primarily to the effects of gravity causing blood to pool in your legs, which reduces the volume of blood returning to your heart. At the same time your heart rate increases. This increase in heart rate when changing to an upright posture is simply an adaptation to maintain the cardiac output, because $\dot{Q} = HR \times SV$.

As you begin your activity, moving from standing to walking, your heart rate increases from about 60 to about 90 beats per minute. With moderate-paced jogging it goes to 140 beats per minute, and can reach 180 beats per minute or more with a fast-paced run. The increase in heart rate when changing positions maintains your cardiac output, but the increase with greater activity allows delivery of substantially more blood to your working muscles to meet the oxygen requirements of increasing activity. Stroke volume also increases with exercise, further increasing cardiac output. These relationships are illustrated in Figure 8.14.

During the initial stages of exercise, increased cardiac output is due to an increase in both heart rate and stroke volume. When the level of exercise exceeds 40% to 60% of the individual's capacity, stroke volume has either plateaued or begun to increase at a much slower rate. Thus further increases in cardiac output are largely the result of increases in heart rate.

Table 8.1 illustrates these relationships. Using three activities (running, cycling, and swimming), it shows the expected changes in heart rate (HR), stroke volume (SV), and cardiac output ($\dot{Q}$) from rest to maximal levels of exercise. It is important to realize that there are very specific responses to each of these modes.

> **■■■ KEY POINT ■■■**
>
> During exercise, cardiac output increases primarily to match the need for increased oxygen supply to the working muscles.

Blood Flow

We now understand the cardiac changes that provide increased cardiac output during exercise, but the

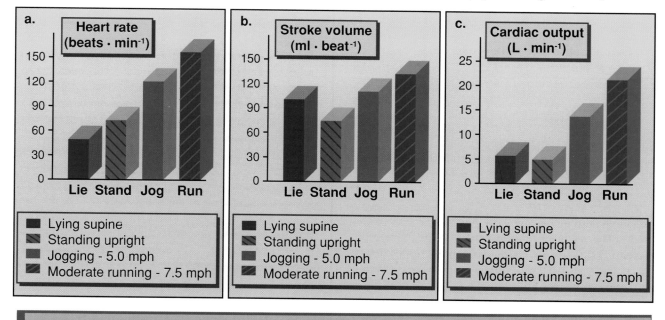

Figure 8.14   Changes in (a) heart rate, (b) stroke volume, and (c) cardiac output with changes in posture and in the level of exercise.

Table 8.1 Changes in Heart Rate, Stroke Volume, and Cardiac Output

Activity	Condition	Heart rate (beats • min⁻¹)	Stroke volume (ml • beat⁻¹)	Cardiac output (L • min⁻¹)
Running	Resting	60	70	4.2
	Maximal exercise	190	130	24.7
Cycling	Resting	60	70	4.2
	Maximal exercise	185	120	22.2
Swimming	Resting[a]	55	95	5.2
	Maximal exercise	170	135	22.9

[a]Measurements taken in the supine position.

cardiovascular system is even more efficient at getting blood to areas where it is needed than what these cardiac adaptations would suggest. Recall from our earlier discussion that the vascular system can redistribute blood so that areas with the greatest need receive more blood than areas with low demands. We now turn our attention to changes in blood flow during exercise.

▬ IN REVIEW . . . ▬

1. As exercise intensity increases, heart rate increases. The heart ejects blood more often, thus speeding up circulation.
2. Stroke volume also increases, so the amount of blood ejected with each contraction increases.
3. Increases in heart rate and stroke volume increase cardiac output. Thus more blood is forced out of the heart during exercise than when at rest, and circulation speeds up. This ensures that adequate supplies of the needed materials— oxygen and nutrients— reach the tissues and that waste products, which build up much more rapidly during exercise, are quickly cleared away.

Redistribution of Blood During Exercise

Blood flow patterns change markedly as you move from rest to exercise. Blood is redirected, through the action of the sympathetic nervous system, away from areas where it is not essential, to those areas that are active during exercise. Only 15% to 20% of the resting cardiac output goes to muscle, but during exhaustive exercise the muscles receive 80% to 85% of the cardiac output. This shift in blood flow to the muscles is accomplished primarily by reducing blood flow to the kidneys, liver, stomach, and intestines.

As the body starts to overheat, either as a direct result of exercise or because of high environmental temperatures, more blood is redirected to the skin to conduct heat away from the body's core to its periphery, where heat is lost to the environment. This increase in skin blood flow means less blood is available for muscles, and it explains why most endurance athletic performances in the heat are well below average.

When considering blood redistribution within the body, it is easy to think of each of these mechanisms separately, but we must remember that they all work together. To illustrate this, we will examine what happens to blood flow during exercise, focusing on the needs of the skeletal muscles.

As exercise begins, the active skeletal muscles rapidly experience an increased need for blood supply. This need is met through a generalized sympathetic stimulation of vessels in those areas in which blood flow is to be reduced (for example, the digestive system and the kidneys). This causes constriction of vessels in those areas and thus diverts blood flow to the skeletal muscles where it is needed. In contrast, in the skeletal muscles, sympathetic stimulation to the constrictor fibers in the vessel walls is reduced and sympathetic stimulation to the vasodilator fibers is increased. Thus these vessels dilate and additional blood flows into the active muscles.

Also, the metabolic rate of the muscle tissue rises during exercise. As a result, metabolic waste products begin to accumulate. Increased metabolism causes an increase in acidity, CO_2, and temperature in the muscle tissue. These local changes trigger vasodilation through autoregulation, increasing blood flow through the local capillaries. Autoregulation is also triggered by the low partial pressure of oxygen (PO_2) in the tissue (increased oxygen demand), the act of muscle contraction, and possibly other vasoactive substances released as a result of contraction.

Regulation of body temperature is controlled in much the same way. During heavy exercise (or even at rest in a hot environment) heat builds up in the body and must be dissipated. To accomplish this, blood is redirected or shunted to the skin through reduced sympathetic stimulation there, leading to dilation of the superficial vessels. This promotes heat loss, because heat from deep in the body can be released when blood moves close to the skin. This allows maintenance of constant body temperature. Conversely, when exposed to a cold environment, the body conserves heat by increasing sympathetic stimulation to vessels in the skin, causing them to constrict to divert blood away from the cold skin.

Cardiovascular Drift

With prolonged exercise or exercise in a hot environment, blood volume is reduced by a loss of water through sweating and a generalized shifting of fluid out of the blood into the tissues. This latter condition is referred to as edema. With the total blood volume gradually decreasing as the duration of exercise increases and with a redistribution of more blood to the periphery for cooling, cardiac filling pressure is reduced. This causes decreased venous return to the right side of the heart. In turn, this reduces stroke volume (EDV is decreased; SV = EDV − ESV). The heart rate compensates for the decreased stroke volume by increasing, in an effort to maintain cardiac output ($\dot{Q}$ = HR × SV).

These alterations are referred to as cardiovascular drift. This response allows you to continue exercising at low to moderate intensities. However, your body is unable to fully compensate for your decreased stroke volume at high intensities because your heart rate attains its maximal value at a much lower exercise intensity, thus limiting your maximal performance capabilities.

Competition for Blood Supply

When the demands of exercise are imposed in addition to all the other demands of the body, competition can occur for the limited volume of blood available. Consider the following research that examined the relationship between the timing of feeding and competition. Working with miniature pigs, McKirnan et al. studied the effects of feeding versus fasting on the distribution of blood flow during exercise.[11] The pigs were divided into two groups. One group fasted for 14 to 17 hr. The other group ate their morning ration distributed in two feedings—half fed 90 to 120 min before exercise, and half fed 30 to 45 min before exercise. Both groups of pigs were run at approximately 65% of their $\dot{V}O_2$ max.

Blood flow to the hindlimb muscles during exercise was 18% lower in the feeding group than in the fasting group. Gastrointestinal blood flow was increased 23% in the fed group. Waaler et al. reported similar results in humans, concluding that the redistribution of gastrointestinal blood flow to the working

muscles is less marked after a meal than before a meal.[18] This suggests that athletes should be very careful in timing their meals before competition, because they want as much blood flow as possible available to the active muscles during exercise.

Redistribution of blood in the body occurs primarily to meet the demands of active tissues. This requires not only that enough blood is supplied to the active tissue, but also that exchange occurs between the blood and the tissue fluid. For the exchange to be effective, it must be an ongoing process, which requires that the blood be constantly flowing, circulating to bring in nutrients and carry away wastes. We next turn our attention to the driving force behind blood flow: blood pressure.

Blood Pressure

When examining differences in blood pressure during exercise, you must distinguish between systolic and diastolic pressure, because they show different changes. With endurance-type, whole-body activity, systolic blood pressure increases in direct proportion to increased exercise intensity. Systolic pressures of 120 mmHg at rest can exceed 200 mmHg at exhaustion. Systolic pressures of 240 to 250 mmHg have been reported in normal, healthy, highly trained athletes at maximal levels of exercise.

Increased systolic blood pressure results from the increased cardiac output ($\dot{Q}$) that accompanies increasing rates of work. It helps drive the blood quickly through the vasculature. Also, blood pressure determines how much fluid leaves the capillaries, entering the tissues and carrying needed supplies. Thus increased systolic pressure facilitates the delivery process.

Diastolic blood pressure changes little if any during endurance exercise, regardless of the intensity. Remember that diastolic pressure reflects the pressure in the arteries when the heart is at rest. None of the changes we have discussed alter this pressure significantly, so there is no reason to expect it to increase. Increases in diastolic pressure of 15 mmHg or more are considered abnormal responses to exercise and are one of several indications for immediately stopping a diagnostic exercise test. Figure 8.15 illustrates a typical blood pressure response to both leg and arm cycling exercise with increasing rates of work.

Blood pressure reaches a steady state during submaximal steady-state endurance exercise. As work intensity increases, so does systolic blood pressure. If steady-state exercise is prolonged, the systolic pressure might start to decrease gradually, but diastolic pressure remains constant. The decrease in systolic blood pressure, if it occurs, is a normal response and simply

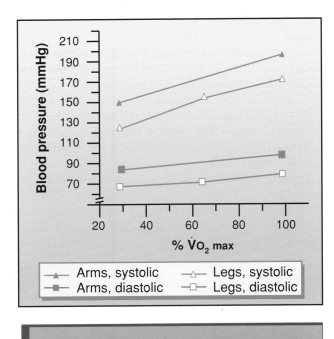

Figure 8.15 Blood pressure response to both leg and arm cycling at the same absolute rates of oxygen consumption. Adapted from Åstrand et al. (1965).

reflects increased arteriole dilation in the active muscles, which decreases the total peripheral resistance (recall from basic physiology that blood pressure = cardiac output × total peripheral resistance).

Blood pressure responses to resistance exercise, such as weight lifting, are exaggerated. With high-intensity resistance training, blood pressure can exceed 480/350 mmHg.[10] In such exercise, use of the Valsalva maneuver is quite common. This maneuver occurs when a person tries to exhale while the mouth, nose, and glottis are closed. This action causes an enormous increase in intrathoracic pressure. Much of the subsequent blood pressure increase results from the body's effort to overcome the high internal pressures created during the Valsalva maneuver.

In exercise of the same absolute rate of energy expenditure, the use of upper body musculature, as opposed to lower body musculature, also causes a greater blood pressure response, as seen in Figure 8.15. This is most likely due to the smaller muscle mass and vasculature of the upper body compared to that of the lower body. This size difference results in more resistance to blood flow and thus an increase in blood pressure to overcome this resistance.

This difference in the systolic blood pressure response to upper and lower body exercise has important implications for the heart. Myocardial oxygen uptake and myocardial blood flow are directly related to the product of heart rate and systolic blood pressure. This value is referred to as the double product (DP = HR × systolic blood pressure). With static or dynamic resistance exercise or upper body work, the double product is elevated, indicating a much higher cost to the heart.

The Blood

We have now examined exercise-induced cardiovascular changes. The remaining component of the cardiovascular system is the blood—the fluid that carries needed substances to the tissues and clears away harmful substances. As metabolism increases during exercise, the functions of the blood become more vital for efficient performance. We will now examine changes that occur within the blood to meet these increased demands.

Oxygen Content

At rest, the blood's oxygen content varies from 20 ml of oxygen per 100 ml of arterial blood to 14 ml of oxygen per 100 ml of venous blood. The difference between these two values (20 ml − 14 ml = 6 ml) is referred to as the arterial-venous oxygen difference (a-$\bar{v}O_2$ diff). This value represents the extent to which oxygen is extracted, or removed, from the blood as it passes through the body.

With increasing rates of exercise, the a-$\bar{v}O_2$ diff increases progressively. The a-$\bar{v}O_2$ diff can increase approximately threefold from rest to maximal levels of exercise (see Figure 8.16). This reflects a decreasing venous oxygen content. More oxygen is required by the active muscles, so more oxygen is extracted from the blood. The venous oxygen content drops, approaching zero in the active muscles, but the mixed venous blood in the right atrium of the heart rarely drops below 2 to 4 ml of oxygen per 100 ml of blood. This is because the blood returning from the active tissues is mixed with blood from inactive areas as it returns to the heart. Oxygen use in the inactive tissues is far lower than in the muscles. Arterial oxygen content remains essentially unchanged; however, there have been reports of decreased arterial oxygen content in highly trained athletes at maximal levels of exercise.[4]

Plasma Volume

With the onset of exercise, there is an almost immediate increase in the loss of blood plasma volume to the interstitial fluid space. This probably results from two factors. As blood pressure increases, the hydrostatic pressure within the capillaries increases. Thus the increase in blood pressure forces water from the vascular compartment to the interstitial compartment. Also, as

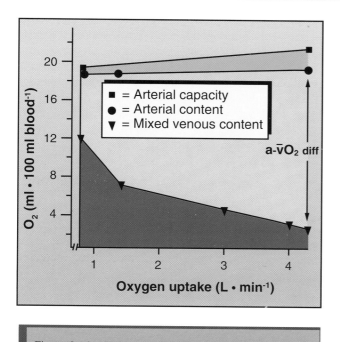

Figure 8.16 Changes in arteriovenous oxygen difference (a-v̄O₂ diff) from low levels to maximal levels of exercise. Adapted from Åstrand and Rodahl (1986).

metabolic waste products build up in the active muscle, intramuscular osmotic pressure increases, and this attracts fluid to the muscle.

A 10% to 20% or greater reduction in plasma volume can occur with prolonged work. Similar 15% to 20% decreases in plasma volume have been observed in 1-min bouts of exhaustive exercise.[15] With resistance training, the plasma volume loss is proportional to the intensity of the effort, with loses of 7.7% when exercising at 40% of the one-repetition maximum up to 13.9% when training at 70%.[2]

If exercise intensity or environmental conditions cause sweating, additional plasma loss can be expected. Although the major source of fluid for sweating is the interstitial fluid, this fluid will be diminished as sweating continues. This increases the osmotic pressure in the interstitial space, which causes even more plasma to move into the tissues. Intracellular fluid volume is impossible to measure directly and accurately, but research suggests that fluid is also lost from the intracellular compartment and even from the red blood cells, which may shrink.

A reduction of plasma volume will likely impair performance. For long-duration activities in which heat loss is a problem, the total flow of blood to active tissues must be reduced to allow increasingly more blood to be diverted to the skin in an attempt to lose body heat. Reduced plasma volume also results in increased blood viscosity, which can impede blood

flow and thus limit oxygen transport, especially if the hematocrit exceeds 60%.

In activities that require several minutes or less, body fluid changes and temperature regulation are of little practical importance. As exercise duration is increased, body fluid changes and temperature regulation become important to efficient performance. For the football player or the marathon runner, these processes are crucial, not only for competition, but also for survival. Deaths have occurred due to dehydration and hyperthermia during or as a result of various sport activities. These issues will be discussed in detail in chapter 11.

Hemoconcentration

When plasma volume is reduced, hemoconcentration occurs. This means that the fluid portion of the blood is reduced, and the cellular and protein portions represent a larger fraction of the total blood volume, as seen in Figure 8.17. Thus they become more concentrated in the blood. This hemoconcentration increases red blood cell concentration substantially—by up to 20% to 25%. Hematocrits increase from 40% to 50%. However, the total number or content of red blood cells is unlikely to change substantially.

As the hematocrit increases, the net effect, even without an increase in the total number of red blood

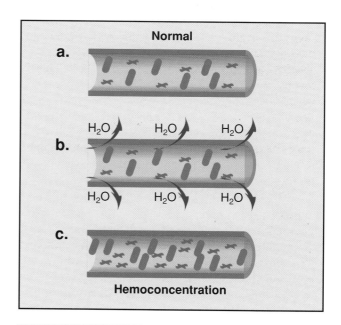

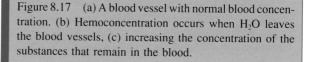

Figure 8.17 (a) A blood vessel with normal blood concentration. (b) Hemoconcentration occurs when H₂O leaves the blood vessels, (c) increasing the concentration of the substances that remain in the blood.

cells, is to increase the amount of red blood cells per unit of blood because the cells are more concentrated. As the red blood cell concentration increases, so does the blood's per unit hemoglobin content. This substantially increases the blood's oxygen-carrying capacity, which is advantageous during exercise.

At one time, the hemoconcentration response was believed to reflect an addition of red blood cells from the spleen to the blood to facilitate oxygen transport. This view assumed that because many animals can increase the number of circulating red blood cells by releasing cells stored in the spleen, humans can also. This explanation was largely discounted in the 1950s and 1960s because limited evidence suggested that the spleen does not serve that function in humans. We now know that the spleen has a storage capacity of

about 50 ml of concentrated red blood cells. Flamm et al., using radionuclide techniques, reported a progressive decrease in the spleen's total blood volume with increasing work rates.[6] The increase in hematocrit paralleled a decrease in the spleen's blood volume. This was confirmed in a subsequent study.[9] The importance of the spleen's role during exercise has yet to be determined.

Blood pH

Finally, blood pH can change considerably with moderate- to high-intensity exercise. Recall that neutral pH is 7.0; greater than 7.0 is alkaline, or basic, and less than 7.0 is acidic (see chapter 9). At rest, arterial blood pH remains constant at about 7.4 — slightly alkaline.

Little change occurs from rest up to an exercise intensity of about 50% of maximal aerobic capacity. As intensity increases above 50%, pH starts to decrease as the blood becomes more acidic. This drop is gradual at first, but becomes more rapid as the body approaches exhaustion. Blood pH values of 7.0 or lower have been reported following maximal sprint-type exercise. The pH in active muscle drops even more, to 6.5 or lower.

The drop in blood pH results primarily from an increased reliance on anaerobic metabolism and corresponds to increases in blood lactate observed with increasing exercise intensity.

IN REVIEW . . .

The changes that occur in the blood during exercise demonstrate that the blood is carrying out its necessary tasks. Here are the major changes seen:

1. The a-$\bar{v}O_2$ diff increases. This happens because the venous oxygen concentration decreases during exercise, reflecting increased extraction of oxygen from the blood for use by the active tissues.

2. Plasma volume decreases during exercise. The fluid (water) is pushed out of the capillaries by increases in hydrostatic pressure as blood pressure increases and is drawn into the muscles by the increased osmotic pressure that results from waste accumulation. However, with prolonged exercise or exercise in hot environments, increasingly more plasma fluid is lost through sweating in an attempt to maintain body temperature, placing the person at risk of dehydration.

3. Hemoconcentration occurs as plasma fluid (water) is lost. Although the actual number of red blood cells might not increase, the net effect of this process is to increase the number of red blood cells per unit of blood, which increases oxygen-carrying capacity.

4. Blood pH can change significantly during exercise, becoming more acidic as it moves from the slightly alkaline resting value of 7.4 down to 7.0 or lower. The muscle pH decreases even further. The decrease in pH primarily results from increased blood lactate accumulation during increased exercise intensity.

In Closing . . .

In this chapter, we have reviewed the structure and function of the cardiovascular system and examined how this system responds during exercise to meet the increased needs of active muscles. We explored its role in transporting and delivering oxygen and nutrients to the active tissues while clearing away metabolic wastes, including carbon dioxide. Knowing how substances are moved within the body, we can now look more closely at the movement of oxygen and carbon dioxide. In the next chapter, we will explore the respiratory system, considering how oxygen is moved into and throughout the body, how it is delivered to the active tissues, and how carbon dioxide is cleared away from them. Then we will examine how respiratory function changes to meet the demands of an active body.

Key Terms

- autoregulation
- cardiac cycle
- cardiac output ($\dot{Q}$)
- cardiovascular drift
- electrocardiogram (ECG)
- end-diastolic volume (EDV)

✓ end-systolic volume (ESV)

✓ extrinsic neural control

Frank-Starling mechanism

✓ hemoglobin

✓ maximum heart rate (HR max)

✓ myocardium

✓ resting heart rate

✓ steady state heart rate

✓ stroke volume (SV)

Study Questions

1. Describe the structure of the heart, the pattern of blood flow through the valves and chambers of the heart, how the heart as a muscle is supplied with blood, and what happens when the resting heart must suddenly supply an exercising body.

2. What events take place that allow the heart to contract, and how is heart rate controlled?

3. What is the difference between systole and diastole, and how does this relate to systolic blood pressure and diastolic blood pressure?

4. How is blood flow to the various regions of the body controlled? How does this vary with exercise?

5. Describe how heart rate, stroke volume, and cardiac output respond to increasing rates of work.

6. How do you determine maximum heart rate? What are alternative methods using indirect estimates? What are the major limitations to these indirect estimates?

7. Describe two important mechanisms for returning blood back to the heart when you are exercising in an upright position.

8. What are the major cardiovascular adjustments made by your body when you are overheated during exercise?

9. What is cardiovascular drift? Why might this be a problem with prolonged exercise?

10. Describe the primary functions of blood.

11. What changes occur in the plasma volume with increasing levels of exercise? With prolonged exercise in the heat?

References

1. Åstrand, P.-O., Cuddy, T.E., Saltin, B., & Stenberg, J. (1964). Cardiac output during submaximal and maximal work. *Journal of Applied Physiology*, **19**, 268-274.

2. Collins, M.A., Cureton, K.J., Hill, D.W., & Ray, C.A. (1989). Relation of plasma volume change to intensity of weight lifting. *Medicine and Science in Sports and Exercise*, **21**, 178-185.

3. Crawford, M.H., Petru, M.A., & Rabinowitz, C. (1985). Effect of isotonic exercise training on left ventricular volume during upright exercise. *Circulation*, **72**, 1237-1243.

4. Dempsey, J.A. (1986). Is the lung built for exercise? *Medicine and Science in Sports and Exercise*, **18**, 143-155.

5. Ekblom, B., & Hermansen, L. (1968). Cardiac output in athletes. *Journal of Applied Physiology*, **25**, 619-625.

6. Flamm, S.D., Taki, J., Moore, R., Lewis, S.F., Keech, F., Maltais, F., Ahmad, M., Callahan, R., Dragotakes, S., Alpert, N., & Strauss, H.W. (1990). Redistribution of regional and organ blood volume and effect on cardiac function in relation to upright exercise intensity in healthy human subjects. *Circulation*, **81**, 1550-1559.

7. Hermansen, L., Ekblom, B., & Saltin, B. (1970). Cardiac output during submaximal and maximal treadmill and bicycle exercise. *Journal of Applied Physiology*, **29**, 82-86.

8. Higginbotham, M.B., Morris, K.G., Williams, R.S., McHale, P.A., Coleman, R.E., & Cobb, F.R. (1986). Regulation of stroke volume during submaximal and maximal upright exercise in normal man. *Circulation Research*, **58**, 281-291.

9. Laub, M., Hvid-Jacobsen, K., Hovind, P., Kanstrup, I.-L., Christensen, N.J., & Nielsen, S.L. (1993). Spleen emptying and venous hematocrit in humans during exercise. *Journal of Applied Physiology*, **74**, 1024-1026.

10. MacDougall, J.D., Tuxen, D., Sale, D.G., Moroz, J.R., & Sutton, J.R. (1985). Arterial blood pressure response to heavy resistance exercise. *Journal of Applied Physiology*, **58**, 785-790.

11. McKirnan, M.D., Gray, C.G., & White, F.C. (1991). Effects of feeding on muscle blood flow during prolonged exercise in miniature swine. *Journal of Applied Physiology*, **70**, 1097-1104.

12. Plotnick, G.D., Becker, L.C., Fisher, M.L., Gerstenblith, G., Renlund, D.G., Fleg, J.L., Weisfeldt, M.L., & Lakatta, E.G. (1986). Use of the Frank-Starling mechanism during submaximal versus maximal upright exercise. *American Journal of Physiology (Heart and Circulation Physiology)*, **251**, H1101-H1105.

13. Poliner, L.R., Dehmer, G.J., Lewis, S.E., Parkey, R.W., Blomqvist, C.G., & Willerson, J.T. (1980). Left

ventricular performance in normal subjects: A comparison of the responses to exercise in the upright and supine position. *Circulation*, **62**, 528-534.

14. Scruggs, K.D., Martin, N.B., Broeder, C.E., Hofman, Z., Thomas, E.L., Wambsgans, K.C., & Wilmore, J.H. (1991). Stroke volume during submaximal exercise in endurance-trained normotensive subjects and in untrained hypertensive subjects with beta-blockade (propranolol and pindolol). *American Journal of Cardiology*, **67**, 416-421.

15. Sejersted, O.M., Vøllestad, N.K., & Medbø, J.I. (1986). Muscle fluid and electrolyte balance during and following exercise. *Acta Physiologica Scandinavica*, **128**(Suppl. 556), 119-127.

16. Stenberg, J., Åstrand, P.-O., Ekblom, B., Royce, J., & Saltin, B. (1967). Hemodynamic response to work with different muscle groups, sitting and supine. *Journal of Applied Physiology*, **22**, 61-70.

17. Turkevich, D., Micco, A., & Reeves, J.T. (1988). Noninvasive measurement of the decrease in left ventricular filling time during maximal exercise in normal subjects. *American Journal of Cardiology*, **62**, 650-652.

18. Waaler, B.A., Eriksen, M., & Janbu, T. (1990). The effect of a meal on cardiac output in man at rest and during moderate exercise. *Acta Physiologica Scandinavica*, **140**, 167-173.

Selected Readings

Åstrand, P.-O., Ekblom, B., Messin, R., Saltin, B., & Stenberg, J. (1965). Intraarterial blood pressure during exercise with different muscle groups. *Journal of Applied Physiology*, **20**, 253-256.

Carlsten, A., & Grimby, G. (1966). *The circulatory response to muscular exercise in man*. Springfield, IL: Charles C Thomas.

Clausen, J.P. (1977). Effect of physical training on cardiovascular adjustments to exercise in man. *Physiological Reviews*, **57**, 779-815.

Costill, D.L., & Fink, W. (1974). Plasma volume changes following exercise and thermal dehydration. *Journal of Applied Physiology*, **37**, 521-525.

Cummin, A.R.C., Iyawe, V.I., Mehta, N., & Saunders, K.B. (1986). Ventilation and cardiac output during the onset of exercise, and during voluntary hyperventilation, in humans. *Journal of Physiology*, **370**, 567-583.

Dowell, R.T. (1983). Cardiac adaptations to exercise. *Exercise and Sport Sciences Reviews*, **11**, 99-117.

Guyton, A.C. (1991). *Textbook of medical physiology* (8th ed.). Philadelphia: Saunders.

Hossack, K.F., Bruce, R.A., Green, B., Kusumi, F., DeRouen, T.A., & Trimble, S. (1980). Maximal cardiac output during upright exercise: Approximate normal standards and variations with coronary heart disease. *American Journal of Cardiology*, **46**, 204-212.

Hossack, K.F., Kusumi, F., & Bruce, R.A. (1981). Approximate normal standards of maximal cardiac output during upright exercise in women. *American Journal of Cardiology*, **47**, 1080-1086.

Laughlin, M.H., & Armstrong, R.B. (1985). Muscle blood flow during locomotory exercise. *Exercise and Sport Sciences Reviews*, **13**, 95-136.

Pivarnik, J.M., Montain, S.J., Graves, J.E., & Pollock, M.L. (1988). Alterations in plasma volume, electrolytes and protein during incremental exercise at different pedal speeds. *European Journal of Applied Physiology*, **57**, 103-109.

Rowell, L.B. (1974). Human cardiovascular adjustments to exercise and thermal stress. *Physiological Reviews*, **54**, 75-159.

Rowell, L.B. (1986). *Human circulation: Regulation during physical stress*. New York: Oxford University Press.

Saltin, B. (1985). Hemodynamic adaptations to exercise. *American Journal of Cardiology*, **55**, 42D-47D.

Saltin, B., & Rowell, L.B. (1980). Functional adaptations to physical activity and inactivity. *Federation Proceedings*, **39**, 1506-1513.

Senay, L.C., Jr., & Pivarnik, J.M. (1985). Fluid shifts during exercise. *Exercise and Sport Sciences Reviews*, **13**, 335-387.

Smith, E.E., Guyton, A.C., Manning, R.D., & White, R.J. (1976). Integrated mechanisms of cardiovascular response and control during exercise in the normal human. *Progress in Cardiovascular Diseases*, **18**, 421-443.

Steingart, R.M., Wexler, J., Slagle, S., & Scheuer, J. (1984). Radionuclide ventriculographic responses to graded supine and upright exercise: Critical role of the Frank-Starling mechanism at submaximal exercise. *American Journal of Cardiology*, **53**, 1671-1677.

Stone, H.L., Dormer, K.J., Foreman, R.D., Thies, R., & Blair, R.W. (1985). Neural regulation of the cardiovascular system during exercise. *Federation Proceedings*, **44**, 2271-2278.

Sullivan, M.J., Cobb, F.R., & Higginbotham, M.B. (1991). Stroke volume increase by similar mechanisms during upright exercise in normal men and women. *American Journal of Cardiology*, **67**, 1405-1412.

Vanoverschelde, J.-L., Essamri, B., Vanbutsele, R., D'Hondt, A.-M., Cosyns, J., Detry, J.-L.R., & Melin, J.A. (1993). Contribution of left ventricular diastolic function to exercise capacity in normal subjects. *Journal of Applied Physiology*, **74**(5), 2225-2233.

Chapter 9
Respiratory Regulation During Exercise

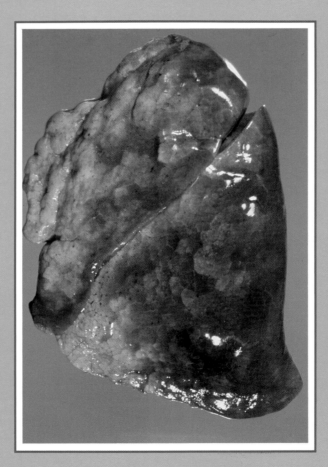

Chapter Overview

We cannot live without oxygen. Our cells depend on it for their survival, and, as we learned in chapter 5, oxygen is essential for the energy production that fuels all of our bodies' activities. Endurance performance depends on the delivery of sufficient amounts of oxygen to our muscles and adequate cellular uptake of this gas once it arrives there. But at the same time, the metabolic processes occurring in our active muscles are generating another gas, carbon dioxide, which, unlike oxygen, is toxic. Normal cellular activity requires oxygen but is impaired when carbon dioxide levels rise.

Our muscles' crucial needs for adequate oxygen supply and carbon dioxide clearance are met by the respiratory system. As we saw in the previous chapter, the cardiovascular system transports these gases. But the respiratory system brings oxygen into our bodies and rids us of excess carbon dioxide. This system will be our focus in this chapter. We will begin with an overview of the steps involved in respiration and gas exchange, then we will examine how these processes are regulated. We will consider how the respiratory system functions when we are exercising and how it can limit performance. Finally, we will consider the respiratory system's unique role in maintaining acid-base balance throughout our bodies and the significance of this balance during physical activity.

Because swimming requires controlled breathing, many competitive swimmers try to improve their breath-holding ability by attempting to swim several pool lengths underwater without breathing. In 1963, while I [DLC] was coaching a high school team, a group of my swimmers tried to see who could swim the farthest underwater. They took repeated deep breaths before diving into the pool and swam until the need to breathe became intolerable. Most were able to make two lengths (total of 50 yd, or 46 m) of the pool. But one swimmer continued on for a third length, made the turn, and headed into a fourth length. Halfway back, and at a depth of 3 or 4 ft (about 1 m), he suddenly stopped swimming and became motionless. One of the other swimmers quickly dove into the pool and recovered his unconscious body. Fortunately, when he reached the surface he began breathing and recovered consciousness within 15 to 20 s. Needless to say, we never used that training ploy again.

The respiratory and cardiovascular systems combine to provide an efficient delivery system that carries oxygen to our body tissues and removes carbon dioxide from them. This transportation involves four separate processes:

1. Pulmonary ventilation (breathing), which is the movement of gases into and out of the lungs
2. Pulmonary diffusion, which is the exchange of gases between the lungs and the blood
3. Transport of oxygen and carbon dioxide via the blood
4. Capillary gas exchange, which is the exchange of gases between the capillary blood and the metabolically active tissues

The first two processes are referred to as external respiration because they involve moving gases from outside the body into the lungs and then the blood. Once the gases are in the blood they must travel to the tissues. When blood arrives at the tissues, the fourth step of respiration occurs. This gas exchange between the blood and the tissues is called internal respiration. Thus external and internal respiration are linked by the circulatory system. In the following sections we will examine all four components of respiration.

Pulmonary Ventilation

Pulmonary ventilation, commonly referred to as breathing, is the process by which we move air into and out of our lungs. The anatomy of the respiratory system is illustrated in Figure 9.1. Air is typically drawn into the lungs through the nose, although the mouth must also be used when the demand for air exceeds the amount that can comfortably be brought in through the nose. Bringing air in through the nose

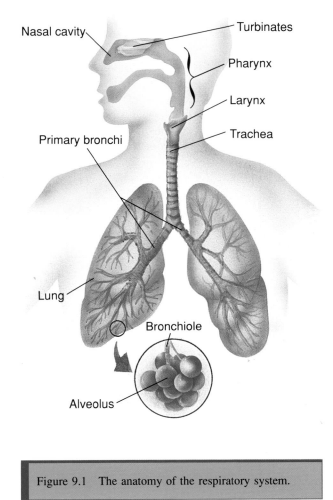

Figure 9.1 The anatomy of the respiratory system.

has certain advantages over mouth breathing. The air is warmed and humidified as it swirls through the irregular surfaces (turbinates) inside the nose. Of equal importance, the turbinates churn the inhaled air, causing dust and other particles to contact and adhere to the nasal mucosa. This filters out all but the tiniest particles, minimizing irritation and the threat of respiratory infections. From the nose and mouth, the air travels through the pharynx, larynx, trachea, bronchi, and bronchioles, until it finally reaches the smallest respiratory units: the alveoli. The alveoli are the sites of gas exchange in the lungs.

KEY POINT

Breathing through the nose helps humidify and warm the air during inhalation and filters out particles from the air.

The lungs are not directly attached to the ribs. Rather, they are suspended by the pleural sacs. These sacs envelop the lungs and contain a thin layer of pleural fluid that reduces friction during respiratory movements. In addition, these sacs are connected to the lungs and to the inner surface of the thoracic cage, causing the lungs to take the shape and size of the cage as the chest expands and contracts.

These relationships between the lungs, the pleural sacs, and the thoracic cage determine air flow into and out of the lungs. Let's examine the two phases involved: inspiration and expiration.

Inspiration

Inspiration is an active process involving the diaphragm and the external intercostal muscles. The dynamics of inspiration are shown in Figure 9.2. Figure 9.2a shows the resting dimensions of the lungs and the thoracic cage. Figure 9.2b indicates the movements that occur during inspiration. The ribs and sternum are moved by the external intercostal muscles. The ribs swing up and out, much like the movement of a bucket handle. The sternum swings up and forward, much like the movement of a pump handle. At the same time, the diaphragm contracts, flattening down toward the abdomen.

These actions expand all three dimensions of the thoracic cage, in turn expanding the lungs. When the lungs are expanded, the air within them has more space to fill, so the pressure within the lungs decreases, as shown in Figure 9.2c. As a result, the pressure in the lungs (intrapulmonary pressure) is less than the pressure of the air outside the body. Because the respiratory tract is open to the outside, air rushes into the lungs to reduce this pressure difference. Thus air is brought into the lungs during inspiration.

During forced or labored breathing, such as during heavy exercise, inspiration is further assisted by the action of other muscles, such as the scalenes (anterior, middle, and posterior) and sternocleidomastoid in the neck and the pectorals in the chest. These help raise the ribs even more than during regular breathing.

The pressure changes required for adequate ventilation at rest are really quite small. For example, at standard atmospheric pressure (760 mmHg), inspiration may decrease the pressure in the lungs (intrapulmonary pressure) by only about 3 mmHg. However, during maximal respiratory effort, such as during exhaustive exercise, the intrapulmonary pressure may decrease by 80 to 100 mmHg!

Expiration

At rest, expiration is usually a passive process involving the relaxation of the inspiratory muscles and elastic recoil of the lung tissue. This is depicted in Figure 9.3a. As the diaphragm relaxes, it returns to its normal upward arched position. As the external intercostal muscles relax, the ribs and sternum lower back into their resting positions. While this happens, the elastic nature of the lung tissue causes it to recoil to its resting size. As shown in Figure 9.3b, this increases the pressure in the thorax, so air is forced out of the lungs. Thus expiration is accomplished.

During forced breathing, expiration becomes a more active process. The internal intercostal muscles can actively pull the ribs down. This action can be assisted by the latissimus dorsi and quadratus lumborum muscles. Contracting the abdominal muscles increases the intra-abdominal pressure, forcing the abdominal viscera upward against the diaphragm and accelerating its return to the domed position. These muscles also pull the rib cage down and inward.

The changes in intra-abdominal and intrathoracic pressure that accompany respiration not only assist in forced breathing, but they also assist in returning venous blood back to the heart. As these pressures increase, they are transmitted to the great veins that transport blood back to the heart through the abdominal and thoracic areas. When the pressures decrease, the veins return to their original size and fill with blood. The changing pressures within the abdomen and thorax squeeze the blood in the veins, assisting its return through a milking action. This is an essential part of venous return. Similarly, muscle contractions during exercise also produce this type of milking action to assist venous return.

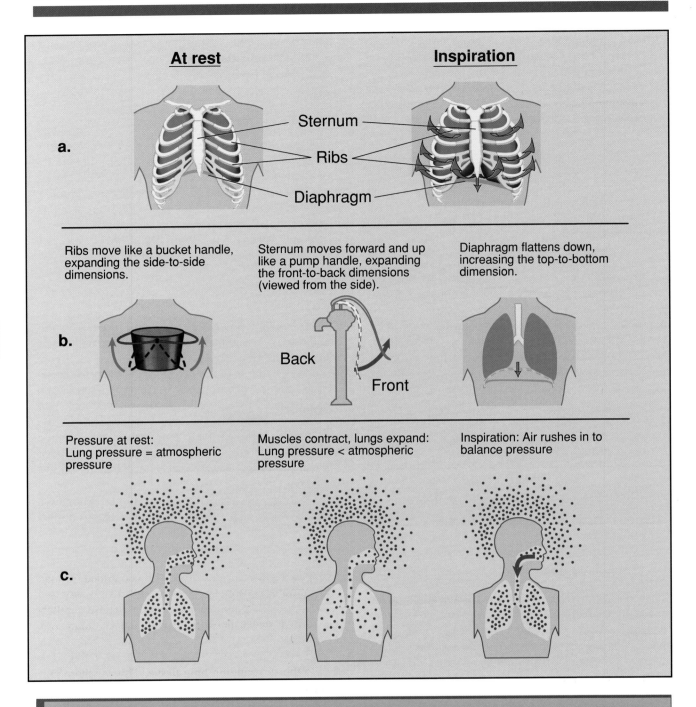

At rest | **Inspiration**

a.

Sternum

Ribs

Diaphragm

Ribs move like a bucket handle, expanding the side-to-side dimensions.

Sternum moves forward and up like a pump handle, expanding the front-to-back dimensions (viewed from the side).

Diaphragm flattens down, increasing the top-to-bottom dimension.

b.

Back

Front

Pressure at rest: Lung pressure = atmospheric pressure

Muscles contract, lungs expand: Lung pressure < atmospheric pressure

Inspiration: Air rushes in to balance pressure

c.

Figure 9.2   The process of inspiration, showing (a) the resting dimensions of the thorax and (b) the increase in its dimensions with muscular contraction. (c) This increase reduces the pressure within the lungs and causes air to rush into them.

Pulmonary Diffusion

Gas exchange in the lungs, called pulmonary diffusion, serves two major functions:

1. It replenishes the blood's oxygen supply that has been depleted at the tissue level where it is used for oxidative energy production.

2. It removes carbon dioxide from returning venous blood.

Pulmonary diffusion has two requirements: air that brings oxygen into the lungs and blood to receive the oxygen and give up carbon dioxide. Air was brought into the lungs during pulmonary ventilation; now gas exchange must occur between this air and the blood.

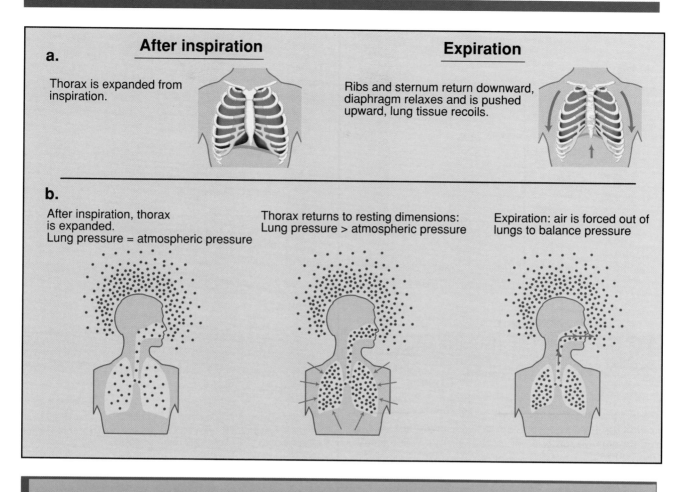

a.

After inspiration

Thorax is expanded from inspiration.

Expiration

Ribs and sternum return downward, diaphragm relaxes and is pushed upward, lung tissue recoils.

b.

After inspiration, thorax is expanded.
Lung pressure = atmospheric pressure

Thorax returns to resting dimensions:
Lung pressure > atmospheric pressure

Expiration: air is forced out of lungs to balance pressure

Figure 9.3   The process of expiration, (a) returning the thorax to its resting dimensions and (b) forcing air out of the lungs.

IN REVIEW . . .

1. Pulmonary ventilation (breathing) is the process by which air is moved into and out of the lungs. It has two phases: inspiration and expiration.
2. Inspiration is an active process through which the diaphragm and the external intercostal muscles increase the dimensions, and thus the volume, of the thoracic cage. This decreases the pressure in the lungs and draws air in.
3. Normal expiration is a passive process. The inspiratory muscles relax and the elastic tissue of the lungs recoils, returning the thoracic cage to its smaller, normal dimensions. This increases the pressure in the lungs and forces air out.
4. Forced or labored inspiration and expiration are active processes, dependent on muscle actions.

Blood from most of the body returns through the venae cava to the pulmonary (right) side of the heart.

From the right ventricle, this blood is pumped through the pulmonary artery to the lungs, ultimately working its way into the pulmonary capillaries. These capillaries form a dense network around the alveolar sacs. These vessels are small enough that the red blood cells must pass through them in single file, exposing each cell to the surrounding lung tissue. This is where pulmonary diffusion occurs.

The Respiratory Membrane

Gas exchange between the air in the alveoli and the blood in the pulmonary capillaries occurs across the respiratory membrane (also called the alveolar-capillary membrane). This membrane, depicted in Figure 9.4, is composed of

- the alveolar wall,
- the capillary wall, and
- their basement membranes.

The respiratory membrane is very thin, measuring only 0.5 to 4.0 μm. As a result, the gases in the nearly 300

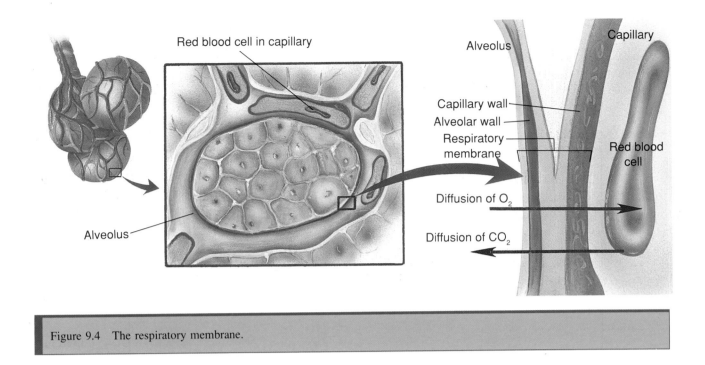

Figure 9.4   The respiratory membrane.

million alveoli are in close proximity to the blood circulating through the capillaries. Nevertheless, this membrane presents a potential barrier for gas exchange. Let's now examine how this exchange occurs.

Partial Pressures of Gases

The air we breathe is a mixture of gases. Each exerts a pressure in proportion to its concentration in the gas mixture. The individual pressures from each gas in a mixture are referred to as partial pressures. According to Dalton's law, the total pressure of a mixture of gases equals the sum of the partial pressures of the individual gases in that mixture.

KEY POINT

The total pressure of a mixture of gases equals the sum of the partial pressures of the individual gases in that mixture.

Consider the air we breathe. It is composed of 79.04% nitrogen (N_2), 20.93% oxygen (O_2), and 0.03% carbon dioxide (CO_2). At sea level, the atmospheric (or barometric) pressure is approximately 760 mmHg, which is also referred to as standard atmospheric pressure. This is considered the total pressure, or 100%. Thus, if the total atmospheric pressure is 760 mmHg, then the partial pressure of nitrogen (P_{N_2}) in air is 600.7

mmHg (79.04% of the total 760 mmHg pressure). Oxygen's partial pressure (P_{O_2}) is 159.0 mmHg (20.93% of 760 mmHg), and carbon dioxide's partial pressure (P_{CO_2}) is 0.3 mmHg (0.03% of 760 mmHg).

Gases in our bodies are dissolved in fluids, such as blood plasma. According to Henry's law, gases dissolve in liquids in proportion to their partial pressures, depending also on their solubilities in the specific fluids and on the temperature. A gas's solubility in blood is a constant, and blood temperature also remains relatively constant. Thus the most critical factor for gas exchange between the alveoli and the blood is the pressure gradient between the gases in the two areas.

Gas Exchange in the Alveoli

Differences in the partial pressures of the gases in the alveoli and the gases in the blood create a pressure gradient across the respiratory membrane. This forms the basis of gas exchange during pulmonary diffusion. If the pressures on each side of the membrane were equal, the gases would be at equilibrium and unlikely to move. But the pressures are not equal. Let's first consider the pressures from oxygen.

Oxygen Exchange

The P_{O_2} of air at standard atmospheric pressure is 159 mmHg. But this drops to 100 to 105 mmHg when air is inhaled and enters the alveoli. The inhaled air mixes with the air in the alveoli, and the alveolar air contains a lot of water vapor and carbon dioxide that contribute to the total pressure there. Fresh air that ventilates the lungs is constantly mixed with the air in the alveoli while some of the alveolar gases are exhaled to the environment. As a result, alveolar gas concentrations remain relatively stable.

The blood, stripped of much of its oxygen by the tissues, typically enters the pulmonary capillaries with a P_{O_2} of 40 to 45 mmHg (see Figure 9.5). This is about 55 to 65 mmHg less than the P_{O_2} in the alveoli. In other words, the pressure gradient for oxygen across the respiratory membrane is typically between 55 and 65 mmHg. As noted earlier, it is this pressure gradient that drives the oxygen from the alveoli into the blood to balance the pressure of the oxygen on each side of the membrane.

The P_{O_2} in the alveoli stays relatively steady at about 104 mmHg. At the arteriole end of the capillary, just as exchange begins, the P_{O_2} in the blood is only about 40 mmHg. But as the blood moves farther along the capillary, more exchange occurs. By the time the venous end of the capillary is reached, the partial pressure of oxygen in the blood will equal that in the alveoli. The P_{O_2} across the membrane equilibrates rapidly so that both the alveoli and the capillary blood have P_{O_2} values of 104 mmHg. Thus the blood leaving the lungs through the pulmonary veins to return to the systemic side of the heart has a rich supply of oxygen to deliver to the tissues.

The rate at which oxygen diffuses from the alveoli into the blood is referred to as the oxygen diffusion

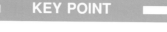

KEY POINT

The greater the pressure gradient across the respiratory membrane, the more rapidly oxygen will diffuse across it.

capacity. At rest, about 23 ml of oxygen diffuse into the pulmonary blood each minute for each 1 mmHg of pressure difference. During maximal effort, oxygen uptake can increase to 45 ml · kg^{-1} · min^{-1} in untrained people to as high as 80 ml · kg^{-1} · min^{-1} in elite endurance athletes. The increase in oxygen diffusion capacity from rest to exercise is due to relatively inefficient, sluggish circulation through the lung at rest, which results primarily from limited perfusion of the upper regions of the lung due to gravity. During maximal exercise, however, blood flow through the lung is greater, primarily due to elevated blood pressure, thereby increasing lung perfusion.

Athletes with large aerobic capacities often also have greater oxygen diffusion capacities. This is likely the combined result of increased cardiac output, increased alveolar surface area, and reduced resistance to diffusion across respiratory membranes.

Carbon Dioxide Exchange

Carbon dioxide exchange, like oxygen exchange, moves along a pressure gradient. As shown in Figure 9.6, the blood passing through the alveoli has a P_{CO_2}

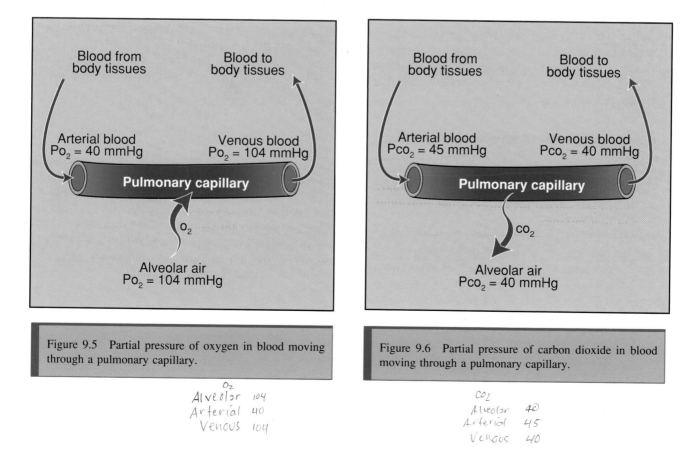

Figure 9.5 Partial pressure of oxygen in blood moving through a pulmonary capillary.

Figure 9.6 Partial pressure of carbon dioxide in blood moving through a pulmonary capillary.

O₂
Alveolar 104
Arterial 40
Venous   104

CO₂
Alveolar 40
Arterial 45
Venous   40

of about 45 mmHg. In the alveoli, air has a P_{CO_2} of about 40 mmHg. Though this results in a relatively small pressure gradient of only about 5 mmHg, it is more than adequate. Carbon dioxide's membrane solubility is 20 times greater than that of oxygen, so CO_2 can diffuse across the respiratory membrane much more rapidly.

The partial pressures of gases involved in pulmonary diffusion are summarized in Table 9.1.

Table 9.1 Partial Pressures of Respiratory Gases at Sea Level

Gas	% in dry air	Partial pressure (mmHg) Dry air	Alveolar air	Venous blood	Diffusion gradient
Total	100.00	760.0	760	760	0
H_2O	0	0	47	47	0
O_2	20.93	159.1	104	40	64
CO_2	0.03	0.2	40	45	5
N_2	79.04	600.7	573	573	0

IN REVIEW . . .

1. Pulmonary diffusion is the process by which gases are exchanged across the respiratory membrane in the alveoli.
2. The amount of gas exchange that occurs across the membrane primarily depends on the partial pressure of each gas, though gas solubility and temperature are also important. Gases diffuse along a pressure gradient, moving from an area of higher pressure to one of lower pressure. Thus oxygen enters the blood and carbon dioxide leaves it.
3. Oxygen diffusion capacity increases as you move from rest to exercise. When your body needs more oxygen, oxygen exchange is facilitated.
4. The pressure gradient for carbon dioxide exchange is less than for oxygen exchange, but carbon dioxide's membrane solubility is 20 times greater than that of oxygen, so carbon dioxide crosses the membrane easily, even without a large pressure gradient.

Transport of Oxygen and Carbon Dioxide

Now we have considered how we bring air into our lungs via pulmonary ventilation and how gas exchange occurs via pulmonary diffusion. Next we must consider how gases are transported in our blood to deliver the oxygen to the tissues and to remove the carbon dioxide that the tissues produce. We will consider separately the transport of each gas.

Oxygen Transport

Oxygen is transported by the blood either combined with hemoglobin (Hb) in the red blood cells (>98%) or dissolved in the blood plasma (<2%). Only about 3 ml of oxygen are dissolved in each liter of plasma. Assuming a total plasma volume of 3 to 5 L, only about 9 to 15 ml of oxygen can be carried in the dissolved state. This limited amount of oxygen cannot adequately meet the needs of even resting body tissues, which generally require more than 250 ml of oxygen per minute (depending on body size). Fortunately, hemoglobin, contained in the body's four to six billion red blood cells, allows the blood to transport nearly 70 times more oxygen than can be dissolved in plasma.

Hemoglobin Saturation

Each molecule of hemoglobin can carry four molecules of oxygen. When oxygen binds to hemoglobin, it forms oxyhemoglobin; hemoglobin that is not bound to oxygen is referred to as deoxyhemoglobin. The binding of oxygen to hemoglobin depends on the P_{O_2} in the blood and the bonding strength, or affinity, between hemoglobin and oxygen. Figure 9.7a shows an oxygen-hemoglobin dissociation curve, which reveals the amount of hemoglobin saturation at different P_{O_2} values. A high blood P_{O_2} results in almost complete hemoglobin saturation, which means the maximum amount of oxygen is bound. But as the P_{O_2} is reduced, so is hemoglobin saturation.

Many factors can influence hemoglobin saturation. If, for example, the blood becomes more acidic, the dissociation curve shifts to the right. This indicates that more oxygen is being unloaded from the hemoglobin at the tissue level. This rightward shift of the curve (see Figure 9.7b) due to a decline in pH is referred to as the Bohr effect.[6] The pH in the lungs is generally high, so hemoglobin passing through the lungs has a strong affinity for oxygen, encouraging high saturation. At the tissue level, however, the pH is lower, causing oxygen to dissociate from hemoglobin, thereby supplying oxygen to the tissues. With exercise, the ability to unload oxygen to the muscle increases as the muscle pH decreases.

Blood temperature also affects oxygen dissociation. As shown in Figure 9.7c, increased blood temperature shifts the dissociation curve to the right, indicating that oxygen is unloaded more efficiently. Because of this, the hemoglobin will unload more oxygen when blood circulates through the metaboli-

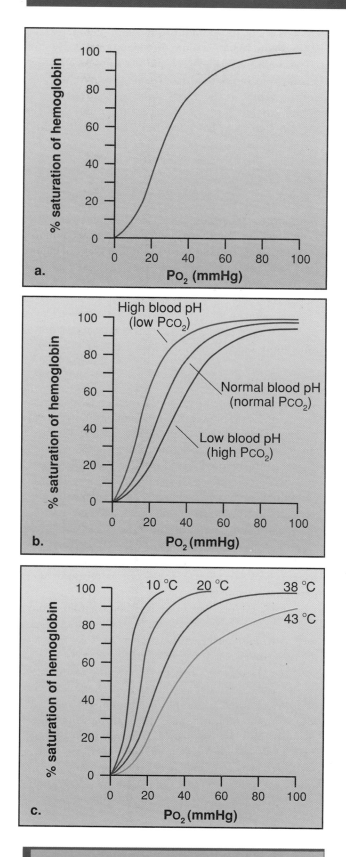

a.

b.

c.

Figure 9.7   (a) The normal oxygen-hemoglobin dissociation curve and the effects of (b) blood pH and (c) blood temperature on its shape.

cally heated active muscles. In the lungs, where the blood might be a bit cooler, hemoglobin's affinity for oxygen is increased. This encourages oxygen binding.

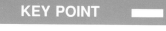

KEY POINT

Increased temperature and hydrogen ion (H^+) concentration in exercising muscle affect the oxygen dissociation curve, allowing more oxygen to be unloaded to supply the active muscle.

Blood Oxygen-Carrying Capacity

Blood oxygen-carrying capacity is the maximum amount of oxygen the blood can transport. It primarily depends on the blood hemoglobin content. Each 100 ml of blood contains an average of 14 to 18 g of hemoglobin in men and 12 to 16 g in women. Each gram of hemoglobin can combine with about 1.34 ml of oxygen, so the blood oxygen-carrying capacity is approximately 16 to 24 ml per 100 ml when blood is fully saturated with oxygen. As the blood passes through the lungs, it is in contact with the alveolar air for approximately 0.75 s. This is sufficient time for hemoglobin to bind nearly all the oxygen it can hold, resulting in 98% saturation.

People with low hemoglobin contents, such as those with anemia, have reduced oxygen-carrying capacities. Depending on the severity of the condition, these people might feel few effects of anemia while they are at rest because their cardiovascular systems can compensate for reduced blood oxygen content by increasing cardiac output. However, during activities in which oxygen delivery can become a limitation, such as in highly intense aerobic effort, reduced blood oxygen content limits their energy production and performance.

Carbon Dioxide Transport

Carbon dioxide also relies on the blood for transportation. Once carbon dioxide is released from the cells, it is carried in the blood primarily in three forms:

1. Dissolved in plasma
2. As bicarbonate ions resulting from the dissociation of carbonic acid
3. Bound to hemoglobin

Let's examine each method of transportation.

Dissolved Carbon Dioxide

Part of the carbon dioxide released from the tissues is dissolved in plasma. But only a small amount, typically just 7% to 10%, is transported this way. This dissolved carbon dioxide comes out of solution where the P_{CO_2} is low, such as in the lungs. There it diffuses out of the capillaries into the alveoli to be exhaled.

Bicarbonate Ion

By far the majority of carbon dioxide is carried in the form of bicarbonate ion. This form accounts for the transport of 60% to 70% of the carbon dioxide in the blood. Carbon dioxide and water molecules combine to form carbonic acid (H_2CO_3). This acid is unstable and quickly dissociates, freeing a hydrogen ion (H^+) and forming a bicarbonate ion (HCO_3^-):

$$CO_2 + H_2O \rightarrow H_2CO_3 \rightarrow H^+ + HCO_3^-$$
$$\text{(carbonic} \qquad \text{(bicarbonate}$$
$$\text{acid)} \qquad \text{ion)}$$

The H^+ subsequently binds to hemoglobin and this binding triggers the Bohr effect, mentioned previously, which shifts the oxygen-hemoglobin dissociation curve to the right. Thus the formation of bicarbonate ion enhances oxygen unloading. Through this mechanism, hemoglobin acts as a buffer, binding and neutralizing the H^+ and thus preventing any significant acidification of the blood. We will discuss the issue of acid-base balance in more detail later in this chapter. When the blood enters the lungs, where the P_{CO_2} is lower, the H^+ and bicarbonate ions rejoin to form carbonic acid, which then splits into carbon dioxide and water:

$$H^+ + HCO_3^- \rightarrow H_2CO_3 \rightarrow CO_2 + H_2O$$

The carbon dioxide that is thus re-formed can enter the alveoli and be exhaled.

▬ KEY POINT ▬

The majority of carbon dioxide produced by the active muscle is transported back to the lung in the form of bicarbonate ions.

Carbaminohemoglobin

Carbon dioxide transport also can occur when the gas binds with hemoglobin, forming a compound called carbaminohemoglobin. The compound is so named because carbon dioxide binds with amino acids in the globin part of the hemoglobin molecule, rather than with the heme group as oxygen does. Because carbon dioxide binding occurs on a different part of the hemoglobin molecule than does oxygen binding, the two processes do not compete. Carbon dioxide binding

depends on the oxygenation of the hemoglobin (deoxyhemoglobin binds carbon dioxide more easily than oxyhemoglobin) and the partial pressure of CO_2 (carbon dioxide is released from hemoglobin when P_{CO_2} is low). Thus in the lungs, where the P_{CO_2} is low, carbon dioxide is readily released from the hemoglobin, allowing it to enter the alveoli to be exhaled.

▬ IN REVIEW . . . ▬

1. Oxygen is transported in the blood primarily bound to hemoglobin (as oxyhemoglobin), though a small part of it is dissolved in blood plasma.
2. Hemoglobin oxygen saturation decreases
   - when P_{O_2} decreases,
   - when pH decreases, and
   - when temperature increases.

   Each of these conditions can reflect increased local oxygen demand. They increase oxygen unloading in the needy area.
3. Hemoglobin is usually about 98% saturated with oxygen. This reflects a much higher oxygen content than our bodies require, so the blood's oxygen-carrying capacity seldom limits performance.
4. Carbon dioxide is transported in the blood primarily as bicarbonate ion. This prevents the formation of carbonic acid, which can cause H^+ to accumulate, decreasing the pH. Smaller amounts of carbon dioxide are carried either dissolved in the plasma or bound to hemoglobin.

Gas Exchange at the Muscles

Now we have considered how our respiratory and cardiovascular systems bring air into our lungs, exchange oxygen and carbon dioxide in the alveoli, and transport oxygen to the muscles (and carbon dioxide away from them). All that remains is for us to consider the delivery of oxygen from the capillary blood to the muscle tissue and the removal of metabolically produced carbon dioxide. This gas exchange between the tissues and the blood in the capillaries is our fourth and final step in gas transportation—internal respiration.

The Arterial-Venous Oxygen Difference

At rest, the oxygen content of arterial blood is about 20 ml of oxygen per 100 ml of blood. As shown in

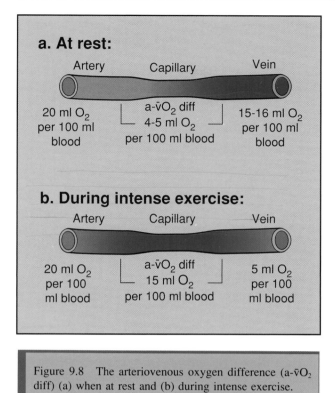

a. At rest:

Artery   Capillary   Vein

20 ml O_2
per 100 ml
blood

a-$\bar{v}O_2$ diff
4-5 ml O_2
per 100 ml blood

15-16 ml O_2
per 100 ml
blood

b. During intense exercise:

Artery   Capillary   Vein

20 ml O_2
per 100
ml blood

a-$\bar{v}O_2$ diff
15 ml O_2
per 100 ml blood

5 ml O_2
per 100
ml blood

Figure 9.8   The arteriovenous oxygen difference (a-$\bar{v}O_2$ diff) (a) when at rest and (b) during intense exercise.

Figure 9.8a, this value drops to 15 or 16 ml of oxygen per 100 ml as the blood passes through the capillaries into the venous system. This difference in oxygen content between arterial and venous blood is referred to as the arterial-venous oxygen difference (a-$\bar{v}O_2$ diff) It reflects the 4 to 5 ml of oxygen per 100 ml of blood taken up by the tissues. The amount of oxygen taken up is proportional to its use for oxidative energy production. Thus as the rate of oxygen use increases, the a-$\bar{v}O_2$ diff also increases. For example, during intense exercise, as shown in Figure 9.8b, the a-$\bar{v}O_2$ diff in contracting muscles can increase to 15 to 16 ml per 100 ml of blood. During such an effort, the blood unloads more oxygen to the active muscles because the Po_2 in the muscles is drastically lower than in arterial blood.

KEY POINT

The a-$\bar{v}O_2$ diff increases from a resting value of about 4 to 5 ml per 100 ml of blood up to values of 15 to 16 ml per 100 ml of blood during intense exercise. This increase reflects an increased extraction of oxygen from arterial blood by active muscle, thus decreasing the oxygen content of the venous blood.

Factors Influencing Oxygen Delivery and Uptake

The rates of oxygen delivery and uptake depend on three major variables:

1. The oxygen content of blood
2. The amount of blood flow
3. The local conditions

As we begin to exercise, each of these variables must be adjusted to ensure increased oxygen delivery to our active muscles. We have discussed the oxygen content of the blood and know that under normal circumstances hemoglobin is 98% saturated with oxygen. Any reduction in the blood's normal oxygen-carrying capacity would hinder oxygen delivery and reduce cellular uptake of oxygen.

As shown in chapter 8, exercise causes increased blood flow through the muscles. As more blood carries oxygen through the muscles, less oxygen must be removed from each 100 ml of blood (assuming the demand is unchanged). Thus increased blood flow improves oxygen delivery and uptake.

Many local changes in the muscle during exercise affect oxygen delivery and uptake. For example, muscle activity increases muscle acidity because of lactate production. Also, muscle temperature and carbon dioxide concentration both increase because of increased metabolism. All of these increase oxygen unloading from the hemoglobin molecule, facilitating oxygen delivery and uptake by the muscles.

During maximal exercise, however, when we push our bodies to the limit, changes in any of these areas can impair oxygen delivery and restrict our abilities to meet oxidative demands. We will discuss these potential limitations later in this chapter.

Carbon Dioxide Removal

Carbon dioxide exits the cells by simple diffusion in response to the partial pressure gradient between the tissue and the capillary blood. For example, muscles generate carbon dioxide through oxidative metabolism, so the Pco_2 in muscles would be relatively high compared to that in the capillary blood. Consequently, CO_2 diffuses out of the muscles and into the blood to be transported to the lungs.

We have completed our discussion of how oxygen is brought into the body and delivered to the tissues and how carbon dioxide is removed from the tissues and delivered to the lungs to be cleared. These processes are summarized in Figure 9.9.

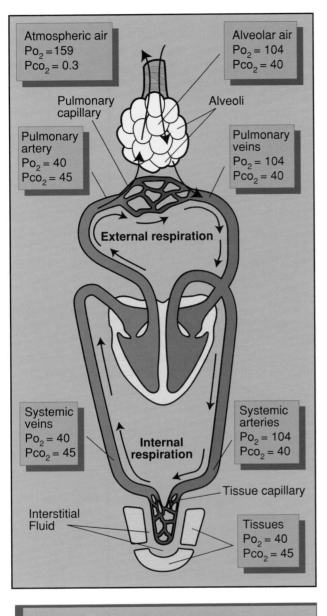

Figure 9.9   A summary of external and internal respiration.

The Mechanisms of Regulation

The respiratory muscles are under the direct control of motor neurons, which are in turn regulated by respiratory centers (inspiratory and expiratory) located within the brainstem (in the medulla oblongata and pons). These centers establish the rate and depth of breathing by sending out periodic impulses to the respiratory muscles.

However, the respiratory centers don't act alone in controlling breathing. Its regulation is also determined by a changing chemical environment in the body. For example, sensitive areas in the brain respond to changes in carbon dioxide and H^+ levels. When these levels increase, signals are sent to the inspiratory center instructing it to increase the rate and depth of respiration, which increases the removal of carbon dioxide and H^+. In addition, chemoreceptors in the aortic arch (the aortic bodies) and in the bifurcation of the common carotid artery (the carotid bodies) are primarily sensitive to blood changes in P_{O_2}, but also respond to changes in H^+ concentration and P_{CO_2}. Overall, of the various stimuli, P_{CO_2} appears to be the strongest stimulus for the regulation of breathing. When carbon dioxide levels become too high, recall that carbonic acid forms, then quickly dissociates, giving off H^+. If this accumulates, the blood will become too acidic (pH drops). Thus an increased P_{CO_2} stimulates the inspiratory center to increase respiration, not to bring in more oxygen, but to rid the body of excess carbon dioxide and minimize pH changes.

In addition to the chemoreceptors, other neural mechanisms influence breathing. The pleurae, bronchioles, and alveoli contain stretch receptors. When these areas are excessively stretched, that information is relayed to the expiratory center. It responds by shortening the duration of an inspiration, which decreases the

The Regulation of Pulmonary Ventilation

Maintaining homeostatic balance in blood P_{O_2}, P_{CO_2}, and pH requires a high degree of coordination between the respiratory and circulatory systems. Much of this coordination is accomplished by involuntary regulation of pulmonary ventilation. This control is not yet fully understood, though many of the intricate neural controls have been identified. Let's examine some of them.

risk of overinflating the respiratory structures. This is known as the Hering-Breuer reflex.

We can exert some voluntary control over our breathing through the cerebral motor cortex. However, this voluntary control can be overridden by the involuntary control of the respiratory center. Try to hold your breath for 5 minutes. At some point, regardless of your conscious decision to suppress breathing, your carbon dioxide and H⁺ levels become quite high, your oxygen level drops, and your inspiratory center decides that breathing is imperative and it forces you to inhale.

So we see that many control mechanisms are involved in the regulation of breathing, as shown in Figure 9.10. Such simple stimuli as emotional distress or an abrupt change in the temperature of your surroundings can have an impact. But all these control mechanisms are essential. The goal of respiration is to maintain appropriate levels of the blood and tissue

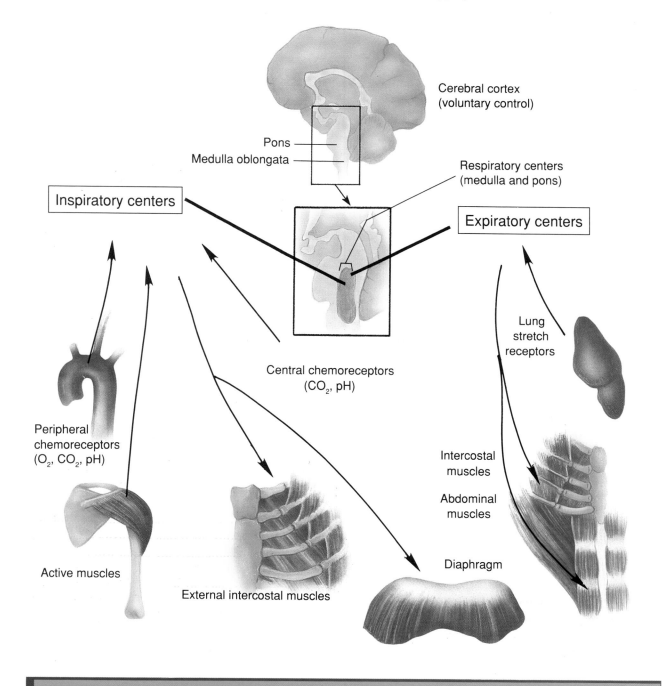

Figure 9.10   An overview of the processes involved in respiratory regulation.

gases and to maintain proper pH for normal cellular function. Even relatively small changes in any of these, if they are not carefully controlled, can impair physical activity and jeopardize health.

Pulmonary Ventilation During Exercise

The onset of physical activity is accompanied by a two-phase increase in ventilation. An almost immediate marked increase occurs, followed by a continued, more gradual rise in the depth and rate of breathing. This is shown in Figure 9.11 for light, moderate, and heavy exercise. This two-phase adjustment suggests that the initial rise in ventilation is produced by the mechanics of body movement. As exercise begins, but before any chemical stimulation occurs, the motor cortex becomes more active and transmits stimulatory impulses to the inspiratory center, which responds by increasing respiration. Also, proprioceptive feedback from the active skeletal muscles and joints provides additional input about the movement, and the respiratory center can adjust its activity accordingly.

The more gradual second phase of the respiratory increase is produced by changes in the temperature and chemical status of the arterial blood. As exercise progresses, increased metabolism in the muscles generates more heat, carbon dioxide, and H^+. All these enhance oxygen unloading in the muscles, which increases the a-$\bar{v}O_2$ diff. Also, more carbon dioxide enters the blood, increasing blood levels of both carbon dioxide and H^+. This is sensed by the chemoreceptors, which in turn stimulate the inspiratory center, increasing rate and depth of respiration. Some researchers have suggested that chemoreceptors in the muscles might also be involved. In addition, data suggest that receptors in the right ventricle of the heart send information to the inspiratory center so that increases in cardiac output can stimulate breathing during the early minutes of exercise.

Pulmonary ventilation increases during exercise, up to near-maximal rates of work, in direct proportion to the body's metabolic needs. At lower exercise intensities, this is accomplished by increases in tidal volume—the amount of air moved in and out of the lungs during regular breathing. At higher intensities, the rate of respiration also increases. Maximal rates of pulmonary ventilation are dependent on body size. Maximal ventilation rates of approximately 100 L · min^{-1} are common for smaller individuals, but rates exceeding 200 L · min^{-1} are found in larger individuals.

At the end of exercise, the muscles' energy demands drop almost immediately to resting levels. But pulmonary ventilation returns to normal at a relatively slow rate. If the rate of breathing perfectly matched the metabolic demands of the tissues, respiration would drop to the resting level within seconds after exercise. But respiratory recovery takes several minutes, which suggests that post-exercise breathing is regulated primarily by acid-base balance, P_{CO_2}, and blood temperature.

Problems Associated With Breathing During Exercise

Ideally, during exercise our breathing will be regulated in a way that maximizes our abilities to perform. Unfortunately this doesn't always occur. Many respiratory problems can accompany exercise and hinder performance. Let's examine a few.

Dyspnea

The sensation of dyspnea (shortness of breath) during exercise is most common among individuals in poor physical condition who attempt to exercise at levels that significantly elevate their arterial carbon dioxide and H^+ concentrations. As noted earlier, both stimuli send strong signals to the inspiratory center to increase the rate and depth of ventilation. Although exercise-induced dyspnea is sensed as an inability to breathe, the underlying cause is an inability to readjust the blood P_{CO_2} and H^+. Failure to reduce these stimuli during exercise appears related to poor conditioning of respiratory muscles. Despite a strong neural drive to ventilate the lungs, the respiratory muscles fatigue

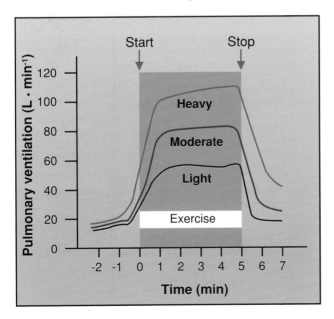

Figure 9.11   The ventilatory response to light, moderate, and heavy exercise.

easily and are unable to reestablish normal homeostasis.

Hyperventilation

The anticipation or anxiety of exercise, as well as some respiratory disorders, can cause a sudden increase in ventilation that exceeds the metabolic need for oxygen. Such overbreathing is termed hyperventilation. At rest, voluntary hyperventilation decreases the normal P_{CO_2} of 40 mmHg in the alveoli and arterial blood to about 15 mmHg. As carbon dioxide levels drop, so do H^+ levels; thus blood pH increases. These effects reduce the ventilatory drive. Because the blood leaving the lungs is nearly always about 98% saturated with oxygen, an increase in the alveolar P_{O_2} does not increase the oxygen content of the blood. Consequently, the reduced desire to breathe and the improved ability to hold one's breath after hyperventilating results from carbon dioxide unloading rather than increased blood oxygen. When performed for only a few seconds, such deep, rapid breathing can lead to lightheadedness and even loss of consciousness. This phenomenon reveals the sensitivity of the respiratory system's regulation of carbon dioxide and pH.

In hope of reducing respiratory distress, swimmers often hyperventilate before competition. Breath holding during competitive swimming offers some advantages to stroke mechanics, so most swimmers hyperventilate immediately before starting sprint events. Although they might feel little desire to breathe during the first 8 to 10 s of the race, their alveolar and arterial oxygen contents can decline to critically low levels because oxygen is being used but not replaced. This can impair muscle oxidation and oxygen delivery to the central nervous system. The benefits of pre-exercise hyperventilation aren't clear, but it may impair performance rather than improve it. Perhaps future studies will provide some insight into the effects of this practice.

Pre-exercise hyperventilation is also common among people who attempt to perform long underwater swims. Hyperventilating before a dive decreases the drive to breathe but doesn't increase the body's oxygen stores. Breath holding usually becomes intolerable when the P_{CO_2} in arterial blood reaches 50 mmHg. Unfortunately, during a dive that is preceded by hyperventilation, the oxygen content of the blood can reach critically low levels long before carbon dioxide accumulation signals the swimmer to surface and breathe. These events can cause a diver to lose consciousness before experiencing a desire to breathe.

The Valsalva Maneuver

A respiratory procedure that is frequently performed in certain types of exercise and which can be potentially dangerous is referred to as the Valsalva maneuver. This occurs when the individual does the following:

1. Closes the glottis (the opening between the vocal cords)
2. Increases the intra-abdominal pressure by forcibly contracting the diaphragm and the abdominal muscles
3. Increases the intrathoracic pressure by forcibly contracting the respiratory muscles

As a result of these actions, air is trapped and pressurized in the lungs. This maneuver is often performed during the lifting of heavy objects as the person attempts to stabilize the chest wall.

The high intra-abdominal and intrathoracic pressures restrict venous return by collapsing the great veins. This maneuver, if held for an extended period of time, can greatly reduce the volume of blood returning to the heart, decreasing cardiac output. Although the Valsalva maneuver can be helpful in certain circumstances, this maneuver can be dangerous and should be avoided by people who have hypertension or known cardiovascular limitations.

▬▬ IN REVIEW . . . ▬▬

1. The respiratory centers in the brainstem set the rate and depth of breathing.
2. Central chemoreceptors in the brain respond to changes in concentrations of carbon dioxide and H^+. When either of these rise, the inspiratory center increases respiration.
3. Peripheral receptors in the arch of the aorta and the bifurcation of the common carotid artery respond primarily to changes in blood oxygen levels, but also to changes in carbon dioxide and H^+ levels. If oxygen levels drop too low, or if the other levels rise, these chemoreceptors relay their information to the inspiratory center, which in turn increases respiration.
4. Stretch receptors in the air passages and lungs can cause the expiratory center to shorten respirations to prevent overinflation of the lungs. In addition, we can exert some voluntary control over our respiration.
5. During exercise, ventilation shows an almost immediate increase, resulting from increased inspiratory center stimulation caused by the muscle activity itself. This is followed by a more gradual increase that results from the rise in temperature and chemical changes in the arterial blood that are caused by the muscular activity.
6. Problems associated with breathing during exercise include dyspnea, hyperventilation, and performance of the Valsalva maneuver.

Ventilation and Energy Metabolism

During long periods of mild steady-state activity, ventilation appears to match the rate of energy metabolism. It tends to vary in proportion to the volume of oxygen consumed and the volume of carbon dioxide produced by the body. Let's examine how closely breathing is matched to the consumption of oxygen.

The Ventilatory Equivalent for Oxygen

The ratio between the volume of air ventilated ($\dot{V}E$) and the amount of oxygen consumed by the tissues ($\dot{V}O_2$) indicates breathing economy. This ratio is referred to as the ventilatory equivalent for oxygen, or $\dot{V}E/\dot{V}O_2$. It is typically measured in liters of air breathed per liter of oxygen consumed.

At rest, the $\dot{V}E/\dot{V}O_2$ can range from 23 to 28 L of air per liter of oxygen consumed. This value changes very little during mild exercise, such as walking. But when work intensity increases to near maximum, the $\dot{V}E/\dot{V}O_2$ can be greater than 30 L of air per liter of oxygen consumed. In general, however, the $\dot{V}E/\dot{V}O_2$ remains relatively constant over a wide range of exercise levels. This indicates that the control systems for breathing are properly matched to the body's need for oxygen. Even in activities such as swimming, where breathing must be synchronized with the arm-stroke cycle, the $\dot{V}E/\dot{V}O_2$ does not differ from that of other free-breathing activities.

The Ventilatory Breakpoint

As exercise intensity increases toward maximum, at some point ventilation increases disproportionately as compared to oxygen consumption. This point is called the ventilatory breakpoint, illustrated in Figure 9.12. When the work rate exceeds 55% to 70% of one's $\dot{V}O_2$ max, oxygen delivery to the muscles can no longer support the oxygen requirements of oxidation. To compensate, more energy is derived from glycolysis. This results in increased lactic acid production and accumulation. This lactic acid combines with sodium bicarbonate (which buffers acid) and forms sodium lactate, water, and carbon dioxide. As we know, the increase in carbon dioxide stimulates chemoreceptors that signal the inspiratory center to increase ventilation. Thus the ventilatory breakpoint reflects the respiratory response to increased carbon dioxide levels. Ventilation increases dramatically beyond the ventilatory breakpoint, as seen in Table 9.2.

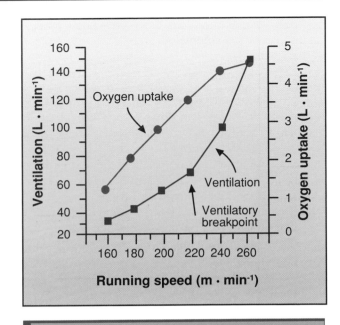

Figure 9.12 Changes in pulmonary ventilation during exercise, illustrating the ventilatory breakpoint.

Table 9.2 Ratio Between Pulmonary Ventilation ($\dot{V}E$) and Oxygen Uptake ($\dot{V}O_2$)

Running speed (m · min⁻¹)	$\dot{V}E/\dot{V}O_2$
160	21.5
180	20.0
200	20.4
220	20.3
240	24.9
260	33.3

Note. Note the sudden rise in $\dot{V}E/\dot{V}O_2$ at ventilatory breakpoint.

KEY POINT

Ventilation increases during exercise in direct proportion to the rate of work being performed, up to the ventilatory breakpoint. Beyond this point, ventilation increases disproportionately as the body tries to clear excess CO_2.

Anaerobic Threshold

The disproportionate increase in ventilation without an increase in oxygen consumption led to early speculation that the ventilatory breakpoint might be related to the lactate threshold (the point at which blood lactate begins to accumulate above resting levels during a graded exercise test). Ventilatory breakpoint reflects an increase in the volume of carbon dioxide produced per minute ($\dot{V}CO_2$). Recall from chapter 5 that the respiratory exchange ratio (RER) is the ratio of carbon dioxide production to oxygen consumption. Thus increased carbon dioxide production also causes RER to increase.

The increased $\dot{V}CO_2$ was thought to result from excess carbon dioxide being released from bicarbonate buffering of lactic acid. Wasserman and McIlroy coined the term anaerobic threshold to describe this phenomenon because they assumed the sudden increase in CO_2 reflected a shift toward more anaerobic metabolism.[10] They used the increase in RER as the marker of anaerobic threshold and believed that this was a good noninvasive alternative to blood sampling for detecting the onset of anaerobic metabolism.

Over the years, this concept has been refined considerably. The most accurate technique for identifying anaerobic threshold now appears to involve monitoring both the ventilatory equivalent for oxygen ($\dot{V}E/\dot{V}O_2$) and the ventilatory equivalent for carbon dioxide ($\dot{V}E/\dot{V}CO_2$), which is the ratio of the amount of air breathed to the amount of carbon dioxide produced. The most specific criterion for estimating anaerobic threshold is a systematic increase in $\dot{V}E/\dot{V}O_2$ without a concomitant increase in $\dot{V}E/\dot{V}CO_2$.[2] This is illustrated in Figure 9.13. The ventilatory equivalent for carbon dioxide remains relatively constant, indicating that ventilation matches the body's need to remove CO_2. The increase in $\dot{V}E/\dot{V}O_2$ indicates that the increase in ventilation to remove CO_2 is disproportionate to the body's need to provide O_2.

Anaerobic threshold has been used as a noninvasive estimate of lactate threshold, and under most conditions the two occur at the same point in time during an incremental exercise bout, or at the same percentage of maximal oxygen uptake. However, there are exceptions.[1] For example, people with McArdle's disease are incapable of increasing blood lactate and H^+ levels during exercise due to a lack of muscle phosphorylase. They demonstrate a clear anaerobic threshold during exercise of increasing intensity even though blood lactate concentration remains at resting levels. Depleting the glycogen stores prior to exercise also alters the relationship between anaerobic threshold and lactate threshold.

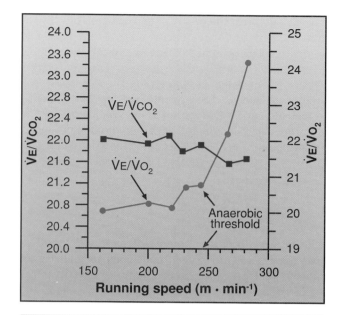

Figure 9.13 Changes in the ventilatory equivalent for carbon dioxide ($\dot{V}E/\dot{V}CO_2$) and the ventilatory equivalent for oxygen ($\dot{V}E/\dot{V}O_2$) during increasing intensities of running.

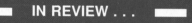

IN REVIEW . . .

1. During mild, steady-state exercise, ventilation accurately reflects the rate of energy metabolism. Ventilation parallels oxygen uptake. The ratio of air ventilated to oxygen consumed is the ventilatory equivalent of oxygen ($\dot{V}E/\dot{V}O_2$).
2. The ventilatory breakpoint is the point at which ventilation abruptly increases, even though oxygen consumption does not. This increase reflects the need to remove excess carbon dioxide.
3. The anaerobic threshold can be determined by identifying the point at which $\dot{V}E/\dot{V}O_2$ shows a sudden increase while $\dot{V}E/\dot{V}CO_2$ stays relatively stable. Anaerobic threshold has been used as a noninvasive estimate of lactate threshold.

Respiratory Limitations to Performance

Like all aspects of tissue activity, lung ventilation and gas transport in the body require energy. Most of this energy is used by the respiratory muscles during pulmonary ventilation. At rest, only about 2% of the total energy used by the body is used by the respiratory

KEY POINT

Anaerobic threshold accurately reflects lactate threshold under most conditions; however, the relationship is certainly not perfect.

muscles for breathing. As the rate and depth of ventilation increase, so do their energy costs. More than 15% of the oxygen consumed during heavy exercise can be used by the diaphragm, the intercostal muscles, and the abdominal muscles for ventilation. During recovery, breathing continues to demand much energy, accounting for 9% to 12% of the total oxygen consumed.

Though the muscles of respiration are heavily taxed during exercise, ventilation is sufficient to prevent a rise in alveolar carbon dioxide or a decline in alveolar PO_2 during activities lasting only a few minutes. Even during maximal effort, ventilation usually is not pushed to the person's maximal capacity to voluntarily move air in and out of the lungs. This capacity is called the maximal voluntary ventilation (MVV). However, recent evidence suggests that pulmonary ventilation might be a limiting factor in highly trained subjects during maximal exhaustive exercise.[3]

Some researchers have suggested that heavy breathing for several hours (such as during marathon running) can cause glycogen depletion and fatigue of the respiratory muscles. However, untrained rats studied during exercise experienced a substantial sparing of their respiratory muscle glycogen, compared to muscle glycogen in their hindlimbs. Unfortunately, similar data are not available for humans, but our respiratory muscles apparently are better designed for long-term activity than are the muscles in our extremities. The diaphragm, for example, has 2 to 3 times more oxidative capacity (oxidative enzymes and mitochondria) and capillary density than other skeletal muscle. Consequently, more energy can be obtained from fat oxidation in the diaphragm than in other muscles.

Airway resistance and gas diffusion in the lungs do not limit exercise in a normal, healthy individual. Although the volume of air inspired can increase 10- to 20-fold with exercise, airway resistance is maintained at near-resting levels by airway dilation (through an increase in the laryngeal aperture and bronchodilation). Blood leaving the lungs remains nearly saturated with oxygen even during maximal effort. Thus the respiratory system is well designed to accommodate the demands of heavy breathing during short- and long-term physical effort. Individuals who consume unusually large amounts of oxygen during exhaustive exercise, however, can face some respiratory limitations.

The respiratory system can also limit performance in people with abnormally restricted or obstructed airways. For example, asthma causes constriction of the bronchial tubes and swelling of their mucous membranes. These effects cause considerable resistance to ventilation and shortness of breath. Exercise is known to have an adverse effect on some people with asthma. The mechanism or mechanisms through which exercise induces airway obstruction in individuals with asthma are unknown despite extensive study. Thorough reviews of this topic have been presented by Sly and Eggleston.[4,9]

IN REVIEW . . .

1. More than 15% of the body's total oxygen consumption during heavy exercise can occur in the respiratory muscles.
2. Pulmonary ventilation is usually not a limiting factor for performance, even during maximal effort, though it can limit performance in a few highly trained people.
3. The respiratory muscles seem to be better designed for avoiding fatigue during long-term activity than muscles of the extremities.
4. Airway resistance and gas diffusion usually do not limit performance in normal, healthy individuals.
5. The respiratory system can limit performance in people with restrictive or obstructive respiratory disorders.

Respiratory Regulation of Acid-Base Balance

As noted earlier, intense muscular activity often results in the production and accumulation of lactate and H^+. This can impair energy metabolism and reduce muscle contractile force. Although the body's regulation of acid-base balance involves more than control of respiration, we include it here because the respiratory system plays a crucial role in rapid adjustment of the body's acid-base status during and immediately after exercise.

Acids, such as lactic acid and carbonic acid, release hydrogen ions (H^+). As noted in chapter 5, the metabolism of carbohydrate, fat, or protein produces

---

KEY POINT

Highly trained distance runners have been shown to have respiratory limitations to their performances. They cannot sufficiently ventilate their lungs to prevent a decrease in arterial blood PO_2, leading to reduced hemoglobin saturation.

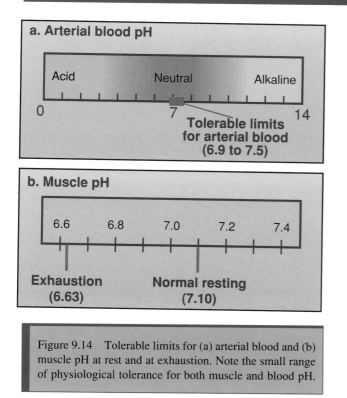

Figure 9.14   Tolerable limits for (a) arterial blood and (b) muscle pH at rest and at exhaustion. Note the small range of physiological tolerance for both muscle and blood pH.

Table 9.3 Buffering Capacity of Blood Components

Buffer	Slykes[a]
Bicarbonate	18.0
Hemoglobin	8.0
Proteins	1.7
Phosphates	0.3
Total	28.0

[a]Milliequivalents of hydrogen ions taken up by each liter of blood from pH 7.4 to 7.0.

inorganic acids that dissociate, increasing the H^+ concentration in body fluids. To minimize the effects of free H^+, the blood and muscles contain base substances that combine with, and thus buffer or neutralize, the H^+:

$$H^+ + Buffer \rightarrow H\text{-}Buffer$$

Under resting conditions, body fluids have more base (as bicarbonate, phosphate, and proteins) than acids, resulting in a tissue pH that ranges from 7.1 in muscle to 7.4 in arterial blood. The tolerable limits for arterial blood pH extend from 6.9 to 7.5, though these extremes can be tolerated only for a few minutes (see Figure 9.14). A H^+ concentration elevated above normal is referred to as acidosis, whereas a decrease in H^+ below the normal concentration is termed alkalosis.

The pH of intra- and extracellular body fluids is kept within a relatively narrow range by

- chemical buffers,
- pulmonary ventilation, and
- kidney function.

The three major chemical buffers in the body are bicarbonate (HCO_3^-), phosphates (P_i), and proteins. In addition to these, the hemoglobin in the red blood cells, as we mentioned earlier, also is a major buffer. Table 9.3 illustrates the relative contributions of these buffers in handling acids in the blood. Recall that bicarbonate combines with H^+ to form carbonic acid, thereby eliminating its acidifying influence. The car-

bonic acid in turn forms carbon dioxide and water in the lungs. The CO_2 is then exhaled and only water remains.

The amount of bicarbonate that combines with H^+ equals the amount of acid buffered. When lactic acid drops the pH from 7.4 to 7.0, more than 60% of the bicarbonate initially present in the blood has been used. Even under resting conditions, the acid produced by the end products of metabolism would eliminate a major portion of the bicarbonate from the blood if there were no other way of removing H^+ from the body. Fortunately, the blood and these buffers are required only to transport metabolic acids from their sites of production (the muscles) to the lungs or kidneys, where they can be removed. Once transportation is completed, the buffer molecules can be used again.

In the muscle fibers and the kidney tubules, H^+ is primarily buffered by phosphates, such as phosphoric acid and sodium phosphate. Unfortunately, less is known about the capacity of the buffers housed in the cells, though we know that the cells contain more protein and phosphates, and less bicarbonate, than the extracellular fluids.

As noted earlier, any increase in free H^+ in the blood stimulates the respiratory center to increase ventilation. This facilitates the binding of H^+ and bicarbonate and the removal of carbon dioxide. The end result is a decrease in the free H^+ and an increase in blood pH. Thus both the chemical buffers and the respiratory system provide temporary means of neutralizing the acute effects of exercise acidosis. To maintain a constant buffer reserve, the accumulated H^+ is removed from the body via the kidneys and urinary system. The kidneys filter H^+ from the blood along with other waste products. This provides a way to eliminate H^+ from the body while maintaining the concentration of extracellular bicarbonate.

During sprint exercise, muscles generate a large amount of lactate and H^+, which lowers the muscle pH from a resting level of 7.08 to less than 6.70. As shown in Table 9.4, an all-out sprint for 400 m results in a drop in leg muscle pH to 6.63 and a rise in muscle

Air Pollution

During the past 20 years, concern has increased about possible problems associated with exercising in polluted air. The air in many cities is contaminated with small quantities of gases and particles not naturally found in the air we breathe. When air becomes stagnant or when a temperature inversion occurs, some of these pollutants reach concentrations that significantly impair athletic performance. The major contaminants of concern are carbon monoxide, ozone, and sulfur oxides.

Carbon monoxide (CO) is an odorless gas that rapidly enters the blood when breathed and can be lethal. Hemoglobin's affinity for carbon monoxide is approximately 240 times greater than its affinity for oxygen, so hemoglobin preferentially binds the carbon monoxide. Blood carbon monoxide levels are directly related to the carbon monoxide levels in the inspired air. Several studies have reported a linear decrease in $\dot{V}O_2$ max with increases in blood levels of carbon monoxide. Literature reviews on this topic have concluded that the reduction in $\dot{V}O_2$ max is not statistically significant until blood carbon monoxide levels exceed 4.3%, although performance time on the treadmill has been reduced at carbon monoxide levels as low as 2.7%.[5,8] Submaximal exercise at less than 60% of $\dot{V}O_2$ max doesn't appear to be affected until blood carbon monoxide levels exceed 15%.

Ozone (O_3) is the most common photochemical oxidant. It produces many subjective complaints when its concentration in inspired air is high. Eye irritation, chest tightness, breathlessness, coughing, and nausea are common complaints. Ozone especially affects the respiratory tract. Decrements in lung function occur with increasing ozone concentrations, as well as with increased exposure and ventilation. $\dot{V}O_2$ max has been found to be significantly decreased following 2 hr of intermittent exercise with exposure to 0.75 ppm of ozone. This decrease in $\dot{V}O_2$ max is likely associated with reduced oxygen transfer at the lung, resulting from reduced alveolar air exchange.

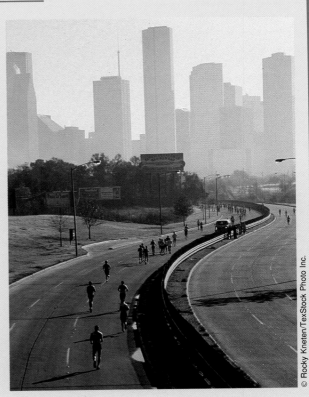

© Rocky Kneten/TexStock Photo Inc.

Sulfur dioxide (SO_2) is another contaminant of concern. Research on sulfur dioxide and exercise is limited, but we know that air levels of this gas above 1.0 ppm cause significant discomfort and are detrimental to performance.[8] Sulfur dioxide is primarily an upper airway and bronchial irritant.

Certain cities have initiated air pollution or smog alerts. These are usually color-coded, with colors indicating pollution severity. Standards need to be established nationally and air monitored accordingly. Increasing evidence points to the wisdom of canceling all games and practices when pollution levels put athletes' health at risk.

Hopefully, current and future research will provide a clearer understanding of the limitations imposed by air pollutants.

---

lactate from a resting value of 1.2 mmol · kg⁻¹ to 19.7 mmol · kg⁻¹ of muscle. As noted earlier, such disturbances in acid-base balance impair muscle contractility and its capacity to generate ATP. Lactate and H^+ accumulate in the muscle, in part because they do not freely diffuse across fiber membranes. Despite the great production of lactate and H^+ during the 60 s required to run 400 m, these by-products diffuse throughout the body fluids and reach equilibrium after only about 5 to 10 min of recovery. Five minutes after the exercise, the runners evaluated for Table 9.4 had blood pH values of 7.10 and blood lactate values of 12.3

Table 9.4 Blood and Muscle pH and Lactate Concentration After a 400-m Run

Runner	Time(s)	Muscle pH	Muscle Lactate (mmol · L⁻¹)	Blood pH	Blood Lactate (mmol · Kg⁻¹)
1	61.0	6.68	19.7	7.12	12.6
2	57.1	6.59	20.5	7.14	13.4
3	65.0	6.59	20.2	7.02	13.1
4	58.5	6.68	18.2	7.10	10.1
Average	60.4	6.63	19.7	7.10	12.3

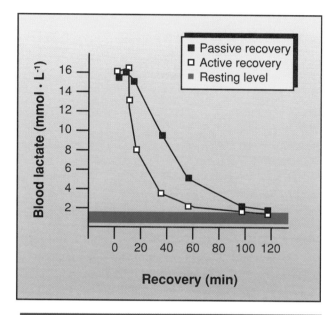

Figure 9.15 Effects of active and passive recovery of blood lactate levels after a series of exhaustive sprint bouts.

━━ IN REVIEW . . . ━━

1. Excess H⁺ (decreased pH) impairs muscle contractility and ATP formation.
2. The respiratory system plays an integral role in maintaining acid-base balance.
3. Whenever H⁺ levels start to rise, the inspiratory center responds by increasing respiration. Removing carbon dioxide is an essential means for reducing the H⁺ concentrations. Carbon dioxide is primarily transported bound to bicarbonate. Once it reaches the lungs, carbon dioxide is formed again and exhaled.
4. Whenever H⁺ levels begin to rise, whether from carbon dioxide or lactate accumulation, bicarbonate ion can buffer the H⁺ to prevent acidosis.

mmol · L⁻¹, compared to a resting pH of 7.40 and a resting lactate level of 1.5 mmol · L⁻¹.

Reestablishing normal resting levels of blood and muscle lactate after such an exhaustive exercise bout is a relatively slow process, often requiring 1 to 2 hr. As shown in Figure 9.15, recovery of blood lactate to the resting level is facilitated by continued lower intensity exercise, called active recovery.[7] After a series of exhaustive sprint bouts, the participants in this study either sat quietly (passive recovery) or exercised at an intensity of 50% $\dot{V}O_{2\,max}$. Blood lactate is removed more quickly during active recovery because the activity maintains elevated blood flow through the active muscles, which in turn enhances both lactate diffusion out of the muscles and lactate oxidation.

Although blood lactate remains elevated for 1 to 2 hr after highly anaerobic exercise, blood and muscle H⁺ concentrations return to normal within 30 to 40 min of recovery. Chemical buffering, principally by bicarbonate, and respiratory removal of excess carbon dioxide are responsible for this relatively rapid return to normal acid-base homeostasis.

In Closing . . .

In chapter 8, we discussed the role of the cardiovascular system during exercise. In this chapter we have looked at the role played by the respiratory system. We have also considered the limitations that these systems can impose on our abilities to perform. In the next chapter, we will examine the physiological adaptations that occur in both the cardiovascular and the respiratory systems when they are exposed to the repeated stimulus of training. We will see how these adaptations improve these systems' abilities to meet our bodies' demands and how they can improve performance.

▌ **Key Terms**

anaerobic threshold
arterial-venous oxygen
  difference (a-v̄O₂ diff)
dyspnea
expiration
external respiration
hemoglobin saturation
hyperventilation
inspiration
internal respiration
oxygen diffusion
  capacity

partial pressures
pulmonary diffusion
pulmonary ventilation
respiratory centers
respiratory membrane
Valsalva maneuver
ventilatory breakpoint
ventilatory equivalent
  for carbon dioxide
  ($\dot{V}E/\dot{V}CO_2$)
ventilatory equivalent
  for oxygen ($\dot{V}E/\dot{V}O_2$)

Study Questions

1. Describe the anatomical structures involved in pulmonary ventilation.
2. Identify the muscles associated with breathing and their function in pulmonary ventilation.
3. What are the partial pressures of oxygen and carbon dioxide in inspired air, alveolar air, and arterial and mixed venous blood?
4. In what forms are oxygen and carbon dioxide transported in the blood?
5. What are the chemical stimuli that control the depth and rate of breathing? How do they control respiration during exercise? How are they affected during voluntary hyperventilation?
6. What other stimuli control ventilation during exercise?
7. What is the ventilatory equivalent for oxygen? What is the ventilatory equivalent for CO_2?
8. Define ventilatory breakpoint and anaerobic threshold.
9. Define lactate threshold and anaerobic threshold. How are these terms related?
10. What role does the respiratory system play in acid-base balance?
11. What is the normal resting pH for arterial blood? For muscle? How are these values changed as a result of exhaustive sprint exercise?
12. What are the primary buffers in the blood? In muscles?
13. How long does it take blood pH and lactate levels to return to normal after an all-out sprint?

References

1. Anderson, G.S., & Rhodes, E.C. (1989). A review of blood lactate and ventilatory methods of detecting transition thresholds. *Sports Medicine*, **8**, 43-55.

2. Davis, J.A. (1985). Anaerobic threshold: Review of the concept and directions for future research. *Medicine and Science in Sports and Exercise*, **17**, 6-18.

3. Dempsey, J.A., Vidruk, E.H., & Mitchell, G.S. (1986). Is the lung built for exercise? *Medicine and Science in Sport and Exercise*, **18**, 143-155.

4. Eggleston, P.A. (1986). Pathophysiology of exercise-induced asthma. *Medicine and Science in Sport and Exercise*, **18**, 318-321.

5. Folinsbee, L.J., & Raven, P.B. (1984). Exercise and air pollution. *Journal of Sports Sciences*, **2**, 57-75.

6. Guyton, A.C. (1991). *Textbook of medical physiology* (8th ed.). Philadelphia: Saunders.

7. Hermansen, L. (1981). Effect of metabolic changes on force generation in skeletal muscle during maximal exercise. In R. Porter and J. Whelan (Eds.), *Human muscle fatigue: Physiological mechanisms* (pp. 75-88). London: Pitman Medical.

8. Raven, P.B. (1979). Heat and air pollution: The cardiac patient. In M.L. Pollock & D.H. Schmidt (Eds.), *Heart disease and rehabilitation*. Boston: Houghton Mifflin.

9. Sly, R. M. (1986). History of exercise-induced asthma. *Medicine and Science in Sports and Exercise*, **18**, 314-317.

10. Wasserman, K., & McIlroy, M.B. (1964). Detecting the threshold of anaerobic metabolism in cardiac patients during exercise. *American Journal of Cardiology*, **14**, 844-852.

Selected Readings

Brooks, G.A. (1985). Response to Davis manuscript. *Medicine and Science in Sports and Exercise*, **17**, 19-21.

Brooks, G.A., & Fahey, T.D. (1985). *Exercise physiology: Human bioenergetics and its applications* (pp. 221-278). New York: Wiley.

Comroe, J.H. (1974). *Physiology of respiration* (2nd ed.). Chicago: Year Book Medical.

Costill, D.L. (1970). Metabolic responses during distance running. *Journal of Applied Physiology*, **28**, 251-255.

Costill, D.L., Barnett, A., Sharp, R., Fink, W.J., & Katz, A. (1983). Leg muscle pH following sprint running. *Medicine and Science in Sport and Exercise*, **15**, 325-329.

Costill, D.L., Verstappen, F., Kuipers, H., Janssen, E., & Fink, W. (1984). Acid-base balance during repeated bouts of exercise: Influence of HCO_3. *International Journal of Sports Medicine*, **5**, 228-231.

Dempsey, J.A., Vidruk, E.H. & Mastenbrook, S.M. (1980). Pulmonary control systems in exercise. *Federation Proceedings*, **39**, 1498-1505.

Dempsey, J.A., Vidruk, E.H., & Mitchell, G.S. (1985). Pulmonary control systems in exercise: Update. *Federation Proceedings*, **44**, 2260-2270.

Dempsey, J.G. (1985). Exercise and chemoreception. *American Review of Respiratory Disease*, **129**, 31-34.

Powers, S.K., & Howley, E.T. (1990). Exercise physiology: Theory and application to fitness and performance. Dubuque, IA: Brown.

Sharp, R.L., Costill, D.L., Fink, W.J., & King, D.S. (1986). Effects of eight weeks of bicycle ergometer sprint training on human muscle buffer capacity. *International Journal of Sports Medicine, 7,* 13-17.

Sutton, J.R., Jones, N.L. & Toews, C.J. (1981). Effect of pH on muscle glycolysis during exercise. *Clinical Science,* **61,** 331-338.

Chapter 10

Cardiorespiratory Adaptations to Training

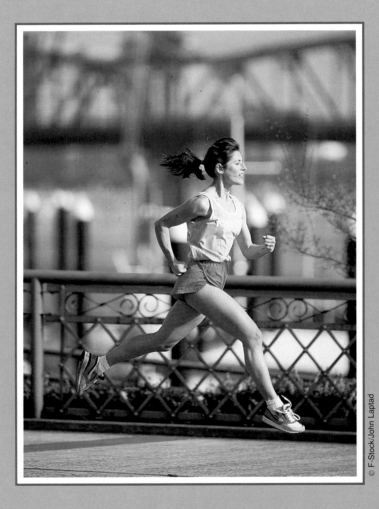

© F-Stock/John Laptad

Chapter Overview

During a single bout of exercise, the human machine is quite adept at adjusting its cardiovascular and respiratory functioning to adequately meet the heightened demands of active muscles. When these systems are faced with these demands repeatedly, such as on a daily basis when training, they adapt in ways that allow the body to improve its performance of endurance activity. For example, the miler can run a faster mile. The physiological and metabolic processes that bring oxygen into the body, distribute it, and allow it to be used by active tissues become and remain highly efficient at these tasks. In this chapter, we will examine adaptations in cardiorespiratory function in response to training, and how such adaptations affect an athlete's endurance capacity and performance.

Chapter Outline

Miguel Indurain of Spain won the 78th Tour de France, the world's most prestigious bicycle race, completing the 21-day, 3,934 km (2,445 mi) ordeal in a total time of 101 hr 1 min 20 s. At an average speed of over 38 kph (24 mph), many considered this contest to be the most grueling endurance event ever. The cyclists who compete have to climb mountains and then ride at breakneck speeds down mountainsides and across valleys. How are these athletes able to compete in this race? They must train specifically to develop their cardiorespiratory endurance capacities.

Cardiorespiratory endurance is probably the least understood component of a total training program. The training programs for many nonendurance athletes completely ignore the endurance factor. This is understandable, because for maximum improvement in performance, training should be highly specific to the particular sport or activity in which the athlete participates, and endurance is frequently not recognized as important to nonendurance activities. The reasoning then is "Why waste valuable training time if the result is not improved performance?"

The problem with this reasoning is that often, although it might not be obvious, a nonendurance sport does indeed have an endurance, or aerobic, component. For example, if you play football, you and your coach might fail to recognize the importance of cardiorespiratory endurance as part of your total training program. From all outward appearances, football is an anaerobic or burst-type activity, consisting of repeated bouts of high-intensity work of short duration. Seldom does a run exceed 40 to 60 yd (37 to 55 m), and even this is followed by a substantial rest interval. The need for endurance is not readily apparent.

What you and your coach might fail to consider is that this burst-type activity must be repeated many times during the game. With a high endurance level, the quality of your burst activity could be maintained throughout the game, and you would still be relatively fresh during the fourth quarter.

Sport scientists are beginning to realize the importance of endurance training for almost all types of sports or activities:

- Burst-type, such as football and basketball
- Moderate-intensity and skilled, such as baseball and golf
- Endurance-type, such as running, cycling, and swimming

Many authorities now believe football teams that fall apart in the final quarter have ignored the endurance component in their training programs. A similar case can be made for athletes in most sports. But before we look specifically at how endurance can improve performance, we must understand what endurance is.

Endurance

Endurance is a term that describes two separate but related concepts: muscular endurance and cardiorespiratory endurance. Each makes a unique contribution to athletic performance, so each differs in importance to different athletes.

For sprinters, endurance is the quality that allows them to sustain a high speed over the full distance of, for example, the 100- or 200-m race. This quality is muscular endurance—the ability of a single muscle or muscle group to sustain high-intensity, repetitive, or static exercise. This type of endurance is also exemplified by the weight lifter, boxer, and wrestler. The exercise or activity can be rhythmical and repetitive in nature, such as the bench-press for the weight lifter and jabbing for the boxer. Or the activity can be more static, such as a sustained muscle action when a wrestler attempts to pin an opponent to the mat. In either case, the resulting fatigue is confined to a specific muscle group and the activity's duration is usually no more than 1 or 2 min. Your muscular endurance is highly related to your muscular strength and anaerobic development.

Whereas muscular endurance refers to the ability of individual muscles, cardiorespiratory endurance relates to the body as a whole. Specifically, it refers to your body's ability to sustain prolonged, rhythmical exercise. This type of endurance is typified by the cyclist, distance runner, or endurance swimmer who can complete long distances at a fairly fast pace. Your cardiorespiratory endurance is highly related to the development of your cardiovascular and respiratory systems, and thus your aerobic development.

In chapter 7 we reviewed training adaptations for muscular endurance. In this chapter we focus on cardiorespiratory endurance. Now that we understand the concept of cardiorespiratory endurance, we are ready to examine the physiological bases for it. We will primarily focus on endurance-type training, but will occasionally refer to burst- and resistance-type training specifically by name.

Evaluating Endurance Capacity

To study training effects on endurance, we need a means for evaluating an individual's endurance capacity which we can easily use to monitor her or his improvement during the training program.

$\dot{V}O_2$ max: Aerobic Power

Most sport scientists regard $\dot{V}O_2$ max, representing aerobic power, as the best objective laboratory measure of cardiorespiratory endurance capacity. Recall from chapter 5 that $\dot{V}O_2$ max is defined as the highest rate of oxygen consumption attainable during maximal or exhaustive exercise. If you increase your exercise intensity beyond the point at which you reach $\dot{V}O_2$ max, your oxygen consumption will either plateau or decrease slightly.

Reaching this plateau means the end of your exercise bout is near because you can't deliver oxygen as quickly as is needed to meet your muscles' demands. Thus this limit, $\dot{V}O_2$ max, dictates the rate of work or the pace that you can sustain. You can continue exercising for a brief period after reaching $\dot{V}O_2$ max by calling on your anaerobic reserves, but these also have a finite capacity.

With endurance training, more oxygen can be delivered and consumed than in an untrained state. Previously untrained subjects show average $\dot{V}O_2$ max increases of 20% or more following a 6-month training program.[30] These improvements allow you to perform endurance activities at a higher work rate or faster pace, improving your performance potential.

Some improvement in cardiorespiratory function can occur with burst-type anaerobic training and with resistance-type training, but improvements in $\dot{V}O_2$ max are small.[21]

The Oxygen Transport System

Cardiorespiratory endurance is intimately related to your body's ability to deliver sufficient oxygen to meet your active tissues' needs. Oxygen transportation and delivery are major functions shared by both your cardiovascular and respiratory systems. All components of these two systems that are related to the transportation of oxygen are collectively referred to as the oxygen transport system.

The functioning of the oxygen transport system is defined by the interaction of the cardiac output and the arterial-venous oxygen difference (a-$\bar{v}O_2$ diff). Cardiac output (stroke volume × heart rate) tells us how much oxygen-carrying blood leaves the heart in 1 min. The arterial-venous oxygen difference, which is the difference between the oxygen content of the arterial blood and the oxygen content of the venous blood, tells us how much oxygen is extracted by the tissues. The product of these values tells us the rate at which oxygen is being consumed by the body tissues.

The active tissues' oxygen demand naturally increases during exercise. Your endurance depends on your oxygen transport system's ability to deliver sufficient oxygen to these active tissues to meet the heightened demands. Endurance training elicits numerous changes in the components of the oxygen transport system that enable it to function more effectively. In the next sections, we'll examine some of these adaptations to training.

Cardiovascular Adaptations to Training

Numerous cardiovascular adaptations occur in response to training. Let's look at changes in the following cardiovascular parameters:

- Heart size
- Stroke volume
- Heart rate
- Cardiac output
- Blood flow
- Blood pressure
- Blood volume

Heart Size

In response to increased work demand, the heart's weight and volume, and the left ventricle's wall thickness and

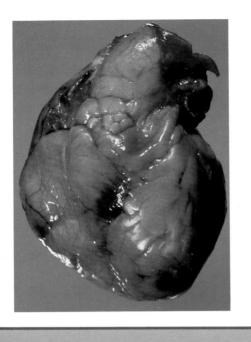

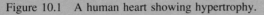

Figure 10.1 A human heart showing hypertrophy.

chamber size all increase as a result of endurance training as seen in Figure 10.1. Cardiac muscle, like skeletal muscle, undergoes hypertrophy as a result of chronic endurance training. At one time, cardiac hypertrophy induced by exercise —"athlete's heart" as it was called — caused great concern because experts generally believed that enlargement of the heart always reflected a pathological state. Fortunately, cardiac hypertrophy is now recognized as a normal adaptation to chronic endurance training.

The left ventricle, the hardest working heart chamber, undergoes the greatest change. It was first thought that the extent and location of changes in heart size depend on the type of exercise performed. Those who held this view reasoned that during resistance-type training, the heart must contract against high blood pressure in the systemic circulation, a situation referred to as a high afterload. To overcome this high afterload, it was postulated that the heart muscle compensates by increasing its size (wall thickness), thereby increasing its contractility.

With endurance-type training, the reasoning continued, left ventricular filling would increase. This would be largely due to a training-induced rise in plasma volume (discussed later in this chapter) that would increase left ventricular end-diastolic volume (an increased preload). It was postulated that the heart would adapt to this by increasing the internal dimensions of the left ventricle, thus increasing chamber size.

At the time, most believed that an increase in chamber size was the only change in the left ventricle

caused by endurance training. Studies have verified that this increase does indeed occur.[25] But more recent research has revealed that myocardial wall thickness also increases with endurance training, rather than just with resistance training.[9,22] Using magnetic resonance imaging, Milliken et al. found that highly trained competitive cross-country skiers, endurance cyclists, and long-distance runners had greater left ventricular masses compared to nonathletic control subjects.[24] They also found that left ventricular mass was highly correlated to $\dot{V}O_{2\,max}$, or aerobic power.

Similar results were found in a study comparing elite bodybuilders and highly trained endurance athletes. Using echocardiography, where sound waves are bounced off various heart structures and monitored, the following measurements were compared:

- Heart volume
- Left ventricular muscle mass
- Left ventricular end-diastolic diameter
- Left ventricular septal and posterior wall thickness

The absolute measurements did not differ significantly between the athletes, which seemed to indicate that the results of the two types of training did not

IN REVIEW ...

1. Cardiorespiratory endurance refers to your body's ability to sustain prolonged, rhythmical exercise. It is highly related to your aerobic development.
2. Most sport scientists regard $\dot{V}O_{2\,max}$—the highest rate of oxygen consumption obtainable during maximal or exhaustive exercise—to be the best indicator of cardiorespiratory endurance.
3. Cardiac output tells how much blood leaves the heart each minute, whereas a-$\bar{v}O_2$ diff indicates how much oxygen is extracted from the blood by the tissues. The product of these tells us the rate of oxygen consumption.

$$\dot{V}O_2 = SV \times HR \times \text{a-}\bar{v}O_2 \text{ diff}$$

4. The left ventricle undergoes the most change in response to endurance training.
5. The internal dimensions of the left ventricle increase, mostly in response to an increase in ventricular filling.
6. Left ventricular wall thickness also increases, increasing the strength potential of that chamber's contractions.

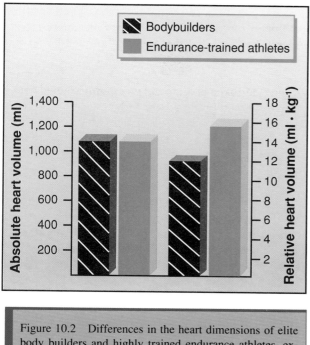

Figure 10.2 Differences in the heart dimensions of elite body builders and highly trained endurance athletes, expressed as absolute heart volume and relative to body weight. Data from Urhausen and Kindermann (1989).

Table 10.1 Typical Stroke Volumes for Different States of Training

Subjects	SV Rest (ml)	Maximal SV (ml)
Untrained	55 - 75	80 - 110
Trained	80 - 90	130 - 150
Highly trained	100 - 120	160 - >220

walls and, by the Frank-Starling law, this results in more elastic recoil.

We know that the posterior and septal walls of the left ventricle hypertrophy with endurance training. Increased ventricular muscle mass can cause more forceful contraction. This increased contractility would cause the end-systolic volume (ESV) to decrease because more blood would be forced out of the heart during the more powerful contractions, leaving less blood in the left ventricle after systole.

Increased contractility coupled with the increased elastic recoil that results from greater diastolic filling increase the ejection fraction in the trained heart. More blood enters the left ventricle, and a greater percentage of what enters is forced out with each contraction, so stroke volume is increased.

These stroke volume changes are well illustrated by a study in which older men were endurance trained for a period of 1 year.[9] Their cardiovascular function was evaluated before and after training. Running, treadmill, and cycle ergometer exercise were performed for an hour each day, 4 days per week. The exercise was performed at intensities of 60% to 80% of $\dot{V}O_{2\,max}$, with brief bouts of exercise exceeding 90% of $\dot{V}O_{2\,max}$.

The results are shown in Figure 10.3. End-diastolic volume increased at rest and throughout submaximal exercise. The ejection fraction increased, and this was associated with a decreased end-systolic volume, both suggesting increased contractility of the left ventricle. $\dot{V}O_{2\,max}$ increased by 23%, indicating a substantial improvement in endurance.

Stroke volume at rest and during exercise is not merely a function of a person's state of training. It

differ significantly.[37] But the bodybuilders weighed an average of 90.1 kg compared to 68.7 kg for the endurance athletes. When these measurements were expressed relative to body mass (ventricular mass and body mass are closely related), the endurance athletes had significantly greater values for each variable, indicating that endurance training results in far greater changes in the left ventricle than does resistance training. These results are illustrated in Figure 10.2.

Stroke Volume

As a result of endurance training, stroke volume (SV) shows an overall increase. Stroke volume at rest is substantially higher after an endurance training program than it is before training. This training-induced increase is also seen during both standardized submaximal exercise and maximal exercise. Typical values for stroke volume at rest and during maximal exercise in untrained, trained, and highly trained athletes are listed in Table 10.1. What causes the increase?

After training, the left ventricle fills more completely during diastole than it does in an untrained heart. As we will discuss later, blood plasma volume increases with training, which means more blood is available to enter the ventricle, causing an increased end-diastolic volume (EDV). More blood entering the ventricle increases the stretching of the ventricular

---

KEY POINT

A stronger heart and the availability of a greater blood volume appear to account for the increases in resting, submaximal, and maximal stroke volumes following an endurance training program.

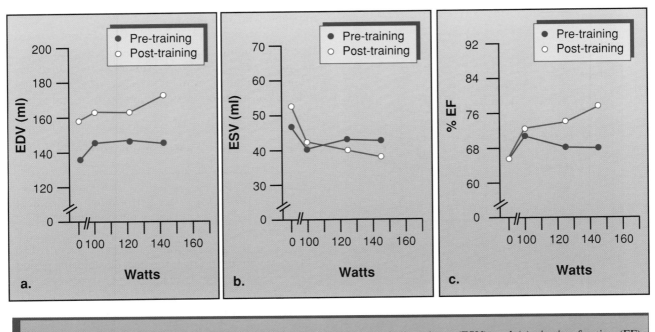

Figure 10.3   Differences in (a) end-diastolic volume (EDV), (b) end-systolic volume (ESV), and (c) ejection fraction (EF) with increasing rates of work in individuals before and after endurance training. Data from Ehsani et al. (1991).

also reflects body size. Larger people typically have greater stroke volumes. This is very important to remember when comparing stroke volumes of different people.

IN REVIEW . . .

1. Following endurance training, stroke volume increases during rest, submaximal levels of exercise, and maximal exertion.
2. A major factor leading to the stroke volume increase is an increased end-diastolic volume, probably caused by an increase in blood plasma.
3. Another major factor is increased left ventricular contractility. This is caused by hypertrophy of the cardiac muscle and increased elastic recoil, which results from increased stretching of the chamber with more diastolic filling.

Heart Rate

Now that we have examined one aspect of cardiac output, we can turn our attention to the other half of the equation: heart rate. Studies in which the oxygen consumption of the heart has been directly monitored have shown that the heart rate, both at rest and during exercise, is a good index of how hard the heart is working. Because active muscle requires more oxygen than resting muscle, it is not surprising that the heart's oxygen consumption, and thus the amount of work it performs, are directly related to the heart's contraction rate. Let's examine how training affects heart rate.

Resting Heart Rate

The heart rate at rest decreases markedly as a result of endurance training. If you are a sedentary individual with an initial resting heart rate of 80 beats per minute, your heart rate will decrease by approximately 1 beat per minute each week for the first few weeks of training. So after ten weeks of moderate endurance training, your resting heart rate should drop from 80 to 70 beats per minute. The actual mechanisms responsible for this decrease are not entirely known, but training appears to increase parasympathetic activity in the heart while decreasing sympathetic activity.

Highly conditioned endurance athletes often have resting heart rates lower than 40 beats per minute, and some have values lower than 30 beats per minute!

Recall from chapter 8 that bradycardia is a clinical term indicating a heart rate of less than 60 beats per minute. In untrained individuals, bradycardia is usually

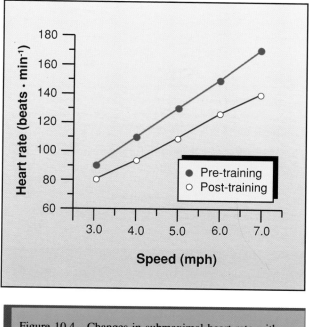

Figure 10.4 Changes in submaximal heart rate with endurance training.

the result of abnormal cardiac function or a diseased heart. Therefore, it is necessary to differentiate between training-induced bradycardia, which is a natural response to endurance training, and pathological bradycardia, which can be a serious cause for concern.

Submaximal Heart Rate

During submaximal exercise, greater aerobic conditioning results in proportionally lower heart rates at a specified rate of work. This is illustrated in Figure 10.4, which shows the heart rate of an individual exercising on a treadmill both before and after training. At each specified work rate, indicated by the speed at which the subject is walking and running, the post-training heart rate is lower than the heart rate before training. Following a 6-month endurance training program of moderate intensity, heart rate decreases of 20 to 40 beats per minute are common at a standardized submaximal rate of work.

These decreases indicate that the heart becomes more efficient through training. In carrying out its necessary functions, a conditioned heart performs less work than an unconditioned heart.

Maximum Heart Rate (HR max)

A person's maximum heart rate (HR max) tends to be stable. At maximal rates of exercise, HR max usually remains relatively unchanged following endurance training. However, several studies have suggested that

in people who have untrained HR max values exceeding 180 beats per minute, HR max might be slightly reduced following training. Also, highly conditioned endurance athletes tend to have lower HR max values than untrained individuals of the same age. Why does it not remain constant for everyone during maximal levels of exercise?

Heart Rate and Stroke Volume Interactions

During exercise, your heart rate combines with your stroke volume to provide an appropriate cardiac output for the rate of work you are performing. At maximal or near-maximal rates of work, your body might adjust your heart rate to provide the optimal combination of heart rate and stroke volume to maximize your cardiac output. If your heart rate is too fast, diastole, the period of ventricular filling, is reduced and your stroke volume might be compromised.[36] For example, if your HR max is 180 beats per minute, your heart beats three times per second. Each cardiac cycle thus lasts for only 0.33 s. Diastole is as short as 0.150 s or less. This allows very little time for your ventricles to fill. As a consequence, your stroke volume could decrease.

However, if your heart rate slows, your ventricles would have longer to fill. Perhaps this is why highly trained endurance athletes tend to have lower HR max values—their hearts have adapted to training by drastically increasing their stroke volumes so lower HR max values can provide optimum cardiac output.

All disciplines have their dilemmas, and this is one for exercise physiology: Which comes first—does increased stroke volume allow a decreased heart rate or does decreased heart rate allow an increased stroke volume? This question remains unanswered. In any event, the combination of increased stroke volume and decreased heart rate is a very efficient way for the heart to meet the body's demands. The heart expends less energy by contracting less often but more forcibly than it would by increasing contraction frequency. Changes in heart rate and stroke volume in response to training go hand-in-hand and share a common goal: to allow the heart to expel the maximum amount of oxygenated blood at the lowest energy cost.

Heart Rate Recovery

During exercise, as discussed in chapter 8, your heart rate must increase to meet the demands of your active muscles. When the exercise bout is finished, your heart rate does not instantly return to its resting level. Instead, it remains elevated for a while, slowly returning to its resting rate. The time it takes for your heart rate to return to its resting rate is called the heart rate recovery period.

Following a period of training, as shown in Figure 10.5, heart rate returns to its resting level much more

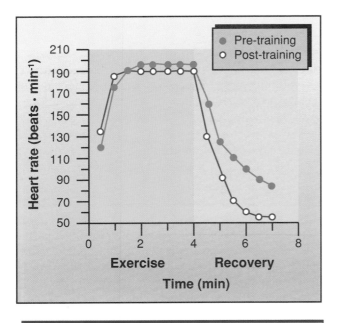

Figure 10.5   Changes in heart rate recovery with endurance training.

tained from endurance training. These changes appear to be dependent on the following characteristics of the resistance training program:[33]

- Training volume
- Training intensity
- Training duration
- Length of rest periods between sets
- Amount of muscle mass used

The mechanisms responsible for this drop in heart rate, when it occurs with resistance training, have not been determined but could be related to changes in heart size and contractility resulting from training, as discussed earlier in this chapter.

IN REVIEW . . .

1. Resting heart rate decreases considerably as a result of endurance training. In a sedentary person the decrease is typically about 1 beat per minute per week during initial training. Highly trained endurance athletes often have resting rates of 40 beats per minute or less.
2. Heart rate during submaximal exercise also decreases, often by about 20 to 40 beats per minute following 6 months of moderate training. A person's submaximal heart rate decreases proportionately with the amount of training completed.
3. Maximal heart rate either remains unchanged or decreases slightly with training. When a decrease occurs, it is probably to allow for optimum stroke volume to maximize cardiac output.
4. The heart rate recovery period decreases with increased endurance, making this value well suited to tracking an individual's progress with training. However, this is not useful for comparing fitness levels of different people.
5. Resistance training can also lead to reduced heart rates; however, these decreases are not as reliable or as large as those seen with endurance training.

quickly after exercise than it does prior to training. This is true after standardized submaximal exercise as well as after maximal exercise.

Because the heart rate recovery period is shortened by endurance training, this measurement can be used as an index of cardiorespiratory fitness. In general, a more fit person recovers faster after a standardized rate of work than a less fit person. However, factors other than training level can affect heart rate recovery time. For example, exercise in hot environments or at high altitudes can prolong heart rate elevation. Some people undergo a stronger sympathetic nervous system response during exercise than others, and this could also prolong heart rate elevation.

The heart rate recovery curve is an excellent tool for tracking a person's progress during a training program. But because of the potential influence of other factors, it should not be used to compare one individual to another.

Resistance Training and Heart Rate

Our discussion about heart rate so far has focused on endurance training. With resistance training, some research has shown that the heart rate at rest and at standardized rates of submaximal exercise can be reduced. But not all studies have confirmed these reductions.

The reductions in heart rate that have been reported are much less than the typical reductions ob-

Cardiac Output

Now we have looked at the effects of training on the two components of cardiac output: stroke volume and heart rate. We have seen that stroke volume increases, but heart rate generally decreases. How does this affect cardiac output?

When at rest or during submaximal exercise at standardized work rates, cardiac output doesn't change much following endurance training. For exercise at the

Maximum Breathing Capacity Test

To better understand the concept of optimizing the heart rate–stroke volume relationship, consider the maximum breathing capacity test. In this test, the objective is to inspire and expire the largest volume of air possible in a fixed period of time, usually 15 s. During the test, you are encouraged to breathe as deeply as possible. But you are also encouraged to breathe in and out as rapidly as possible. Try it! It is impossible to simultaneously breathe both deeply and rapidly. Obviously an optimal combination of respiratory rate and depth will produce the greatest ventilation volume in a given period of time. The same principle is thought to apply to heart rate and stroke volume. At an optimal heart rate, your stroke volume is maximized to provide the greatest cardiac output.

same submaximal metabolic rate (meaning at a specific oxygen consumption rate, such as 1.5 L $O_2 \cdot min^{-1}$) cardiac output might decrease slightly. This could be the result of an increase in the a-$\bar{v}O_2$ diff, reflecting greater oxygen extraction by the tissues.

However, cardiac output increases considerably at maximal rates of work, as seen in Figure 10.6. This results primarily from the increase in maximal stroke volume because HR max changes little, if any. Maximal cardiac output ranges from 14 to 16 L · min^{-1} in untrained people, 20 to 25 L · min^{-1} in trained people, and 40 L · min^{-1} or more in large, highly conditioned endurance athletes.

IN REVIEW . . .

1. Cardiac output at rest or during submaximal levels of exercise remains unchanged or decreases slightly after training.
2. Cardiac output at maximal levels of exercise increases considerably. This is largely the result of the substantial increase in maximal stroke volume.

Blood Flow

Now that we have discussed training-induced changes in cardiac structure and function, we next turn our attention to changes in the vasculature, beginning with blood flow.

We know that active muscles need much more oxygen and nutrients. To meet these needs, more blood must be brought into these muscles during exercise. As the muscles become better trained, the cardiovascular system adapts to increase blood flow to them. Three factors account for this enhanced muscle blood supply following training:

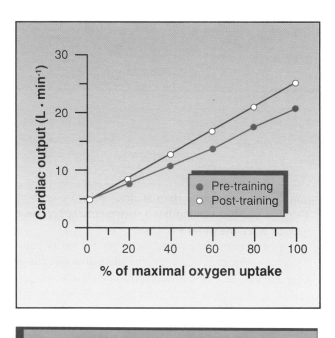

Figure 10.6 Changes in cardiac output with endurance training.

1. Increased capillarization of trained muscles
2. Greater opening of existing capillaries in trained muscles
3. More effective blood redistribution

To permit increased blood flow, new capillaries develop in trained muscles. This allows the blood to more fully perfuse the tissues. This increase in capillaries is usually expressed as an increase in the number of capillaries per muscle fiber, or the capillary to fiber ratio. Table 10.2 illustrates the differences in capillary to fiber ratios between well-trained and untrained men.

The existing capillaries in trained muscles can open up more, which increases blood flow through the capillaries and into the muscles. Because endurance

Table 10.2 Capillaries and Muscle Fibers per mm², Capillary to Fiber Ratio, and Diffusion Distance in Well-Trained and Untrained Men

Groups	Capillaries per mm²	Muscle fibers per mm²	Capillary to fiber ratio	Diffusion distance[a]
Well-trained				
Pre-exercise	640	440	1.5	20.1
Post-exercise	611	414	1.6	20.3
Untrained				
Pre-exercise	600	557	1.1	20.3
Post-exercise	599	576	1.0	20.5

Note. This table illustrates the larger size of the muscle fibers in the well-trained men in that they had fewer fibers for a given area (fibers per mm²). They also had an approximately 50% higher capillary to fiber ratio.

[a]Diffusion distance is expressed as the average half distance between capillaries on the cross sectional view, expressed in μm.

Adapted from Hermansen and Wachtlova (1971).

training also increases blood volume, this adaptation is easily accomplished because more blood is present in the system to begin with, so shifting more into the capillaries will not severely compromise venous return.

Blood flow to the active muscles can also be increased by a more effective redistribution of the cardiac output. Blood flow is directed to the active musculature and shunted away from areas that don't need high flow. Venous compliance can also be decreased with endurance training as a result of increased venous tone. That means that the veins are not as easily distended by the blood, so less blood pools in the venous system, thereby increasing the amount of arterial blood available for working muscles.

Blood flow can even be increased to the more active areas in a specific muscle group. Armstrong and Laughlin demonstrated that during exercise, endurance-trained rats could redistribute blood flow to their most active tissues better than untrained rats could.[1] The researchers used radiolabeled microspheres—radioactive particles that are injected into the blood stream. By using a counter to monitor the distribution of these microspheres, the scientists could trace their distribution throughout the body. The total blood flow to the hindlimbs did not differ between the trained and untrained rats during exercise. However, the trained rats distributed more of their blood to the most active muscle fibers.

Blood Pressure

Following endurance training, arterial blood pressure changes very little during standardized submaximal exercise or at maximal work rates.[5] But resting blood pressure is generally lowered in people who are borderline or moderately hypertensive before training. This reduction occurs in both systolic and diastolic blood pressure. Decreases average approximately 11 mmHg for systolic pressure and 8 mmHg for diastolic pressure.[14,35] The mechanisms underlying this reduction are unknown.

Although resistance-type exercise can cause large increases in both systolic and diastolic blood pressure during lifting of heavy weights (see chapter 8), chronic exposure to these high pressures does not result in elevations of resting blood pressure.[33] Hypertension is not common in high-level weight lifters, or in strength and power athletes. In fact, the cardiovascular system can respond to resistance training by lowering resting blood pressure. Hagberg et al. followed a group of borderline-hypertensive adolescents through 5 months of weight training.[15] The subjects' resting systolic blood pressures decreased significantly. These reductions were somewhat greater than those resulting from endurance training.

IN REVIEW . . .

1. Blood flow to muscles is increased by endurance training.
2. Increased blood flow results from three factors:
   - Increased capillarization
   - Greater opening of existing capillaries
   - More effective blood redistribution
3. Resting blood pressure is generally reduced by endurance training in those with borderline or moderate hypertension.
4. Endurance training has little or no effect on blood pressure during standardized submaximal or maximal exercise.

Blood Volume

Endurance training increases blood volume. This effect is greater with more intense levels of training. This increased blood volume, as mentioned earlier, actually results from an increase in blood plasma volume. This is thought to be primarily caused by two mechanisms. First, exercise increases the release of antidiuretic hormone (ADH) and aldosterone. Recall from chapter 6 that these cause the kidneys to retain water, which increases blood plasma. Second, exercise increases the amount of plasma proteins, particularly albumin. Recall from basic physiology that plasma proteins are the major basis for the blood's osmotic pressure. As plasma protein concentration increases, so does osmotic pressure; the result is that more fluid is retained in the blood. Thus both mechanisms work together to increase the fluid portion of the blood—the blood plasma.

Red Blood Cells

An increase in red blood cell volume might also contribute to the overall increase in blood volume, but this increase has not been found consistently.[13] When red blood cell volume has been shown to increase, plasma volume usually has increased much more. Because of this, although the actual number of red blood cells is increased, the hematocrit—the ratio of the red blood cell volume to the total blood volume—actually decreases. Figure 10.7 illustrates the increase in plasma volume and total blood volume with endurance training. Notice that the hematocrit is reduced even though there has been a slight increase in red blood cells. In a trained athlete, the hematocrit can decrease to a level where the person appears to be anemic on the basis of a relatively low concentration of red cells and hemoglobin (pseudoanemia).

This change in the ratio of plasma to cells resulting from an increase in the fluid portion reduces the blood's viscosity. That may facilitate blood movement through the blood vessels, particularly through the smallest vessels, such as the capillaries. Research has shown that low blood viscosity enhances oxygen delivery to the active muscle mass.

Both the total amount (absolute values) of hemoglobin and the total number of red blood cells are typically above normal in highly trained athletes even though the relative values are below normal. This ensures that the blood has more than ample oxygen-carrying capacity to meet the body's needs at all times. Table 10.3 shows the differences in total blood volume,

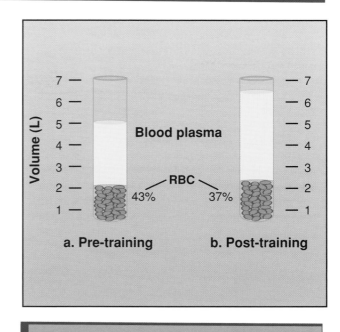

Figure 10.7   Increases in total blood volume and plasma volume with endurance training. Note that, although the hematocrit (% red blood cells) has decreased from 43% to 37%, the total volume of red blood cells has slightly increased.

plasma volume, blood cell volume, and hematocrit between a highly trained athlete and an untrained person.

Plasma Volume, Stroke Volume, and $\dot{V}O_{2\,max}$

An increase in plasma volume is one of the most significant changes that occurs with endurance training. Recall from our previous discussion that the increase in plasma volume is a major factor in the increase of stroke volume resulting from training. Stroke volume, in turn, affects oxygen consumption.

As plasma volume increases, so does blood volume. Consequently, more blood enters the heart. As more blood enters the heart, stroke volume increases. At maximal rates of work, HR max generally remains relatively stable, so an increased stroke volume allows

Table 10.3 Differences in Total Blood Volume, Plasma Volume, Blood Cell Volume, and Hematocrit Between a Highly Trained Athlete and an Untrained Individual

Subjects	Age (yr)	Height (cm)	Weight (kg)	Total blood volume (L)	Plasma volume (L)	Blood cell volume (L)	Hematocrit (%)
Highly trained male athlete	25	180	80.1	7.4	4.8	2.6	35.1
Untrained male	24	178	80.8	5.6	3.2	2.4	42.9

maximal cardiac output to increase. Increasing maximal cardiac output makes more oxygen available to working muscles, thus allowing $\dot{V}O_2$ max to increase.

This sequence of events—a plasma volume increase leading to a stroke volume increase, which, in turn, leads to an increase in $\dot{V}O_2$ max—has also been demonstrated in untrained individuals who have had their plasma volumes expanded using a 6% dextran infusion.[18] This sequence also works in reverse: A plasma volume reduction by detraining highly trained athletes, or by placing healthy men in a position of head-down tilt ($-5°$) for 20 hr results in significant decreases in stroke volume, and equivalent decreases in $\dot{V}O_2$ max.[6,12]

IN REVIEW . . .

1. Blood volume increases as a result of endurance training.
2. The increase is primarily caused by an increase in blood plasma volume.
3. Red blood cell count can increase, but the gain in plasma is typically much higher, resulting in a relatively greater fluid portion of the blood.
4. Increased plasma volume causes decreased blood viscosity, which can improve circulation.
5. Research has shown that plasma volume changes are highly correlated with changes in stroke volume and $\dot{V}O_2$ max, making the training-induced increase in plasma volume one of the most significant training effects.

Respiratory Adaptations to Training

No matter how efficient the cardiovascular system is at supplying adequate amounts of blood to tissues, endurance would be hindered if the respiratory system didn't bring in enough oxygen to meet oxygen demands. Respiratory system functioning usually does not limit performance because ventilation can be increased to a greater extent than cardiovascular function. But, as with the cardiovascular system, the respiratory system undergoes specific adaptations to endurance training to maximize its efficiency. Let's consider some of them.

Lung Volumes

In general, lung volumes and capacities change little with training. Vital capacity (the amount of air that can be expelled after maximal inspiration) increases slightly. At the same time, residual volume (the amount of air that cannot be moved out of the lungs) shows a slight decrease, and the changes in these two volumes may be related. Overall, total lung capacity remains essentially unchanged. Following endurance training, tidal volume (the amount of air breathed in and out during normal respiration) is unchanged at rest and at standardized submaximal levels of exercise. However, it appears to be increased at maximal levels of exercise.

Respiratory Rate

After training, the respiratory rate is usually lowered at rest and during standardized submaximal exercise. This reduction is small and probably reflects greater pulmonary efficiency caused by training. However, respiratory rate is generally increased at maximal levels of exercise following training.

Pulmonary Ventilation

After training, pulmonary ventilation is essentially unchanged or slightly reduced at rest, and it is slightly reduced at standardized submaximal work rates. But maximal pulmonary ventilation is substantially increased. Typical increases in untrained subjects are from a beginning rate of about $120 \text{ L} \cdot \text{min}^{-1}$ to a rate of about $150 \text{ L} \cdot \text{min}^{-1}$ following training. Pulmonary ventilation rates typically increase to about $180 \text{ L} \cdot \text{min}^{-1}$ in highly trained athletes. Two factors can account for the increase in maximal pulmonary ventilation following training: increased tidal volume and increased respiratory rate at maximal exercise.

Large, highly trained endurance athletes, such as rowers, can have maximal pulmonary ventilation rates in excess of $240 \text{ L} \cdot \text{min}^{-1}$—fully twice the rate typical of untrained individuals!

Ventilation is usually not considered a limiting factor for endurance exercise performance. However, some evidence suggests that at some point in a highly trained person's adaptation, the pulmonary system's capacity for oxygen transport won't be able to meet the demands of the limbs and the cardiovascular system.[7]

Pulmonary Diffusion

Pulmonary diffusion, which is the gas exchange occurring in the alveoli, is unaltered at rest and during standardized submaximal exercise following training. However, it is increased during maximal exercise. Pulmonary blood flow (blood coming from the heart to the lungs) appears to be increased following training, particularly the flow to the upper regions of the lung when a person is sitting or standing. This increases lung perfusion. More blood is brought into the lungs for gas exchange, and at the same time ventilation is increased so more air is brought into the lungs. This means that more alveoli will be actively involved in pulmonary diffusion. The net result is that pulmonary diffusion increases.

Arterial-Venous Oxygen Difference

The oxygen content of arterial blood changes very little with training. Even though total hemoglobin is increased, the amount of hemoglobin per unit of blood is the same or even slightly reduced. The arterial-venous oxygen difference (a-$\bar{v}O_2$ diff), however, does increase with training, particularly at maximal levels of exercise. This increase results from a lower mixed venous oxygen content. That means the blood returning to the heart, which is a mixture of venous blood from all body parts, not just the active tissues, contains less oxygen than it would in an untrained person. This reflects both greater oxygen extraction at the tissue level and a more effective distribution of total blood volume (more goes to the active tissues).

In summary, the respiratory system is quite adept at bringing adequate amounts of oxygen into the body. For this reason, the respiratory system is seldom a limiter of endurance performances. Not surprisingly, the major training adaptations noted in the respiratory system are apparent during maximal exercise when all systems are being maximally stressed.

Metabolic Adaptations

Now that we have discussed training changes occurring in both the cardiovascular and respiratory systems, we are ready to look at how these systems integrate with metabolism in the active tissues. Because metabolic adaptations to training were discussed in chapter 7, our discussion will briefly focus on

- lactate threshold,
- respiratory exchange ratio, and
- oxygen consumption.

Lactate Threshold

Endurance training increases lactate threshold. In other words, after training you can perform at a higher rate of work and at a higher absolute rate of oxygen consumption without raising your blood lactate above resting levels (see Figure 10.8). Even though $\dot{V}O_2$ max also increases, the lactate threshold occurs at a higher percentage of $\dot{V}O_2$ max after training. Thus, blood lactate

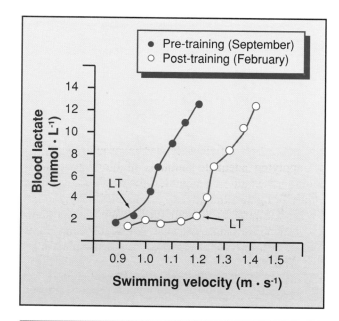

Figure 10.8 The relationship between lactate threshold (LT) and swimming velocity before and after 5 months of training. After training, lactate threshold occurs at a higher rate of work (velocity).

IN REVIEW . . .

1. Most static lung volumes remain essentially unchanged after training. Tidal volume, though unchanged at rest and during submaximal exercise, increases with maximal exertion.
2. Respiratory rate remains steady at rest, can decrease slightly with submaximal exercise, but increases considerably with maximal exercise after training.
3. The combined effect of increased tidal volume and respiration rate is an increase in pulmonary ventilation at maximal effort following training.
4. Pulmonary diffusion at maximal work rates increases, probably because of increased ventilation and increased lung perfusion.
5. The a-$\bar{v}O_2$ diff increases with training, most notably at maximal levels of work, reflecting an increased oxygen extraction by the tissues and more effective blood distribution.

concentrations at each level of a standardized graded exercise test above lactate threshold are lower following endurance training.

This increase in lactate threshold appears to be due to several factors. These include a greater ability to clear lactate produced in the muscle, and an increase in skeletal muscle enzymes coupled with a shift in metabolic substrate as a result of training. The net result is less lactate production for the same work rate.

Maximal blood lactate concentration at the point of exhaustion is increased slightly following endurance training. This increase is relatively small, particularly when compared to the magnitude of increase seen with sprint-type training.

Respiratory Exchange Ratio

Recall from chapter 4 that the respiratory exchange ratio (RER) is the ratio of the carbon dioxide released to the oxygen consumed during nutrient metabolism. It reflects the type of substrates being used as an energy source.

After training, the RER is decreased at both absolute and relative submaximal rates of work. These changes are due to a greater utilization of free fatty acids instead of carbohydrate at these work rates in trained individuals. This shift in substrate utilization was discussed in chapter 7.

However, at maximal levels of work the RER increases in trained individuals. This increase results from the ability to perform at maximal levels for longer periods of time than possible before training. It reflects a sustained hyperventilation with excessive CO_2 release and results from a better all-out maximal performance, which most likely reflects an increased psychological drive.

Resting and Submaximal Oxygen Consumption

Oxygen consumption at rest is either slightly increased or unaltered following endurance training. Several recent studies suggest that resting metabolic rates are elevated in highly trained endurance athletes.[27] At submaximal levels of exercise, $\dot{V}_{O_2}$ is either unchanged or slightly reduced in endurance-trained athletes. A decrease in $\dot{V}_{O_2}$ during submaximal exercise could result from an increase in metabolic efficiency, an increase in mechanical efficiency (performing the same physical work with less extraneous movement), or a combination of both.

Although this possible reduction in submaximal $\dot{V}_{O_2}$ has been postulated, research findings are divided as to whether this change does, in fact, occur. In those

studies that demonstrate a reduced $\dot{V}_{O_2}$ for standardized submaximal work, researchers might have observed a practice effect in their subjects. If you were one of the subjects and you were placed on an ergometer—a treadmill or cycle ergometer, for example—with which you had no prior experience, you would likely feel awkward on the device the first time you used it. As a result, you might expend more energy during the first trial, then perform at a lower energy cost the second or third time you exercised on that device simply because you became more familiar with using it.

Another potential problem could arise if the exercise device is weight dependent, that is, the work performed is dependent on your body weight. In this case, any weight loss from training decreases your $\dot{V}_{O_2}$ because you are doing less work without necessarily reflecting changes in efficiency. Thus, any observed change in submaximal $\dot{V}_{O_2}$ with endurance training might not be the result of cardiovascular or metabolic adaptations to training.

Maximal Oxygen Consumption

As we pointed out early in the chapter, most researchers regard $\dot{V}_{O_2\,max}$ as the best indicator of cardiorespiratory endurance capacity. Now that we have gone through the various physiological adaptations that occur, it is not surprising to find that $\dot{V}_{O_2\,max}$ increases substantially in response to endurance training. Increases of from 4% to 93% have been reported.[28] An increase of 15% to 20% is more typical for an average person who was sedentary prior to training and who trains at 75% of his or her capacity 3 times per week, 30 min per day, for 6 months.[28] The $\dot{V}_{O_2\,max}$ of a sedentary individual can increase from an initial value of 35 ml $\cdot$ kg^{-1} $\cdot$ min^{-1} to 42 ml $\cdot$ kg^{-1} $\cdot$ min^{-1} as a result of such a program. This is far below the values we see in world-class endurance athletes, whose values generally range from 70 to 94 ml $\cdot$ kg^{-1} $\cdot$ min^{-1}.

Level of Conditioning and $\dot{V}_{O_2\,max}$

The higher the initial state of conditioning, the smaller will be the relative improvement for the same program of training. In other words, if two people, one sedentary and the other partially trained, undergo the same endurance training program, the sedentary person will show the greatest relative improvement. You can look at this in terms of how well trained the people are when they begin the program—those who are less trained have the most room for improvement.

It appears that in fully mature athletes, the highest attainable $\dot{V}_{O_2\,max}$ is reached within 8 to 18 months of heavy endurance training, indicating that each athlete has a finite level of oxygen consumption that can be attained. This finite range is potentially influenced by training in early childhood.[11] The latter observation is conjecture at this time; it needs to be substantiated by experimental research.

Reasons for Increased $\dot{V}_{O_2 max}$

The factors responsible for increased $\dot{V}_{O_2 max}$ have been identified, and we have discussed many in this chapter. But at one time, much controversy surrounded their importance. Two theories were proposed to explain these increases with training.

Limitation of Oxidative Enzymes.   One theory held that endurance performance is usually limited by the lack of sufficient amounts of oxidative enzymes in the mitochondria. Proponents of this theory provided impressive evidence that endurance training programs substantially increase the amount of these oxidative enzymes. This would allow active tissue to utilize more of the available oxygen, resulting in a higher $\dot{V}_{O_2 max}$. In addition, proponents supported their case by pointing out that endurance training results in increases in both the size and number of muscle mitochondria. Thus, this theory argues, the main limitation of maximal oxygen consumption is an inability of the existing mitochondria to utilize the available oxygen beyond a certain rate. This has been referred to as the utilization theory.

Limitation of Oxygen Delivery.   The second theory proposed that central and peripheral circulatory factors limited endurance capacity. This would preclude delivery of sufficient amounts of oxygen to the active tissues. According to this theory, improvement in $\dot{V}_{O_2 max}$ following endurance training results from increases in blood volume, cardiac output (via stroke volume), and a better perfusion of active muscle with blood. This has been referred to as the presentation theory.

Again, impressive research evidence strongly supported this theory. In one study, subjects breathed a mixture of carbon monoxide and air during exercise to exhaustion.[26] $\dot{V}_{O_2 max}$ decreased in direct proportion to the percentage of carbon monoxide breathed. The carbon monoxide molecules were bonded to approximately 15% of the total hemoglobin; this percentage agreed with the percentage reduction in $\dot{V}_{O_2 max}$. In another study, approximately 15% to 20% of each subject's total blood volume was removed. $\dot{V}_{O_2 max}$ decreased by approximately the same relative amount.[10] Reinfusion of the subjects' packed red blood cells approximately 4 weeks later resulted in an increase in $\dot{V}_{O_2 max}$ above baseline or control conditions. In both studies, the reduction in the oxygen-carrying capacity of the blood—by either blocking hemoglobin or removing whole blood—resulted in less oxygen being delivered to the active tissues. This resulted in a

corresponding reduction in $\dot{V}_{O_2 max}$. Similarly, studies have shown that breathing oxygen-enriched mixtures, where the partial pressure of oxygen in the inspired air is substantially increased, results in increased endurance capacity.

These and subsequent studies indicate that the available oxygen supply is the major limiter of endurance performance. Saltin and Rowell, in an excellent review article, conclude that it is the oxygen transport to the working muscles, not the available mitochondria and oxidative enzymes, that limits $\dot{V}_{O_2 max}$.[32] They argue that increases in $\dot{V}_{O_2 max}$ with training are largely attributable to increased maximal blood flow and increased muscle capillary density in the active tissues. The major skeletal muscle adaptations (including increased mitochondrial content and respiratory capacity of the muscle fibers) appear more closely related to the ability to perform prolonged high-intensity submaximal exercise.[17]

Table 10.4 provides a summary of the physiological changes that occur with endurance training, illustrating the expected changes pre- to post-training in a previously inactive male, compared to values for a world-class endurance athlete.

IN REVIEW . . .

1. Lactate threshold increases with endurance training, which allows you to perform at higher rates of work and levels of oxygen consumption without increasing your blood lactate above resting levels. Maximal blood lactate levels can be increased slightly.
2. The respiratory exchange ratio decreases at submaximal work rates, indicating a greater utilization of free fatty acids, but increases at maximal effort.
3. Oxygen consumption can be increased slightly at rest and decreased slightly or unaltered during submaximal exercise.
4. $\dot{V}_{O_2 max}$ increases substantially following training, but the amount of increase possible is limited in each individual. The major limiting factor appears to be oxygen delivery to the active muscles.

Long-Term Improvement in Endurance

Although the highest attainable $\dot{V}_{O_2 max}$ is usually reached within 18 months of intense endurance

Table 10.4 Summary of the Physiological Alterations Resulting From Endurance Training, Illustrating the Expected Changes Pre- to Post-Training in a Previously Inactive Male, Compared to Values for a World-Class Endurance Athlete

Variables	Sedentary normal		World-class endurance runner
	Pre-training	Post-training	
Cardiovascular			
HR at rest (beats per minute)	71	59	36
HR max (beats per minute)	185	183	174
SV at rest (ml^2)	65	80	125
SV max (ml^2)	120	140	200
$\dot{Q}$ at rest (L $\cdot$ min^{-1})	4.6	4.7	4.5
$\dot{Q}$ max (L $\cdot$ min^{-1})	22.2	25.6	34.8
Heart volume (ml)	750	820	1,200
Blood volume (L)	4.7	5.1	6.0
Systolic BP at rest (mmHg)	135	130	120
Systolic BP max (mmHg)	210	205	210
Diastolic BP at rest (mmHg)	78	76	65
Diastolic BP max (mmHg)	82	80	65
Respiratory			
VE at rest (L $\cdot$ min^{-1})	7	6	6
VE max (L $\cdot$ min^{-1})	110	135	195
TV at rest (L)	0.5	0.5	0.5
TV max (L)	2.75	3.0	3.5
VC (L)	5.8	6.0	6.2
RV (L)	1.4	1.2	1.2
Metabolic			
a-$\bar{v}O_2$ diff at rest (ml $\cdot$ 100 ml^{-1})	6.0	6.0	6.0
a-$\bar{v}O_2$ diff max (ml $\cdot$ 100 ml^{-1})	14.5	15.0	16.0
$\dot{V}O_2$ at rest (ml $\cdot$ kg^{-1} $\cdot$ min^{-1})	3.5	3.5	3.5
$\dot{V}O_2$ max (ml $\cdot$ kg^{-1} $\cdot$ min^{-1})	40.5	49.8	76.7
Blood lactate at rest (mmol $\cdot$ L^{-1})	1.0	1.0	1.0
Blood lactate max (mmol $\cdot$ L^{-1})	7.5	8.5	9.0
Body composition			
Weight (kg)	79	77	68
Fat weight (kg)	12.6	9.6	5.1
Fat-free weight (kg)	66.4	67.4	62.9
Relative fat, %	16.0	12.5	7.5

Note. HR = heart rate; SV = stroke volume; $\dot{Q}$ = cardiac output; BP = blood pressure; $\dot{V}E$ = ventilatory volume; TV = tidal volume; VC = vital capacity; RV = residual volume; a-$\bar{v}O_2$ diff = arterial venous oxygen difference; $\dot{V}O_2$ = oxygen consumption.

conditioning, endurance performance continues to improve with continued training for many additional years. Improvement in endurance performance without improvements in $\dot{V}O_2$ max is probably due to the body's ability to perform at increasingly higher percentages of $\dot{V}O_2$ max for extended periods.

Consider, for example, a young male runner who starts training with an initial $\dot{V}O_2$ max of 52.0 ml $\cdot$ kg^{-1} $\cdot$ min^{-1}. He reaches his genetically determined peak $\dot{V}O_2$ max of 71 ml $\cdot$ kg^{-1} $\cdot$ min^{-1} 2 years later and is unable to increase it further, even with more intensive workouts. At this point, as shown in Figure 10.9, the young runner is able to run at 75% of his $\dot{V}O_2$ max (0.75 × 71.0 = 53.3 ml $\cdot$ kg^{-1} $\cdot$ min^{-1}) in a 6-mi (9.7-km) race. Following an additional 2 years of intensive training, his $\dot{V}O_2$ max is unchanged, but he is now able

to compete at 88% of his $\dot{V}O_2$ max (0.88 × 71.0 = 62.5 ml $\cdot$ kg^{-1} $\cdot$ min^{-1}). Obviously, by being able to sustain an oxygen uptake of 62.5 ml $\cdot$ kg^{-1} $\cdot$ min^{-1} he is able to run at a much faster pace.

This increase in performance without an increase in $\dot{V}O_2$ max is the result of an increase in lactate threshold, because race pace is directly related to the $\dot{V}O_2$ value at lactate threshold, as we have seen in previous chapters.

Factors Affecting the Response to Aerobic Training

We have discussed general trends in adaptations occurring in response to endurance training. However,

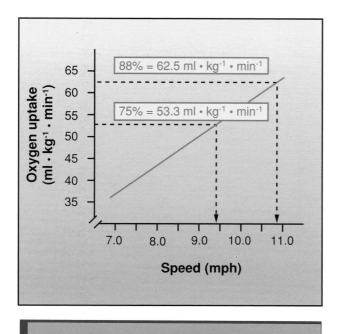

Figure 10.9   Change in race pace with continued training when maximal oxygen uptake fails to continue to increase.

we must always remember that we are talking about adaptations in individuals, so not everyone will respond in the same manner. Several factors must be considered that can affect individual response to aerobic training. Let's consider them now.

Heredity

Maximum oxygen consumption levels depend on genetic limits. You should not take this to mean that each individual has an exact $\dot{V}_{O_2 max}$ that cannot be exceeded. Rather, a range of $\dot{V}_{O_2 max}$ values seems to be predetermined by an individual's genetic makeup, and his or her highest attainable $\dot{V}_{O_2 max}$ should fall in that range.

The genetic basis of $\dot{V}_{O_2 max}$ has been studied by Klissouras in a series of studies conducted in the late 1960s and early 1970s, and more recently by Bouchard and his colleagues.[4,19] Research has found that identical (monozygous) twins have nearly identical $\dot{V}_{O_2 max}$ values, whereas the variability for dizygous (fraternal) twins is much greater. Figure 10.10 illustrates this.

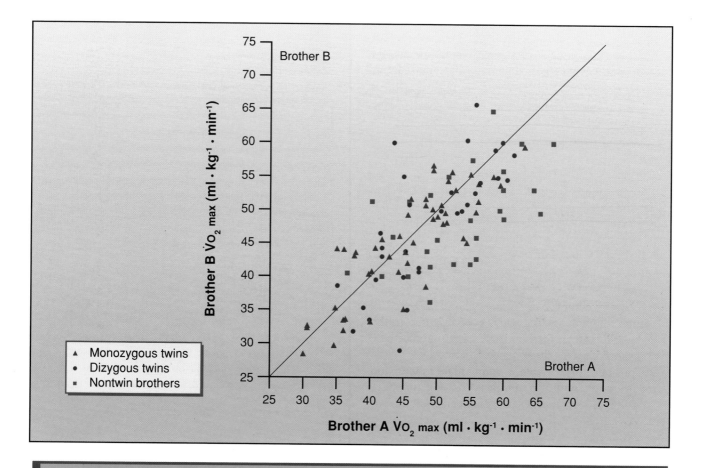

Figure 10.10   Comparisons of $\dot{V}_{O_2 max}$ in twin (monozygous and dizygous) and nontwin brothers. Adapted from Bouchard et al. (1986).

Each symbol represents a pair of brothers. Brother A's $\dot{V}O_2$ max value is indicated by the symbol's position on the x-axis, and Brother B's $\dot{V}O_2$ max value is indicated by the symbol's position on the y-axis. Similarity in the siblings' $\dot{V}O_2$ max values is noted by comparing the x- and y-coordinates of the symbol. Similar results were found for endurance capacity, determined by the maximum amount of work performed in an all-out 90-min ride on a cycle ergometer.

Bouchard et al. have concluded that heredity accounts for between 25% and 50% of the variance in $\dot{V}O_2$ max values.[3] This means that of all factors influencing $\dot{V}O_2$ max, heredity alone is responsible for one quarter to one half of the total influence. World-class athletes who have stopped endurance training continue for many years to have high $\dot{V}O_2$ max values in their sedentary, deconditioned state. Their $\dot{V}O_2$ max values may decrease from 85 ml · kg^{-1} · min^{-1} to 65 ml · kg^{-1} · min^{-1}, but this deconditioned value is still very high.

Thus, both genetic and environmental factors influence $\dot{V}O_2$ max values. The genetic factors probably establish the boundaries for the athlete, but endurance training can push $\dot{V}O_2$ max to the upper limit of these boundaries. Dr. Per-Olof Åstrand, one of the most recognized exercise physiologists during the second half of the 20th century, has stated on numerous occasions that the best way to become a champion Olympic athlete is to be selective when choosing your parents!

Age

Age can also influence $\dot{V}O_2$ max. However, $\dot{V}O_2$ max values that have been reported in the research literature could lead to an improper interpretation of true age differences if compared across ages. Figure 10.11 illustrates the $\dot{V}O_2$ max values of two groups of older endurance athletes—those who maintained their training intensity and those who reduced it.[29] For those men who continued to train at the same intensity, the rate of decline in $\dot{V}O_2$ max was attenuated. This indicates that age-related decreases might partly result from an age-related decrease in activity levels. This decrease is not an absolute trend—endurance training of untrained elderly subjects results in substantial $\dot{V}O_2$ max increases.[20] This will be discussed in greater detail in chapter 18.

Gender

Healthy untrained girls and women have much lower $\dot{V}O_2$ max values (20% to 25% lower) than healthy untrained boys and men. However, highly conditioned female endurance athletes have values much closer to those of highly trained male endurance athletes (about

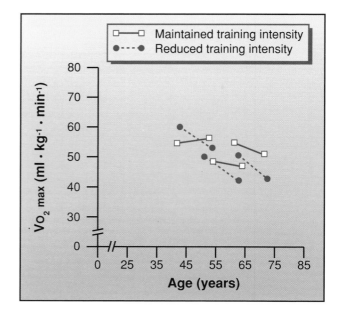

Figure 10.11 Changes in $\dot{V}O_2$ max with age in a group of athletes who maintained training intensity and in a group that reduced training intensity. Individual data points represent longitudinal data from men followed for 10 years. Data from Pollock et al. (1987).

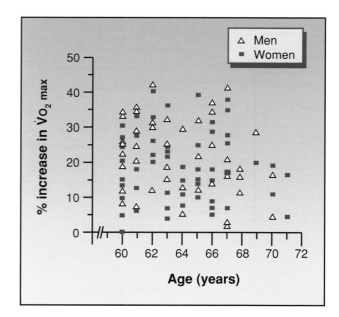

Figure 10.12 Variations in the improvements in $\dot{V}O_2$ max with training in older men and women, showing that individuals respond differently to training even when following the same program. Data from Kohrt et al. (1991).

Table 10.5 Maximal Oxygen Uptake Values ($ml \cdot kg^{-1} \cdot min^{-1}$) for Nonathletes and Athletes

Group or Sport	Age	Males	Females
Nonathletes	10-19	47-56	38-46
	20-29	43-52	33-42
	30-39	39-48	30-38
	40-49	36-44	26-35
	50-59	34-41	24-33
	60-69	31-38	22-30
	70-79	28-35	20-27
Baseball/softball	18-32	48-56	52-57
Basketball	18-30	40-60	43-60
Bicycling	18-26	62-74	47-57
Canoeing	22-28	55-67	48-52
Football	20-36	42-60	—
Gymnastics	18-22	52-58	36-50
Ice hockey	10-30	50-63	—
Jockey	20-40	50-60	—
Orienteering	20-60	47-53	46-60
Racquetball	20-35	55-62	50-60
Rowing	20-35	60-72	58-65
Skiing:			
Alpine	18-30	57-68	50-55
Cross-country	20-28	65-95	60-75
Ski jumping	18-24	58-63	—
Soccer	22-28	54-64	—
Speed skating	18-24	56-73	44-55
Swimming	10-25	50-70	40-60
Track and field			
Runners	18-39	60-85	50-75
	40-75	40-60	—
Discus	22-30	42-55	—
Shot put	22-30	40-46	—
Volleyball	18-22	—	40-56
Weight lifting	20-30	38-52	—
Wrestling	20-30	52-65	—

10% lower). This will be discussed in greater detail in chapter 19. $\dot{V}O_2$ max values for athletes and nonathletes are presented in Table 10.5 by age, gender, and sport.

Responders and Nonresponders

For years, researchers have found wide variations in improvement in $\dot{V}O_2$ max with aerobic training. This is illustrated in Figure 10.12, where a group of older men and women were endurance trained for 9 to 12 months.[20] Improvement in $\dot{V}O_2$ max ranged from 0% to 43%, even though all the subjects completed the same training program.

Scientists have assumed that these variations result from differing degrees of compliance with the training program. Good compliers should have the highest percentage of improvement and poor compliers

should show little or no improvement. Now, the idea of comparing compliers with noncompliers has been replaced with the concept of comparing responders with nonresponders. Given the same training stimulus, implying full compliance with the program, substantial fluctuations occur in the percentage improvements in $\dot{V}O_2$ max values of different people.

Bouchard has now clearly established that the response to a training program is also genetically determined.[2] This is illustrated in Figure 10.13. Ten pairs of identical twins completed a 20-week endurance training program; the improvements in $\dot{V}O_2$ max, expressed in $ml \cdot kg^{-1} \cdot min^{-1}$ and in percent improvement, are plotted for each twin pair, Twin A on the x-axis and Twin B on the y-axis. Notice the similarity in response for each twin pair. These results, and those from other studies, indicate that there will be responders (large improvement) and nonresponders (little or no improvement) among groups of people who experience identical training programs.

It is now clear that this is a genetic phenomenon, not a result of compliance or noncompliance. This important point must be considered when conducting training studies and when designing training programs. You must allow for individual differences.

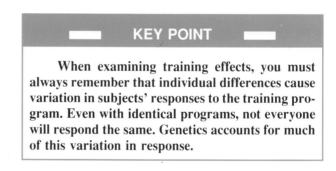

KEY POINT

When examining training effects, you must always remember that individual differences cause variation in subjects' responses to the training program. Even with identical programs, not everyone will respond the same. Genetics accounts for much of this variation in response.

Specificity of Training

Physiological adaptations in response to physical training are highly specific to the nature of the training activity. Furthermore, the more specific the training program is to a given sport or activity, the greater the improvement in performance. The concept of specificity of training is very important for cardiorespiratory adaptations. This concept, as mentioned earlier, is also important in testing athletes.

To accurately measure endurance improvements, athletes should be tested while engaged in an activity similar to the sport or activity they usually participate in. Consider one study of highly trained rowers, cyclists, and cross-country skiers. They were tested for $\dot{V}O_2$ max while performing two types of work: uphill running on a treadmill and maximal performance of

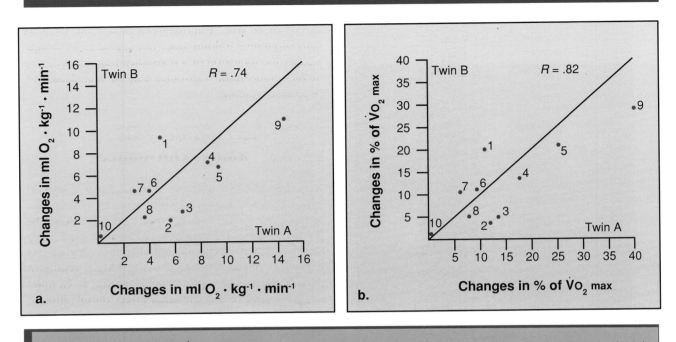

Figure 10.13 Variations in $\dot{V}O_2$ max for identical twins undergoing the same 20-week training program, expressed (a) in absolute values and (b) in relative change. Adapted from Bouchard (1990).

their specific sport activity.[34] The important finding, as indicated in Figure 10.14, was that the $\dot{V}O_2$ max values attained by all the athletes during their sport-specific activity were as high as or higher than the values obtained on the treadmill. For many of these athletes, $\dot{V}O_2$ max values were substantially higher during their sport-specific activity.

In nonathletes, uphill running had previously been shown to consistently produce the highest $\dot{V}O_2$ max values. The widespread assumption was that this result would hold true for athletes, but that assumption is not correct.

The concept of training specificity is further illustrated in a study by Magel and his associates.[23] They studied $\dot{V}O_2$ max improvements with swim training (1 hr per day, 3 days per week, for 10 weeks). Subjects performed maximal treadmill running and tethered swimming tests both before and after training. The swimming $\dot{V}O_2$ max increased by 11.2% following the 10-week training period. However, the running $\dot{V}O_2$ max increased by only 1.5%, not a statistically significant change from the pre-training value. If the treadmill alone had been used for testing, the researchers would have concluded that swim training had no influence on cardiorespiratory endurance capacity!

One of the most elegant designs to study the concept of specificity of training involves one-legged exercise training, where the untrained opposite leg is used as the control. In one study, subjects were placed in three

groups: one group sprint trained one leg and endurance trained the other leg; one group sprint trained one leg, and the other leg remained untrained; and the last group endurance trained one leg, and the other leg remained untrained.[31] Improvement in $\dot{V}O_2$ max and lowered heart rate and blood lactate response at submaximal work rates were found only when exercise was performed with the endurance-trained leg.

Much of the training response occurs in the specific muscles that have been trained, possibly even in individual motor units in a specific muscle. From the studies conducted in this area, it appears that this involves both metabolic and cardiorespiratory responses to training.

▬▬ KEY POINT ▬▬

Close attention must be given to selecting the appropriate training program. It must be carefully matched with the athlete's individual needs to maximize the physiological adaptations to training, thereby optimizing the athlete's performance.

Cross-Training

Cross-training refers to training for more than one sport at the same time, or training for several different fitness components (such as endurance, strength, and

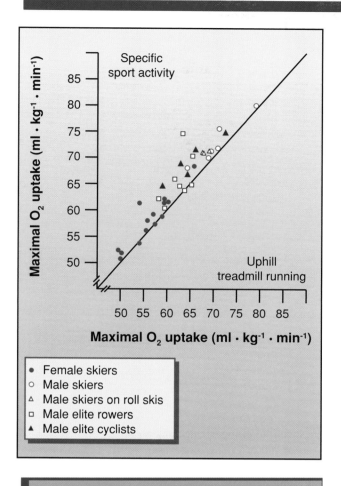

Figure 10.14 $\dot{V}O_2$ max values during uphill treadmill running versus sport-specific activities in selected groups of athletes. Adapted from Strømme et al. (1977).

appear to be true: Improvement of aerobic capacity with endurance training does not appear to be attenuated by the inclusion of a resistance training program. In fact, short-term endurance can be increased with resistance training.[16]

Cardiorespiratory Endurance and Performance

Cardiorespiratory endurance is regarded by many people as the most important component of physical fitness. It is an athlete's major defense against fatigue. Low endurance capacity leads to fatigue, even in the more sedentary sports or activities. For any athlete, regardless of the sport or activity, fatigue represents a major deterrent to optimal performance. Even minor fatigue can have a detrimental effect on the athlete's total performance:

- Muscular strength is decreased.
- Reaction and movement times are prolonged.
- Agility and neuromuscular coordination are reduced.
- Whole-body movement speed is slowed.
- Concentration and alertness are reduced.

The decline in concentration and alertness associated with fatigue is particularly important. The athlete can become careless and more prone to serious injury, especially in contact sports. Even though these decrements in performance might be small, they can be just enough to cause an athlete to miss the critical free throw in basketball, the strike zone in baseball, or the 20-ft putt in golf.

All athletes can benefit from maximizing their endurance. Even golfers, whose sport is relatively sedentary, can improve. Improved endurance can allow golfers to complete a round of golf with less fatigue and to better withstand long periods of walking and standing.

For the sedentary middle-aged adult, numerous health factors indicate that cardiovascular endurance should be the primary emphasis of training. This will be discussed at length in Part G of this book.

The extent of endurance training needed varies considerably from one athlete to the next. It depends on the athlete's current endurance capacity and the endurance demands of the chosen activity. The marathon runner uses endurance training almost exclusively, with limited attention to strength, flexibility, and speed. The baseball player, however, places very limited demands on endurance capacity, so endurance conditioning is not as highly emphasized. Nevertheless, baseball players could gain substantially from endurance running, even if only at a moderate pace

flexibility) at one time. The athlete who trains by swimming, running, and cycling in preparation for competing in a triathlon is an example of the former, and the athlete involved in heavy resistance training and high-intensity cardiorespiratory training at the same time is an example of the latter.

Very little research data are available concerning multisport training. In any cross-training program of this nature, it will be important to determine how best to partition the available training time to optimize performance in each of the sports. Although certain aspects of training are the same for all endurance activities, most training is highly specific to a particular sport.

For the athlete training for cardiorespiratory endurance and strength at the same time, the few studies conducted to date indicate that gains in strength, power, and endurance can result. However, the gains in muscular strength and power are less when strength training is combined with endurance training than when strength training alone is done.[8] The opposite does not for 3 mi (5 km) per day for 3 days per week. As a benefit of training, baseball players would have little or no leg trouble (a frequent complaint), and they would be able to complete a doubleheader with little or no fatigue.

Adequate cardiovascular conditioning must be the foundation of any athlete's general conditioning program. Many athletes in nonendurance activities have never incorporated even moderate endurance training into their training programs. Those who have done so are well aware of their improved physical condition and its impact on their athletic performance.

IN REVIEW . . .

1. Although $\dot{V}O_2$ max has an upper limit, endurance performance can continue to improve for years with continued training.
2. An individual's genetic makeup predetermines a range for his or her $\dot{V}O_2$ max, accounting for 25% to 50% of the variance in $\dot{V}O_2$ max values. Heredity also largely explains individual variations in response to identical training programs.
3. Age-related decreases in aerobic capacity might partly result from decreased activity.
4. Highly conditioned female endurance athletes have $\dot{V}O_2$ max values only about 10% lower than those of highly conditioned male endurance athletes.
5. To maximize cardiorespiratory gains from training, the training should be specific to the type of activity that an athlete usually performs.
6. Resistance training in combination with endurance training does not appear to restrict improvement in aerobic capacity and may increase short-term endurance.
7. All athletes can benefit from maximizing their endurance.

In Closing . . .

In this chapter, we have examined how the cardiovascular and respiratory systems adapt to chronic exposure to the stress of training. We have concentrated on how these adaptations can improve cardiorespiratory endurance. This chapter concludes our review of how body systems respond to both acute and chronic exercise. Now that we have completed our examination of how the body responds to internal changes, we can turn our attention to the external world. In the next part, we will focus on the body's adaptations to varying environmental conditions, beginning in the next chapter by considering how external temperature can affect performance.

Key Terms

a-$\bar{v}O_2$ diff
capillary to fiber ratio
cardiorespiratory
  endurance
cross-training
heart rate recovery
  period
nonresponders
oxygen transport system

residual volume
respiratory exchange
  ratio
responders
specificity of training
tidal volume
vital capacity
$\dot{V}O_2$ max

Study Questions

1. Differentiate between muscular endurance and cardiovascular endurance.
2. What is maximal oxygen uptake ($\dot{V}O_2$ max)? How is it defined physiologically, and what determines its limits?
3. Of what importance is $\dot{V}O_2$ max to endurance performance?
4. Describe those changes in the oxygen transport system that occur with endurance training.
5. What is possibly the most important adaptation the body makes in response to endurance training which allows for an increase in both $\dot{V}O_2$ max and performance?
6. What metabolic adaptations occur in response to endurance training?
7. Explain the two theories that had been proposed to account for improvements in $\dot{V}O_2$ max with endurance training. Which of these has the greatest validity today? Why?
8. How important is genetic potential in developing a young athlete?
9. Why would cardiovascular endurance conditioning be important for athletes in nonendurance sports?

References

1. Armstrong, R.B., & Laughlin, M.H. (1984). Exercise blood flow patterns within and among rat muscles after training. *American Journal of Physiology*, **246**, H59-H68.

2. Bouchard, C. (1990). Discussion: Heredity, fitness, and health. In C. Bouchard, R.J. Shephard, T. Stephens, J.R. Sutton, & B.D. McPherson (Eds.), *Exercise, fitness, and health* (pp. 147-153). Champaign, IL: Human Kinetics.

3. Bouchard, C., Dionne, F.T., Simoneau, J.-A., & Boulay, M.R. (1992). Genetics of aerobic and anaerobic performances. *Exercise and Sport Sciences Reviews*, **20**, 27-58.

4. Bouchard, C., Lesage, R., Lortie, G., Simoneau, J.A., Hamel, P., Boulay, M.R., Pérusse, L., Thériault,

G., & Leblanc, C. (1986). Aerobic performance in brothers, dizygotic and monozygotic twins. *Medicine and Science in Sports and Exercise*, **18**, 639-646.

5. Clausen, J.P. (1977). Effect of physical training on cardiovascular adjustments to exercise in man. *Physiological Reviews*, **57**, 779-816.

6. Coyle, E.F., Hemmert, M.K., & Coggan, A.R. (1986). Effects of detraining on cardiovascular responses to exercise: Role of blood volume. *Journal of Applied Physiology*, **60**, 95-99.

7. Dempsey, J.A. (1986). Is the lung built for exercise? *Medicine and Science in Sports and Exercise*, **18**, 143-155.

8. Dudley, G.A., & Fleck, S.J. (1987). Strength and endurance training: Are they mutually exclusive? *Sports Medicine*, **4**, 79-85.

9. Ehsani, A.A., Ogawa, T., Miller, T.R., Spina, R.J., & Jilka, S.M. (1991). Exercise training improves left ventricular systolic function in older men. *Circulation*, **83**, 96-103.

10. Ekblom, B., Goldbarg, A.M., & Gullbring, B. (1972). Response to exercise after blood loss and reinfusion. *Journal of Applied Physiology*, **33**, 175-180.

11. Fahey, T.D., Del Valle-Zuris, A., Oehlsen, G., Trieb, M., & Seymour, J. (1979). Pubertal stage differences in hormonal and hematological responses to maximal exercise in males. *Journal of Applied Physiology*, **46**, 823-827.

12. Gaffney, F.A., Nixon, J.V., Karlsson, E.S., Campbell, W., Dowdey, A.B.C., & Blomqvist, C.G. (1985). Cardiovascular deconditioning produced by 20 hours of bedrest with head-down tilts ($-5°$) in middle-aged healthy men. *American Journal of Cardiology*, **56**, 634-638.

13. Green, H.J., Sutton, J.R., Coates, G., Ali, M., & Jones, S. (1991). Response of red cell and plasma volume to prolonged training in humans. *Journal of Applied Physiology*, **70**, 1810-1815.

14. Hagberg, J.M. (1990). Exercise, fitness, and hypertension. In C. Bouchard, R.J. Shephard, T. Stephens, J.R. Sutton, & B.D. McPherson (Eds.), *Exercise, fitness, and health* (pp. 455-466). Champaign, IL: Human Kinetics.

15. Hagberg, J.M., Ehsani, A.A., Goldring, D., Hernandez, A., Sinacore, D.R., & Holloszy, J.O. (1984). Effect of weight training on blood pressure and hemodynamics in hypertensive adolescents. *Journal of Pediatrics*, **104**, 147-151.

16. Hickson, R.C., Dvorak, B.A., Gorostiaga, E.M., Kurowski, T.T., & Foster, C. (1988). Potential for strength and endurance training to amplify endurance performance. *Journal of Applied Physiology*, **65**, 2285-2290.

17. Holloszy, J.O., & Coyle, E.F. (1984). Adaptations of skeletal muscle to endurance exercise and their metabolic consequences. *Journal of Applied Physiology*, **56**, 831-838.

18. Hopper, M.K., Coggan, A.R., & Coyle, E.F. (1988). Exercise stroke volume relative to plasma-volume expansion. *Journal of Applied Physiology*, **64**, 404-408.

19. Klissouras, V. (1971). Adaptability of genetic variation. *Journal of Applied Physiology*, **31**, 338-344.

20. Kohrt, W.M., Malley, M.T., Coggan, A.R., Spina, R.J., Ogawa, T., Ehsani, A.A., Bourey, R.E., Martin, W.H. III, & Holloszy, J.O. (1991). Effects of gender, age and fitness level on response of $\dot{V}O_{2\,max}$ to training in 60-71 yr olds. *Journal of Applied Physiology*, **71**, 2004-2011.

21. Kraemer, W.J., Deschenes, M.R., & Fleck, S.J. (1988). Physiological adaptations to resistance exercise: Implications for athletic conditioning. *Sports Medicine*, **6**, 246-256.

22. Landry, F., Bouchard, C., & Dumesnil, J. (1985). Cardiac dimension changes with endurance training. *Journal of the American Medical Association*, **254**, 77-80.

23. Magel, J.R., Foglia, G.F., McArdle, W.D., Gutin, B., Pechar, G.S., & Katch, F.I. (1975). Specificity of swim training on maximum oxygen uptake. *Journal of Applied Physiology*, **38**, 151-155.

24. Milliken, M.C., Stray-Gundersen, J., Peshock, R.M., Katz, J., & Mitchell, J.H. (1988). Left ventricular mass as determined by magnetic resonance imaging in male endurance athletes. *American Journal of Cardiology*, **62**, 301-305.

25. Morrison, D.A., Boyden, T.W., Pamenter, R.W., Freund, B.J., Stini, W.A., Harrington, R., & Wilmore, J.H. (1986). Effects of aerobic training on exercise tolerance and echocardiographic dimensions in untrained postmenopausal women. *American Heart Journal*, **112**, 561-567.

26. Pirnay, F., Dujardin, J., Deroanne, R., & Petit, J.M. (1971). Muscular exercise during intoxication by carbon monoxide. *Journal of Applied Physiology*, **31**, 573-575.

27. Poehlman, E.T., Melby, C.L., & Goran, M.I. (1991). The impact of exercise and diet restriction on daily energy expenditure. *Sports Medicine*, **11**, 78-101.

28. Pollock, M.L. (1973). Quantification of endurance training programs. *Exercise and Sport Sciences Reviews*, **1**, 155-188.

29. Pollock, M.L., Foster, C., Knapp, D., Rod, J.L., & Schmidt, D.H. (1987). Effect of age and training on aerobic capacity and body composition of master athletes. *Journal of Applied Physiology*, **62**, 725-731.

30. Pollock, M.L., & Wilmore, J.H. (1990). *Exercise in health and disease: Evaluation and prescription for prevention and rehabilitation* (2nd ed.). Philadelphia: Saunders.

31. Saltin, B., Nazar, K., Costill, D.L., Stein, E., Jansson, E., Essén, B., & Gollnick, P.D. (1976). The nature of the training response; peripheral and central adaptations to one-legged exercise. *Acta Physiologica Scandinavica*, **96**, 289-305.

32. Saltin, B., & Rowell, L.B. (1980). Functional adaptations to physical activity and inactivity. *Federation Proceedings*, **39**, 1506-1513.

33. Stone, M.H., Fleck, S.J., Triplett, N.T., & Kraemer, W.J. (1991). Health- and performance-related potential of resistance training. *Sports Medicine*, **11**, 210-231.

34. Strømme, S.B., Ingjer, F., & Meen, H.D. (1977). Assessment of maximal aerobic power in specifically trained athletes. *Journal of Applied Physiology*, **42**, 833-837.

35. Tipton, C.M. (1991). Exercise, training and hypertension: An update. *Exercise and Sport Sciences Reviews*, **19**, 447-505.

36. Turkevich, D., Micco, A., & Reeves, J.T. (1988). Noninvasive measurement of the decrease in left ventricular filling time during maximal exercise in normal subjects. *American Journal of Cardiology*, **62**, 650-652.

37. Urhausen, A., & Kindermann, W. (1989). One- and two-dimensional echocardiography in body builders and endurance-trained subjects. *International Journal of Sports Medicine*, **10**, 139-144.

Selected Readings

Dowell, R.T. (1983). Cardiac adaptations to exercise. *Exercise and Sport Sciences Reviews*, **11**, 99-117.

Fisher, A.G., Adams, T.D., Yanowitz, F.G., Ridges, J.D., Orsmond, G., & Nelson, A.G. (1989). Noninvasive evaluation of world class athletes engaged in different modes of training. *American Journal of Cardiology*, **63**, 337-341.

George, K.P., Wolfe, L.A., & Burggraf, G.W. (1991). The "athletic heart syndrome:" A critical review. *Sports Medicine*, **11**, 300-331.

Gergley, T.J., McArdle, W.D., DeJesus, P., Toner, M.M., Jacobowitz, S., & Spina, R.J. (1984). Specificity of arm training on aerobic power during swimming and running. *Medicine and Science in Sports and Exercise*, **16**, 349-354.

Ginzton, L.E., Conant, R., Brizendine, M., & Laks, M.M. (1989). Effect of long-term high intensity aerobic training on left ventricular volume during maximal upright exercise. *Journal of the American College of Cardiology*, **14**, 364-371.

Hermansen, L., & Wachtlova, M. (1971). Capillary density of skeletal muscle in well-trained and untrained men. *Journal of Applied Physiology*, **30**, 860-863.

Hudlicka, O. (1977). Effect of training on macro- and microcirculatory changes in exercise. *Exercise and Sport Sciences Reviews*, **5**, 181-230.

MacRae, H.S.-H., Dennis, S.C., Bosch, A.N., & Noakes, T.D. (1992). Effects of training on lactate production and removal during progressive exercise in humans. *Journal of Applied Physiology*, **72**, 1649-1656.

Rowell, L.B. (1986). *Human circulation regulation during physical stress*. New York: Oxford University Press.

Sexton, W.L., Korthuis, R.J., & Laughlin, M.H. (1988). High-intensity exercise training increases vascular transport capacity of rat hindquarters. *American Journal of Physiology*, **254**, H274-H278.

Environmental Influences on Performance

In the previous sections of the book, we have discussed how the various body systems coordinate their activities to allow us to perform physical activity. We have also seen how these systems adapt when exposed to the stress of various types of training. In Part D, we turn our attention to how the body responds and adapts when challenged to exercise under unusual environmental conditions. In chapter 11, Thermal Regulation and Exercise, we will examine mechanisms by which the body can regulate its internal temperature both at rest and during exercise. Then we will consider how the body responds to and adapts to exercise in the heat and cold along with health risks that are associated with physical activity in each environment. In chapter 12, Exercise in Hypobaric, Hyperbaric, and Microgravity Environments, we will discuss the unique challenges the body faces when performing physical activity under conditions of low atmospheric pressure (altitude), high atmospheric pressure (diving), and low gravity (space travel).

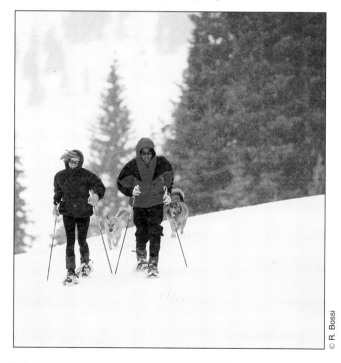

© R. Bossi

Chapter 11

Thermal Regulation and Exercise

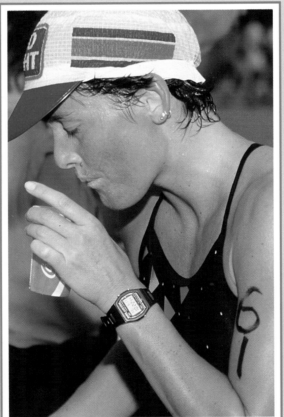

© Dan Holmes/TexStock Photo Inc.

Chapter Overview

In the preceding chapters, we have discussed how the various body systems enable us to perform physical activity. We have seen how different parts of the body communicate and function together. We have examined the body's physiological responses to acute exercise as well as its adaptations to training, all of which make it a more efficient performer. Yet our discussion thus far has focused only on the internal environment and how one body system responds to the demands of another.

Beginning with this chapter, we will change our focus. Now that we know how the body meets the demands of exercise, we are ready to see how it meets them when these demands are coupled with the demands imposed by the external environment. In this chapter, we will examine the impact of extreme temperatures on performance.

Chapter Outline

On a clear, sunny September day in 1979, President Jimmy Carter entered the 10-km Catoctin Mountain Park Run, near Camp David. The course was quite challenging—the initial mile was all uphill and the remainder took the runners over several hills. Although he had trained diligently for this race, President Carter made the mistake of trying to beat his personal best by running faster than his training pace. As the president passed the course's only water station, he was unable to grab a cup, yet he, in his black socks, continued to run up the hill while many opted to walk. His faster pace and the environmental stress combined to raise his body temperature to a critical level by the time he had reached the hill's top. The staggering, ashen, dazed president was forced to drop out before completing 6 km.

The stresses of physical exertion are often complicated by environmental thermal conditions. Performing in the extremes of heat and cold places a heavy burden on the mechanisms that regulate body temperature. Although they are amazingly effective in regulating body heat, these mechanisms of thermoregulation can be inadequate when we are subjected to extremes of heat or cold. Fortunately, our bodies are able to adapt to such environmental stresses with continued exposure over time.

In the following discussion, we focus on the physiological responses to acute and chronic exercise in both hot and cold environments. Specific health risks are associated with exercise in both temperature extremes, so we will also discuss the prevention of temperature-related illness and injuries during exercise.

Mechanisms of Body Temperature Regulation

Humans are homeothermic, which means that internal body temperature is kept nearly constant throughout life. Although your temperature varies from day to day, and even from hour to hour, these fluctuations are usually no more than about 1.0 °C (1.8 °F). Only during prolonged heavy exercise, illness, or extreme conditions of heat and cold do body temperatures deviate outside the normal range of 36.1 to 37.8 °C (97.0 to 100.0 °F).

Body temperature reflects a careful balance between heat production and heat loss. Whenever this balance is disturbed, your body temperature changes. Recall from chapter 5 that a large part of the energy your body generates is degraded to heat, the lowest form of energy. All metabolically active tissues produce heat that can be used to maintain the internal temperature of your body. But if your body's heat production exceeds its heat loss, your internal temperature rises. Your ability to maintain a constant internal temperature depends on your ability to balance the heat you gain from metabolism and from the environment with the heat that your body loses. This balance is depicted in Figure 11.1. Now let's examine the mechanisms by which heat is transferred between you and your surroundings.

The Transfer of Body Heat

For your body to transfer heat to the environment, the heat produced in your body must have access to the outside world. The heat from deep in your body (the core) is moved by the blood to your skin (the shell). Once heat nears your skin, it can be transferred to the environment by any of four mechanisms:

1. Conduction
2. Convection
3. Radiation
4. Evaporation

These are illustrated in Figure 11.1 and Figure 11.2.

Conduction and Convection

Heat conduction involves the transfer of heat from one material to another through direct molecular contact. As an example, heat generated deep in your body can be conducted through adjacent tissue until it reaches your body's surface. It can then be conducted to your clothing or to the air that is in direct contact with your skin. Conversely, if the air around you is hotter than your skin, heat from the air will be conducted to your skin, warming it.

Convection involves transferring heat from one place to another by the motion of a gas or a liquid across the heated surface. Though we're not always aware of it, the air around us is in constant motion. As it circulates around us, passing over the skin, it sweeps away the air molecules that have been warmed by their contact with the skin. The greater the move-

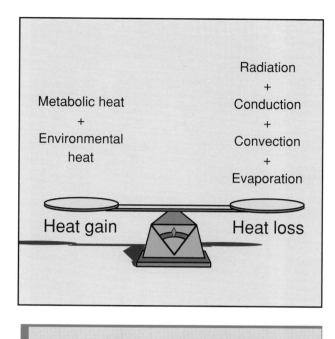

Radiation
+
Conduction
+
Convection
+
Evaporation

Metabolic heat
+
Environmental heat

Heat gain   Heat loss

Figure 11.1   The balance of body heat gain and loss (at temperatures below 92 °F).

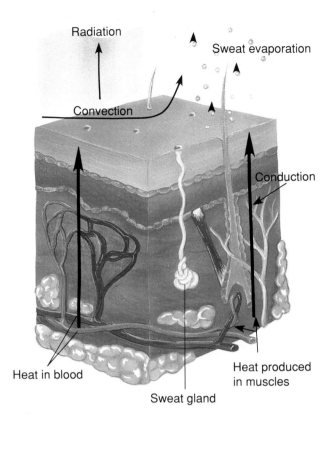

Radiation

Sweat evaporation

Convection

Conduction

Heat in blood

Sweat gland

Heat produced in muscles

Figure 11.2   The removal of heat from the skin. Heat is delivered to the body surface via the arterial blood and also by conduction through the subcutaneous tissue.

ment of the air (or liquid, such as when we are in water), the greater the rate of heat removal by convection. When combined with conduction, convection can also cause the body to gain heat in a very hot environment.

Although conduction and convection constantly remove body heat when the air temperature is lower than your skin temperature, their contribution to your body's total heat loss in air is relatively small—only about 10% to 20%. However, if you are submerged in cold water, the amount of heat dissipated by conduction is nearly 26 times greater than when you are exposed to a similar air temperature.

Radiation

At rest, radiation is the primary method for discharging the body's excess heat. At normal room temperature (typically 21 to 25 °C, or 69.8 to 77 °F), the nude body loses about 60% of its excess heat by radiation. The heat is given off in the form of infrared rays, which are a type of electromagnetic wave. Figure 11.3 shows two infrared thermograms of an individual.

Your body constantly radiates heat in all directions to the objects around it, such as clothing, furniture, and walls, but it can also receive radiational heat from surrounding objects that are warmer. If the temperature of the surrounding objects is greater than that of your body, you'll experience a net body heat gain via radiation. A tremendous amount of radiational heat is received from exposure to the sun.

Evaporation

Evaporation is the primary avenue for heat dissipation during exercise. It accounts for about 80% of the total heat loss when you are physically active, but for only about 20% of body heat loss at rest. Some evaporation occurs without our awareness, and as the fluid evaporates, heat is lost. This is referred to as insensible heat loss, which happens wherever body fluid is brought into contact with the external environment, such as in your lungs, at the mucosa (such as that lining your mouth), and at your skin.

Insensible heat loss removes about 10% of the total metabolic heat produced by the body. But insensible heat loss is relatively constant, so when your body needs to lose more heat, this mechanism cannot help. Instead, as body temperature rises, sweat production increases. As sweat reaches the skin, it is converted from a liquid to a vapor by heat from the skin. Thus sweat evaporation becomes increasingly important as body temperature increases.

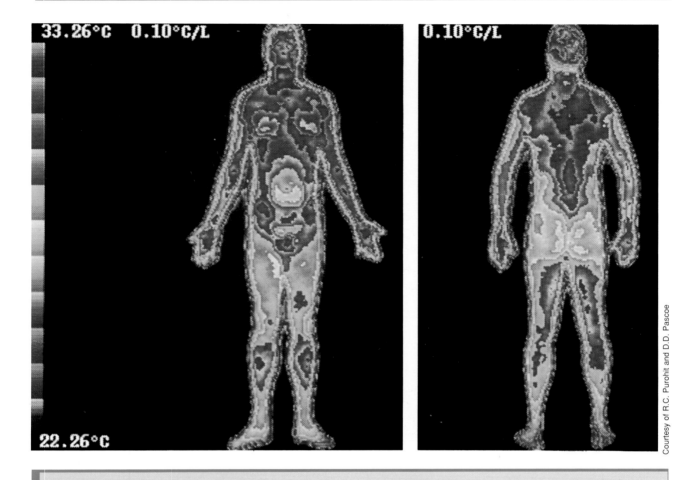

33.26°C 0.10°C/L

0.10°C/L

22.26°C

Courtesy of R.C. Purohit and D.D. Pascoe

Figure 11.3   Thermograms of the body showing the variations in radiant heat over the front and back of the body surface.

KEY POINT

The four avenues by which we lose heat are convection, conduction, radiation, and evaporation. During exercise, evaporation becomes the predominant avenue of heat loss, particularly as the environmental temperature approaches the body's skin temperature.

The relative contributions of each of these four heat loss mechanisms are summarized in Table 11.1. The data presented are taken both at rest, when the body produces about 1.5 kcal of heat per minute, and during prolonged exercise at 70% of $\dot{V}O_2$ max, when heat production is 10 times higher, or about 15 kcal per minute. These values are simple averages, because individual metabolic heat production varies with body size, composition, and temperature. Figure 11.4 shows the complex interaction between the mechanisms of body heat balance (production and loss) and environmental conditions.

Humidity and Heat Loss

The water vapor content, or humidity, of the air plays a major role in heat loss, especially by evaporation. When the humidity is high, the air already contains many water molecules. This decreases its capacity to accept more water because the concentration gradient is decreased. Thus high humidity limits sweat evaporation and heat loss. Low humidity, on the other hand, offers an ideal opportunity for sweat evaporation and heat loss. But this too can pose problems. If water evaporates from the skin more rapidly than sweat is produced, the skin can become too dry.

Humidity affects our perception of thermal stress. Consider two situations: exposure to dry desert air at 32.2 °C (90.0 °F) with 10% relative humidity, compared to the same air temperature with 90% relative humidity. You sweat profusely in the dry desert, but evaporation occurs so rapidly that you are not aware that you are sweating. But in the latter situation, little sweat can evaporate because the air is already 90% saturated with water. The result is a continuous bath of sweat that drips from your skin. Very little heat is removed and you feel very uncomfortable.

Table 11.1 Estimated Caloric Heat Loss at Rest (About 1.5 kcal • min⁻¹ Heat Production) and During Prolonged Exercise at 70% $\dot{V}O_{2\,max}$ (About 15 kcal • min⁻¹ Heat Production)

Mechanism of heat loss	Rest		Exercise	
	% total	kcal • min⁻¹	% total	kcal • min⁻¹
Conduction and convection	20	0.3	15	2.2
Radiation	60	0.9	5	0.8
Evaporation	20	0.3	80	12.0

▬ KEY POINT ▬

Sweat must evaporate to provide cooling. Sweat that drips off the skin provides little or no cooling.

▬ IN REVIEW . . . ▬

1. Humans are homeothermic, meaning that they maintain a constant internal body temperature, usually in the range of 36.1 to 37.8 °C (97.0 to 100.0 °F).
2. Body heat is transferred by conduction, convection, radiation, and evaporation. At rest, most heat is lost via radiation, but during exercise, evaporation becomes the most important avenue of heat loss.
3. Higher humidity decreases the capacity to lose heat by evaporation.

During exercise, humidity is a primary concern because evaporation is the major method of heat loss. If the air is saturated with water, almost no evaporation can occur, even at lower environmental temperatures. Your body might not be able to shed all its excess heat when faced with high temperature, high humidity, and prolonged intense exercise. Consequently, your body temperature can rise to critical levels, seriously jeopardizing your health.

Fortunately, the mechanisms for heat transfer to the skin and for sweat production are well developed. Generally speaking, except under extreme conditions, the removal of heat from the body is dependent on the gradient between the skin temperature and the environment.

Control of Heat Exchange

Internal body temperature (rectal) when at rest is kept at approximately 37 °C (99 °F). But during exercise, because the body is often unable to dissipate heat as rapidly as it is produced, a person can develop an internal temperature exceeding 40 °C (104 °F), with a muscle temperature above 42 °C (107.6 °F). The muscles' energy systems become more chemically efficient with a small rise in muscle temperature. But internal body temperatures above 40 °C (104 °F) can adversely affect the nervous system and reduce further

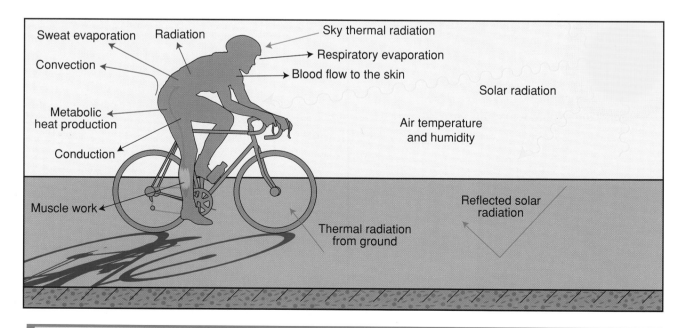

Figure 11.4   The complex interaction between the body's mechanisms for heat balance and environmental conditions.

efforts to unload excess heat. How can your body regulate its internal temperature?

The Hypothalamus: Your Thermostat

The mechanisms that control body temperature are analogous to the thermostat that controls the air temperature in your home, though your body's mechanisms function in a more complex manner and generally with greater precision than your home heating and cooling system. Sensory receptors, called thermoreceptors, detect changes in your body temperature and relay this information to your body's thermostat: the hypothalamus. In response, the hypothalamus acti-

vates mechanisms that regulate the heating or cooling of your body. Like your home thermostat, the hypothalamus has a predetermined temperature, or set point, that it tries to maintain. This is your normal body temperature. The smallest deviation from this set point signals your thermoregulatory center, located within your hypothalamus, to readjust your body temperature. This process of thermoregulation is depicted in Figure 11.5.

Changes in your body temperature are sensed by two sets of thermoreceptors: central receptors and peripheral receptors. Central receptors are located in your hypothalamus and monitor the temperature of

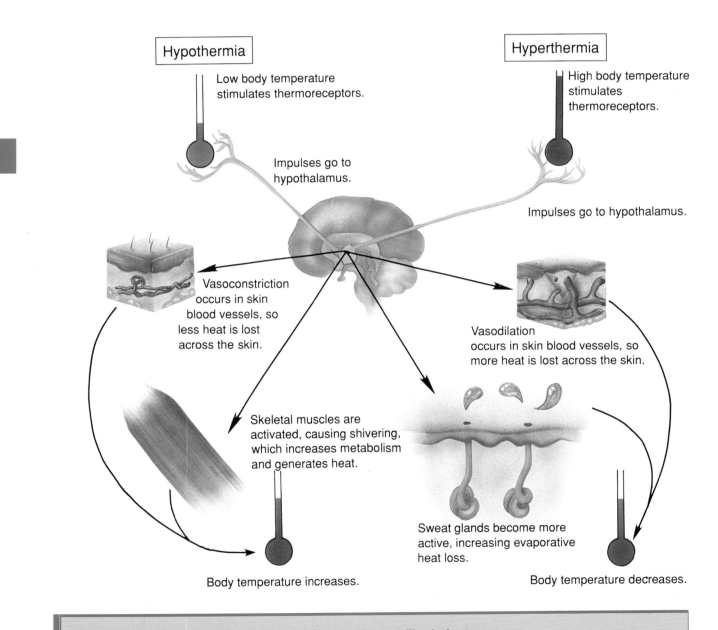

Figure 11.5   An overview of the role of the hypothalamus in controlling body temperature.

your blood as it circulates through your brain. These central receptors are sensitive to blood temperature changes as small as 0.01 °C. Changes in the temperature of the blood passing through the hypothalamus trigger reflexes that help you conserve or eliminate body heat as needed.

Peripheral receptors, located in your skin, monitor the temperature around you. They provide information to the hypothalamus and also to your cerebral cortex, allowing you to consciously perceive temperature so you can voluntarily control your exposure to heat or cold. You might decide to go to a more temperate environment or to select appropriate clothing. However, during sweat evaporation, your skin can feel cold while the interior of your body is hyperthermic (overheated). In this case your skin receptors would incorrectly notify your hypothalamus and your cerebral cortex that you are chilled when in fact you might be nearing a critically high temperature.

Effectors That Alter Body Temperature

When your body temperature fluctuates, your normal temperature can usually be restored by the actions of four effectors:

1. Sweat glands
2. Smooth muscle around the arterioles
3. Skeletal muscles
4. Several endocrine glands

Let's examine how each of these can alter your temperature.

Sweat Glands.   When either your skin or your blood is heated, your hypothalamus sends impulses to your sweat glands, commanding them to actively secrete sweat that moistens the skin. The hotter you are, the more sweat you produce. The evaporation of this moisture, as discussed earlier, removes heat from your skin's surface.

Smooth Muscle Around Arterioles.   When your skin and blood are heated, your hypothalamus sends signals to the smooth muscle in the walls of the arterioles that supply your skin, causing them to dilate. This increases blood flow to your skin. The blood carries heat from the deeper parts of your body to your skin, where the heat dissipates to the environment through conduction, convection, radiation, or evaporation.

Skeletal Muscle.   Skeletal muscle is called into action when you need to generate more body heat. In a cold environment, the thermoreceptors in your skin relay signals to your hypothalamus. Similarly, whenever your blood temperature drops, the change is noted by the central receptors in the hypothalamus. In response to this neural input, your hypothalamus activates the brain centers that control muscle tone. These centers stimulate shivering, which is a rapid, involuntary cycle of contraction and relaxation of skeletal muscles. This increased muscle activity generates heat to either maintain or increase your body temperature.

Endocrine Glands.   The effects of several hormones cause your cells to increase their metabolic rates. This affects heat balance because increased metabolism increases heat production. Cooling the body stimulates thyroxine release (from the thyroid gland). Thyroxine can elevate the metabolic rate throughout the body by more than 100%. Also, recall that epinephrine and norepinephrine (the catecholamines) mimic and enhance the activity of the sympathetic nervous system. Thus they directly affect the metabolic rate of virtually all body cells.

Assessing Mean Body Temperature

Your temperature can be assessed in many ways. We are all accustomed to the oral thermometer, but not all body tissues have the same temperature. Because of this, we often consider the mean body temperature, or T_{body}, which takes into account temperature variations found throughout the body. The mean body temperature is a weighted average of skin and internal body temperatures, so you must know both of these to calculate T_{body}.

Calculating Skin Temperature

Your skin is generally cooler than the central core of your body because your skin is affected by evaporation and air temperature. To determine the average skin temperature (T_{skin}), temperature sensors are placed on the skin at different areas of the body. The weighted average of the resulting values can then be calculated. If, for example, temperature sensors (also called thermistors) were placed on the arm (T_a), trunk (T_t), leg (T_l), and head (T_h), T_{skin} could be calculated as follows:

$$T_{skin} = (0.1 \times T_a) + (0.6 \times T_t) + (0.2 \times T_l) + (0.1 \times T_h)$$

The constants in the equation represent the fraction of the total skin area represented by each region from which a temperature is recorded. Now, for the sake of illustration, let's put some numbers into the equation:

$$T_{skin} = (0.1 \times 32.0 \ °C) + (0.6 \times 33.0 \ °C)$$
$$+ (0.2 \times 32.5 \ °C) + (0.1 \times 31.5 \ °C)$$
$$T_{skin} = 32.7 \ °C$$

Calculating Mean Body Temperature

Several methods are used to measure the temperature of the body's deep tissues. These include using sensors to measure the temperature in the rectum, on the tympanic membrane, and in the esophagus. Although some controversy exists about what site is best for monitoring internal body temperature, rectal temperature (T_r) has been the most widely used because it is believed to best represent the temperature of the blood and internal body mass.

Once you have the skin temperature and the internal body temperature, T_{body} can be calculated by using the following equation:

$$T_{body} = (0.4 \times T_{skin}) + (0.6 \times T_r)$$

Here, the constants reflect the relative parts of the total body that the temperature represents. Using the T_{skin} from our example above, and assuming the average T_r of 37.0 °C, these calculations reveal that

$$T_{body} = (0.4 \times 32.7 \text{ °C}) + (0.6 \times 37.0 \text{ °C})$$
$$T_{body} = 35.3 \text{ °C}$$

KEY POINT

$$T_{body} = (0.4 \times T_{skin}) + (0.6 \times T_r)$$

Heat Content of the Body

Once mean body temperature has been calculated and body weight (W_{tb}) is known, body heat content (HC) can be approximated. Heat content represents the total calories of heat contained in the body tissues. To calculate this value, we must know the specific heat of body tissues.

The specific heat of a substance is the amount of heat required to change the temperature of that substance by 1 °C. As noted in chapter 5, the kilocalorie is the unit of measure for heat energy, representing the heat required to raise the temperature of 1 kg of water 1 °C. Thus the specific heat of water is 1.0 kcal · kg^{-1}· °C^{-1}. Other components of the body have different specific heats. Body tissues have an average specific heat of 0.83 kcal · kg^{-1}· °C^{-1}. Thus if the T_{body} of a 50-kg (110-lb) person were increased by 1 °C, the amount of heat gained would be 0.83 kcal for each kilogram of body weight, a total of 41.5 kcal (0.83 kcal · kg^{-1} × 50 kg).

Knowing that the average specific heat of body tissues is 0.83 kcal · kg^{-1}· °C^{-1} allows us to calculate the caloric content of the human body as follows:

$$HC = 0.83 (W_{tb} \times T_{body})$$

Let's try an example. Assume a 50-kg person has a mean body temperature of 35.3 °C (about 95.5 °F).

This person's body heat content would be calculated as follows:

$$HC = 0.83 (50 \text{ kg} \times 35.3 \text{ °C})$$
$$HC = 1,465 \text{ kcal}$$

Thus, the body of this 50-kg individual contains 1,465 kcal of heat.

Rate of Heat Exchange

Calculations of body heat content are useful for estimating the body's rate of heat exchange. If, for example, your heat content remains constant during a long period of exercise, we can assume that your thermoregulatory system is 100% efficient—it dissipates as much heat as your muscles produce. Assume, instead, that your internal body temperature rises while your skin temperature and body weight remain constant. Increasing your internal body temperature increases your mean body temperature. This, in turn, increases your body heat content.

Under resting conditions, an average body generally produces 1.25 to 1.50 kcal of heat per minute. Completely blocking the body's ability to dissipate heat would increase its heat content by about 75 to 90 kcal per hour. Thus the ability to unload excess metabolic heat is crucial, even when at rest. Without this ability, body heat content would quickly increase to levels incompatible with life.

During exercise, heat production can exceed 15 kcal per minute (900 kcal per hr). The mechanisms for heat dissipation are heavily taxed. Such quantities of heat can be dissipated only by evaporating a large amount of sweat. Each liter of evaporated sweat removes 580 kcal, so the body would have to lose 1.55 L of sweat per hour if all the sweat was evaporated and all the metabolic heat was removed by evaporation (900 kcal of heat produced / 580 kcal removed per liter of sweat = 1.55 L).

Physiological Responses to Exercise in the Heat

Heat production is beneficial when you exercise in a cold environment. It helps maintain normal body temperature. However, even when you exercise in a thermally neutral environment, such as 21 to 26 °C (70 to 80 °F), the metabolic heat load places a considerable burden on the mechanisms that control body temperature. In this section we examine some physiological changes that occur in response to exercise while the body is exposed to heat stress, and the impact these

IN REVIEW . . .

1. The hypothalamus houses your thermoregulatory center. It acts like a thermostat, monitoring your temperature and accelerating heat loss or heat production as needed.

2. Two sets of thermoreceptors provide temperature information to your thermoregulatory center. The peripheral receptors in the skin relay information about the temperature of your skin and the environment around it. Central receptors in your hypothalamus transmit information about your internal body temperature.

3. Effectors can alter your body temperature. Increased skeletal muscle activity increases your temperature by increasing metabolic heat production. Increased sweat gland activity decreases your temperature by increasing evaporative heat loss. Smooth muscle in the arterioles can dilate to direct blood to the skin for heat transfer, or constrict to retain heat deep in the body. Metabolic heat production can be increased by the actions of hormones like thyroxine and the catecholamines.

4. Your mean body temperature is a weighted average of your skin temperature and your internal body temperature.

5. Your body's heat content is the total amount of heat in kilocalories that it contains.

changes can have on performance. For this discussion, heat stress means any environmental condition that causes an increase in body temperature and jeopardizes homeostasis.

Cardiovascular Function

As we learned in chapter 8, exercise increases the demands on the cardiovascular system. When the need to regulate body temperature is added, the cardiovascular system can become burdened during exercise in the heat. The circulatory system transports the heat generated in the muscles to the surface of the body, where the heat can be transferred to the environment. To accomplish this during exercise in the heat, a large part of the cardiac output must be shared by the skin and the working muscles. Because blood volume is limited, exercise poses a complex problem: Increased blood flow to one of these areas automatically decreases flow to the others.

Consider what happens when you are running at a fast pace on a hot day. The exercise increases the demand for more blood flow and oxygen delivery to your muscles. It also increases metabolic heat production. This excess heat can be dissipated only if blood flow increases to your skin, transferring the heat to your body's surface. However, blood flow to your skin cannot increase as much as necessary if your muscles receive all the blood flow that they need. So the demands of muscles impair heat transfer to the skin.

At the same time, your thermoregulatory center instructs your cardiovascular system to direct more blood flow to your skin. The superficial blood vessels dilate to bring more of the warm blood to your body's surface. This restricts the amount of blood available to your active muscles, limiting their endurance capacity. Thus the cardiovascular demands of exercise and those of thermoregulation compete for the limited blood supply.

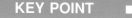

KEY POINT

Exercising in hot environments sets up a competition between the active muscles and the skin for the limited blood supply. The muscles need blood and the oxygen it delivers to sustain activity; the skin needs blood to facilitate heat loss to keep the body cool.

To maintain a constant cardiac output with the shunting of blood to the periphery, the cardiovascular system must make some noticeable adjustments. The redistribution of blood reduces the volume of blood that returns to the heart, which reduces the end-diastolic volume. This, in turn, reduces the stroke volume. Cardiac output remains reasonably constant throughout a 27-min exercise bout in warm (36 °C, 96.8 °F) and temperate (20 °C, 68 °F) environments, despite a steady decrease in stroke volume. The drop in stroke volume throughout the exercise is compensated for by a gradual upward drift in heart rate. This is known as cardiovascular drift.

At some point, though, your body can no longer compensate for the increasing demands of exercise: Neither your muscles nor your skin can receive adequate blood flow. Consequently, any factor that tends to overload the cardiovascular system or to interfere with heat dissipation can drastically impair your performance and increase your risk of overheating. Not surprisingly, this means that the best endurance performances are achieved in cool conditions. Seldom are records set in, for example, distance running events when the environmental heat stress is great.

Energy Production

Studies by Fink et al. demonstrated that, in addition to raising body temperature and heart rate, exercise in the heat also increases oxygen uptake, causing the working muscles to use more glycogen and to produce more lactate compared to exercise in the cold.[6] As shown in Figure 11.6a, repeated bouts (15 min) of exercise in the heat (40 °C, 104 °F) increased the subjects' heart rates and oxygen uptakes significantly compared to exercise in a cooler environment (9 °C, 48 °F). As described earlier, a warmer environment places greater stress on the cardiovascular system, which raises the heart rate. Also, increased sweat production and respiration demand more energy, which requires a higher oxygen uptake. As seen in Figure 11.6b, the compromised blood flow to the muscles during exercise in the heat leads to a greater use of muscle glycogen and production of more lactic acid. Thus exercise in the heat can hasten glycogen depletion and increase muscle lactate, both of which are known to contribute to the sensations of fatigue and exhaustion.

Body Fluid Balance: Sweating

Under some conditions, the temperature of the environment approaches and can exceed both the skin and deep body temperatures. As mentioned earlier, this makes evaporation far more important for heat loss because radiation, convection, and conduction are less effective as environmental temperature rises. In fact, these mechanisms can lead to heat gain in extreme environmental conditions. Increased dependence on evaporation means an increased demand for sweating.

The sweat glands are controlled by stimulation of the hypothalamus. Elevated blood temperature causes the hypothalamus to transmit impulses through the sympathetic nerve fibers to the millions of sweat glands distributed over the body's surface. The sweat glands are tubular structures extending through the dermis and epidermis, opening onto the skin, as illustrated in Figure 11.7.

Sweat is formed by the filtration of plasma. As the filtrate passes through the duct of the gland, sodium and chloride are gradually reabsorbed back into the surrounding tissues and then into the blood. During light sweating, the filtrate sweat travels slowly through the tubules, allowing time for almost complete reabsorption of sodium and chloride. Thus the sweat that forms during light sweating contains very little of these

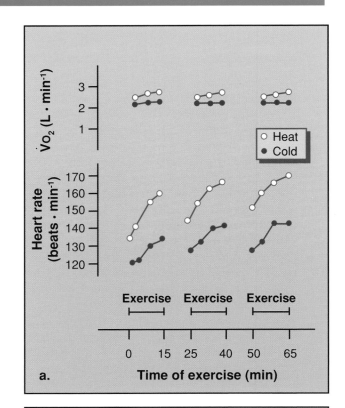

a.

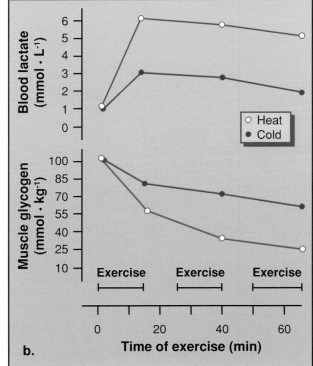

b.

Figure 11.6   (a) Oxygen uptake and heart rate responses during exercise in hot (40 °C, 15% humidity) and cold (9 °C, 55% humidity) conditions; (b) changes in blood lactate and muscle glycogen during cycling in the same conditions. Adapted from Fink et al. (1975).

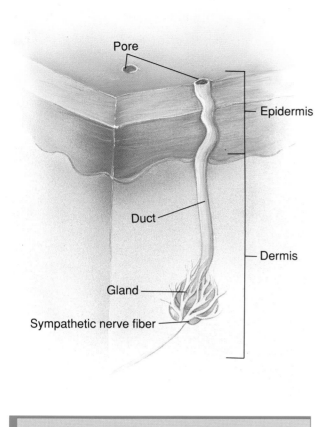

Figure 11.7   An eccrine sweat gland innervated by a sympathetic nerve.

Table 11.2 Sodium and Chloride Concentrations in the Sweat of Trained and Untrained Subjects During Exercise

Subjects	Sweat Na⁺ (mmol • L⁻¹)	Sweat Cl⁻ (mmol • L⁻¹)	Sweat K⁺ (mmol • L⁻¹)
Untrained males	90	60	4
Trained males	35	30	4
Untrained females	105	98	4
Trained females	62	47	4

Data from the Human Performance Laboratory, Ball State University.

2% to 4% of body weight each hour. A person can lose a critical amount of body water in only a few hours of exercise in these conditions.

Sweat rates as high as 2 to 3 L per hr have been observed, but these rates cannot be sustained for more than several hours. Maximal daily sweat rates are in the range of 10 to 15 L.

A high rate of sweating reduces blood volume. This limits the volume of blood available to supply the needs of the muscles and to prevent heat buildup, which, in turn, reduces performance potential, particularly for endurance activities. In long-distance runners, sweat losses can approach 6% to 10% of body weight. Such severe dehydration can limit subsequent sweating and make the individual susceptible to heat-related illnesses. Chapter 15 provides a detailed discussion of dehydration and the value of fluid replacement.

Loss of both minerals and water by sweating triggers the release of aldosterone and antidiuretic hormone (ADH). Recall that aldosterone is responsible for maintaining appropriate sodium levels and ADH maintains fluid balance. As mentioned in chapter 6, aldosterone is released from the adrenal cortex in response to stimuli such as decreased blood sodium content, reduced blood volume, or reduced blood pressure. During acute exercise in the heat and during repeated days of exercise in the heat, this hormone limits sodium excretion from the kidneys. More sodium is retained by the body, which in turn promotes water retention. Because of this, plasma and interstitial fluid volumes can increase 10% to 20%. This allows the body to retain water and sodium in preparation for additional exposures to the heat and subsequent sweat losses.

Similarly, exercise and body water loss stimulate the posterior pituitary gland to release ADH. This hormone stimulates water reabsorption from the kidneys, which further promotes fluid retention in the body. Thus the body attempts to compensate for mineral and

minerals by the time it reaches the skin. However, when the sweating rate increases during exercise, the filtrate moves more quickly through the tubules, allowing less time for reabsorption. As a result, the sodium and chloride content of the sweat can be considerably higher.

As seen in Table 11.2, the mineral content of each subject's sweat is significantly different in trained and untrained subjects. With training and repeated heat exposure, aldosterone can strongly stimulate the sweat glands, causing them to reabsorb more sodium and chloride. Unfortunately, the sweat glands apparently do not have a similar mechanism for conserving other electrolytes. Potassium, calcium, and magnesium, for example, are normally found in the same concentrations in both sweat and plasma.

While performing heavy exercise in hot conditions, the body can lose more than 1 L of sweat per hour per square meter of body surface. This means that during intense effort on a hot and humid day (high level of heat stress), an average-sized individual (50 to 75 kg) might lose 1.5 to 2.5 L of sweat, or about water loss during periods of heat stress and heavy sweating by reducing their losses in urine.

■■■   IN REVIEW . . .   ■■■

1. During exercise in the heat, the heat loss mechanisms compete with the active muscles for more of the limited blood volume. Thus neither area is adequately supplied under extreme conditions.
2. Though cardiac output may remain reasonably constant, stroke volume may decline, resulting in a gradual upward drift in heart rate.
3. Oxygen uptake also increases during constant-rate exercise in the heat.
4. Sweating increases during exercise in the heat, and this can quickly lead to dehydration and excessive electrolyte loss. To compensate, the release of aldosterone and ADH increases, causing sodium and water retention, which can expand the plasma volume.

Health Risks During Exercise in the Heat

Air temperature alone is not an accurate index of the total physiological stress imposed on the body in a hot environment. At least four variables must be taken into account:

1. Air temperature
2. Humidity
3. Air velocity
4. The amount of radiation

All these influence the degree of heat stress experienced by the person. The contributions of each of these factors to the total heat stress are not clearly understood, because the contributions vary with changing environmental conditions.

With an air temperature of 23 °C (73.4 °F), an individual exercising on a bright, sunny day with no measurable wind experiences considerably more heat stress than someone exercising in the same air temperature but under cloud cover and with a slight breeze. At temperatures above 30 to 32 °C (86 to 89.6 °F), radiation, conduction, and convection substantially add to the body's heat load rather than acting as avenues for heat loss. How, then, can we judge the amount of heat stress to which you may be exposed?

■■■   KEY POINT   ■■■

Heat stress is not accurately reflected by air temperature alone. Humidity, air velocity (or wind), and thermal radiation also contribute to the total heat stress that you experience when exercising in the heat.

Measuring Heat Stress

Through the years, efforts have been made to quantify atmospheric variables into a single index. In the 1970s, the wet bulb globe temperature (WBGT) was devised to simultaneously account for conduction, convection, evaporation, and radiation. It provides a single temperature reading to estimate the cooling capacity of the surrounding environment.

The WBGT apparatus is depicted in Figure 11.8. It consists of three parts:

1. Dry bulb
2. Wet bulb
3. Black globe

The dry bulb measures the actual air temperature (T_{DB}). The wet bulb is kept moist. As water evaporates from this bulb, its temperature (T_{WB}) will be cooler than the dry bulb's, simulating the effect of sweat evaporating from your skin. The difference between the wet and dry bulb temperatures indicates the environment's capacity for cooling by evaporation. In still air with 100% humidity, these two bulb temperatures are the same because evaporation is impossible. Lower humidity and moving air both promote evaporation, increasing the difference between these two bulb temperatures. The black globe absorbs radiated heat. Thus its temperature (T_G) is a good indicator of the environment's capacity for transmitting radiated heat.

The temperatures from these three bulbs can be put together to estimate the overall atmospheric challenge to body temperature in that specific environment by using the following equation:

$$WBGT = 0.1 \, (T_{DB}) + 0.7 \, (T_{WB}) + 0.2 \, (T_G)$$

This measurement of thermal stress has received considerable attention in recent years, and is now used by coaches and athletic trainers to anticipate the health risks associated with athletic competitions in thermally stressful environments.

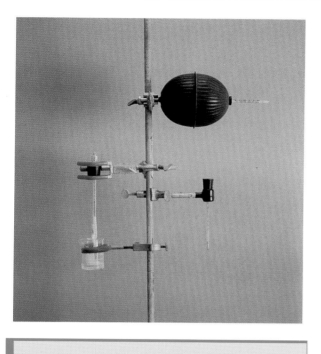

Figure 11.8   A wet bulb globe temperature apparatus.

KEY POINT

$$WBGT = 0.1 (T_{DB}) + 0.7 (T_{WB}) + 0.2 (T_G)$$

Heat-Related Disorders

Exposure to the combination of external heat stress and the inability to dissipate metabolically generated heat can lead to three heat-related injuries:

1. Heat cramps
2. Heat exhaustion
3. Heat stroke

Heat Cramps

Heat cramps, the least serious of the three heat disorders, is characterized by severe cramping of the skeletal muscles. It primarily involves the muscles that are most heavily used during exercise. This disorder is probably brought on by the mineral losses and dehydration that accompany high rates of sweating, but a cause and effect relationship has not been fully established. Heat cramps are treated by moving the stricken individual to a cooler location and administering fluids or a saline solution.

Heat Exhaustion

Heat exhaustion is typically accompanied by such symptoms as extreme fatigue, breathlessness, dizziness, vomiting, fainting, cold and clammy or hot and dry skin, hypotension (low blood pressure), and a weak, rapid pulse. It is caused by the cardiovascular system's inability to adequately meet the body's needs. Recall that during exercise in heat, your active muscles and your skin, through which excess heat is lost, compete for their fair share of your total blood volume. Heat exhaustion results when these simultaneous demands are not met. The disorder typically occurs when your blood volume is reduced, either by excessive fluid loss or by mineral loss from sweating.

With heat exhaustion, the thermoregulatory mechanisms are functioning but cannot dissipate heat quickly enough because there is insufficient blood volume to allow adequate distribution to the skin. Although the condition often occurs during mild to moderate exercise in the heat, it is not generally accompanied by a high rectal temperature. Some people who collapse from heat stress exhibit symptoms of heat exhaustion, but have internal temperatures below 39 °C (102.2 °F). People who are poorly conditioned or unacclimatized to the heat are more susceptible to heat exhaustion.

Treatment for victims of heat exhaustion involves rest in a cooler environment with their feet elevated to avoid shock. If the person is conscious, administration of salt water is usually recommended. If the person is unconscious, medically supervised intravenous administration of saline solution is recommended. If allowed to progress, heat exhaustion can deteriorate to heat stroke.

Heat Stroke

Heat stroke is a life-threatening heat disorder that requires immediate medical attention. It is characterized by

- a rise in internal body temperature to values exceeding 40 °C (104 °F),
- cessation of sweating,
- hot and dry skin,
- rapid pulse and respiration,
- usually hypertension (high blood pressure),
- confusion, and
- unconsciousness.

If left untreated, heat stroke progresses to coma, and death quickly follows. Treatment involves rapidly cooling the person's body in a bath of cold water or ice, or wrapping the body in wet sheets and fanning the victim.

This disorder is caused by failure of the body's thermoregulatory mechanisms. Body heat production during exercise is dependent on exercise intensity and body weight, so heavier athletes run a higher risk of overheating than lighter athletes when exercising at the same rate, assuming both have about equal heat acclimatization.

For the athlete, heat stroke is not a problem associated only with extreme conditions. Studies have reported rectal temperatures above 40.5 °C (105 °F) in marathon runners who successfully completed races conducted under relatively moderate thermal conditions (for example, 70 °F and 30% relative humidity).[4,18] Even in shorter events, the body's core temperature can reach life-threatening levels. As early as 1937, Robinson observed rectal temperatures of 41 °C (105.8 °F) in runners competing in events lasting only about 14 minutes, such as the 5,000-m race. Following a 10,000-m race conducted with an air temperature of 29.5 °C (85 °F), 80% relative humidity, and bright sun, one runner who collapsed had a rectal temperature of 43 °C (109.4 °F)![3] Without proper medical attention, such fevers can result in permanent central nervous system damage or death. Fortunately, this runner was rapidly cooled with ice and recovered without complications.

KEY POINT

When exercising in the heat, if you suddenly feel chilled and goose bumps form on your skin, stop exercising, get into a cool environment, and drink plenty of cool fluids. The body's thermoregulation system has become confused and thinks that the body temperature needs to increase even more! Left untreated, this condition can lead to heat stroke and death.

Prevention of Hyperthermia

We can do little about environmental conditions. Thus, in threatening conditions, athletes must decrease their effort in order to reduce their heat production and their risk of developing hyperthermia (high body temperature). All athletes, coaches, and sports organizers should be able to recognize the symptoms of hyperthermia. Fortunately, our subjective sensations are well correlated

with our body temperatures, as indicated in Table 11.3. Although there is generally little concern when rectal temperature remains below 40 °C (104 °F) during prolonged exercise, athletes who experience throbbing pressure in their head and chills should realize that they are rapidly approaching a dangerous situation that could prove fatal if they continue to exercise.

To prevent heat disorders, several simple precautions should be taken. Competition and practice outdoors should not be held when the WBGT is over 28 °C (82.4 °F). As mentioned earlier, because the wet bulb temperature reflects the humidity as well as the absolute temperature, it reflects the true physiological heat stress more accurately than does standard air temperature. Scheduling practices and contests either in the early morning or at night avoids the severe heat stress of midday. Fluids should be readily available and athletes should be required to drink as much as they can, stopping every 10 to 20 minutes for a fluid break when in warm temperatures.

Clothing is another important consideration. Obviously, the more clothing worn, the less body area that is exposed to the environment to allow heat exchange. The foolish practice of exercising in a rubberized suit to promote weight loss is an excellent illustration of how a dangerous microenvironment (the isolated environment inside the suit) can be created in which temperature and humidity can reach a sufficiently high level to block all heat loss from the body. This can rapidly lead to heat exhaustion or heat stroke. Football uniforms are another example. Areas that are covered by sweat-soaked clothing and padding are exposed to 100% humidity and higher temperatures, reducing the gradient between the body surface and the environment.

Athletes should wear as little clothing as possible when heat stress is a potential limitation to thermoregu-

Table 11.3 Subjective Symptoms Associated With Overheating

Rectal temperature	Symptoms
(104 °F– 105 °F)	sensation over stomach and back, with piloerection ("goose bumps")
40.5 °C–41.1 °C (105 °F– 106 °F)	Muscular weakness, disorientation and loss of postural equilibrium
41.1 °C–41.7 °C (106 °F– 107 °F)	Diminished sweating, loss of consciousness and hypothalamic control
42.2 °C (108 °F– above)	Death

Adapted from Costill (1986).

lation. The athlete should always under dress because the metabolic heat load will soon make extra clothing an unnecessary burden. When clothing is needed or required, it should be loosely woven to allow the skin to unload as much heat as possible and light colored to reflect heat back to the environment.

The American College of Sports Medicine has provided guidelines to help distance runners prevent these heat-related injuries.[2] A modified list of these recommendations appears in Table 11.4.

Acclimatization to Exercise in the Heat

How can we prepare for prolonged activity in the heat? Does training in the heat make us more tolerant of thermal stress? Many studies have investigated these questions and have concluded that repeated exercise in the heat causes a gradual adjustment that enables us to perform better in hot conditions.

Table 11.4 ACSM Guidelines for Distance Runners Competing Under Conditions of Heat Stress

1. Distance races of greater than 10 km should not be conducted when the combination of air temperature, humidity, and sun raise the WBGT temperature above 28° C (82° F).

2. Summer events should be scheduled for early morning, ideally before 8:00 a.m., or in the evening after 6:00 p.m., to minimize solar radiation.

3. An adequate supply of water or other fluids should be available before the race and at 2- to 3-km intervals throughout the race course. Runners should drink 100 to 200 ml at each feeding station.

4. Runners should train adequately for fitness and become heat acclimatized.

5. Runners should be aware of the early symptoms of heat injury, including
   • dizziness,
   • chilling,
   • headache, and
   • awkwardness.

6. Race sponsors should make prior arrangements with medical personnel to care for heat injuries. Responsible and informed personnel should supervise each feeding station.

7. Organizational personnel should reserve the right to stop runners who exhibit clear signs of heat stroke or heat exhaustion.

Reprinted from American College of Sports Medicine (1987).

Effects of Heat Acclimatization

Repeated prolonged exercise bouts in the heat cause gradual improvement in your ability to eliminate excess body heat, which reduces your risk of heat exhaustion and heat stroke. This process, termed heat acclimatization, results in many adjustments in sweating and blood flow. Though the total amount of sweat produced during exercise in the heat might not change with heat acclimatization, the amount of sweat produced often increases in the most exposed body areas and in the areas that are most effective at dissipating body heat. At the beginning of exercise, sweating starts earlier in an acclimatized person, which improves heat tolerance. As a result, skin temperatures are lower. This increases the temperature gradient from deep in the body to the skin and the environment. Because heat loss is facilitated, less blood must flow to the skin for body heat transfer, so more blood is available for the active muscles. In addition, the sweat produced is more dilute following training in the heat, so the body's mineral stores are conserved more efficiently.

Because the body's heat loss capacity for a specified level of work is enhanced by training, body

---

IN REVIEW . . .

1. Heat stress involves more than just the air temperature. Perhaps the most accurate means for measuring it is the wet bulb globe temperature, which measures air temperature and accounts for the heat exchange potential through conduction, convection, evaporation, and radiation in a specific environment.

2. Heat cramps are probably caused by losses of fluids and minerals that result from excessive sweating.

3. Heat exhaustion results from the inability of the cardiovascular system to adequately meet the needs of the active muscles and the skin. It is brought on by a reduced blood volume, typically caused by excessive loss of fluids and minerals through prolonged heavy sweating. Though it is not in itself life-threatening, heat exhaustion can deteriorate to heat stroke if untreated.

4. Heat stroke is caused by failure of the body's thermoregulatory mechanisms. If untreated it will progress and be fatal.

5. Several precautions must be taken when planning to exercise in the heat. These include canceling the event if the environmental heat stress is too high (WBGT above 28 °C, 82.4 °F), wearing proper clothing, being alert to the signs of hyperthermia, and ensuring adequate fluid intake.

temperatures are lower following training in the heat than they are before training (Figure 11.9a). Also, after training, as shown in Figure 11.9b, heart rate increases less in response to standardized submaximal exercise. This adaptation results from an increased blood volume, reduced blood flow to the skin, or both. Either of these changes increases the stroke volume. Although some investigators have found that an increase in blood volume accompanies heat acclimatization, this change is temporary and

probably relates to the body's efforts to retain sodium, thereby expanding the plasma volume.

In addition, following heat acclimatization, more work can be done before the onset of fatigue or exhaustion. Recall that exercise at a given intensity in the heat requires the use of more muscle glycogen than the same effort done in cooler air. As a result, repeated days of training in the heat can rapidly deplete muscle glycogen and cause chronic fatigue in unacclimatized people. Heat acclimatization reduces the rate of muscle glycogen use by as much as 50% to 60%, reducing this risk.

Achieving Heat Acclimatization

Heat acclimatization requires more than mere exposure to a hot environment. It is dependent on

- the environmental conditions during each exercise session,
- the duration of heat exposure, and
- the rate of internal heat production (exercise intensity).

Although the research literature is not in total agreement on this point, apparently an athlete must exercise in a hot environment to attain acclimatization that carries over to exercise in the heat. Simply sitting in a hot environment, such as a sauna, for long periods each day will not prepare the individual for physical exertion in the heat.

How can the athlete maximize heat acclimatization? Although most individuals must be exposed to the heat to gain full adjustment, they can gain partial heat tolerance simply by training, even if it is done in a cooler environment. Interestingly, when athletes become acclimatized to a given level of heat stress, they can also perform better in cooler environments. But to gain maximum benefits, athletes who train in environments cooler than those in which they will be competing should achieve heat acclimatization prior to the contest or event. This will improve their performances and reduce the associated physiological stress and risk of heat injury.

If athletes must compete in hot weather, at least part of their training should be conducted in the warmest part of the day. Early morning and evening training will not fully prepare an athlete to tolerate the midday heat. Normal workouts in the heat for 5 to 10 days should provide nearly total heat acclimatization. Workout intensity should be reduced to 60% to 70% during the first few days to prevent excessive heat stress. Of course, care must be taken to guard against heat injuries such as heat stroke and heat exhaustion. Those in training should be alert to any symptoms and should consume as much fluid as possible.

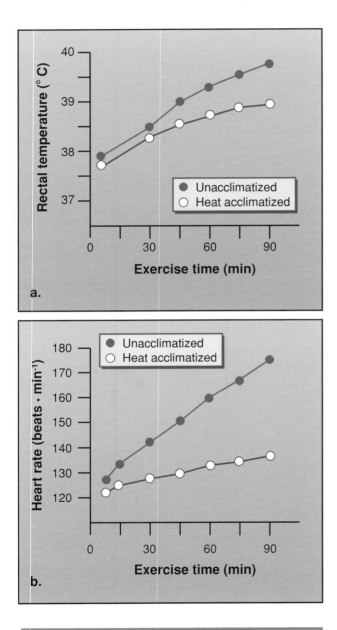

Figure 11.9   Differences in (a) rectal temperature and (b) heart rate before training in the heat (unacclimatized) and after training in the heat (heat acclimatized). Adapted from King et al., (1985).

KEY POINT

You can adapt to heat (undergo heat acclimatization) by exercising in the heat for up to an hour or more each day for 5 to 10 days. Cardiovascular changes generally occur in the first 3 to 5 days, but changes in the sweating mechanisms generally take much longer, up to 10 days.

IN REVIEW . . .

1. Repeated exposure to heat stress causes a gradual improvement in your ability to lose excess heat. This process of adaptation is called heat acclimatization.
2. The rate of sweating increases in areas that are well exposed and are the most efficient at promoting heat loss. This reduces skin temperature, increasing the thermal gradient from the internal to external body, promoting heat loss.
3. Stroke volume increases with heat acclimatization. This aids the delivery of more blood to the active muscles and skin when necessary.
4. Heat acclimatization reduces the rate of muscle glycogen use, delaying the onset of fatigue.
5. Heat acclimatization requires exercise in a hot environment, not merely exposure to heat.
6. The amount of heat acclimatization attained depends on the conditions to which you are exposed during each session, the duration of the exposure, and the rate of internal heat production.

Exercise in the Cold

Increasing year-round participation in such sporting activities as the triathlon, scuba diving, running, cycling, and long-distance swimming has sparked new interest in, and concerns about, exercise in the cold. In addition, some occupations require employees to work in cold conditions that can limit their performance. For these reasons, understanding the physiological responses and health risks associated with cold stress are important issues in exercise science. We define cold stress here as any environmental condition that causes a loss of body heat that threatens homeostasis. In the following discussion we will focus on the two major cold stressors: air and water.

The hypothalamus has a temperature set point of about 37 °C (99 °F), but daily fluctuations in the body temperature can be as much as 1 °C. A decrease in either skin or blood temperature provides feedback to the thermoregulatory center (hypothalamus) to activate the mechanisms that will conserve body heat and increase heat production. The primary means by which our bodies avoid excessive cooling are

- shivering,
- nonshivering thermogenesis, and
- peripheral vasoconstriction.

Because these mechanisms of heat production and conservation are often inadequate, we must also rely on clothing and subcutaneous fat to help insulate our deep body tissues from the environment.

Shivering—the uncontrolled muscular contractions discussed earlier—can cause a four- to five-fold increase in the body's resting rate of heat production. Nonshivering thermogenesis involves stimulation of metabolism by the sympathetic nervous system. Increasing the metabolic rate increases the amount of internal heat production.

Peripheral vasoconstriction occurs as a result of sympathetic stimulation to the smooth muscle surrounding the arterioles in the skin. This stimulation causes the muscle to contract, which constricts the arterioles and reduces the blood flow to the shell of the body and prevents unnecessary heat loss. The metabolic rate of the skin cells also decreases as the skin's temperature falls, so the skin requires less oxygen.

Factors Affecting Body Heat Loss

As in the case of heat stress, the body's ability to meet the demands of thermoregulation is limited when exposed to extreme cold. Too much heat loss can occur. Those factors (conduction, convection, radiation, and evaporation) that usually perform so effectively in dissipating metabolically produced heat during exercise in warm conditions, can, in a cold environment, dissipate heat faster than the body produces it.

Pinpointing the exact conditions that permit excessive body heat loss and eventual hypothermia (low body temperature) is difficult. Thermal balance depends on a wide variety of factors that affect the gradient between body heat production and heat loss. Generally speaking, the larger the difference between the temperature of the skin and the cold environment, the greater the heat loss. However, a number of anatomical and environmental factors can influence the rate of heat loss. Let's consider a few.

When exercising in the cold, do not overdress. When you overdress, your body can become hot and initiate sweating. As the sweat soaks through the clothing, evaporation rapidly removes the heat and you become chilled.

Body Size and Composition

Insulating the body against the cold is the most obvious protection against hypothermia. Subcutaneous fat is an excellent source of insulation.[7] Skinfold measurements of subcutaneous fat thickness are a good indicator of an individual's tolerance for cold exposure. The thermal conductivity of fat (its capacity for transferring heat) is relatively low, so it impedes heat transfer from the deep tissues to the body surface. People who have more fat mass conserve heat more efficiently in the cold.

The body's insulative shell consists of two regions: the superficial skin together with subcutaneous fat, and the underlying muscle. When skin temperatures drop below normal, constriction of the blood vessels supplying the skin and contraction of the skeletal muscles increase the shell's insulative properties. In fact, it is estimated that vasoconstricted inactive muscle can provide as much as 85% of the body's total insulation during exposure to extreme cold. This represents a resistance to heat loss that is two to three times greater than that of the overlying fat and skin.[13,15]

The rate of heat loss is also affected by the ratio of body surface area to body mass. Tall, heavy individuals have a small surface-area-to-body-mass ratio, which makes them less susceptible to hypothermia. As shown in Table 11.5, small children tend to have a large area-to-mass ratio compared to adults. This makes it more difficult for them to maintain normal body temperature in the cold.

True gender differences in cold tolerance are minimal. Women tend to have more body fat than men. Some studies have shown that the added subcutaneous fat in females might give them an advantage during cold water immersion.[8] When males and females of similar body fat mass, size, and fitness are compared, little difference is noted in body temperature regulation with exposure to the cold.

Windchill

As with heat, the air temperature alone is not a valid index of the amount of thermal stress experienced by the individual. Wind creates a chill factor, known as the windchill, by increasing the rate of heat loss via convection and conduction. Also, the more humid the air, the greater the physiological stress. A dry, still day at 10 °C (50 °F) in the direct sun can be comfortable. Yet on a moist, windy day with complete cloud cover, the cold at this same temperature can be quite penetrating. Table 11.6 lists equivalent temperatures for various ambient air temperatures and wind velocities.

Table 11.5 An Example of Body Weight, Height, Surface Area, and the Surface Area to Mass Ratios for an Averaged-Size Adult and Child

Person	Weight (kg)	Height (cm)	Surface area (cm²)	Area: mass ratio
Adult	85	183	210	2.47
Child	25	100	79	3.16

Heat Loss in Cold Water

More research has been conducted on cold exposure in water than air, so we will focus on the effects of immersion in cold water. Whereas radiation and sweat evaporation are the primary mechanisms for heat loss in air, conduction allows the greatest heat transfer during immersion in water. As mentioned earlier in this chapter, water has a thermal conductivity about 26 times greater than air. This means that heat loss by conduction is 26 times faster in water than it is in air. When all factors are considered (radiation, conduction, convection, and evaporation), the body generally loses heat from the body four times faster in water than it does in air of the same temperature.

Humans generally maintain a constant internal temperature when they remain inactive in water at temperatures down to about 32 °C (about 90 °F). But when the water temperature drops lower, they become hypothermic at a rate proportional to either the duration of their exposure or the thermal gradient.[10,11] Because of the large drain of heat from a body immersed in cold water, prolonged exposure or unusually cold conditions can lead to extreme hypothermia and death. Individuals immersed in water at 15 °C (59 °F) experience a decrease in rectal temperature of about 2.1 °C (3.8 °F) per hour. If the water temperature were lowered to 4 °C (39 °F), rectal temperature would decrease at a rate of 3.2 °C (5.8 °F) per hour.[12] The rate of heat loss is further accelerated if the cold water is moving around the individual, because heat loss by convection increases. As a result, survival time in cold water is quite brief. The victim would become weak and lose consciousness within minutes.

In a 3-year study of factors limiting long-distance swimmers, Pugh and Edholm observed a variety of responses to cold water immersion (water temperature below 21 °C, or 69.8 °F).[14] Subcutaneous fat appeared to play an important role in thermal insulation against the cold water, because subjects with obesity (about 30% body fat) could swim for 6 hr 50 min in water at 11.8 °C (56.8 °F) with virtually no change in rectal temperature. But swimmers with relatively low body fatness (about 10%) experienced severe discomfort and their rectal temperatures dropped to 33.7 °C (92.7 °F)

Table 11.6 Wind-Chill Factor Chart

Estimated wind speed (mph)	Actual thermometer reading (°F)											
	50	40	30	20	10	0	-10	-20	-30	-40	-50	-60
	Equivalent temperature (°F)											
Calm	50	40	30	20	10	0	-10	-20	-30	-40	-50	-60
5	48	37	27	16	6	-5	-15	-26	-36	-47	-57	-68
10	40	28	16	4	-9	-24	-33	-46	-58	-70	-83	-95
15	36	22	9	-5	-18	-32	-45	-58	-72	-85	-99	-112
20	32	18	4	-10	-25	-39	-53	-67	-82	-96	-110	-124
25	30	16	0	-15	-29	-44	-59	-74	-88	-104	-118	-133
30	28	13	-2	-18	-33	-48	-63	-79	-94	-109	-125	-140
35	27	11	-4	-20	-35	-51	-67	-82	-98	-113	-129	-145
40	26	10	-6	-21	-37	-53	-69	-85	-100	-116	-132	-148
	Green			**Yellow**				**Red**				
(Wind speeds >40 mph have little additional effect.)	LITTLE DANGER for properly clothed person. Maximum danger of false sense of security.			INCREASING DANGER Danger from freezing of exposed flesh.			GREAT DANGER					

Adapted from *Runner's World* (1973).

after only 30 min of swimming in the same water temperature.

If the metabolic rate is low, such as when at rest, then even a moderately cool water temperature can cause hypothermia. But exercise increases the metabolic rate and offsets some of the heat loss. For example, although heat loss increases when swimming at high speeds (because of convection), the swimmer's accelerated rate of metabolic heat production more than compensates for the greater heat transfer. As shown in Figure 11.10a, subjects with low body fat (about 8%) maintained constant internal temperature during exercise in water as cold as 17.4 °C (63.3 °F) when their metabolic rate was increased to about 15 kcal per min. As shown in Figure 11.10b, this was true even though their skin temperatures averaged about 17 °C (31 °F) below their internal temperature! When the exercise ended, however, the skin was warmed rapidly and the body core began to cool. For competition, water temperatures between 23.9 to 27.8 °C (75 to 82 °F) seem appropriate.

Physiological Responses to Exercise in the Cold

We have seen how the body must struggle to maintain its internal temperature when exposed to a cold environment. Now we can consider what happens when you add the demands of physical performance to that struggle. How does the body respond to exercise when it is also dealing with exposure to the cold?

Muscle Function

Cooling muscle causes it to become weaker. The nervous system responds to muscle cooling by altering the normal muscle fiber recruitment patterns.[5] Some researchers have suggested that this change in fiber selection for force development decreases the efficiency of the muscle's actions. Both muscle shortening velocity and power decrease significantly when temperature is lowered. If people attempt to work at the same velocity and power output when the muscle is at 25 °C (77 °F) as when it is at 35 °C (95 °F), they experience fatigue earlier. Thus, they have the choice of either performing an activity at a decreased velocity or expending more energy.

If clothing insulation and exercise metabolism are sufficient to maintain the athlete's body temperature in the cold, then exercise performance may be unimpaired. However, as fatigue sets in and muscle activity slows, body heat production gradually decreases. Long-distance running, swimming, and skiing in the cold can expose the participant to such conditions. At the beginning of these activities, the athlete can exercise at a rate that generates sufficient internal heat to maintain body temperature. However, late in the activity, when the energy reserves have diminished, exercise intensity declines and this reduces metabolic

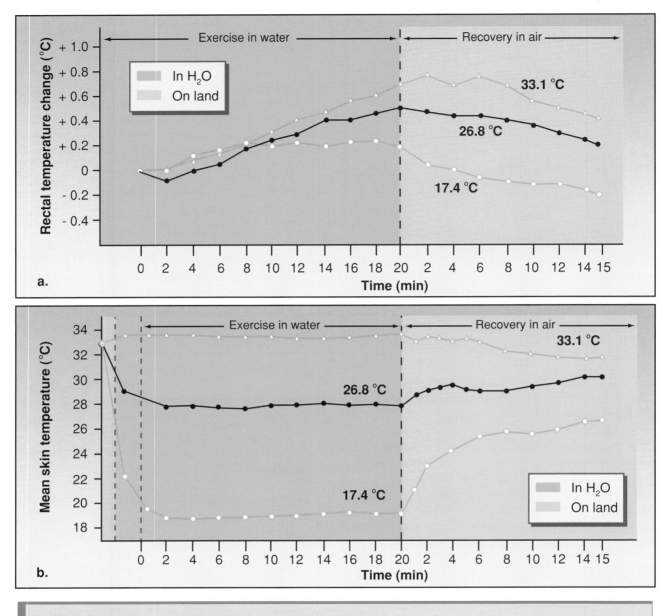

Figure 11.10   Changes in (a) rectal temperature and (b) mean skin temperature during and following swimming in three different water temperatures. Adapted from Costill et al., (1967).

heat production. Subsequent hypothermia causes the individual to become even more fatigued and less capable of generating heat. In these conditions the athlete is confronted with a potentially dangerous situation.

Metabolic Responses

As we learned earlier, prolonged exercise increases the mobilization and oxidation of free fatty acids (FFA). The primary stimulus for this increased lipid metabolism is the release of the catecholamines (epinephrine and norepinephrine) into the vascular system. Exposure to cold triggers a marked increase in epinephrine and norepinephrine secretion, but FFA levels rise substantially less than during prolonged exercise in warmer conditions. Cold exposure triggers vasoconstriction in the vessels supplying the skin and subcutaneous tissues. The subcutaneous tissue is the major storage site for lipids (adipose tissue), so this vasoconstriction reduces the blood flow to the area from which the FFA would be mobilized. Thus FFA levels do not increase as much as the elevated levels of epinephrine and norepinephrine would indicate.

Blood glucose plays an important role in cold tolerance and exercise endurance. Hypoglycemia (low blood sugar), for example, suppresses shivering and significantly reduces rectal temperature. The reasons for these changes are unknown. Fortunately, the blood glucose level is maintained reasonably well during cold exposure. Muscle glycogen, on the other hand, is used at a somewhat higher rate in cold water than it is in warmer conditions.[19] However, studies on exercise metabolism in the cold are limited, and our knowledge regarding hormonal regulation of metabolism in the cold is too limited to support any definitive conclusions.

IN REVIEW . . .

1. Shivering (involuntary muscle contractions) increases metabolic heat production to help us maintain or increase our temperature.
2. Nonshivering thermogenesis accomplishes the same goal, but through stimulation of the sympathetic nervous system and by the action of hormones such as thyroxine and the catecholamines.
3. Peripheral vasoconstriction decreases the transfer of core heat to the skin, thus decreasing heat loss to the environment.
4. Body size is an important consideration for heat loss. Both increased surface area and reduced subcutaneous fat facilitate the loss of body heat to the environment. So those who have a small surface-area-to-body-mass ratio and those with more fat are less susceptible to hypothermia.
5. Wind increases heat loss by convection and conduction, so this effect, known as windchill, must be considered along with air temperature during cold exposure.
6. Immersion in cold water tremendously increases heat loss through conduction. Exercise generates metabolic heat to offset some of this loss.
7. When muscle is cooled, it is weakened, and fatigue occurs more rapidly.
8. During prolonged exercise in the cold, as energy supplies diminish and exercise intensity declines, a person becomes increasingly susceptible to hypothermia.
9. Exercise triggers release of the catecholamines, which increase the mobilization and use of free fatty acids for fuel. But in the cold, vasoconstriction impairs circulation to the subcutaneous fat tissue, so this process is attenuated.

Health Risks During Exercise in the Cold

If humans had retained the ability of lower animals, like reptiles, to tolerate low body temperatures, we could survive extreme hypothermia. Unfortunately, in humans, the evolution of thermoregulation has been accompanied by a loss in the ability of vital tissues to function when they are cooled by more than a few degrees. Let's briefly examine what happens during hypothermia and frostbite.

Hypothermia

Data from the infamous Dachau experiments, collected by Alexander after World War II, show that people who were immersed in near-freezing water died when their rectal temperatures fell to 24.2 to 25.7 °C (75.6 to 78.3 °F).[1] Cases of accidental hypothermia and data obtained from surgical patients who are intentionally made hypothermic reveal that the lethal lower limit of body temperature is usually between 23 and 25 °C (72.4 to 77 °F), although patients have recovered after having rectal temperatures below 18 °C (64.4 °F).[11] As early as 1958, a woman deliberately cooled to a rectal temperature of 9 °C (48.2 °F) under anaesthesia was satisfactorily revived despite a cardiac arrest lasting for more than 60 min.[12]

Once the body temperature falls below 34.5 °C (94 °F), the hypothalamus begins to lose its ability to regulate body temperature. This ability is completely lost when the internal temperature falls to about 29.5 °C (85 °F). This loss of function is associated with slowing of metabolic reactions to one half their normal rates for each 10 °C decline in cellular temperature. As a result, cooling the body can cause drowsiness and even coma.

Cardiorespiratory Effects

The hazards of excessive cold exposure include potential injury to both peripheral tissues and the life-supporting cardiovascular and respiratory systems. The most important effect of hypothermia is on the heart. Death from hypothermia has resulted from cardiac arrest while respiration was still functional. Cooling primarily influences the SA node—the heart's pacemaker. As early as 1912, Knowlton and Starling demonstrated that cooling heart-lung preparations of dogs leads to a progressive decline of heart rate followed by cardiac arrest.[9] The combined decrements in core temperature and heart rate result in a rapid decline in cardiac output.

Many people have questioned whether rapid, deep breathing of cold air can cause freezing or damage to the respiratory tract. In fact, the cold air that passes into the mouth and trachea is rapidly warmed, even when the inhaled air is at less than −25 °C (−13 °F).[17] Even at this temperature, the air has been warmed to about 15 °C (59 °F) by the time it has traveled about 5 cm (2 in.) into the nasal passage. As shown in Figure 11.11, extremely cold air entering the nose is quite warm by the time it reaches the rear of the nasal passage, thereby posing no threat of damage to the throat, trachea, or lungs. But excessive cold exposure

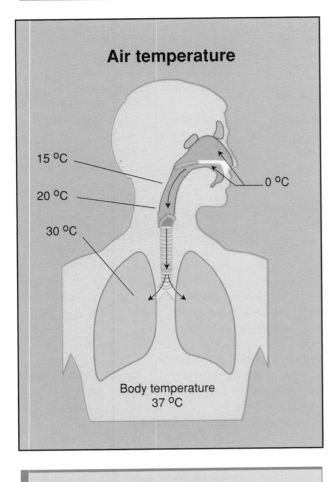

Air temperature

15 °C

20 °C

30 °C

0 °C

Body temperature
37 °C

Figure 11.11   The warming of inspired air as it moves through the respiratory tract.

does affect respiratory function: It decreases the respiratory rate and volume.

Treatment for Hypothermia

Mild hypothermia can be treated by giving a person protection from the cold and providing dry clothing and warm beverages. Moderate to severe cases of hypothermia require gentle handling to avoid initiating a cardiac arrhythmia. This requires slowly rewarming the victim. Severe cases of hypothermia require hospital facilities and medical care.

Frostbite

Exposed skin can freeze when its temperature is lowered just a few degrees below the freezing point (0 °C, 32 °F). Because of the warming influence of circulation and metabolic heat production, the environmental air temperature (including windchill) required to freeze one's exposed fingers, nose, and ears is about −29 °C (−20 °F). Recall from our earlier discussion that periph-

eral vasoconstriction helps the body retain heat. Unfortunately, during exposure to extreme cold, the circulation in the skin can decrease to the point that the tissue dies from the lack of oxygen and nutrients. This is commonly called frostbite. If not treated early, frostbite injuries can be serious, leading to gangrene and loss of tissue. Frostbitten parts should be left untreated until they can be thawed, preferably in a hospital, without risk of refreezing.

■■■   IN REVIEW . . .   ■■■

1. The hypothalamus begins to lose its ability to regulate body temperature if that temperature drops below 34.5 °C (94.1 °F).
2. The heart's SA node is primarily affected by hypothermia, causing the heart rate to drop, which in turn reduces cardiac output.
3. Breathing cold air does not freeze the respiratory passages or the lungs.
4. Exposure to extreme cold does decrease respiratory rate and volume.
5. Frostbite occurs as a consequence of the body's attempts to prevent heat loss. Vasoconstriction to the skin causes reduced blood flow, so the skin rapidly cools. This, combined with the lack of oxygen and nutrients, causes the skin tissue to die.

Cold Acclimatization

Information about cold acclimatization is limited, but some data suggest that chronic daily exposure to cold water increases subcutaneous body fat.[8] Much of our information regarding habituation to the cold has been obtained from observations on the aborigines, natives of the Australian outback, where they are normally exposed to low temperatures at night and high temperatures during the day.[16] Compared to unacclimatized Europeans, the aborigines were able to sleep more comfortably in the cold with little protection, and they experienced only minor changes in their metabolism and rectal temperatures. The Europeans, on the other hand, experienced significant distress and considerable difficulty in maintaining normal body temperature.

Although some data suggest that repeated exposure to the cold alters peripheral blood flow and skin temperatures, these changes are small and the findings are inconclusive. Field studies have shown that chronic exposure of some areas of the skin, such as the hands, can provide greater cold tolerance. For example, fishermen who must work with their hands in cold water for many hours develop increased vasodilation and local warming of this exposed skin. The rate and degree of adjustment to these conditions have not been fully explained. Thus, acclimatization to cold is not as thoroughly understood as acclimatization to environmental heat stress.

◼◼ IN REVIEW . . . ◼◼

1. Cold acclimatization is not well studied, so our knowledge is limited.
2. Repeated exposure to the cold may alter peripheral blood flow and skin temperatures, allowing greater cold tolerance.

In Closing . . .

In this chapter, we began our examination of how the external environment affects the body's ability to perform physical work. We have looked at the effects of extreme heat and cold stress and the body's responses to them. We considered the health risks associated with these temperature extremes and how the body can try to adapt to these conditions through acclimatization.

Now, in the next chapter, we are ready to examine still more environmental extremes: hypobaric, hyperbaric, and microgravity environments.

Key Terms

acclimatization
conduction
convection
evaporation
frostbite
heat content
heat cramps
heat exhaustion
heat stroke
hyperthermia
hypothermia

mean body temperature (T_{body})
nonshivering thermogenesis
radiation
shivering
thermoreceptors
thermoregulation
thermoregulatory center
wet bulb globe temperature (WBGT)

Study Questions

1. What are the four major avenues for loss of body heat?
2. Which of these four pathways is most important for controlling body temperature when at rest? During exercise?
3. What happens to the body temperature during exercise, and why?
4. Why is humidity an important factor when performing in the heat? Why are wind and cloud cover important?
5. What is the purpose of the wet bulb globe temperature (WBGT)? What does it measure?
6. Differentiate between heat cramps, heat exhaustion, and heat stroke.
7. What physiological adaptations occur allowing one to acclimatize to exercise in the heat?
8. How does the body minimize excessive heat loss during cold exposure?
9. What dangers are associated with cold water immersion?
10. What factors should be considered to provide maximum protection when exercising in the cold?

References

1. Alexander, L. (1946). *Treatment of shock from prolonged exposure to cold especially in water* (Item No. 24, File No. 26-37). Washington, DC: Combined Intelligence Objectives Sub-committee.

2. American College of Sports Medicine. (1987). Prevention of thermal injuries during distance running. *Medicine and Science in Sports and Exercise*, **19**, 529-533.

3. Costill, D.L. (1986). *Inside running: Basics of sports physiology*. Indianapolis: Benchmark Press.

4. Costill, D.L., Kammer, W.F., & Fisher, A. (1970). Fluid ingestion during distance running. *Archives of Environmental Health*, **21**, 520-525.

5. Faulkner, J.A., Claflin, D.R., & McCully, K.K. (1987). Muscle function in the cold. In J.R. Sutton, C.S. Houston, & G. Coates (Eds.), *Hypoxia and cold* (pp. 429-437). New York: Praeger.

6. Fink, W., Costill, D.L., Van Handel, P., & Getchell, L. (1975). Leg muscle metabolism during exercise in the heat and cold. *European Journal of Applied Physiology*, **34**, 183-190.

7. Hayward, M.G., & Keatinge, W.R. (1981). Roles of subcutaneous fat and thermoregulatory reflexes in determining ability to stabilize body temperature in water. *London Journal of Physiology*, **320**, 229-251.

8. Kang, B.S., Song, S.H., Suh, C.S., & Hong, S.K. (1963). Changes in body temperature and basal metabolic rate of the ama. *Journal of Applied Physiology*, **18**, 483-488.

9. Knowlton, F.P., & Starling, E.H. (1912). The influence of variations in temperature and blood-pressure on the performance of the isolated mammalian heart. *Journal of Physiology*, **44**, 206-219.

10. Molnar, G.W. (1946). Survival of hypothermia by man immersed in the ocean. *Journal of the American Medical Association*, **131**, 1046-1050.

11. Newburgh, L.H. (1949). *Physiology of heat regulation*. Philadelphia: Saunders.

12. Niazi, S.A., & Lewis, F.J. (1958). Profound hypothermia in man. *Annals of Surgery*, **147**, 264-266.

13. Pendergast, D.R. (1988). The effect of body cooling on oxygen transport during exercise. *Medicine and Science in Sports and Exercise*, **20**(Suppl.), S171-S176.

14. Pugh, L.G., & Edholm, D.G. (1955). The physiology of channel swimmers. *Lancet*, **2**, 761-767.

15. Rennie, D.W. (1988). Tissue heat transfer in water: Lessons from the Korean divers. *Medicine and Science in Sports and Exercise*, **20**, S177.

16. Scholander, P.F., Hammel, H.T., Hart, J.S., Lemessurier, D.H. & Steen, J. (1958). Cold adaptation in Australian aborigines. *Journal of Applied Physiology*, **13**, 211-218.

17. Webb, P. (1951). Air temperature in respiratory tracts of resting subjects in the cold. *Journal of Applied Physiology*, **4**, 378-382.

18. Wyndham, C.H. (1973). The physiology of exercise under heat stress. *Annual Review of Physiology*, **35**, 193-220.

19. Young, A.J., Sawka, M.N., Neufer, P.D., Muza, S.R., Askew, E.W., & Pandolf, K.B. (1989). Thermoregulation during cold water immersion is unimpaired by low muscle glycogen levels. *Journal of Applied Physiology*, **66**, 1809-1816.

Selected Readings

Armstrong, L.E., & Dziados, J.E. (1986). Effects of heat exposure on the exercising adult. In D.B. Bernhardt (Ed.), *Sports physical therapy*. New York: Churchill Livingstone.

Armstrong, L.E., & Maresh, C.M. (1991). The induction and decay of heat acclimatisation in trained athletes. *Sports Medicine*, **12**, 302-312.

Clarke, R.S.J., Hellon, R.F., & Lind, A.R. (1958). The duration of sustained contractions of the human forearm at different muscle temperatures. *Journal of Physiology*, **143**, 454-473.

Doubt, T.J. (1991). Physiology of exercise in the cold. *Sports Medicine*, **11**, 367-381.

Edwards, R.H.T., Harris, R.C., Hultman, E., Kaijser, L., Koh, D., & Nordesjo, L.O. (1972). Effect of temperature on muscle energy metabolism and endurance during successive isometric contractions, sustained to fatigue, of the quadriceps muscle in man. *Journal of Physiology*, **220**, 335-352.

Ferretti, G., Veicsteinas, A., & Rennie, D.W. (1988). Regional heat flows of resting and exercising men immersed in cool water. *Journal of Applied Physiology*, **64**, 1239-1248.

Fox, E.L., Bowers, R.W., & Foss, M.L. (1993). *The physiological basis for exercising and sport* (5th ed.) (pp. 795). Philadelphia: Saunders.

Gisolfi, C.V., & Wenger, C.B. (1984). Temperature regulation during exercise: Old concepts, new ideas. *Exercise and Sport Sciences Reviews*, **12**, 339-372.

Greenleaf, J.E. (1979). Hyperthermia in exercise. In D. Robertshaw (Ed.), *International review of physiology: Environmental physiology III: Vol. 20*. Baltimore: University Park Press.

Keatinge, W.R. (1969). *Survival in cold water* (p. 131). Oxford: Blackwell Scientific.

Kenney, W.L., & Anderson, R.K. (1988). Response of older and younger women in dry and humid heat without fluid replacement. *Medicine and Science in Sports and Exercise*, **20**, 155.

King, D.S., Costill, D.L., Fink, W.J., Hargreaves, M., & Fielding, R.A. (1985). Muscle metabolism during exercise in the heat in unacclimatized and acclimatized humans. *Journal of Applied Physiology*, **59**, 1350-1354.

Laufman, H. (1951). Profound accidental hypothermia. *Journal of the American Medical Association*, **147**, 1201-1212.

Nadel, E.R. (Ed.) (1977). *Problems with temperature regulation during exercise*. New York: Academic Press.

Neuffer, P.D. (1986). Effects of exercise and carbohydrate conposition on gastric emptying. *Medicine and Science in Sports and Exercise*, **18**, 656.

Sawaka, M.N., & Wegner, C.B. (1988). Physiological responses to acute-exercise heat stress. In K.B. Pandolf (Ed.), *Human performance physiology and environmental medicine at terrestrial extremes*. Indianapolis: Benchmark Press.

Siple, P.A. & Passel, C.F. (1945). Measurement of dry atmospheric cooling in subfreezing temperatures. *Proceedings of The American Physiological Society*, **89**, 177-199.

Toner, M.M., & McArdle, W.D. (1988). Physiological adjustments of a man to cold. In K.B. Pandolf (Ed.), *Human performance physiology and environmental medicine at terrestrial extremes*. Indianapolis: Benchmark Press.

Wegner, C.B. (1988). Human heat acclimatization. In K.B. Pandolf (Ed.), *Human performance physiology and environmental medicine at terrestrial extremes*. Indianapolis: Benchmark Press.

Young, A.J. (1990). Energy substrate utilization during exercise in extreme environments. In K. Pandolf & J.O. Holloszy (Eds.), *Exercise and sport sciences reviews: Vol. 18*. Baltimore: Williams & Wilkins.

Chapter 12

Exercise in Hypobaric, Hyperbaric, and Microgravity Environments

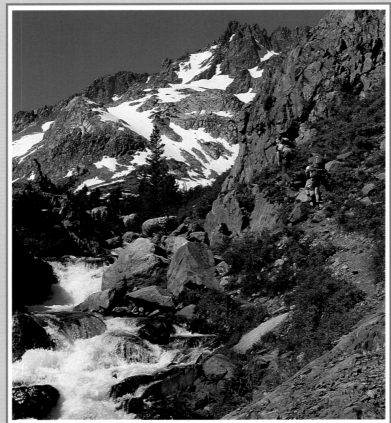

© Rene Laursen/Photo Network

Chapter Overview

We have heard accounts of grueling attempts to scale Mount Everest. We have heard of the bitter cold, the avalanches, and the failures. In contrast, most of us have, from our armchairs, joined in the undersea adventures of Jacques Cousteau, exploring the magnificent beauty under the ocean along with the team from his ship, the *Calypso*. And we have followed the journeys of our astronauts as they have ventured into space.

The physical conditions of each of these environments are so different from those to which we are accustomed that exposure to these extreme environments alters our bodies' functioning. Our bodies must deal with low pressure at altitude, high pressure underwater, and weightlessness in space.

In this chapter we will examine the conditions experienced in these specialized environments, how these conditions affect our bodies, and how they affect performance. We will also consider health risks associated with each environment and how we can adapt to these extreme conditions.

Chapter Outline

Sports competition at altitude has traditionally been associated with performance impairment. As a result, there were many complaints when it was announced that the site of the 1968 Olympic Games would be Mexico City, at an altitude of 2,290 m (7,500 ft) above sea level. At least two athletes who participated in those games were glad to perform in the rarified air at that moderate altitude. Bob Beamon soared more than 2 ft farther than the world record in the long jump, and Lee Evans beat the world record in the 400-m run by nearly a full second. These records stood for nearly 20 years, indicating that conditions at the altitude of Mexico City contributed to the stellar performances in these relatively short, explosive events.

Our previous discussions of the physiological responses to exercise were based on the conditions that exist at or near sea level, where the barometric pressure averages about 760 mmHg, the partial pressure of oxygen (P_{O_2}) is about 159 mmHg, and we experience normal gravitational force. Although the human body tolerates reasonable fluctuations in these conditions, large variations from these values pose special problems. This is evident when mountain climbers ascend to higher altitudes, when divers are exposed to pressurized conditions underwater, or when astronauts are in space. Any of these situations can seriously impair physical performance and can even jeopardize life.

Barometric pressure is reduced at altitude. This situation is referred to as a hypobaric environment (low atmospheric pressure). The lower atmospheric pressure also means a lower partial pressure of oxygen, which limits pulmonary diffusion and oxygen transport to the tissues. This reduces oxygen delivery to the body tissues, resulting in hypoxia (oxygen deficiency). On the other hand, when immersed in water, the body is exposed to greater pressure. Thus the underwater world is a hyperbaric environment (high atmospheric pressure). Gases breathed under these conditions must be pressurized to equal the force of water against the chest wall. This means the lung and body tissues are presented with gas pressures well in excess of those experienced at sea level. Breathing pressurized gases has little effect on the transport of oxygen and carbon dioxide in the body, but the increased partial pressure of several gases can lead to life-threatening complications.

Our third environment of concern is microgravity, in which the body experiences a reduced gravitational force. Though athletes certainly do not compete in space, space exploration has revealed some physiological challenges that are relevant to exercise and sport physiology.

In the following discussion, we will examine the special characteristics of hypobaric, hyperbaric, and microgravity environments and how these conditions alter our physiological responses to physical activity. We will focus on the impact of these environments on oxygen transport and examine health risks associated with each.

Hypobaric Environments: Exercising at Altitude

Clinical problems associated with altitude were reported as early as 400 B.C.[40] However, most of the early concerns about ascent to high altitudes focused on the cold conditions at altitude rather than the limitations imposed by rarefied air. The initial discoveries that led to our current understanding of the reduced oxygen pressure at altitude can be credited to three scientists. Torricelli (ca. 1644) developed the mercury barometer, an instrument that permits accurate measurement of atmospheric gas pressures. A few years later (1648), Pascal demonstrated a reduction in barometric pressure at high altitudes.[40] Nearly 130 years later (1777), Lavoisier described oxygen and the other gases that contribute to the total barometric pressure.[40]

The deleterious effects of high altitude on humans that are caused by low oxygen tension (hypoxia) were subsequently recognized by Bert in the late 1800s.[1] More recently, the selection of Mexico City, with an elevation of 2,290 m (1.4 mi) above sea level, for the 1968 Olympic Games drew considerable attention to the effects of altitude on physical performance. For our discussion, the term altitude will refer to elevations above 1,500 m (4,921 ft) because few physiological effects on performance are reported below that level.

Conditions at Altitude

Before examining how altitude affects performance, we must consider what special conditions exist in such hypobaric environments. Let's look at how the atmosphere differs at altitude from what we are accustomed to near sea level.

Atmospheric Pressure at Altitude

Air has weight. The barometric pressure at any place on Earth is related to the weight of the air in the atmosphere above that point. At sea level, for example, the air extending to the outermost reaches of the Earth's atmosphere (approximately 24 mi or 38.6 km) exerts a pressure equal to 760 mmHg. At the summit of Mount Everest, the highest point on Earth (8,848 m, or 29,028 ft), the pressure exerted by the air above is only about 250 mmHg. These (and other) differences are depicted in Figure 12.1.

The barometric pressure on Earth does not remain constant. Rather it varies with changes in climatic conditions, time of year, and the specific site at which the measurement is taken. On Mount Everest, for example, the mean atmospheric pressure varies from 243 mmHg in January to nearly 255 mmHg in June and July. Also, the Earth's atmosphere bulges outward slightly at the equator, which increases the atmospheric pressure there by a few mmHg above standard pressure. These points, of little interest to people living near sea level, are of considerable physiological import

for anyone attempting to climb Mount Everest without supplemental oxygen.

Though atmospheric pressure varies, the percentages of gases in the air that we breathe remain unchanged from sea level to high altitude. At any elevation, the air always contains 20.93% oxygen, 0.03% carbon dioxide, and 79.04% nitrogen. Only the partial pressures change. As shown in Table 12.1, the pressure that oxygen molecules exert at various altitudes is directly affected by the barometric pressure,

Table 12.1 Changes in Barometric Pressure (P_b) and Partial Pressure of Oxygen (P_{O_2}) at Different Altitudes

Altitude (m)	P_b (mmHg)	P_{O_2} (mmHg)
0 (sea level)	760	159.2
1,000	674	141.2
2,000	596	124.9
3,000	526	110.2
4,000	462	96.9
9,000	231	48.4

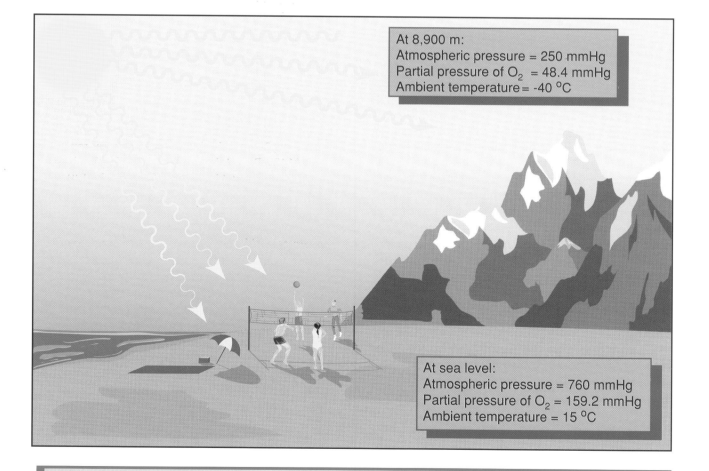

At 8,900 m:
Atmospheric pressure = 250 mmHg
Partial pressure of O_2 = 48.4 mmHg
Ambient temperature = -40 °C

At sea level:
Atmospheric pressure = 760 mmHg
Partial pressure of O_2 = 159.2 mmHg
Ambient temperature = 15 °C

Figure 12.1 Differences in atmospheric conditions at sea level and at an altitude of 8,900 m.

Table 12.2 Changes in Air Temperature at Different Altitudes

Altitude (m)	Temperature (°C)
0 (sea level)	15.0
1,000	8.5
2,000	2.0
3,000	-4.5
4,000	-10.9
9,000	-43.4

and a change in the partial pressure of oxygen has a significant effect on the partial pressure gradient between the blood and the tissues. This point will be discussed later in this chapter.

Air Temperature at Altitude

Air temperature drops at a rate of about 1 °C for every 150 m (about 490 ft) of ascent, as shown in Table 12.2. The average temperature near the summit of Mount Everest is estimated to be about –40 °C, whereas at sea level the temperature would be about 15 °C. The combination of low temperatures and high winds at altitude poses a serious risk of cold-related disorders, such as hypothermia and windchill injuries.

Because of the cold temperatures at altitude, the absolute humidity is extremely low. Cold air holds very little water. Thus, even if it is fully saturated with water (100% relative humidity), the actual amount of water contained in the air is small. The partial pressure of water at 20 °C is about 17 mmHg. But at –20 °C, this pressure drops to only about 1 mmHg. The very low humidity at high altitude promotes dehydration. In fact, a large volume of body water is lost through respiratory evaporation due to the dry air and increased respiration rate (discussed later) experienced at altitude. The dry air also increases evaporative water loss through sweating during exercise at altitude.

Solar Radiation at Altitude

The intensity of solar radiation increases at high altitude for two reasons. First, because you are positioned higher in the atmosphere, light travels through less of the atmosphere before reaching you. For this reason, less of the sun's radiation, especially the ultraviolet rays, is absorbed by the atmosphere at altitude. Second, because atmospheric water normally absorbs a substantial amount of the sun's radiation, the limited water vapor found at altitude also increases your exposure. Solar radiation is further amplified if you are also exposed to reflective light from snow, which is usually found at higher elevations.

━━ KEY POINT ━━

The mixture of gases in the air we breathe at altitude is identical to that at sea level—O_2 is 20.93%, CO_2 is 0.03%, and N_2 is 79.04% of the total air. The partial pressure of each gas, however, is reduced in direct proportion to the increase in altitude. The reduced partial pressure of O_2 leads to decreased performance at altitude, due to a reduced pressure gradient that hinders oxygen transport to the tissues.

Air temperature decreases as altitude increases. This drop in temperature is accompanied by a decrease in the amount of water vapor in the air. As a result, this drier air can lead to dehydration through increased insensible water loss.

━━ IN REVIEW . . . ━━

1. Altitude presents a hypobaric environment—one in which the atmospheric pressure is reduced. Altitudes of 1,500 m (4,921 ft) or more have a notable physiological impact on the human body.
2. Though the percentages of the gases in the air we breathe remain constant regardless of altitude, the partial pressures of each of these gases varies with atmospheric pressure.
3. Air temperature drops as altitude increases. Cold air can hold little water, so the air at altitude is dry. These two factors increase your susceptibility to cold-related disorders and dehydration when at altitude.
4. Because the atmosphere is thinner and drier at altitude, solar radiation is more intense at higher elevations.

Physiological Responses to Altitude

We have looked at some of the unique environmental conditions associated with altitude. Now we can examine how exposure to these conditions affects you. In this section we will examine how your body responds to altitude, emphasizing those responses that can affect performance. Our main concerns will be

- respiratory responses,
- cardiovascular responses, and
- metabolic responses.

Most of this discussion deals with the physiological responses of unacclimatized males at altitude. Unfortunately, few studies on the effects of altitude have included females or children, populations whose sensitivity to the conditions of altitude might differ from what is described here.

Respiratory Responses to Altitude

Adequate oxygen delivery to the muscles is essential to physical performance, and, as we saw in chapter 9, depends on bringing an adequate supply of oxygen into the body and transporting it to the muscles and on adequate oxygen uptake by the muscles. Any deficiency in these steps can impair performance. Let's see how altitude affects these processes.

Pulmonary Ventilation.   Pulmonary ventilation (breathing) increases at higher altitudes, when at rest and during exercise. Because the number of oxygen molecules in a given volume of air is less at higher altitudes, more air must be inspired there to supply as much oxygen as during normal breathing at sea level. Ventilation increases to bring in a larger volume of air.

> ## KEY POINT
>
> **You ventilate greater volumes of air at altitude because air is less dense.**

Increased ventilation acts much the same as hyperventilation at sea level. The amount of carbon dioxide in the alveoli is reduced. Carbon dioxide follows the pressure gradient so more diffuses out of the blood, where its pressure is relatively high, and into the lungs to be exhaled. Such increased carbon dioxide clearance allows blood pH to increase, a condition known as respiratory alkalosis. In an effort to prevent this condition, the kidneys excrete more bicarbonate ion. Recall that bicarbonate ions buffer the carbonic acid formed from carbon dioxide. Thus, a reduction in bicarbonate ion concentration reduces the blood's buffering capacity. More acid remains in the blood and the alkalosis can be reversed.

Pulmonary Diffusion and Oxygen Transport.   Pulmonary diffusion is unlimited in a resting subject at sea level. If it were limited, less oxygen would enter the blood, so the arterial P_{O_2} would be lower than the alveolar P_{O_2}. Instead, these two values are about equal. For a resting person at sea level, the amount of oxygen entering the blood is determined by the alveolar P_{O_2} and the rate of blood flow through the pulmonary capillaries.

Recall that the partial pressure of oxygen at sea level is 159 mmHg. But it drops to 125 mmHg at an elevation of 2,439 m (8,000 ft). As a result, the partial pressures of oxygen within the alveoli and the pulmonary capillaries also decrease. Consequently hemoglobin satu-

ration drops from about 98% at sea level to approximately 92% at an elevation of 2,439 m (8,000 ft). This small drop in the hemoglobin saturation was once believed to reduce $\dot{V}_{O_2\,max}$ by approximately 15%, and thus restrict performance at this altitude. However, as we will soon see, this $\dot{V}_{O_2\,max}$ reduction is really the result of the low P_{O_2} that accompanies the drop in barometric pressure at altitude.

Gas Exchange at the Muscles.   Arterial P_{O_2} at sea level is about 94 mmHg, and the partial pressure of oxygen in body tissues is consistently about 20 mmHg, so the difference, or the pressure gradient, between the arterial P_{O_2} and the tissue P_{O_2} at sea level is about 74 mmHg. However, when you move to an elevation of 2,439 m (8,000 ft), your arterial P_{O_2} drops to about 60 mmHg, while your tissue P_{O_2} remains at 20 mmHg. Thus the pressure gradient decreases from 74 mmHg to only 40 mmHg. This is a nearly 50% reduction in the diffusion gradient! Because the diffusion gradient is responsible for driving the oxygen from your blood into your tissues, this change in arterial P_{O_2} at altitude is an even greater consideration than the small 5% reduction in hemoglobin saturation that occurs.

Maximal Oxygen Uptake.   Maximal oxygen uptake decreases as altitude increases (see Figure 12.2). $\dot{V}_{O_2\,max}$ decreases little until the atmospheric P_{O_2} drops below 125 mmHg. This generally occurs at an altitude of

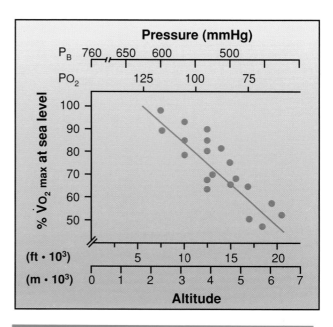

Figure 12.2   Reductions in the maximal oxygen uptake ($\dot{V}_{O_2\,max}$) with the decreased barometric pressure (P_B) and decreased partial pressure of oxygen (P_{O_2}) experienced at increasing altitude. Data from Buskirk et al., (1967).

1,600 m (5,248 ft)—about the elevation of Denver, Colorado. Although this illustration suggests a steady linear decline in $\dot{V}O_2$ max as altitude increases, $\dot{V}O_2$ max is more accurately related to the decrease in barometric pressure.[41] Specifically, $\dot{V}O_2$ max decreases at a progressively greater rate (exponentially) as the partial pressure of oxygen drops with increasing altitude.

Below an altitude of 1,600 m (5,248 ft), altitude appears to have little effect on $\dot{V}O_2$ max and endurance performance. However, above 1,600 m $\dot{V}O_2$ max decreases approximately 11% for every 1,000 m (3,281 ft) increase.

As shown in Figure 12.3, men climbing Mount Everest in a 1981 expedition experienced a change in $\dot{V}O_2$ max from about 62 ml · kg⁻¹ · min⁻¹ at sea level to only about 15 ml · kg⁻¹ · min⁻¹ near the mountain's peak. Normal resting oxygen requirements are about 5 ml · kg⁻¹ · min⁻¹, so, without supplemental oxygen, these men had little capacity for physical effort at this elevation. A study by Pugh et al. showed that men with $\dot{V}O_2$ max values of 50 ml · kg⁻¹ · min⁻¹ at sea level would be unable to exercise, or even to move, near the peak of Mount Everest because their $\dot{V}O_2$ max values at that altitude would drop to 5 ml · kg⁻¹ · min⁻¹. In fact, most normal people with sea level $\dot{V}O_2$ max values below 50 ml · kg⁻¹ · min⁻¹ would not be able to survive without supplemental oxygen at the summit of Mount Everest because their $\dot{V}O_2$ max at such altitude would be too low to sustain their body tissues. Only enough oxygen would be consumed to meet their resting requirements.

Cardiovascular Responses to Altitude

As the respiratory system becomes increasingly stressed at altitude, so does the cardiovascular system, which undergoes substantial changes to compensate for the decrease in the partial pressure of oxygen that accompanies increased altitude. Let's examine a few of these changes.

Blood Volume. Soon after arriving at altitude, a person's plasma volume begins to progressively decrease, then plateaus by the end of the first few weeks. The result of this plasma loss is an increase in the number of red blood cells per unit of blood, allowing more oxygen to be delivered to the muscles for a given cardiac output. Initially, this reduction in plasma volume occurs with little or no change in the total red blood cell count, which results in a higher hematocrit, but a smaller total blood volume, than at lower altitudes. The diminished plasma volume is eventually restored to normal levels. In addition, continued exposure to high altitude triggers increased red blood cell production, so the total number of red blood cells increases. These adaptations ultimately result in a greater total blood volume, which allows the person to partially compensate for the lower P_{O_2} experienced at altitude.

Cardiac Output. As we have seen, the amount of oxygen carried to the muscles by a given volume of blood is limited at altitude because the reduced P_{O_2} causes a reduced diffusion gradient. A logical means to compensate for this is to increase the volume of blood delivered to the active muscles. At rest and during submaximal exercise, this is accomplished by increasing cardiac output. Recall that cardiac output is the product of stroke volume and heart rate, so increasing either of these will increase cardiac output.

Standardized submaximal work levels performed during the first few hours at altitude result in an increased heart rate but decreased stroke volume (due to the reduced plasma volume). Fortunately, the rise in heart rate is sufficient to compensate for the drop in stroke volume and to slightly increase cardiac output. However, making the heart take on this extra work load for prolonged periods is not an efficient way to ensure sufficient oxygen delivery to the body's active tissues. Consequently, after a few days at altitude, the muscles begin extracting more oxygen from the blood (increasing the a-$\bar{v}O_2$ diff), which reduces the demand for an increased cardiac output, in turn reducing the need for an elevated heart rate. It has been shown that, after 10 days at high altitude, cardiac

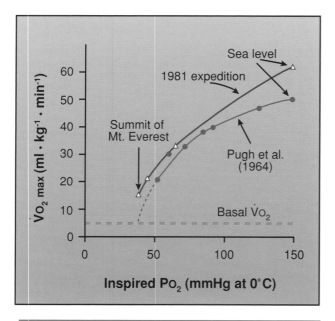

Figure 12.3 $\dot{V}O_2$ max relative to the P_{O_2} of the inspired air. Adapted from West et al. (1983) and Powers and Edwards (1994).

output during a given exercise bout is lower than it was at sea level before these adaptations to altitude occurred.[15]

At maximal or exhaustive work levels, both maximal stroke volume and maximal heart rate are decreased at higher altitudes. The effect is obvious—maximal cardiac output decreases. With a decreased diffusion gradient to push oxygen from the blood into the muscles coupled with this reduction in maximal cardiac output, we can easily understand why both $\dot{V}O_2$ max and aerobic performance are hindered at altitude. Thus, hypobaric conditions significantly limit oxygen delivery to the muscles, reducing your capacity to perform high-intensity aerobic activities.

Pulmonary Hypertension.   Blood pressure in the pulmonary arteries increases during exercise at altitude. These pressure changes are observed in both acclimatized and unacclimatized subjects.[16,23] The cause for this pulmonary hypertension is not fully understood, but this condition is presumed to indicate some structural changes in the pulmonary arteries in addition to hypoxic vasoconstriction.[16]

Metabolic Adaptations to Altitude

Given the hypoxic conditions at altitude, we would expect anaerobic metabolism to increase during exercise to meet the body's energy demands at altitude because oxidation would be limited. If this occurs, we would expect lactic acid production to increase at any given work rate. This is in fact the case except at maximal effort, during which lactate accumulation in the muscles and blood is lower.[14,36] Some researchers propose that this depression in lactic acid accumulation at maximal effort is due to the body's inability to reach a work rate that fully taxes the energy systems. Debate on this topic continues.

Performance at Altitude

The difficulty of exercise at high altitude has been described by many climbers. In 1924, E.G. Norton gave the following account of climbing without supplemental oxygen at 8,600 m (28,208 ft): "Our pace was wretched. My ambition was to do 20 consecutive paces uphill without a pause to rest and pant elbow on bent knee, yet I never remember achieving it—13 was nearer the mark."[27] In this section we will briefly consider how performance is affected by altitude.

Endurance Activity

Obviously, activities of long duration that place considerable demands on oxygen transport and the aerobic energy system are the most severely affected by the hypobaric conditions at altitude. At the summit

---

■■■ IN REVIEW . . . ■■■

1. The hypoxic conditions (diminished oxygen supply) at altitude alter many of the body's normal physiological responses. Pulmonary ventilation increases, resulting in a hyperventilation state in which too much carbon dioxide can be cleared, leading to respiratory alkalosis. In response, the kidneys excrete more bicarbonate ion, so less acid can be buffered.

2. Pulmonary diffusion is not hindered by altitude, but oxygen transport is slightly impaired because hemoglobin saturation at altitude is reduced, although by only a small amount.

3. The diffusion gradient that allows oxygen exchange between the blood and active tissue is substantially reduced at elevation, thus oxygen uptake is impaired. This is partially compensated for by a decrease in plasma volume, concentrating the red blood cells and allowing more oxygen to be transported per unit of blood.

4. Maximal oxygen consumption decreases along with atmospheric pressure. As the partial pressure of oxygen decreases, $\dot{V}O_2$ max decreases at a progressively greater rate.

5. During submaximal work at altitude, the body increases its cardiac output, by increasing the heart rate, to compensate for the decrease in the pressure gradient that drives oxygen exchange.

6. During maximal work, stroke volume and heart rate are both lower, resulting in a reduced cardiac output. This combined with the decreased pressure gradient severely impairs oxygen delivery and uptake.

7. Because oxygen delivery is restricted at altitude, oxidative capacity is decreased. More anaerobic energy production must occur, as evidenced by increased blood lactate levels for a given submaximal work rate. However, at maximal work rates, lactate levels are lower, perhaps because the body must work at a rate that cannot fully stress the energy systems.

---

of Mount Everest, $\dot{V}O_2$ max is reduced to 10% to 25% of its value at sea level. This severely limits the body's exercise capacity. Because $\dot{V}O_2$ max is reduced by a certain percentage, individuals with larger aerobic capacities can perform a standard work task with less perceived effort and with less cardiovascular stress at altitude than those with lower $\dot{V}O_2$ max values. This may explain how Messner and Habeler were able to reach the summit of Everest without supplemental oxygen in 1978. They obviously possessed high sea-level $\dot{V}O_2$ max values.

KEY POINT

Athletes that are typically not highly endurance-trained can prepare themselves for competition at altitude through high-intensity endurance training at sea level, or at whatever elevation they live, for the purpose of increasing their $\dot{V}O_2$ max. Then, on arrival at altitude, competition at any given rate of work can be performed at a lower percentage of their $\dot{V}O_2$ max.

IN REVIEW . . .

1. Endurance activity suffers the most in hypobaric conditions because oxidative energy production is limited.
2. Anaerobic sprint activities that last less than one minute are generally not impaired at moderate altitude.
3. The thinner air at altitude provides less resistance to movement, which is a major reason for the amazing performances of sprint runners and long jumpers at the 1968 Olympic Games in Mexico City.

Anaerobic Sprint Activity

Whereas endurance events are impaired at altitude, anaerobic sprint activities that last less than a minute (such as swimming sprints) are generally not impaired by moderate altitude. Such activities place minimal demands on the oxygen transport system and aerobic metabolism. Instead, most of the energy is provided through the ATP-PCr and glycolytic systems.

In addition, the thinner air of altitude also provides less aerodynamic resistance to athletes' movements. At the 1968 Olympic Games, for example, the thinner air of Mexico City clearly aided the performances by the sprint runners and the long jumpers, as we saw at the beginning of this chapter.

Exhaustive Activity

Exhaustive exercise at high altitude produces lower lactate levels in the blood and muscle than exercise performed at sea level. As mentioned earlier, with limited oxygen uptake and increased reliance on anaerobic energy production, we would expect the muscles to produce more, rather than less, lactate for a given all-out effort. But studies in the 1930s showed remarkable changes in peak blood lactate values (7.9 mmol · L^{-1} at sea level compared to 1.9 mmol · L^{-1} at 5,340 m, or 17,515 ft) during exhaustive exercise at high altitude. This phenomenon might be related to decreased muscle enzyme activities and reduced total work performance that occurs in an all-out effort at altitude rather than at sea level.

Acclimatization: Prolonged Exposure to Altitude

A number of investigations have examined human habituation to altitude. When people are exposed to altitude for days and weeks, their bodies gradually adjust to the lower oxygen tension in the air. But, however well they acclimatize to the conditions at high altitude, these people never fully compensate for hypoxia. Even endurance-trained athletes who live at altitude for years never attain the level of performance or the $\dot{V}O_2$ max values that they might achieve at sea level.

In the following sections, we will examine some of the adaptations that occur with prolonged altitude exposure. We will focus on

- blood adaptations,
- muscle adaptations, and
- cardiorespiratory adaptations.

Blood Adaptations

During the first weeks at altitude there is an increase in the number of circulating erythrocytes (red blood cells). The lack of oxygen at altitude stimulates the release of erythropoietin, the hormone responsible for stimulating erythrocyte production. Within the first 3 hr of arriving at a high elevation, the blood's erythropoietin concentration increases, reaching a maximum within 24 to 48 hr.[44] After living at 4,000 m (13,120 ft) for about 6 months, a person's total blood volume increases by about 9% to 10% as a result not only of this altitude-induced stimulation of erythrocyte production but also of plasma volume expansion (discussed later).[28]

The percentage of total blood volume composed of erythrocytes is referred to as the hematocrit. Residents in the central Andes of Peru (4,540 m or 14,891 ft) have an average hematocrit of 65%. This is considerably higher than the average hematocrit of sea-level residents, which is only 48%. However, during 6 weeks of exposure to the Peruvian altitude, sea-level residents have shown remarkable increases in their hematocrits, up to an average of 59%.

As the volume of erythrocytes increases, so does the blood's hemoglobin content. As noted in Figure 12.4, blood hemoglobin concentration tends to increase

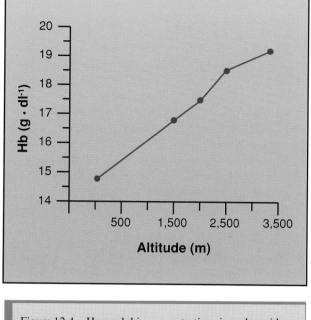

Figure 12.4 Hemoglobin concentrations in male residents at various altitudes.

Table 12.3 Changes in Muscle Structure and Metabolic Potential During 4 to 6 Weeks of Chronic Hypoxia

Parameter	Change	% change
Muscle area	Decreased	11-13
Slow-twitch fiber area	Decreased	21-25
Fast-twitch fiber area	Decreased	19
Capillary density (capillaries per mm²)	Increased	13
Succinate dehydrogenase	Decreased	25
Citrate synthase	Decreased	21
Phosphorylase	Decreased	32
Phosphofructokinase	Decreased	48

exponentially among residents at various elevations. These adaptations improve the oxygen-carrying capacity of a fixed volume of blood.

Plasma volume decreases within a few hours of arrival at altitude as a result of fluid shifts and respiratory water loss. Recall that more water is lost by evaporation during respiration at altitude because the air entering the lungs is very dry. This causes dehydration, which decreases the plasma volume. This reduction in plasma volume concentrates the erythrocytes, even further increasing the blood's oxygen-carrying capacity.

KEY POINT

At altitude, plasma volume initially decreases, resulting in more red blood cells, and thus hemoglobin, for a given volume of blood. This increases the oxygen-carrying capacity of a given volume of blood. This adaptation is beneficial at rest and during low levels of exercise, but it reduces endurance capacity at near-maximal and maximal levels of exercise.

Muscle Adaptations

Although few attempts have been made to study muscular changes that occur during exposure to altitude, sufficient muscle biopsy data indicate that muscles undergo significant structural and metabolic changes during ascent to altitude. Table 12.3 summarizes some of the muscle adaptations that accompanied 4 to 6 weeks of chronic hypoxia during expeditions to Mount Everest and Mount McKinley. Muscle fiber areas decreased, thus decreasing total muscle area. Capillary density in the muscles increased, which allowed more blood and oxygen to be delivered to them. The cause for these changes is currently being debated. Muscles' inability to meet exercise demands at high altitude might be related to a decrease in their mass and their ability to generate ATP.

Prolonged exposure to high altitude frequently causes a loss of appetite and a noticeable weight loss. During a 1992 expedition to climb Mount McKinley, six men experienced an average weight loss of 6 kg (13.2 lb). Although part of this loss represents a general decrease in body weight and extracellular water, all the men experienced a noticeable decrease in muscle mass. As shown in Table 12.3, this is associated with a significant decrease in the cross-sectional area of both the slow-twitch (ST) and the fast-twitch (FT) muscle fibers. It seems logical to assume that this decrease in muscle mass is associated with loss of appetite and a wasting of muscle protein. Perhaps future studies on nutrition and body composition in mountain climbers will provide a more thorough explanation of the incapacitating influences of high altitude on muscle.

Several weeks at high altitude (above 2,500 m, or 8,200 ft) reduces the metabolic potential of muscle. Though this may not occur at lower elevations, at the higher elevations of Mount McKinley and Mount Everest, the mitochondria and glycolytic enzyme activities of the leg muscles (vastus lateralis and gastrocnemius) are significantly reduced after 3 to 4 weeks. This suggests that in addition to receiving less oxygen, muscles lose some of their capacity to perform oxidative phosphorylation and to perform both aerobic and anaerobic exercise. Unfortunately, no muscle biopsy data have been obtained from residents at high altitudes to determine whether these individuals experience any muscular adaptations as a consequence of living at these elevations.

Cardiorespiratory Adaptations

One of the most important adaptations to altitude is an increase in pulmonary ventilation, both at rest and during exercise. Ventilation is stimulated by the decreased oxygen content of the inspired air at altitude. At an elevation of 4,000 m (13,100 ft), ventilation can be increased by 50% at rest and during submaximal exercise. However, as noted earlier, such hyperventilation also promotes the unloading of CO_2 and the alkalization of blood. To prevent the blood from becoming abnormally alkaline, the amount of blood bicarbonate decreases rapidly during the first few days at altitude and remains depressed throughout the stay at high elevations.

The decrements in $\dot{V}O_2$ max upon first reaching higher altitude improves little during several weeks of exposure to hypoxia. The lack of improvement in aerobic capacity at altitude has been studied in endurance-trained runners. Aerobic capacity remained unchanged after 18 to 57 days at altitude.[4,15] Although the runners who had previously been exposed to altitude were more tolerant of hypoxia, their $\dot{V}O_2$ max and running performance were not significantly improved with acclimatization. Because of the blood changes that occur during these relatively long visits to altitude, finding no improvement in aerobic endurance is somewhat unexpected. Perhaps these trained subjects had already attained maximal training adaptations and were unable to further adapt as a consequence of altitude exposure. Or perhaps the reduced PO_2 of altitude made it more difficult for them to train at the same intensity and with the same volume as at sea level.

Physical Training and Performance

We have considered the major changes that occur as the human body becomes acclimatized to altitude and how these adaptations affect performance at altitude. But what happens when physical training is combined with altitude?

Altitude Training for Sea-Level Performance

Can altitude training improve sea-level performance? Most studies have shown no improvement in sea-level performance following altitude training. In the few studies where altitude training was found to influence postaltitude-sea-level performance, the subjects were not well trained before going to altitude. This makes it difficult to determine how much of their postaltitude improvement was due solely to training, independent of altitude.

Studying athletes at altitude poses a difficult problem because they are often unable to train at the same volume and intensity of effort as when at sea level. In addition, the conditions at moderate to high altitude often cause them to dehydrate and to lose fat-free mass. These and other conditions tend to diminish the athletes' fitness and their tolerance for intense training. As a result, previous studies are difficult to interpret, and the debate over the value of altitude training for optimal performance continues.

> ### ◼ KEY POINT ◼
>
> **Altitude training has been used in an attempt to improve the endurance performance of athletes. This form of training, however, is expensive (due to transportation, housing, food, and other costs), and its effectiveness is not fully supported by the existing research conducted on endurance athletes.**

A strong theoretical argument can be made for altitude training. First, altitude training evokes a substantial tissue hypoxia (reduced oxygen supply). This is thought to be essential for initiating the conditioning response. Second, the altitude-induced increase in red blood cell count and hemoglobin levels improves oxygen delivery upon return to sea level. Although evidence suggests these latter changes are transient, lasting only several days, this still should provide an advantage for the athlete.

We might anticipate that all these adaptations would give the athlete a distinct advantage upon returning to sea level. Anecdotal reports from athletes who train at moderate altitude and compete at sea level tend to support this concept, but to resolve this issue we must await more definitive results. Most authorities agree that highly trained athletes can benefit little from additional training at altitude. However, though this concept of training is still under debate, many coaches and athletes are convinced that altitude training enhances performance (such as competitive swimming).

Training for Performance at Altitude

What about athletes who normally train at sea level but must compete at altitude? What can they do to prepare most effectively for competition? Although research thus far has not been conclusive, it appears that athletes have two options. One option is to compete within 24 hr of arrival at higher altitudes. This does not provide much acclimatization, but the altitude exposure is brief enough that the classic symptoms of altitude sickness have not yet become totally manifest. After the first 24 hr, the athlete's physical condition worsens because of physiological responses to altitude, such as dehydration and sleep disturbances.

The other option is to train at higher altitudes for at least 2 weeks before competing. But not even 2 weeks is sufficient for total acclimatization—that would require a minimum of 4 to 6 weeks. For team sports requiring considerable endurance (such as basketball, volleyball, or football), several weeks of intense aerobic training at sea level to increase the athletes' $\dot{V}O_2$ max levels will let them compete at altitude at a lower relative intensity than those who haven't prepared in a similar manner.

Training for optimal adaptations at altitude requires an elevation between 1,500 m (4,921 ft), which is considered the lowest level at which an effect will be noticed, and 3,000 m (9,843 ft), which is the highest level for efficient conditioning. Work capacity will be reduced during the initial days at altitude. For this reason, when first reaching higher altitudes, workout intensity should be reduced to between 60% and 70% of sea-level intensity, gradually working up to full intensity within 10 to 14 days.

Adaptations to altitude are generally responses to the hypoxia experienced there, so we might anticipate that similar adaptations could be achieved by simply breathing gases with a low P_{O_2}. But no evidence supports the idea that brief periods (1 to 2 hr per day) of breathing hypobaric gases will induce even a partial adaptation similar to that observed at altitude. On the other hand, Daniels and Oldridge observed that alternate periods of training at 2,287 m (7,503 ft) and at sea level adequately stimulated altitude acclimatization.[12] Staying at sea level for up to 11 days did not interfere with the usual adjustments to altitude as long as training was maintained.

Clinical Problems of Acute Exposure to Altitude

In addition to the cold, wind, and solar radiation that confronts those who ascend to moderate and high altitudes, some people can experience symptoms of altitude (mountain) sickness. This is characterized by such symptoms as headache, nausea, vomiting, dyspnea (difficult breathing), and insomnia. These symptoms typically begin 6 to 96 hr after arriving at high altitude. Although medically not life threatening, acute altitude sickness can be incapacitating for several days or longer. In some cases, conditions can worsen. The victim can develop the more lethal altitude illnesses of high-altitude pulmonary edema or high-altitude cerebral edema. Let's examine these conditions, their causes, and precautions that can be taken to avoid them.

IN REVIEW . . .

1. Hypoxic conditions stimulate the release of erythropoietin, which increases erythrocyte (red blood cell) production. More red blood cells means more hemoglobin. Although plasma volume decreases initially, which also concentrates the hemoglobin, it eventually returns to normal. Normal plasma volume plus additional red blood cells increases total blood volume. All of these changes increase blood oxygen-carrying capacity.

2. Total muscle mass decreases when at altitude, as does total body weight. Part of this is from dehydration and appetite suppression, which leads to protein breakdown in the muscles.

3. Other muscle adaptations include decreased fiber area, increased capillary supply and decreased metabolic enzyme activities.

4. The decrease in $\dot{V}O_2$ max with initial exposure to altitude does not improve much during several weeks of exposure.

5. Most studies show that training at altitude leads to no significant improvement of sea-level performance. The physiological changes that do occur, such as increased red blood cell production, are transient but could offer an advantage during the first few days after returning to sea level. This is still an area of debate.

6. Athletes who must perform at altitude should do so within the first 24 hr of arrival while the detrimental changes that occur have not yet become too great.

7. Alternatively, athletes who must perform at altitude could train at an altitude of 1,500 m (4,921 ft) to 3,000 m (9,843 ft) for at least 2 weeks prior to performing. This allows their bodies time to adapt to hypoxic and other environmental conditions at altitude.

Acute Altitude Sickness

The incidence of acute altitude sickness varies with the altitude, rate of ascent, and the individuals' susceptibility.[17] Several studies have been conducted to determine the frequency of acute altitude sickness in groups of hikers. Reports vary widely, ranging from a frequency of 0.1% to 53% at altitudes of 3,000 m to 5,500 m (9,840 ft to 18,044 ft). Forster, however, reported that 80% of those who ascended to the top of Mauna Kea (4,205 m, or 13,796 ft) on the island of Hawaii experienced some symptoms of acute altitude sickness.[13] The symptoms vary widely at 2,500 m to 3,500 m (8,200 to 11,480 ft), altitudes commonly experienced by most recreational skiers and hikers. At these elevations the incidence of acute altitude sickness is about 6.5% for men and 22.2% for women (the reason for this gender difference is unclear).[35]

Though the underlying cause of acute altitude sickness is not fully understood, several studies indicate that those people who experience the greatest distress also have a low ventilatory response to hypoxia.[18,22,25] Some people experience reduced breathing rate and depth during acute exposures to moderate and high altitude. This reduced ventilation allows carbon dioxide to accumulate in the tissues, and this may induce most of the symptoms associated with altitude sickness.

Another side effect of acute altitude sickness is an inability to sleep despite marked fatigue. Studies have shown that the inability to achieve satisfying sleep at altitude is associated with an interruption in the sleep stages.[42] In addition, some people suffer interrupted breathing, called Cheyne-Stokes breathing, which prevents them from relaxing and falling to sleep. Cheyne-Stokes breathing is characterized by alternating rapid breathing and slow, shallow breathing, usually including intermittent periods in which breathing completely stops. The incidence of this irregular breathing pattern increases with altitude, occurring 24% of the time at 2,440 m (8,005 ft), 40% of the time at 4,270 m (14,009 ft), and 100% of the time at altitudes above 6,300 m (20,669 ft).[39,43]

How can athletes avoid acute altitude sickness? We would like to think that well-trained individuals would be less susceptible to this disorder than poorly trained individuals, but no evidence indicates that physical conditioning prevents the symptoms of altitude sickness. The athlete who is highly endurance-trained prior to altitude exposure seems to have little protection against the effects of hypoxia, because the percentage by which $\dot{V}O_2$ max is reduced is the same in both trained and untrained people.

The prevention and treatment of acute altitude sickness can usually be accomplished by a gradual ascent to altitude, spending periods of a few days at lower elevations. A gradual ascent of no more than 300 m (984 ft) per day above an elevation of 3,000 m (9,843 ft) has been suggested to minimize the risks of altitude illness. Two drugs have been used to reduce the symptoms of those who develop acute altitude sickness: acetazolamide and dexamethasone. Both drugs must be used with medical supervision. Of course the definitive treatment for severe acute mountain sickness is a retreat to lower altitude.

High-Altitude Pulmonary Edema

Unlike acute mountain sickness, pulmonary edema, which is the accumulation of fluids in the lungs, is life threatening. The cause of high-altitude pulmonary edema (HAPE) is unknown. It seems to occur most frequently in people who rapidly ascend to altitudes above 2,700 m (8,858 ft). This disorder occurs in otherwise healthy people and has been reported more often in children and young adults. The fluid accumulation interferes with air movement into and out of the lungs, leading to shortness of breath and excessive fatigue. Disruption of normal breathing impairs blood oxygenation, causing blueness of the lips and fingernails, mental confusion, and loss of consciousness. HAPE is treated by administering supplemental oxygen and moving the victim to a lower altitude.

High-Altitude Cerebral Edema

Some rare cases of high-altitude cerebral edema (HACE), which is fluid accumulation in the cranial cavity, have been reported. This condition is characterized by mental confusion, progressing to coma and death. Most cases have been reported at altitudes greater than 4,300 m (14,106 ft). The cause of HACE is unknown, but the treatment is administration of supplemental oxygen and descent to a lower altitude.

IN REVIEW . . .

1. Acute altitude sickness typically causes symptoms such as headaches, nausea, vomiting, dyspnea, and insomnia. These usually appear in 6 to 96 hr after arrival at altitude.
2. The exact cause of acute altitude sickness is not known, but many researchers suspect the symptoms may result from carbon dioxide accumulation in the tissues.
3. Acute altitude sickness can usually be avoided by a gradual ascent to altitude, climbing no more than 300 m (984 ft) per day at elevations above 3,000 m (9,843 ft). Medications can also be used to reduce the symptoms.
4. Pulmonary edema and cerebral edema, which involve accumulation of fluid in the lungs and cranial cavity, respectively, are life-threatening conditions. Both are treated by oxygen administration and descent.

Hyperbaric Conditions: Exercising Underwater

The popularity of recreational scuba diving and snorkel diving presents a unique challenge to human physiology. Aside from the thermal effects of water (chapter 11), the body must endure the effects of a hyperbaric environment—an environment in which the pressure is greater than at sea level. This environment increases the pressure of the gases contained in the paranasal sinuses, the respiratory tract, and the gastrointestinal tract and dissolved in body fluids. In the following discussion we will consider the physiological effects you experience when submerged underwater.

Water Immersion and Gas Pressures

A balloon filled with air above water shrinks rapidly when it is pushed only a few feet below the water's surface. Even above water, the air we breathe is under the pressure of the weight of the atmosphere (1 atmosphere, or 760 mmHg at sea level). When you descend to a depth of 10 m (33 ft), water exerts an additional 760 mmHg pressure on you. Because water is more dense than air, the pressure at this depth—under 10 m of water—equals the pressure experienced with a 6,000 m (19,685 ft) descent into a mine shaft.

Recall that volume and pressure are inversely related, so as pressure increases, volume decreases. As shown in Figure 12.5, the air you breathe into your lungs at the surface will be compressed to one half its volume when you descend to a depth of 10 m. If you continue to descend to greater depths, the gas volume becomes progressively smaller. At a depth of 30 m (98.4 ft), for example, your lung volume will be reduced to 25% of its volume at the surface.

Conversely, air taken into your lungs at a depth of 10 m will expand to twice its original volume by the time you reach the water's surface. Let's consider an example of a diver breathing from a self-contained underwater breathing apparatus (scuba). It would be extremely dangerous for you to take in a deep breath at a depth of 10 m (33 ft) and then to hold this breath as you ascend to the surface. As you ascend, the air would expand in your lungs. Before you reached the surface, your lungs would overdistend, rupturing the alveoli and causing pulmonary hemorrhage and lung collapse (this condition, known as spontaneous pneumothorax, is discussed later). If air bubbles enter the circulatory system as a result of this extensive damage, emboli develop and can block major vessels, leading to extensive tissue damage, if not death. Thus it is important for divers to always exhale as they ascend to the surface.

Whereas the gases in the body are compressible, water and body fluids are noncompressible and thus are not measurably affected by either water depth or increased pressure. Nevertheless, we cannot ignore the pressure exerted by water on the gases (oxygen, nitrogen, and carbon dioxide) dissolved in body fluids. Breathing air at a depth of 10 m doubles the partial pressure of each of the gases (Table 12.4). At depths approaching 30 m, the partial pressures of the dissolved gases are four times greater than on the surface. This increase in their partial pressures causes more molecules of these gases to dissolve in the body fluids. If the pressure is decreased too rapidly during ascent, the partial pressures of the gases in the body fluids will exceed the water pressure. As a result, the tissue gases can come out of solution, forming bubbles. We will discuss this condition later.

━━ IN REVIEW . . . ━━

1. Submersion in water exposes the human body to a hyperbaric environment—one in which the external pressure is greater than at sea level.
2. Because volume decreases as pressure increases, air that is in the body before it goes underwater is compressed when the body is submerged. Conversely, the air taken in at depth expands during ascent.
3. More molecules of gas are forced into solution when the body is submerged, but with a rapid ascent they come out of solution and can form bubbles.

Cardiovascular Response to Water Immersion

Water immersion reduces the stress on the cardiovascular system. Immersing the body to the neck applies pressure to the lower body, which tends to minimize blood pooling and facilitate blood return to the heart, reducing the cardiovascular system's work. In addition, plasma volume tends to increase, as seen by a reduction in hemoglobin and hematocrit. As a result, resting heart rate can drop by 5 to 8 beats per minute with only partial body immersion. In addition, placing the face in the water lowers the heart rate even further. This is the result of a facial reflex common to many mammals.

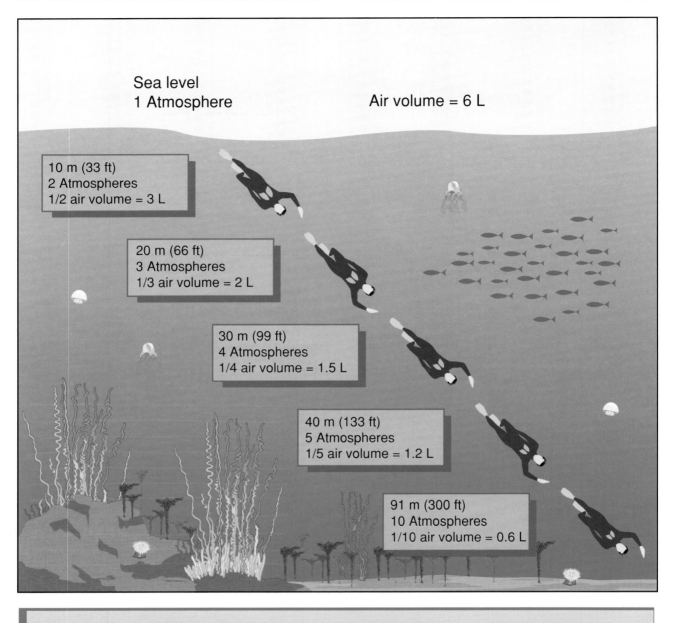

Figure 12.5   The relationship between varied depths of water submersion and the volume of air in the diver's lungs.

Table 12.4 Effects of Water Depth on the Partial Pressure of Inspired Oxygen (Po_2) and Nitrogen (Pn_2)

Depth (m)	Total pressure (mmHg)	Po_2 (mmHg)	Pn_2 (mmHg)
0	760	159	600
10	1,520	318	1,201
20	2,280	477	1,802
30	3,040	636	2,402

In some diving animals (such as beavers, seals, and whales) heart rate can be reduced (bradycardia) by 90% during diving. In humans, bradycardia is typically more than 50% of the predive heart rate.[34] For example, if your predive heart rate is 70 beats per minute, it might drop to only 40 to 45 beats per minute during submersion. Cold water can exaggerate the drop in both resting and exercise heart rate during immersion.[21] From a clinical point of view, the incidence of irregularities in cardiac conduction increases significantly

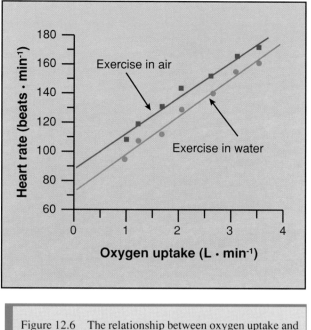

Figure 12.6   The relationship between oxygen uptake and heart rate during exercise in air and water.

when the water temperature is low. In other words, diving in cold water is associated with greater bradycardia and a higher incidence of cardiac arrythmias. Of greatest importance is the fact that at a given exercise effort in the water, such as at a certain $\%\dot{V}O_2\ _{max}$, a person's heart rate can be 10 to 12 beats per minute lower than during similar effort on land, as seen in Figure 12.6.

Breath-Hold Diving

Breath-hold diving is the oldest form of diving and is still used for recreation and work. The length of time that swimmers can hold their breath is determined by the breakpoint at which the stimulus to breathe becomes too strong to resist. The urge to breathe while underwater results from a buildup of arterial carbon dioxide, which, you should recall from chapter 9, is the greatest breathing stimulus. Voluntarily increasing either the rate or depth of breathing, such as by hyperventilating, before a dive increases carbon dioxide removal from the body tissues. This can lengthen the time that you can hold your breath before you must breathe.[26] Remember, though, that hyperventilation does not increase the oxygen content of the blood. Thus, although hyperventilation may increase your breath-holding ability, it does not increase your oxygen reserves. Arterial oxygen levels can drop to critically low levels in some individuals, causing them to lose consciousness before the carbon dioxide buildup in their blood forces them to the surface to breathe.[11]

Generally, swimming at the surface poses no pressure problems for the body's air compartments (lungs, respiratory passages, sinuses, middle ear, etc.), but breath-hold diving a meter or two below the surface can quickly pressurize these compartments. This can cause some discomfort to the ears and sinuses unless the gases trapped in these compartments are equalized to the pressure of the water by holding your nose closed and blowing air into the middle ear and sinuses.

As a breath-hold diver descends, the chest wall is squeezed and the volume of air in the lungs is reduced because of the increasing water pressure surrounding the diver. Eventually, lung volume can be reduced to the residual volume of the lung, but no smaller. Recall that the residual volume is the amount of air that remains in the lungs after maximal exhalation, so it is the amount that cannot be exhaled. If the diver attempts to descend below that depth, the blood vessels in the lungs and respiratory tract can rupture because the blood pressure in the vessels exceeds the air pressure. Because of this, the depth limit to breath-hold diving is determined by the ratio between the diver's total lung volume (TLV) and residual volume (RV).

On the average, adults have a TLV:RV ratio of 4:1 or 5:1. Water pressure at 20 to 30 m is usually sufficient to compress the volume of the chest and lungs to that of the residual volume. But people with large total lung volumes and small residual volumes can descend to greater depths before this point is reached. The ama (Japanese pearl divers) work daily at depths near the limits predicted by the TLV:RV ratio. The world breath-hold record depth of 73 m was set by a man who dove approximately 12 m below the limits predicted by the TLV:RV ratio.[32]

Gases trapped in the body are not the diver's only concern when facing changing water pressures with depth. The air trapped in the diver's goggles or mask is also compressed. Compression of this air can limit the maximum depth for unassisted diving because blood vessels in the eyes and face can rupture if the air is too compressed. To minimize this problem, pearl divers who regularly descend to depths of at least 5 m (16 ft) wear goggles that trap only a very small air volume or that can be equalized with air from the nose or the mouth. Goggles with a small volume reduce the amount of air that can be compressed and minimize the risk of injury to the blood vessels of the eye.

Scuba Diving

Drawing air into the lungs when the chest is submerged under only a few feet of water requires that the gases being breathed are pressurized to equal the water pressure. Scuba is the most popular apparatus for accomplishing this task. This equipment, created by Jacques Cousteau in 1943, is illustrated in Figure 12.7, and consists of the following four components:

1. One or more tanks of air compressed to about 5.74 to 8.61 N · m^{-2} (2,000 to 3,000 psi)
2. A first-stage regulator valve for reducing the pressure from the tank to a lower breathable pressure (about 0.40 N · m^{-2}, 140 psi)
3. A second-stage regulator valve that releases air on demand at a pressure equal to that of the water
4. A one-way breathing valve that allows the pressurized air to be drawn into the lungs and to be expelled into the water during expiration

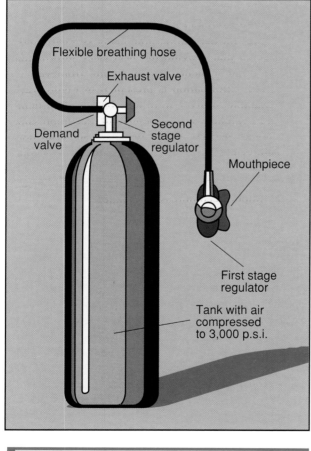

Figure 12.7 The open-circuit demand type of scuba system.

Because expired air does not return to the tanks, this form of scuba is referred to as an open-circuit–demand type. How long the diver can remain underwater depends on the depth of the dive: Deeper dives demand greater air flow to compensate for the water pressure. Because the amount of air the diver needs varies with depth, the supply of air from a scuba tank is limited by the depth of the dive. The contents of a single air tank, for example, can be exhausted in only a few minutes at a depth of 60 to 70 m (197 to 230 ft), but can last for 30 to 40 minutes when the diver is at a depth of 6 to 7 m (20 to 23 ft).

━━ IN REVIEW . . . ━━

1. Water reduces the stress on the cardiovascular system, reducing its work load. When the body is submerged, plasma volume also increases. Because of these factors, resting heart rate drops even when the body is only partially submerged. This effect is enhanced by cold water.
2. Hyperventilation is often practiced before breath-hold diving to increase how long you can hold your breath. But this can lead to dangerously low oxygen levels, which can cause you to lose consciousness underwater.
3. During breath-hold diving, the gases in your body can become pressurized even when swimming at a depth of only 1 to 2 m (3 to 6 ft) below the surface. At greater depths, the volume of air in the lungs can be reduced to the residual volume, but no smaller.
4. The depth limit to breath-hold diving is determined by the ratio of your total lung volume and your residual volume. Those with large TLV:RV ratios can safely dive deeper than those with smaller ratios.
5. Scuba diving can alleviate many of the problems faced during breath-hold diving because you breathe pressurized air while submerged.

Health Risks of Hyperbaric Conditions

The development of the underwater breathing apparatus increased divers' capacities for deeper and longer duration dives. However, this also presented them with additional health risks. As a diver descends, the air in the breathing apparatus must be pressurized to equal the pressure exerted by the water. In turn, this increases the partial pressures of all gases in the mixture. This increases the pressure gradient that drives oxygen and nitrogen into the body tissues, and the increased alveolar partial pressure of carbon dioxide decreases the pressure gradient that allows it to be cleared by the lungs. Thus breathing oxygen, carbon dioxide, and nitrogen under pressure can cause the body tissues to accumulate toxic levels of these gases.

Oxygen Poisoning

Exposure to a partial pressure of oxygen ranging from 318 mmHg to 1,500 mmHg has been shown to have severe effects, particularly on the lungs and the central nervous system.[5,33] A high P_{O_2} in inspired air can force enough oxygen into solution in the plasma that the dissolved oxygen can supply the metabolic needs of the diver, resulting in less oxygen unloading from hemoglobin at the tissues. Because of this, the hemoglobin in the venous blood will still remain highly saturated with oxygen.

Carbon dioxide does not bind as well to hemoglobin that is fully saturated with oxygen, so this impairs carbon dioxide elimination via hemoglobin. In addition, when the diver breathes oxygen at a P_{O_2} greater than 318 mmHg (twice the normal atmospheric P_{O_2}), cerebral blood vessels can become constricted, severely restricting the circulation to the central nervous system. This can result in such symptoms as visual distortion, rapid and shallow breathing, and convulsions. In some cases, this high P_{O_2} can irritate the respiratory tract, eventually leading to pneumonia. This condition, resulting from excessive oxygen, is referred to as oxygen poisoning.

Decompression Sickness

The high partial pressure of nitrogen experienced during diving forces more nitrogen into the blood and tissues. If the diver attempts to ascend too rapidly, this additional nitrogen cannot be delivered to and released from the lungs quickly enough, and it becomes trapped as bubbles in the circulatory system and the tissues. This causes severe discomfort and pain, and is referred to as decompression sickness, or the bends. Typically, this disorder is characterized by aching in the elbows, shoulders, and knees where nitrogen bubbles accumulate. If bubbles become emboli in the blood, they can interfere with normal circulation, and this can be fatal.

Treatment involves placing the diver in a recompression chamber (see Figure 12.8). The air pressure is increased in the chamber (recompression) to simulate that experienced while diving, and then it is gradually returned to the ambient pressure. Recompression

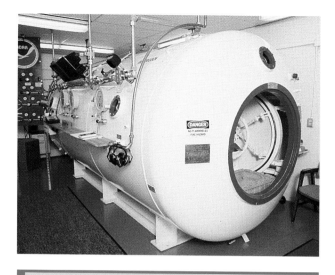

Figure 12.8   A recompression chamber.

forces the nitrogen back into solution, then a gradual decrease in pressure allows the nitrogen to escape through the respiratory system.

To prevent decompression sickness, charts have been created that provide the necessary information about the time sequence for ascending from various depths. This information is presented in Figure 12.9. If, for example, a diver were to submerge to a depth of about 50 ft (about 15 m) for an hour, decompression would not be needed. But if the diver spent an hour at a depth of about 100 ft (about 30 m), slow decompression would be necessary. Strict adherence to the timetable for a specific diving depth allows a safe ascent without decompression sickness.

Nitrogen Narcosis

Although nitrogen is not metabolically active, meaning it doesn't participate in biological processes in our bodies, at high pressures, such as during deep dives, it can act much like an anaesthetic gas. The resulting condition is referred to as nitrogen narcosis, or rapture of the deep. The effect worsens as depth, and consequently pressure, increases. The diver develops symptoms similar to alcohol intoxication. In fact, research suggests that for every 15-m increase in depth this effect equals that of one martini ingested on an empty stomach.

Divers at depths of 30 m or more have impaired judgment, but might not recognize the problem. Poor judgment during diving can be life threatening, so most divers who descend below 30 m breathe a specialized gas mixture containing mostly helium.

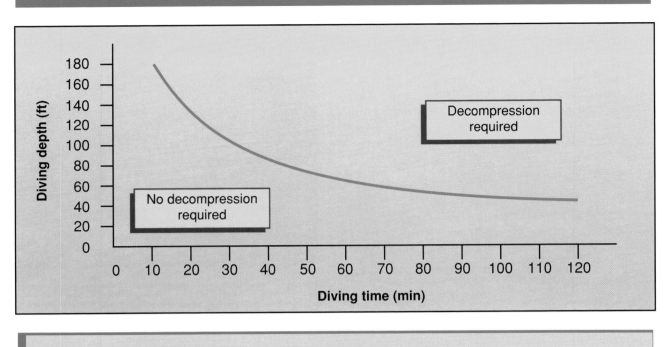

Figure 12.9   The need for decompression during diving at various depths and durations.

Spontaneous Pneumothorax

Breathing pressurized gas at a depth of more than a meter or two below the surface can create a major problem if the gas is not expelled during ascent. A full breath taken at 2 m and held will expand enough during ascent to overdistend the lungs. This can rupture alveoli, allowing gas to enter the pleural space, in turn collapsing the lung. This is known as a spontaneous pneumothorax, depicted in Figure 12.10. At the same time, small air bubbles can enter the pulmonary blood and form air emboli, which can become trapped in the vessels of other tissues, blocking circulation to those tissues. Severe blockage of the vessels supplying the lungs, myocardium, and central nervous system can cause death. Fortunately, this condition can be pre-

Staying Underwater

A series of SEALAB projects conducted by the U.S. Navy have enabled divers to live at depths of from 60 to 260 m for up to 30 days. To allow these long stays, the Navy developed a technique called saturation diving. This technique is based on the fact that, at a given depth, the amount of metabolically inactive gases (such as nitrogen) that can dissolve in body tissues is limited. While living in a pressurized housing for about 24 h, the body tissues become saturated with nitrogen gas. After saturation is reached, the tissues do not absorb significantly more nitrogen no matter how long the diver stays at that depth. For time-consuming underwater work, it is far more efficient to stay at depth and complete the job than to repeatedly return to the surface, spending hours in decompression before each return.

Although brief ascents and descents to depths of nearly 100 m are possible with adequate precautions and decompression, the Navy's saturation diving program with SEALAB I, II, and III has brought to light some pathological problems associated with prolonged habitation in hyperbaric conditions. These problems generally relate to the narcotic effects of nitrogen. Substituting helium for nitrogen appears to cause far fewer effects, though it is difficult for divers to talk (helium causes the voice to sound like Donald Duck). Studies conducted before, during, and after the SEALAB project show that prolonged exposure to hyperbaric conditions will have metabolic and cardiovascular consequences.[19] These findings are outside the scope of this discussion, but can be considered in greater detail in a paper by Hochachka and one by Hochachka and Storey.[19,20]

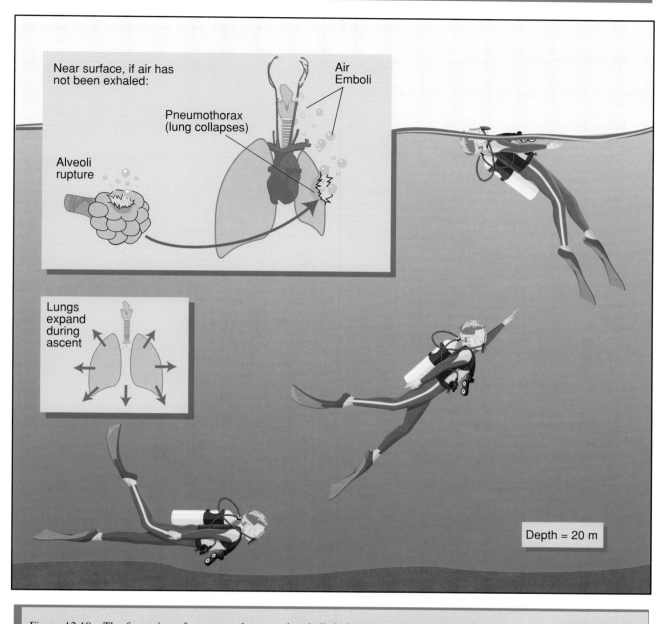

Figure 12.10   The formation of a pneumothorax and emboli during ascent from scuba diving.

vented simply by keeping the mouth open and exhaling, allowing the compressed air in the respiratory passageways to escape during ascent.

Ruptured Eardrum

In addition to the risk of spontaneous pneumothorax and air embolism, not equalizing the air pressure in the sinuses and middle ear during ascent and descent can rupture the small blood vessels and membranes that line these cavities. Pressure in the middle ear is normally allowed to equalize through the eustachian tube (which connects the middle ear to the throat). Inability to equalize the pressure in the middle ear creates unequal force against the eardrum, causing considerable pain. Under severe conditions, as during ascent or descent in deep water, an inability to equalize this pressure can rupture the eardrum.

During diving, the middle ear and the sinuses can usually be equalized by blowing with moderate pressure against the closed nostrils. But because upper respiratory infections and sinusitis can cause swelling of the membranes in the sinuses and eustachian tube, scuba and breath-hold diving is not recommended for people suffering from these conditions.

Some of the health risks associated with hyperbaric conditions are depicted in Figure 12.11. This section is not meant to cover all of the health risks.

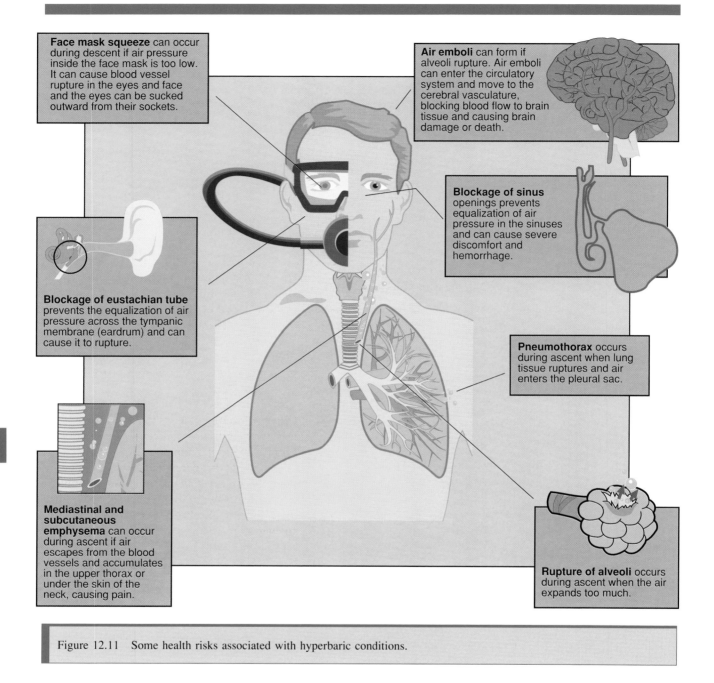

Face mask squeeze can occur during descent if air pressure inside the face mask is too low. It can cause blood vessel rupture in the eyes and face and the eyes can be sucked outward from their sockets.

Air emboli can form if alveoli rupture. Air emboli can enter the circulatory system and move to the cerebral vasculature, blocking blood flow to brain tissue and causing brain damage or death.

Blockage of sinus openings prevents equalization of air pressure in the sinuses and can cause severe discomfort and hemorrhage.

Blockage of eustachian tube prevents the equalization of air pressure across the tympanic membrane (eardrum) and can cause it to rupture.

Pneumothorax occurs during ascent when lung tissue ruptures and air enters the pleural sac.

Mediastinal and subcutaneous emphysema can occur during ascent if air escapes from the blood vessels and accumulates in the upper thorax or under the skin of the neck, causing pain.

Rupture of alveoli occurs during ascent when the air expands too much.

Figure 12.11   Some health risks associated with hyperbaric conditions.

Rather, we have provided only an overview of some common and more serious risks. Diving can be dangerous for the inexperienced, and even the most experienced divers can get into trouble if they don't follow proper procedures or if they ignore the health risks associated with this sport.

Microgravity Environments: Exercising in Space

The human body has a tremendous capacity to adapt to considerable environmental variations. In this and the previous chapter, we have discussed adaptations in response to heat, cold, humidity, and hypobaric (altitude) and hyperbaric (diving) conditions. Now we shift our focus to an unusual condition that most of us will never experience: prolonged microgravity.

Earth's gravity produces a standard acceleration force of 1 g (g is the symbol used for gravitational force). Microgravity refers to reduced gravity, so the term is used to define conditions where the gravitational force is less than on the Earth's surface (less than 1 g). For example, the moon's gravitational pull is only about 17% of that experienced here on Earth, or 0.17 g. The term microgravity is often used to

▬ IN REVIEW . . . ▬

1. Breathing gases under pressure can cause the body to accumulate gases in toxic levels, so precautions must be taken when diving with pressurized gases.
2. Oxygen poisoning occurs when P_{O_2} values are above 318 mmHg. Less oxygen will be removed from the hemoglobin for use by the tissues. This impairs the binding of carbon dioxide to the hemoglobin, so less carbon dioxide is removed by this route. Also, high P_{O_2} causes vasoconstriction in the cerebral vessels, which decreases blood flow to the brain.
3. Decompression sickness (the bends) results from ascending too rapidly. The nitrogen dissolved in the body cannot be removed by the lungs quickly enough, so it forms bubbles. The bubbles can form emboli, which can be fatal. To treat this, the diver must undergo recompression to force the nitrogen back into solution, then undergo gradual decompression at a rate that allows the nitrogen to be removed during normal breathing. Tables have been formulated that specify how much time must be allowed for ascension from various depths, and divers must adhere strictly to these.
4. Nitrogen narcosis (rapture of the deep) results from the narcotic effects of nitrogen when its partial pressure is high, such as during depth diving. The symptoms are similar to alcohol intoxication. Judgment is impaired, which can lead to fatal mistakes.
5. Spontaneous pneumothorax and ruptured eardrum are other health risks associated with the changing pressures experienced when diving.

▬ KEY POINT ▬

Most physiological changes that occur as a result of extended periods of exposure to microgravity conditions during spaceflight are similar to those seen with detraining in athletes and with reduced activity in the aging population.

Physiological Alterations With Chronic Microgravity Exposure

Microgravity presents a challenge to normal body functions. An object's weight, which reflects the strength of the gravitational force pulling on it, decreases as the object moves away from the Earth's surface. At a distance of 8,000 mi (12,872 km), for example, body weight is only about 25% of its value on Earth. At 210,000 mi (337,890 km), the body becomes weightless because the gravitational force is 0 g. If your body is weightless, your weight-bearing bones and antigravitational muscles (those that maintain your posture) are unloaded. Reducing the stress on both bone and muscle eventually leads to their deterioration and reduces their ability to function. Similar effects are seen in cardiovascular function.

But what might be perceived as maladaptation might, in fact, be a needed adaptation to microgravity. In this section we will briefly review physiological changes that occur with chronic exposure to microgravity, focusing on

- muscle,
- bone,
- cardiovascular function, and
- body weight and composition.

Whenever possible, actual data from spaceflight will be used. Otherwise, the data will be representative of that obtained in simulated microgravity.

Muscle

Immobilization studies have shown very rapid changes in muscle structure and function when limbs are immobilized in casts or when hindlimbs of four-legged animals are suspended. Muscle atrophy results primarily from decreased protein synthesis.[30] The protein synthesis rate decreases approximately 35% in the first several hours and up to 50% in the first several days of immobilization, leading to a net loss of muscle protein.[2,37] The resulting muscle atrophy can be substantial over time. These studies were conducted on growing rats, so the time course and magnitude of

describe conditions in space, because the body might not always be in a weightless or 0 g state.

Interestingly, most physiological changes that accompany exposure to microgravity mimic, in many respects, detraining responses seen in athletes during periods of inactivity or immobilization, or the changes associated with aging that likely result from reduced activity. This link is substantiated by evidence that exercise training during periods of exposure to microgravity has become a successful countermeasure against the physiological deterioration that occurs in space. For these reasons, and because space exploration is ongoing, the effects of microgravity on physical activity is an area of increasing interest for exercise and sports physiologists.

change might differ in humans. Also, there is a major difference between immobilization and microgravity. With immobilization, the immobilized muscle undergoes little or no activation. But with microgravity the muscles are activated, but they are loaded to a lesser extent due to the loss of the effects of gravity.

Bed-rest studies that simulate microgravity have found major decreases, both in the strength and the cross-sectional area, of both slow-twitch and fast-twitch muscle fibers, with the fast-twitch fibers tending to be the most affected.[8] These relationships are illustrated in Figure 12.12. From Figure 12.12a, note the close agreement for changes in leg strength, leg volume, and body weight between a 30-day–bed-rest trial to simulate microgravity and the 28-day *Skylab 2* spaceflight.

KEY POINT

Strength and the cross-sectional areas of slow-twitch and fast-twitch muscle fibers decrease with exposure to simulated and actual microgravity.

So we must recognize the potential for muscle atrophy and loss of strength when exposed to microgravity. But results from the Skylab missions suggest that a well-designed exercise program can greatly attenuate the loss of muscle size and function.[38] More effective resistance training programs need to be developed for periods of microgravity to minimize the loss of muscle function. Astronauts could be faced with emergency situations in space or on their return to Earth that might require high levels of strength. Because the postural muscles are the most affected, creative exercise devices must be devised to allow an adequate stress to be placed on these muscles.

Bone

Most of the body's larger bones are dependent on the daily loading of gravitational forces. There has been great concern that extended space explorations of 18 months or longer could result in significant skeletal degeneration and calcium loss, increasing the risk of bone fracture upon return to Earth.[9] Calcium balance studies from the Gemini, Apollo, and Skylab missions indicated a negative calcium balance, due largely to increases in both urinary and fecal calcium excretion. Urinary excretion of hydroxyproline also increased, and this is indicative of bone resorption.

Early studies of the Gemini astronauts produced remarkable estimates of bone mineral loss:

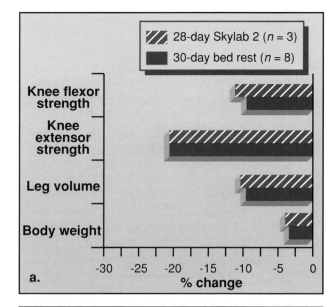

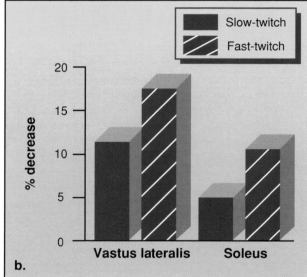

Figure 12.12 (a) Leg strength, leg volume, and body weight changes with 30 days of bed rest and a 28-day spaceflight. (b) Changes in cross-sectional area of slow-twitch and fast-twitch muscle fibers following 30 days of bed rest. Adapted from Convertino (1991).

- 2% to 15% in the calcaneus (heel)
- 3% to 25% in the radius
- 3% to 16% in the ulna

These estimates were later scaled down when it was discovered that technical error had caused an overestimation of bone mineral loss. Conversely, no bone mineral losses were reported in the same bones following the flights of *Apollo 14* and *Apollo 16*, and only slight calcaneal losses of 5% to 6% were reported in two *Apollo 15* crew members.[29] With the Skylab missions, no bone mineral loss was observed in the radius or ulna, but calcaneal losses were approximately 4%, similar to what occurs during bed rest. The calcaneus is a weight-bearing bone, but the radius and ulna are not.

KEY POINT

Microgravity generally results in bone mineral losses approximating 4% from the weight-bearing bones.

The mechanisms responsible for these bone changes have not been resolved. Bone formation could be retarded, bone resorption could be increased, or both. Furthermore, long-term consequences of these changes have not been established. It is not yet clear whether these bone mineral losses will be regained, or whether repeated exposures to microgravity are cumulative so that the astronauts would lose additional bone with each subsequent mission. It is reasonably clear, however, that those changes that have been observed in bone with microgravity or bed rest result from the mechanical unloading of bone, such that the bone is no longer exposed to the normal gravitational or muscular forces experienced on Earth.

Cardiovascular Function

One of the first changes that occurs in response to microgravity or simulated microgravity is a reduction in plasma volume. When the body is in microgravity, blood no longer pools in the lower extremities as it does at 1.0 g, because there is less hydrostatic pressure. As a consequence, more blood returns to the heart, which leads to a transient increase in cardiac output and arterial blood pressure. These increases are accompanied by an increase in the arterial pressure in the kidneys, which, in turn, causes the kidneys to excrete the excess volume. This response to increased blood pressure is referred to as pressure diuresis. Antidiuretic hormone, aldosterone, angiotensin, and atrial natriuretic factor also play roles in blood volume control, but pressure diuresis exerts the greatest control over blood volume in the microgravity state. These adaptations are essential to allow the body to regain its control over blood pressure regulation.

The reduced blood volume serves astronauts well while they remain in microgravity. But it presents a serious problem on their return to a 1-g environment, where the body is again subjected to the hydrostatic

pressure effect but now has a smaller blood volume. Astronauts have experienced postural (orthostatic) hypotension and fainting during their first few hours back in a normal 1-g environment because their blood volume was insufficient to meet all their circulatory needs.

KEY POINT

Microgravity removes most of the effects of hydrostatic pressure experienced in a 1-g environment, resulting in the body's dumping a large percentage of its plasma volume. While this allows excellent regulation of cardiovascular function at rest and during exercise in space, it presents major orthostatic hypotension problems on return to Earth's atmosphere.

Soviet cosmonauts' preflight and in-flight resting cardiac functions and blood pressures were assessed for both the 23-day *Salyut-1* mission and the 63-day *Salyut-4* mission. The in-flight measurements were made between Days 13 and 21, and at Day 56. There were no differences between preflight and in-flight values for heart rate, stroke volume, and cardiac output, although in-flight systolic blood pressure was slightly elevated (see Table 12.5). Also, during the longer *Salyut-4* mission, the in-flight heart rate response to a 5-min standardized exercise bout on a cycle ergometer was not significantly different from the preflight, Earth-based value. For the three Skylab missions, where astronauts exercised at a constant submaximal work rate, the heart rate and blood pressure responses, preflight and in-flight, did not differ.[7]

Preflight and in-flight submaximal exercise data from the 140-day flight of the orbital station *Salyut-6* are presented in Table 12.6. The cosmonauts exercised at a constant work rate for 5 min. No change from preflight values was noted for any of the variables during the first month, but stroke volume, cardiac output, and systolic blood pressure all decreased and heart rate increased through 119 days. These variations were relatively small and could reflect an inadequate in-flight exercise program.

It could be argued that the results of these in-flight tests indicate that the adaptations made in response to microgravity are precise and appropriate for the environment. This is confirmed by the studies of the *Skylab 4* astronauts, who all increased their $\dot{V}O_2\text{max}$ from preflight through the completion of their 84-day mission (see Figure 12.13).[31] These increases in $\dot{V}O_2\text{max}$ were at least

Table 12.5 Cardiovascular Function at Rest, Preflight, and During the Salyut-1 and Salyut-4 Missions

Variables	Salyut-1 23-day mission		Salyut-4 63-day mission	
	Preflight	Inflight Days 13–21	Preflight	Inflight Day 56
Heart rate (beats · min⁻¹)	64 ± 5	65 ± 5	65 ± 3	65 ± 3
Stroke volume (ml)	94 ± 3	96 ± 9	84 ± 5	90 ± 2
Cardiac output (L · min⁻¹)	6.0 ± 0.5	6.1 ± 0.1	5.5 ± 0.3	5.9 ± 0.3
Systolic blood pressure (mmHg)	113 ± 7	122 ± 4[a]	120 ± 5	130 ± 6[a]
Diastolic blood pressure (mmHg)	73 ± 3	80 ± 2[a]	86 ± 4	86 ± 1
Mean arterial pressure (mmHg)	86 ± 4	94 ± 2[a]	97 ± 4	101 ± 2
Aortic pulse wave propagation velocity (m · s⁻¹)	4.4 ± 0.4	4.9 ± 0.1[a]	6.5 ± 0.6	6.4 ± 0.6
Systemic peripheral resistance (units)	15.0 ± 2.7	16.9 ± 2.0[a]	18.6 ± 1.7	16.9 ± 1.2

Note. Values represent mean ± SE.

[a]All cosmonauts changed in the same direction compared to preflight values.

Data from Convertino (1987).

Table 12.6 Cardiovascular Function at a Standardized Rate of Work (750 k · min⁻¹) Preflight and During the 140-Day Soviet Salyut-6 Mission

Variables	Preflight	Inflight days				
		29	41	62	97	119
Heart rate (beats · min⁻¹)	113 ± 5	113 ± 4	124 ± 12[a]	116 ± 8	122 ± 7[a]	128 ± 13[a]
Stroke volume (ml)	136 ± 19	133 ± 20	134 ± 30	120 ± 26[a]	131 ± 34[a]	112 ± 20[a]
Cardiac output (L · min⁻¹)	15.3 ± 1.5	15.0 ± 1.7	16.2 ± 2.2[a]	13.7 ± 2.1[a]	15.8 ± 3.2	14.1 ± 1.2[a]
Systolic blood pressure (mmHg)	156 ± 2	157 ± 9	156 ± 1	149 ± 2[a]	144 ± 4[a]	146 ± 3[a]
Diastolic blood pressure (mmHg)	70 ± 4	69 ± 2	70 ± 3	68 ± 5	73 ± 2	69 ± 1
Aortic pulse wave propagation velocity (m · s⁻¹)	7.5 ± 0.6	7.2 ± 0.8	7.5 ± 0.9	7.9 ± 0.9[a]	7.8 ± 0.7[a]	8.5 ± 1.5[a]
Systemic peripheral resistance (units)	13.6 ± 2.1	12.8 ± 0.9	10.7 ± 2.0[a]		12.4 ± 2.9[a]	

Note. Values represent mean ± SE ($N = 2$).

[a]All cosmonauts changed in the same direction compared to preflight values.

Data from Convertino (1987).

partially due to the training that took place each day during the mission (see Figure 12.14). The important point, however, is that these astronauts did not experience cardiorespiratory deconditioning during this extended period of microgravity.

The crew's ability to adapt successfully and quickly on their return to Earth is a concern with any space mission. We already mentioned the possibility of postural hypotension upon return. Furthermore, echocardiograms from seven members of four space shuttle crews indicated increases in heart rate, mean arterial pressure, and systemic vascular resistance, and a decrease in end-diastolic volume and stroke volume within 1 hr postflight.[3] End-diastolic volume remained depressed 7 to 14 days postflight. These changes can be at least partially explained by reduced plasma volume.

Convertino et al., however, suggest other factors might be involved.[10] They reported that increased leg

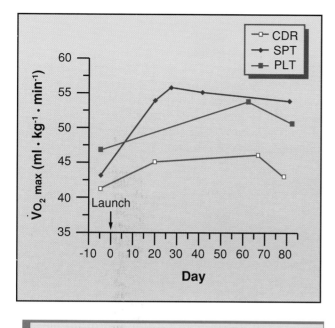

Figure 12.13 Changes in $\dot{V}O_2$ max from preflight through 83 days in space for the three astronauts aboard Skylab 4. Data from Sawin et al. (1975).

venous compliance, in which the veins of the legs can hold more blood, may contribute to the decreased end-diastolic volume. With simulated microgravity, they found a decrease in calf muscle size, which allowed greater distension of the veins. The resulting blood pooling in the legs would decrease blood return to the heart, decreasing end-diastolic volume. Countermeasures during flight that are designed to minimize atrophy of the postural muscles might help prevent this.

Body Weight and Composition

Body weight and composition have been found to change substantially as a result of both bed rest and microgravity during space flight. The 33 Apollo crew members lost an average of 3.5 kg, and the 9 Skylab crew members lost an average of 2.7 kg. Individual weight change varied considerably, from a gain of 0.1 kg to a loss of 5.9 kg.[24] The weight loss in flights of 1 to 3 days appears to be largely due to fluid loss. In flights of 12 days or longer, fluid loss accounts for approximately 50% of the weight loss and the remaining loss is primarily from fat and protein. The Skylab missions provided a comprehensive analysis of the composition of the weight loss.[24] The average 2.7-kg weight loss included

- 1.1 kg from total body water,
- 1.2 kg from fat,
- 0.3 kg from protein, and
- 0.1 kg from other sources.

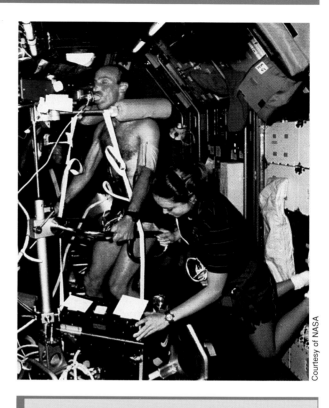

Courtesy of NASA

Figure 12.14 The Skylab 4 astronauts trained on a treadmill, but the process was difficult. A cycle ergometer, shown above, is also used for exercising in microgravity. The padded bars (blue) are placed over the shoulders to keep the subject seated.

The fat loss most likely resulted from an inadequate energy intake.

Exercise as a Countermeasure to Microgravity

Spaceflight and exposure to both short and long periods of microgravity are reasonably well tolerated. The astronaut has the remarkable ability to adapt to this unique environment, allowing normal, or near-normal, function in microgravity. But several of these adaptations pose potential problems when the astronaut returns to Earth, as we briefly described earlier in this section. The primary areas of concern are the reductions in muscle, bone, and cardiovascular regulation of blood pressure. Possible decreases in strength and the increased risk of postural hypotension are of major concern due to the potential problems they present during landing—what if the astronauts couldn't get out of their space vehicle in the event of a crash or a fire? This has led space scientists to search for appropriate countermeasures to increase the crew's likelihood of completing a successful mission.

In-flight exercise training is one of the proposed countermeasures that seems an obvious choice. Data from the Skylab missions have clearly shown that increasing exercise time and providing a variety of exercise equipment greatly attenuates muscle strength losses and even increases $\dot{V}O_2$ max.[31,38] In addition, inflight bouts of maximal exercise might be important in preparing astronauts for return to a 1.0 g environment.[6] Research suggests that even a single maximal bout of exercise can cause a transient increase in plasma volume and increased sensitivity of the arterial receptors that monitor blood pressure, allowing $\dot{V}O_2$ max to be maintained.

Finally, more attention must be focused on the design of equipment that will allow more effective resistance training in microgravity as a means to preserve muscle function. Convertino has suggested that equipment that has an eccentric component might be important because the muscle and bone can be loaded with higher resistances using eccentric-type action.[8] Training against higher resistances might also assist in preserving the calcium content of weight-bearing bones.

KEY POINT

Exercise may be one of the most effective countermeasures during spaceflight to prepare astronauts for successful adaptation on their return to Earth.

The importance of applying exercise physiology to space physiology is just now being realized. Unfortunately, research opportunities for exploring the physiological effects of microgravity are limited, and research on simulated microgravity is not as accurate as research conducted in space. Nonetheless, this promises to be an exciting area of future research for many exercise physiologists.

In Closing . . .

Activities are seldom conducted under ideal environmental conditions. Heat, cold, humidity, altitude, and the underwater environment each present unique problems for humans that impact the physiological demands of exercise. Space exploration has revealed that the body faces unique challenges during exposure to microgravity. This and the preceding chapter have attempted to summarize the nature of these various environmental stresses and how we can cope with these conditions.

Much of our discussion thus far has dealt with how physiological variables and environmental stress can hinder our performance. In the next part, we will examine various ways to optimize performance. We will begin by looking at the importance of the amount of training, considering what happens when we train either too much or too little.

Key Terms

acute altitude (mountain) sickness
decompression sickness (bends)
erythropoietin
high-altitude cerebral edema (HACE)
high-altitude pulmonary edema (HAPE)
hyperbaric environment
hypobaric environment
hypoxia
hypoxic vasoconstriction
microgravity
nitrogen narcosis
oxygen poisoning
respiratory alkalosis
scuba
spontaneous pneumothorax
TLV:RV ratio

Study Questions

1. Describe the conditions at altitude that limit physical activity.
2. What types of activities are detrimentally influenced by exposure to high altitude?
3. Describe the physiological adjustments that accompany acclimatization to altitude.
4. Would an endurance athlete who trained at altitude be able to perform better during subsequent sea-level performance? Why or why not?
5. What environmental conditions are unique to underwater diving?
6. What effect does immersion have on heart rate? What causes this effect?
7. What are some of the health risks associated with diving and using scuba?
8. Describe the physiological and pathological problems that face divers who descend to 30 m or more using scuba.
9. Under what conditions should a diver consider the need for decompression?
10. Define microgravity. What does 1.0 g represent?
11. What happens to muscle during the first few days of casting, hindlimb suspension, or microgravity? Which muscles are most vulnerable to microgravity, and why?
12. What happens to bone when exposed to simulated microgravity? Which bones are most vulnerable?

13. What physiological alterations occur with exposure to microgravity that lead to a reduced plasma volume when exposed to microgravity?

14. How does $\dot{V}O_{2\,max}$ change with prolonged exposure to microgravity? Consider preflight, inflight, and postflight values.

15. What are likely to be productive countermeasures to assist the astronaut on his or her return to Earth?

References

1. Bert, P. (1943). *La pression barometrique*. (M.A. Hitchcock & F.A. Hitchcock, Trans.). Columbus, OH: College Book Co.

2. Booth, F.W. (1982). Effect of limb immobilization on skeletal muscle. *Journal of Applied Physiology*, **52**, 1113-1118.

3. Bungo, M.W., Goldwater, D.J., Popp, R.L., & Sandler, H. (1987). Echocardiographic evaluation of space shuttle crewmembers. *Journal of Applied Physiology*, **62**, 278-283.

4. Buskirk, E.R., Kollias, J., Piconreatique, E., Akers, R., Prokop, E., & Baker, P. (1967). In R.F. Goddard (Ed.), *The effects of altitude on physical performance* (pp. 65-71). Chicago: Athletic Institute.

5. Clark, J.M., & Lambertsen, C.J. (1971). Pulmonary oxygen toxicity: A review. *Pharmacology Review*, **23**, 37-133.

6. Convertino, V.A. (1987). Potential benefits of maximal exercise just prior to return from weightlessness. *Aviation, Space, and Environmental Medicine*, **58**, 568-572.

7. Convertino, V.A. (1990). Physiological adaptations to weightlessness: Effects on exercise and work performance. *Exercise and Sport Sciences Reviews*, **18**, 119-166.

8. Convertino, V.A. (1991). Neuromuscular aspects in development of exercise countermeasures. *The Physiologist*, **34**, S125-S128.

9. Convertino, V.A., & Adams, W.C. (1991). Enhanced vagal baroreflex response during 24 h after acute exercise. *American Journal of Physiology*, **260**, R570-R575.

10. Convertino, V.A., Doerr, D.F., & Stein, S.L. (1989). Changes in size and compliance of the calf after 30 days of simulated microgravity. *Journal of Applied Physiology*, **66**, 1509-1512.

11. Cotes, J.E. (1968). Lung function: Assessment and application in medicine (2nd ed.). Philadelphia: Davis.

12. Daniels, J., & Oldridge, N. (1970). Effects of alternate exposure to altitude and sea level on world-class middle-distance runners. *Medicine and Science in Sports*, **2**, 107-112.

13. Forster, P.J.G. (1985). Effect of different ascent profiles on performance at 4200 m elevation. *Aviation, Space, and Environmental Medicine*, **56**, 785-764.

14. Green, H.J., Sutton, J., Young, P., Cymerman, A., & Houston, C.S. (1989). Operation Everest II: Muscle energetics during maximal exhaustive exercise. *Journal of Applied Physiology*, **66**, 142-150.

15. Grover, R., Reeves, J., Grover, E., & Leathers, J. (1967). Muscular exercise in young men native to 3,100 m altitude. *Journal of Applied Physiology*, **22**, 555-564.

16. Groves, B.M., Reeves, J.T., Sutton, J.R., Wagner, P.D., Cymerman, A., Malconian, M.K., Rock, P.B., Yound, P.M., & Houston, C.S. (1987). Operation Everest II: Elevated high-altitude pulmonary resistance unresponsive to oxygen. *Journal of Applied Physiology*, **63**, 521-530.

17. Hackett, P.H., Rennie, D., & Levine, H.D. (1976). The incidence, importance, and prophylaxis of acute mountain sickness. *Lancet*, **2**, 1149-1154.

18. Hackett, P.H., Roach, R.C., Schoene, R.B., Harrison, G.L., & Mills, Jr., W.J. (1988). Abnormal control of ventilation in high-altitude pulmonary edema. *Journal of Applied Physiology*, **64**, 1268-1272.

19. Hochachka, P.W. (1981). Brain, lung, and heart functions during diving and recovery. *Science*, **212**, 509-514.

20. Hochachka, P.W., & Storey, K.B. (1975). Metabolic consequences of diving in animals and man. *Science*, **187**, 613-621.

21. Hong, S.K., Song, S.H., Kim, P.K., & Suh, C.S. (1967). Seasonal observations on the cardiac rhythm during diving in the Korean ama. *Journal of Applied Physiology*, **23**, 18-22.

22. King, A.B., & Robinson, S.M. (1972). Ventilation response to hypoxia and acute mountain sickness. *Aerospace Medicine*, **43**, 419-421.

23. Kronenberg, R.S., Safar, P., Lee, J., Wright, F., Noble, W., Wahrenbrock, E., Hickey, R., Nemoto, E., & Severinghaus, J.W. (1971). Pulmonary artery pressure and alveolar gas exchange in man during acclimatization to 12,470 ft. *Journal of Clinical Investigation*, **50**, 827-837.

24. Leonard, J.I., Leach, C.S., & Rambaut, P.C. (1983). Quantitation of tissue loss during prolonged space flight. *American Journal of Clinical Nutrition*, **38**, 667-679.

25. Mathews, L., Gopinathan, P.M., & Purkayastha, S.S. (1983). Chemoreceptor sensitivity and maladap-

tion to high altitude in man. *European Journal of Applied Physiology*, **51**, 137-144.

26. Mithoefer, J.C. (1965). Breath-holding. In W.O. Fenn & H. Rahn (Eds.), *Handbook of Physiology: Section 3, Vol. II* (pp. 1011-1025). Washington, DC: American Physiological Society.

27. Norton, E.G. (1925). *The fight for Everest: 1924*. London: Arnold.

28. Pugh, L.C.G.E. (1964). Muscular exercise at great altitudes. *Journal of Applied Physiology*, **19**, 431.

29. Rambaut, P.C., Smith, M.C., Mack, P.B., & Vogel, J.M. (1975). Skeletal response. In R.S. Johnston, L.F. Dietlein, & C.A. Berry (Eds.), *Biomedical results of Apollo* (pp. 303-322) (NASA SP-368). Washington, DC: National Aeronautics and Space Administration.

30. Rennie, M.J., Edwards, R.H.T., Emery, P.W., Halliday, D., Lundholm, K., & Millward, D.J. (1983). Depressed protein synthesis is the dominant characteristic of muscle wasting and cachexia. *Clinical Physiology*, **3**, 387-398.

31. Sawin, C.F., Rummel, J.A., & Michel, E.L. (1975). Instrumented personal exercise during long-duration space flights. *Aviation, Space, and Environmental Medicine*, **46**, 394-400.

32. Schaefer, K.E., Allison, R.D., Dougherty, Jr., J.H., Carey, C.R., Walker, R., Yost, F., & Parker, D. (1968). Pulmonary and circulatory adjustments determining the limits of depth in breath-hold diving. *Science*, **162**, 1020-1023.

33. Smith, J.L. (1899). The pathological effects due to increase of oxygen tension in the air breathed. *London Journal of Physiology*, **24**, 19-35.

34. Song, S.H., Lee, W.K., Chung, Y.A., & Hong, S.K. (1969). Mechanism of apneic bradycardia in man. *Journal of Applied Physiology*, **27**, 323-327.

35. Sutton, J., & Lazarus, L. (1973). Mountain sickness in the Australian Alps. *Medical Journal of Australia*, **1**, 545-546.

36. Sutton, J.R., Reeves, J.T., Wagner, P.D., Groves, B.M., Cymerman, A., Malconian, M.K., Rock, P.B., Young, P.M., Walter, S.D., & Houston, C.S. (1988). Operation Everest II: Oxygen transport during exercise at extreme simulated altitude. *Journal of Applied Physiology*, **64**, 1309-1321.

37. Thomason, D.B., & Booth, F.W. (1990). Atrophy of the soleus muscle by hindlimb unweighting. *Journal of Applied Physiology*, **68**, 1-12.

38. Thornton, W.E., & Rummel, J.A. (1977). Muscular deconditioning and its prevention in space flight. In R.S. Johnston & S.F. Dietlein (Eds.), *Biomedical results from Skylab* (pp. 191-197) (NASA SP-377).

Washington, DC: National Aeronautics and Space Administration.

39. Waggener, T.B., Brusil, P.J., Kronauer, R.E., Gabel, R.A., & Inbar, G.F. (1984). Strength and cycle time of high altitude ventilation patterns in unacclimatized humans. *Journal of Applied Physiology*, **56**, 576-581.

40. Ward, M.P., Milledge, J.S., & West, J.B. (1989). *High altitude medicine and physiology*. Philadelphia: University of Pennsylvania Press.

41. West, J.B., Boyer, S.J., Graber, D.J., Hackett, P.H., Maret, K.H., Milledge, J.S., Peters, Jr., R.M., Pizzo, C.J., Samaja, M., Sarnquist, F.H., Schoene, R.B., & Winslow, R.M. (1983). Maximal exercise at extreme altitudes on Mount Everest. *Journal of Applied Physiology*, **55**, 688-698.

42. West, J.B., Lahiri, S., Gill, M.B., Milledge, J.S., Pugh, L.G.C.E., & Ward, M.P. (1962). Arterial oxygen saturation during exercise at high altitude. *Journal of Applied Physiology*, **17**, 617-621.

43. West, J.B., Peters, R.M., Aksnes, G., Maret, K.H., Milledge, J.S., & Schoene, R.B. (1986). Nocturnal periodic breathing at altitudes of 6300 and 8050 m. *Journal of Applied Physiology*, **61**, 280-287.

44. Wolfel, E.E., Groves, B.M., Brooks, G.A., Butterfield, G.E., Mazzeo, R.S., Moore, L.G., Sutton, J.R., Bender, P.R., Dahms, T.E., McCullough, R.E., McCullough, R.G., Huang, S-Y., Sun, S.-F., Grover, R.F., Hultgren, H.N., & Reeves, J.T. (1991). Oxygen transport during steady-state submaximal exercise in chronic hypoxia. *Journal of Applied Physiology*, **70**, 1129-1136.

Selected Readings

Adams, W.C., Bernauer, E.M., Dill, D.B., & Bomar, J.B. (1975). Effects of equivalent sea level and altitude training on $\dot{V}O_2$ and running performance. *Journal of Applied Physiology*, **39**, 262-266.

Balke, B. (1968). Variation in altitude and its effect on exercise performance. In H.B. Falls (Ed.), *Exercise physiology*. New York: Academic Press.

Bender, P.R., Grove, B.M., McCullough, R.E., McCullough, R.G., Trad, L., Young, A.J., Cymerman, A., & Reeves, J.T. (1989). Decreased exercise muscle lactate release after high altitude acclimatization. *Journal of Applied Physiology*, **67**, 1456-1462.

Blomqvist, C.G. (1983). Cardiovascular adaptation to weightlessness. *Medicine and Science in Sports and Exercise*, **15**, 428-431.

Bungo, M.W., & Johnson, P.C. (1983). Cardiovascular examinations and observations of deconditioning during the space shuttle orbital flight test program. *Aviation, Space, and Environmental Medicine*, **54**, 1001-1004.

Buskirk, E.R., Kollias, J., Akers, R., Prokop, E., & Picon-Reategue, E. (1967). Maximal performance at altitude and on return from altitude in conditioned runners. *Journal of Applied Physiology*, **23**, 259-266.

Cerretelli, P. (1980). Gas exchange at high altitude. In J.B. West (Ed.), *Pulmonary gas exchange: Vol. II*. New York: Academic Press.

Convertino, V.A. (1991). Carotid-cardiac baroreflex: Relation with orthostatic hypotension following simulated microgravity and implications for development of countermeasures. *Acta Astronautica*, **23**, 9-17.

Convertino, V.A. (1992). Effects of exercise and inactivity on intravascular volume and cardiovascular control mechanisms. *Acta Astronautica*, **24**, 1-7.

Convertino, V.A., Goldwater, D.J., & Sandler, H. (1986). Bedrest-induced peak $\dot{V}O_2$ reduction associated with age, gender, and aerobic capacity. *Aviation, Space, and Environmental Medicine*, **57**, 17-22.

Fulco, C.S., & Cymerman, A. (1990). Human performance and acute hypoxia. In K. Pandolf, M. Sawka, & R. Gonzalez (Eds.), *Human performance physiology and environmental medicine at terrestrial extremes* (pp. 467-495). Indianapolis: Benchmark Press.

Gaffney, F.A., Nixon, J.V., Karlsson, E.S., Campbell, W., Dowdey, A.B.C., & Blomqvist, C.G. (1985). Cardiovascular deconditioning produced by 20 hours of bedrest with head-down tilt ($-5°$) in middle-aged healthy men. *American Journal of Cardiology*, **56**, 634-638.

Greenleaf, J.E. (1986). Mechanism for negative water balance during weightlessness: An hypothesis. *Journal of Applied Physiology*, **60**, 60-62.

Greenleaf, J.E., Bulbulian, R., Bernauer, E.M., Haskell, W.L., & Moore, T. (1989). Exercise-training protocols for astronauts in microgravity. *Journal of Applied Physiology*, **67**, 2191-2204.

Grover, R.F., Weil, J.V., & Reeves, J.T. (1986). Cardiovascular adaptation to exercise at high altitude. *Exercise and Sport Sciences Reviews*, **14**, 269-302.

Harrison, M.H. (1986). Athletes, astronauts and orthostatic tolerance. *Sports Medicine*, **3**, 428-435.

Heath, D., & Williams, D.R. (1989). *High-altitude medicine and pathology*. London: Butterworths.

Herbison, G.J., & Talbot, J.M. (1985). Muscle atrophy during space flight: Research needs and opportunities. *The Physiologist*, **28**, 520-527.

Hoffler, G.W., Wolthuis, R.A., & Johnson, R.L. (1974). Apollo space crew cardiovascular evaluations. *Aerospace Medicine*, **45**, 807-820.

Johnson, P.C., Leach, C.S., & Rambaut, P.C. (1973). Estimates of fluid and energy balances of Apollo 17. *Aerospace Medicine*, **44**, 1227-1230.

Johnston, R.S., Dietlein, L.F., & Berry, C.A. (Eds.) (1975). *Biomedical results of Apollo*. (NASA SP-368). Washington, DC: National Aeronautics and Space Administration.

Kirby, C.R., Ryan, M.J., & Booth, F.W. (1992). Eccentric exercise training as a countermeasure to non-weight-bearing soleus muscle atrophy. *Journal of Applied Physiology*, **73**, 1894-1899.

Lenfant, C., & Sullivan, K. (1971). Adaptation to high altitude. *New England Journal of Medicine*, **284**, 1298-1309.

Margaria, R. (Ed.) (1967). *Exercise at altitude*. Amsterdam: Excerpta Medica Foundation.

Mizuna, M., Juel, C., Bro-Rasmussen, T., Mygind, E., Schibye, B., Rasmussen, B., & Saltin, B. (1990). Limb skeletal muscle adaptation in athletes after training at altitude. *Journal of Applied Physiology*, **68**, 496-502.

Musacchia, X.J., Steffen, J.M., & Fell, R.D. (1988). Disuse atrophy of skeletal muscle: Animal models. *Exercise and Sport Sciences Reviews*, **16**, 61-87.

Muza, S.R. (1990). Hyperbaric physiology and human performance. In K. Pandolf, M. Sawka, & R. Gonzalez (Eds.), *Human performance physiology and environmental medicine at terrestrial extremes* (pp. 565-589). Indianapolis: Benchmark Press.

Nicogossian, A.E., Huntoon, C.L., & Pool, S.L. (Eds.) (1989). *Space physiology and medicine* (2nd ed.). Philadelphia: Lea & Febiger.

Pigman, E.C. (1991). Acute mountain sickness: Effects and implications for exercise at intermediate altitude. *Sports Medicine*, **12**, 71-79.

Saltin, B., Blomqvist, G., Mitchell, J.H., Johnson, Jr., R.L., Wildenthal, K., & Chapman, C.B. (1968). Response to submaximal and maximal exercise after bed rest and training. *Circulation*, **38** (Suppl. 7), 75.

Stegemann, J., Essfeld, D., & Hoffmann, U. (1985). Effects of a 7-day headdown tilt ($-6°$) on the dynamics of oxygen uptake and heart rate adjustment in upright exercise. *Aviation, Space, and Environmental Medicine*, **56**, 410-414.

Thompson, C.A., Tatro, D.L., Ludwig, D.A., & Convertino, V.A. (1990). Baroreflex responses to acute changes in blood volume in humans. *American Journal of Physiology*, **259**, R792-798.

Torricelli, E. (1981). Letter of Torricelli to Michelangelo Ricci. In J.B. West (Ed.), *High altitude physiology*. Stroudsburg, PA: Hutchinson Ross. (Letter written 1644)

Volicer, L., Jean-Charles, R., & Chobanian, A.V.

(1976). Effects of headdown tilt on fluid and electrolyte balance. *Aviation, Space, and Environmental Medicine*, **47**, 1065-1068.

West, J.B. (1984). Spacelab—the coming of age of space physiology research. *Journal of Applied Physiology*, **57**, 1625-1631.

West, J.B. (1992). Life in space. *Journal of Applied Physiology*, **72**, 1623-1630.

Wronski, T.J., & Morey, E.R. (1983). Alterations in calcium homeostasis and bone during actual and simulated space flight. *Medicine and Science in Sports and Exercise*, **15**, 410-414.

Young, A.J., & Young, P.M. (1990). Human acclimatization to high terrestial altitude. In K. Pandolf, M. Sawaka, & R. Gonzalez (Eds.), *Human performance physiology and environmental medicine at terrestrial extremes* (pp. 497-543). Indianapolis: Benchmark Press.

Zernicke, R.F., Vailas, A.C., & Salem, G.J. (1990). Biomechanical response of bone to weightlessness. *Exercise and Sport Sciences Reviews*, **18**, 167-192.

Zuntz, N., Loewy, A., Muller, F., & Caspari, W. (1906). *Hohenklima und Bergwanderrungen in ihret Wirkung auf den Menschen*. Berlin: Bong.

PART E

Optimizing Performance in Sport

We now understand how the body responds to an acute bout of exercise, how it adapts to chronic training, and how it adjusts to environmental extremes. Now that we can predict the body's response, we can apply that knowledge to athletic performance. In part E, we shift our focus to how athletes can best prepare for competition. In chapter 13, Quantifying Sports Training, we will discuss the effects of differing the amount of training stress, exploring how either too much or too little training can impair performance. In chapter 14, Ergogenic Aids and Performance, we will discuss various pharmacological agents, hormonal agents, and physiological agents that have been proposed to improve performance. We will examine the potential benefits, proven effects, and health risks associated with their use. In chapter 15, Nutrition and Nutritional Ergogenics, we will evaluate the athlete's dietary needs and consider how nutritional supplementation and diet manipulation have been proposed to improve performance. In chapter 16, Optimal Body Weight for Performance, we will address the issues of assessing body composition, relating body composition to sport performance, and using weight standards in competitions. We will also determine the most effective means for successfully losing body fat while maintaining fat-free body mass, enabling an athlete to achieve optimal competitive weight and likely improve performance.

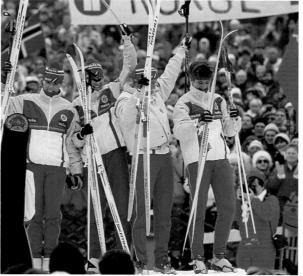

© F-Stock/John Plummer

Chapter 13
Quantifying Sports Training

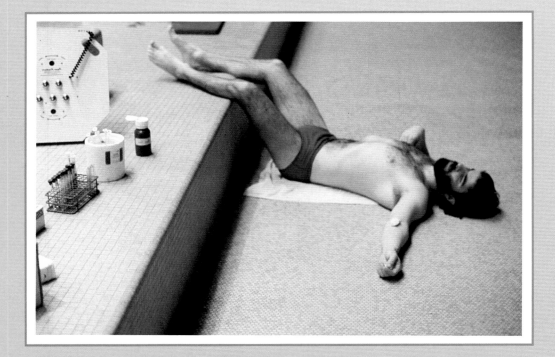

Chapter Overview

In the never-ending quest for performance perfection, many athletes devote as much time as possible to training, believing that the more they train, the better they will perform. For others, the end of the competitive season marks the beginning of a period of rest and relaxation during which training abruptly comes to a halt. These people often are sure that when the season rolls around again, they will still be well conditioned. People who are injured and undergo immobilization while they heal might worry that the performance improvements they have trained so hard to achieve will be lost by the time they are again allowed to perform. Yet none of these beliefs are totally correct. The athlete who relentlessly pushes harder eventually sees his or her performance suffer, not improve. Likewise, both the seasonal athlete who takes a break from training and the injured person who has a limb immobilized will suffer some performance loss but most will be able to rebound quickly.

In this chapter, we will try to quantify training. We will consider the effects of both too much training and too little training, as well as training to regain performance losses that might occur from a temporary interruption of training. We will learn that more is not always better as we explore the complexities of quantifying training to maximize performance.

Chapter Outline

Throughout his college career, Eric had trained at swimming 4 hr each day, covering as much as 8.5 mi (13.7 km) per day. Despite this effort his performance time for the 200-yd (183-m) butterfly event had not improved since his freshman year. With a best performance of 2 min 15 s for the event, he was seldom given a chance to compete because several teammates could perform the event in less than 2 min 5 s. In 1985, his coach made a major change in the team's training plan. The swimmers trained only 2 hr and swam an average of 2.8 to 3.0 mi (4.5 to 4.8 km) per day. Suddenly Eric's performance began to improve. After 3 months, his time had dropped to 2 min 10 s, still not good enough to make him a major contender. But as a reward for Eric's improvement, the coach chose him to swim the 200-yd butterfly event at the conference championship meet, which was preceded by 3 weeks of reduced training with only 1 mi per day. Now, with less training than in previous years and well-rested after the taper, Eric was able to make the finals of the event at the championship meet. His preliminary time was 2 min 1 s. In the finals he improved even further, posting a third-place finish with a time of 1 min 57.7 s, an impressive performance for a swimmer who performed better with "less" training.

Repeated days and weeks of training can be considered positive stress because it improves your capacity for energy production, physical stress tolerance, and exercise performance. The major physical changes associated with training occur in the first 6 to 10 weeks. The magnitude of these adaptations is generally controlled by the volume of exercise performed during training, which has led many coaches and athletes to believe that the athlete who does the greatest volume and intensity of training will be the best performer. As a result, we often consider quantity and quality of training to be synonymous. Too often, training sessions are judged by how many calories have been burned, but this philosophy has resulted in many nonspecific training programs that often impose unrealistic demands on the athlete.

The rate at which an individual can adapt to training is limited and cannot be forced beyond the body's capacity for development. Too much training can yield only small improvements, and, in some cases, can cause a breakdown in adaptation processes.

KEY POINT

A person's rate of adaptation to training is limited and cannot be forced beyond his or her body's capacity for development. Unfortunately, each individual responds differently to the same training stress, so what might be excessive training for one person might be well below the capacity of another. For this reason, it is important that individual differences be recognized and accounted for when designing training programs.

Although the volume of work performed in training is an important stimulus for physical conditioning, it can be overdone, leading to problems of chronic fatigue, illness, overtraining syndrome, or performance decrements. In contrast, proper rest and reductions in training volume can enhance performance. Much effort has been directed toward determining how much training is required to achieve optimal adaptation. Exercise physiologists have tested numerous training regimens to determine both the minimal and maximal stimuli needed for cardiovascular and muscular improvements. Let's examine how the quantity of training can affect your performance, beginning with what happens when the maximum required training is exceeded.

Excessive Training

All well-designed training programs incorporate the principle of progressive overload. In general, this principle holds that to maximize the benefits of training, the training stimulus must be progressively increased as the body adapts to the current stimulus. Your body responds to training by adapting to the stress of the training stimulus. If the amount of stress remains constant, you will eventually adapt fully to that level of stimulation and your body won't need further adaptation. The only way to continue to improve with training is to progressively increase the training stimulus, or stress.

Excessive training refers to training in which the volume, the intensity, or both are increased too quickly, without proper progression. Such training, with too high a volume or intensity, produces no additional improvement in conditioning or performance and can lead to a chronic state of fatigue that is associated with muscle glycogen depletion. Nevertheless, some coaches and athletes believe that maximum improvements with training can be achieved only with highly intense training. The idea that short periods of very intense training will induce a supercompensation in conditioning has been used in a variety of sports. For example, many swimmers train for 4 to 6 hr per day, believing that these overload periods hasten their adaptation or raise their fitness to levels that can't be achieved with less-intense training. In the following sections, we will examine the limits of excessive training.

Volume of Training

Most of the research on excessive training has been conducted on swimmers. For that reason, most of the material in the following sections is derived from research conducted on swimmers, but the information has applications to most other forms of training.

Training volume can be increased by increasing either the duration or the frequency of training bouts. Research shows that swim training 3 to 4 hr per day, 5 or 6 days each week, provides no greater benefits than when training is limited to only 1 to 1-1/2 hr per day.[6] In fact, such excessive training has been shown to significantly decrease muscle strength and sprint swimming performance.

Few studies have compared the physical conditioning and performance benefits of single verses multiple daily training sessions.[5,20,25] Studies conducted thus far reveal no scientific evidence that multiple daily training sessions enhance fitness and performance more than a single daily session. This is illustrated by the data in Figure 13.1, which show the responses of two groups of swimmers who trained once per day (Group 1) or twice per day (Group 2) for a period of 6 weeks during a 25-week training program. All swimmers began the program following the same training regimen—one time per day. But during Weeks 5 through 10, Group 2 increased its training to twice per day. After 6 weeks on the different regimens, both groups returned to the one-time-per-day program.[5] All the swimmers' heart rates and blood lactate values decreased dramatically with the initiation of training, and no significant differences were seen in the two groups' results in response to the change in training volume. The swimmers who trained twice per day showed no additional improvements over those who trained only once per day.

Most research on excessive training has considered only short-term effects. To determine the influence of long-term excessive training, performance improvements in swimmers who trained twice daily for a total distance of more than 10,000 m (10,936 yd)

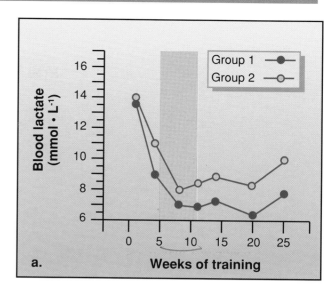

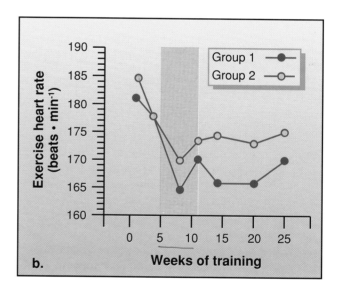

Figure 13.1 Changes in (a) blood lactate levels and (b) heart rate, during a standardized 366-m (400-yd) swim, for swimmers who trained once per day (Group 1) or twice per day (Group 2). Changes are reported for the 5th through 10th weeks of training.

per day were compared to improvements in those who swam approximately half that distance in a single session each day. The results are indicated in Figure 13.2. Changes in performance time for the 100-yd (91-m) front crawl were examined over a 4-year period for both groups—those who swam more than 10,000 m (10,936 yd) per day (LS, or long swim, group) and those who trained at no more than 5,000 m (5,468 yd) per day (SS, or short swim, group). The LS swimmers experienced an average improvement of 0.8% per year, which was identical to that observed for the SS group.

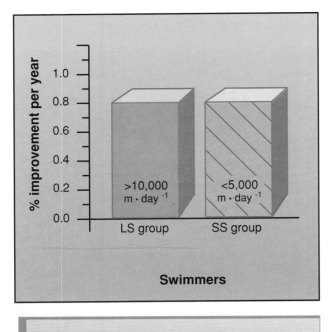

Figure 13.2   Percentages of improvement in performance for swimmers who trained at more than 10,000 m per day (LS group) and those who swam about 5,000 m per day (SS group).

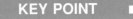

The need for long daily workouts is being seriously questioned by researchers. For certain sports, it appears that training volume could be reduced significantly, possibly by as much as one half in some sports, without reducing the benefits and with less risk of overloading the athletes.

Similar findings were also observed for competitors in other events, such as the 200-, 500-, and 1,650-yd front crawl. Thus, elite swimmers who trained with greater volume—twice each day—showed no greater improvements in performance than less-talented swimmers who trained less and with only one session per day.

Finally, the concept of training specificity implies that several hours of daily training won't provide the adaptations needed for athletes who participate in events of short duration. Most competitive swimming events last less than 2 minutes. How can training for 3 to 4 hr per day at speeds that are markedly slower than competitive pace prepare the swimmer for the maximal efforts of competition? Such a large training volume prepares the athlete to tolerate a high volume of training but likely does little to benefit actual performance.

Intensity of Training

Training intensity relates to both the force of muscle action and the stress placed on the cardiovascular system. With respect to muscle action, intensity is highest, for example, when the muscles exert maximal tension. Repeated days and weeks of such maximal effort improves muscle strength but does little or nothing to enhance cardiovascular endurance—the muscles get stronger but their aerobic capacity remains unchanged.

On the other hand, when the intensity of muscle force is reduced and the number of muscle actions is increased, as in sprint running and swimming, the muscles' energy and oxygen transport systems are stimulated to improve. Whereas strength training involving repeated maximal muscle actions leads to no improvement in aerobic capacity, repeated sprint bouts of 30-s duration have been found to increase $\dot{V}_{O_2\,max}$ by about 8%.

As intensity is reduced, the volume of work that can be tolerated is increased. Whereas only a few maximal muscle actions can be performed during a training bout, many repeated actions can be generated when the force developed by muscle is reduced below maximum.

From a practical point of view, we typically relate the intensity of effort to the capacity to generate energy or to a percentage of the person's $\dot{V}_{O_2\,max}$. When muscle force is low, the energy demand is low (about 10% to 20% of $\dot{V}_{O_2\,max}$) and neither strength nor endurance will improve. As training intensity increases, greater demands are placed on the aerobic system, and this stimulates improvements in oxygen transport and oxidative metabolism. Studies have shown that, for most people, training intensities between 50% and 90% of $\dot{V}_{O_2\,max}$ generate significant improvements in aerobic capacity. As intensity is increased to energy levels that equal or exceed $\dot{V}_{O_2\,max}$, the body gains strength but shows less improvement in aerobic capacity. Although the precise relationship between training intensity and aerobic and strength gains has not been defined, the relationship is assumed to be as indicated in Figure 13.3.

We must also remember the strong interaction between training intensity and training volume—as intensity is reduced, training volume must be increased to achieve adaptation. Training at very high intensities requires substantially less training volume, but the adaptations that occur will be significantly different from those achieved with low-intensity, high-volume training.

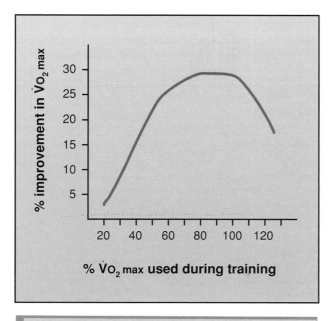

Figure 13.3   Percentages of improvement in $\dot{V}O_2$ max with various training intensities (represented by % $\dot{V}O_2$ max used during training). Strength gains likely show a similar curve when plotted against training intensity.

Attempts to perform large amounts of high-intensity training can have negative effects on adaptation. The energy needs of high-intensity exercise place greater demands on the glycolytic system, rapidly depleting muscle glycogen. If such training is attempted too often, such as daily, the muscles can become chronically depleted of their energy reserves and the person might demonstrate signs of chronic fatigue or overtraining (discussed in the next section).

Although hard training can offer psychological advantages, negative factors must also be considered.[19] Training for 3 to 4 hr per day might exceed the psychological and physical tolerance of some athletes who possess the potential to reach the elite level. As a result, they might drop out of the sport before achieving their best performance. Thus we are faced with a question: How many good athletes have failed because they burned out before realizing their full potential?

Overtraining

Many athletes are obsessed with training. Some attempt to do more work than they can physically tolerate. This is called overtraining. When this happens, the stress of excessive training can exceed the body's ability to recover and adapt, which results in more catabolism (breakdown) than anabolism (buildup).

IN REVIEW . . .

1. Excessive training refers to training that is done with an unnecessarily high training volume, training intensity, or both. It leads to no additional improvements in conditioning or performance and can lead to chronic fatigue and decreased performance because of muscle glycogen depletion.
2. Training volume can be increased by increasing the duration or frequency of training bouts. But numerous studies comparing athletes training with typical training volumes to those training with twice the volume (training conducted once a day instead of twice a day) have shown no significant differences in improvement.
3. Training intensity can determine the specific adaptations that occur in response to the training stimulus. High-intensity, low-volume training can be tolerated only for brief periods, so, although it does increase muscle strength, aerobic capacity will not be improved. Conversely, low-intensity, high-volume training stresses the oxygen transport and oxidative metabolism systems, causing greater gains in aerobic capacity.
4. Training intensities of between 50% to 90% of $\dot{V}O_2$ max produce marked improvement in aerobic capacity for most people.

KEY POINT

Few athletes are undertrained, but, unfortunately, many are overtrained, often erroneously believing that more training will always produce more improvement. We cannot overstress the importance of designing training programs to include both rest and variation in the training intensity and volume in an effort to avoid overtraining.

Athletes experience varied levels of fatigue during repeated days and weeks of training, so not all situations can be classified as overtraining. Fatigue that often follows one or more exhaustive training sessions is usually corrected by a few days of rest and a carbohydrate-rich diet. Such acute, readily correctable conditions of fatigue are generally caused by excessive training, as we just discussed. Overtraining, on the other hand, is characterized by a sudden decline in performance that cannot be remedied by a few days of rest and dietary manipulation.

Effects of Overtraining: Overtraining Syndrome

Most of the symptoms that result from overtraining, collectively referred to as overtraining syndrome, are subjective and identifiable only after the individual's performance has suffered. Unfortunately, these symptoms can be highly individualized, which can make it very difficult for athletes, trainers, and coaches to recognize that performance decrements are brought on by overtraining. The first indication of overtraining syndrome is a decline in physical performance. The athlete can sense a loss in muscle strength, coordination, and maximal working capacity. Other symptoms of overtraining syndrome include

- decreased appetite and body weight loss;
- muscle tenderness;
- head colds, allergic reactions, or both;
- occasional nausea;
- sleep disturbances;
- elevated resting heart rate; and
- elevated blood pressure.

The underlying causes of overtraining syndrome are often a combination of emotional and physiological factors. Hans Selye has noted that a person's stress tolerance can break down as often from a sudden increase in anxiety as from an increase in physical distress.[23] The emotional demands of competition, the desire to win, the fear of failure, unrealistically high goals, and others' expectations can be sources of intolerable emotional stress. Because of this, overtraining is typically accompanied by a loss in competitive desire and a loss in enthusiasm for training.

KEY POINT

The symptoms of overtraining syndrome are highly individualized and subjective, so they cannot be universally applied. The presence of one or more of these symptoms is sufficient to alert the coach or trainer that an athlete might be overtrained.

The physiological factors responsible for the detrimental effects of overtraining are not fully understood. However, many abnormal responses have been reported that suggest that overtraining is associated with alterations in the neurological, hormonal, and immune systems. Though a cause-and-effect relationship between these changes and the symptoms of overtraining has not been established, these symptoms can often help determine if an individual is overtrained.

In the following discussion, we will focus on some of the observed changes associated with overtraining and on potential causes of overtraining syndrome.

Autonomic Nervous System Overtraining

Some studies suggest that overtraining is associated with abnormal responses in the autonomic nervous system. Physiological symptoms accompanying the decline in performance often reflect changes in the neural or endocrine systems that are controlled by either the sympathetic or the parasympathetic nervous systems. Sympathetic overtraining can lead to

- increased resting heart rate,
- increased blood pressure,
- loss of appetite,
- decreased body mass,
- sleep disturbances,
- emotional instability, and
- elevated basal metabolic rate.

Other studies suggest that the parasympathetic nervous system might be dominant in some cases of overtraining.[16] In these cases, athletes show the same performance failures but have markedly different responses than those with sympathetic overtraining. Signs of parasympathetic overtraining include

- early onset of fatigue,
- decreased resting heart rate,
- rapid heart rate recovery after exercise, and
- decreased resting blood pressure.

Some of the symptoms associated with autonomic nervous system overtraining are also seen in people who are not overtrained. For this reason, we cannot always assume that the presence of these symptoms confirms overtraining.

Of the two conditions, symptoms of sympathetic overtraining are the most frequently observed. Nilson et al. have proposed that young athletes are more prone to the symptoms of sympathetic overtraining, but older athletes are more likely to show signs of parasympathetic overtraining.[21]

Hormonal Responses to Overtraining

Measurements of various blood hormone levels during periods of intensified training suggest that the excessive stress is accompanied by marked disturbances in endocrine function. As shown in Figure 13.4, when athletes increase their training 1.5- to 2-fold, their blood levels of thyroxine and testosterone usually decrease, and their blood levels of cortisol increase.[14,15] The ratio of testosterone to cortisol is thought to regulate anabolic processes in recovery, so a change in this

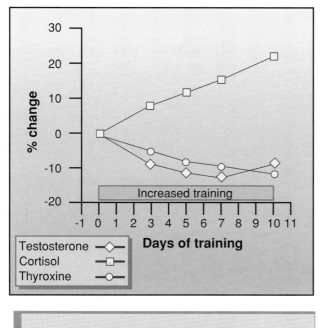

Figure 13.4   Changes in blood levels of thyroxine, testosterone, and cortisol with training.

ratio is considered an important indicator, and perhaps a cause, of overtraining syndrome.[16] Decreased testosterone coupled with increased cortisol might lead to more protein catabolism than anabolism in the cells. Overtrained athletes often have higher blood levels of urea, and because urea is produced by the breakdown of protein, this indicates increased protein catabolism. This mechanism is thought to be responsible for the loss in body mass seen in overtrained athletes.

Resting blood levels of epinephrine and norepinephrine are elevated during periods of intensified training.[14] These two hormones can elevate heart rate and blood pressure. Some suggest that the blood levels of these hormones should be measured to confirm overtraining. Unfortunately, measurement of these hormones is expensive, complex, and time consuming, so this is not a test that can be widely used.

Hard training often produces most of the same endocrine changes reported in overtrained athletes. For this reason, measuring these and other hormones might not provide valid confirmation of overtraining. Athletes whose hormone levels appear abnormal may simply be experiencing the normal effects of hard training. These endocrine changes simply might reflect the stress of training, rather than a breakdown in the adaptive process.

Immunity and Overtraining

Your immune system provides a line of defense against invading bacteria, parasites, viruses, and tumor cells. This system depends on the actions of specialized cells (such as lymphocytes, granulocytes, and macrophages) and antibodies. These function primarily to eliminate or neutralize foreign invaders that might cause illness (pathogens). Unfortunately, one of the most serious consequences of overtraining is the negative effect it has on the body's immune system.

Recent studies confirm that excessive training suppresses normal immune function, increasing the overtrained athlete's susceptibility to infections.[17,18] Numerous studies show that short bouts of intense exercise can temporarily impair the immune response, and successive days of heavy training can amplify this suppression.[1] Several investigators have reported an increased incidence of illness following a single, exhaustive exercise bout. Such immune suppression is characterized by abnormally low levels of both lymphocytes and antibodies. Invading organisms or substances are more likely to cause illness when these levels are low. Also, intense exercise during illness might decrease your ability to fight off the infection and increase your risk of even greater complications.

KEY POINT

Overtraining syndrome appears to be associated with depressed immune function. This places the athlete at an increased risk for infection.

Predicting Overtraining Syndrome

We must remember that the underlying causes of overtraining syndrome are not fully known, though it is likely that physical or emotional overload, or a combination of the two, might trigger this condition. Trying not to exceed an athlete's stress tolerance by regulating the amount of physiological and psychological stress experienced during training is difficult. Most coaches employ intuition to determine training volume and intensity, but few can accurately assess the true impact the workout has on the athlete. No preliminary symptoms warn athletes that they are on the verge of becoming overtrained. By the time coaches realize that they have pushed an athlete too hard, it is too late. The damage done by repeated days of excessive training or stress can only be repaired by days, and in some cases weeks, of reduced training or complete rest.

Numerous investigators have tried to objectively diagnose overtraining syndrome in its early stages by using assorted physiological measurements. Unfortunately none has proven totally effective. It is often difficult to determine whether the measurements obtained are related to overtraining or if they simply reflect normal responses to heavy training. In the following sections, we will examine some of the physiological changes that have been considered as potential means for diagnosing overtraining syndrome.

Blood Enzyme Levels

Measurements of blood enzyme levels have been used with only limited success to diagnose overtraining syndrome. Such enzymes as CPK (creatine phosphokinase), LDH (lactate dehydrogenase), and SGOT (serum glutamic oxalic transaminase) are important in muscle energy production. These enzymes are generally confined to the inside of cells, so the presence of large amounts of these enzymes in the blood suggests that muscle cell membranes have suffered some damage, allowing the enzymes to escape. Following periods of heavy training, blood levels of such enzymes have been reported to increase 2 to 10 times above normal. Recent studies support the idea that these changes might reflect varied degrees of muscle tissue breakdown. As noted in chapter 4, examination of tissue from the leg muscles of marathon runners has shown remarkable damage to the muscle fibers after training and marathon competition, and the onset and timing of these muscle changes paralleled the degree of muscle soreness experienced by the runners.

The performance effects of muscle damage are not fully understood, but experts generally agree that muscle damage might be partly responsible for the localized pain, tenderness, and swelling associated with muscle soreness. Still, no evidence links this condition to overtraining syndrome. Researchers suspect that blood enzyme levels rise and muscle fiber damage occurs frequently during eccentric exercise, regardless of the state of training. For these reasons, and because measuring blood enzyme levels is both difficult and expensive, blood enzyme levels do not appear to be suitable indicators of overtraining syndrome.

Oxygen Consumption

As athletes become overtrained, they often show a loss of skill, which decreases their performance efficiency. As their movement becomes less efficient, their oxygen consumption typically increases. Because of this, measurement of oxygen consumption during standardized exercise is often used to monitor the athlete's loss of skill during overtraining. For example, Figure 13.5 compares the submaximal oxygen consumption rate of a college cross-country runner who performed well during the early season but experienced symptoms of overtraining in late season. You can see that while experiencing the symptoms, the runner's submaximal

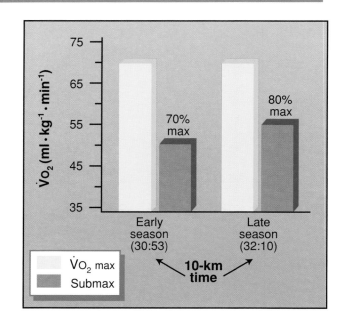

Figure 13.5 Oxygen consumption and 10-km times of a cross-country runner during the early season, while performing well, and in late season, while he was experiencing symptoms of overtraining. Adapted from Costill (1986).

oxygen consumption rate increased by 10%. Unfortunately, such tests are of little value to the coach or athlete because they are too complex, time consuming, and impractical for field use.

ECG

Early studies reported abnormal resting electrocardiograms (ECGs) in athletes who showed signs of overtraining syndrome. Specifically, people who showed sudden decrements in performance often exhibited T wave inversions. Recall from chapter 8 that the T wave represents ventricular repolarization. Such ECG changes are, then, associated with abnormal repolarization of the ventricles. Some researchers suggested that these changes among training athletes might reveal signs of overtraining syndrome, but a number of the athletes who clearly exhibited symptoms of overtraining syndrome had normal ECGs, so this is also not a reliable predictor.

Heart Rate

Current technology allows the coach to monitor the athlete's heart-rate response during a standardized exercise bout. For example, the data presented in Figure 13.6 illustrate a runner's heart-rate response during a 1-mi run performed at a fixed pace of 6 minutes per

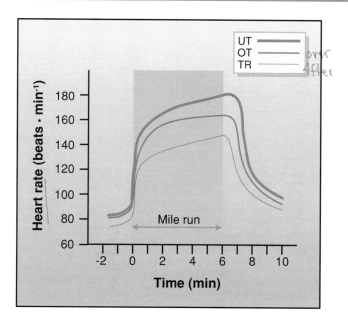

Figure 13.6   A runner's heart rate responses during a standard treadmill run performed before training (UT), after training (TR), and when the runner showed symptoms of overtraining (OT). Adapted from Costill (1986).

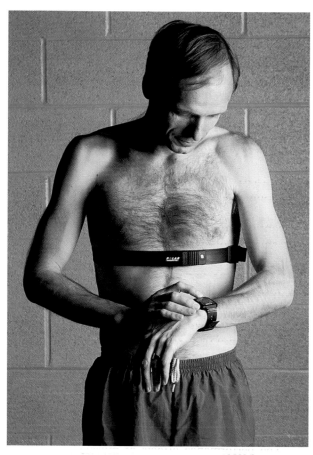

Figure 13.7   A runner outfitted with a heart rate monitor. The chest strap picks up and transmits electrical impulses from the heart to the memory device worn on the wrist. After the run, the recordings are played back for interpretation.

mile (10 mph). This response was monitored when the runner was untrained (UT), after the runner had trained (TR), and during a period when the runner demonstrated symptoms of overtraining syndrome (OT). This figure shows that heart rate is higher in the overtrained state than it is when the runner is responding well to training. Similar findings have been reported for swimmers.[5]

The advantage of this test is that it provides an easily obtained objective measurement of the athlete's cardiovascular response to a given rate of work. Also, measurements of blood lactate (which reflects the body's level of conditioning) taken after this test correlate very closely with heart rate. Heart rates are relatively simple to record (see Figure 13.7) and provide immediate information for the athlete and coach. Such a test provides an objective way to monitor training and can provide a warning signal of overtraining syndrome.[24]

KEY POINT

The best predictors of overtraining syndrome appear to be heart rate, oxygen uptake, and blood lactate responses to a standardized bout of work. Performance decrements are also good indicators.

Treatment of Overtraining Syndrome

Though the causes for performance deterioration with overtraining syndrome are not clear, apparently training intensity or speed is a more potent stressor than training volume. Recovery from overtraining syndrome is possible with a marked reduction in training intensity or complete rest. Although most coaches recommend a few days of easy training, overtrained athletes recover more quickly if they rest completely for 3 to 5 days or if they change to low-intensity exercise. In some cases, counseling might be needed to help the athletes cope with other stress in their lives that might be contributing to this condition.

The best way to minimize the risk of overtraining is to follow cyclic training procedures, alternating easy, moderate, and hard periods of training.

Although individual tolerance varies tremendously, even the strongest athletes have periods when they are susceptible to overtraining syndrome. As a rule, 1 or 2 days of intense training should be followed by an equal number of easy aerobic training days. Likewise, a week or two of hard training should be followed by a week of reduced effort with little or no emphasis on anaerobic exercise.

Endurance athletes (such as swimmers, cyclists, and runners) must pay particular attention to their carbohydrate intake. Repeated days of hard training cause a gradual reduction of muscle glycogen. Unless these athletes consume extra carbohydrate during these periods, their muscle and liver glycogen reserves can be depleted. As a consequence, the most heavily recruited muscle fibers would not be able to generate the energy needed for exercise.

■■■   IN REVIEW . . .   ■■■

1. Overtraining is attempting to do more work than you are physically capable of doing. Overtraining leads to decreased performance capacity.
2. The symptoms of overtraining syndrome are subjective, and many also accompany regular training, which makes prevention or diagnosis of overtraining syndrome difficult.
3. Possible explanations for overtraining syndrome include changes in the functioning of the divisions of the autonomic nervous system, altered endocrine responses, and suppressed immune function.
4. Signs looked at in hopes of being able to diagnose overtraining include

   • changes in blood levels of enzymes normally found inside the cells,
   • increased oxygen consumption at a fixed rate of work as performance becomes less efficient,
   • abnormal ECGs showing T wave inversions, and
   • increased heart rate and blood lactate responses to a fixed rate of work.

   Only heart-rate response can provide a somewhat reliable warning of overtraining.
5. Overtraining syndrome is treated by a marked reduction in training intensity or complete rest. Prevention can best be accomplished by using cyclic training procedures that vary training intensity and, for endurance athletes, ensuring adequate carbohydrate intake to meet energy needs.

Tapering for Peak Performance

Peak performance requires maximal physical and psychological tolerance for the stress of the activity. But periods of intense training reduce muscle strength, decreasing the athletes' performance capacity. For this reason, to compete at their peak, many athletes reduce their training intensity prior to a major competition to give their bodies and their minds a break from the rigors of intense training. This practice is referred to as tapering. The taper period, during which intensity is reduced, should provide adequate time for healing of tissue damage caused by intense training, and time for the body's energy reserves to be fully replenished. Research suggests that, for example, the taper period for swimmers might need to last for at least 2 weeks to maximize performance.

The most notable change during the taper period is a marked increase in muscle strength, which explains at least part of the performance improvement that occurs. It is difficult to determine whether strength improvements result from changes in the muscles' contractile mechanisms or improved muscle fiber recruitment. However, examination of individual muscle fibers taken from swimmers' arms before and after 10 days of intensified training did show that the fast-twitch fibers exhibit a significant reduction in their maximal shortening velocity.[10] This change has been attributed to changes in the fibers' myosin molecules. In these cases, the myosin in the FT fibers became more like that in the ST fibers. We assume from this that such changes in the muscle fibers cause the power loss that is experienced by swimmers and runners during prolonged periods of intense training. We can then also assume that the recovery of strength and power that occurs with tapering might be linked to modifications of the muscles' contractile mechanisms.

■■■   KEY POINT   ■■■

Tapering for competition is crucial to your best performance. Training damages the body, so reduced training volume and intensity, coupled with quality rest, are needed to allow your body time to repair itself and to restore its energy reserves to prepare you for competition.

Although tapering is widely practiced in a variety of sports, many coaches fear that reduced training for such a long period before a major competition will cause a loss of conditioning and poorer performance. But numerous studies clearly show that this fear is unwarranted. Developing optimum maximal oxygen consumption initially requires a considerable amount of training, but once it has been developed, much less training is needed to maintain $\dot{V}O_2$ max at its highest level. In fact, the training level of $\dot{V}O_2$ max can be maintained even when training frequency is reduced by two thirds.[11]

Runners and swimmers who reduce their training by about 60% for 15 to 21 days show no losses in $\dot{V}O_2$ max or endurance performance.[4,13] For swimmers, one study found that blood lactate levels after a standard swim were lower after a taper period than before. More importantly, the swimmers experienced a 3.1% improvement in performance as a result of the reduced training and demonstrated a 17.7% to 24.6% increase in arm strength and power.[4]

Tapering produces less improvement in distance runners than in swimmers.[12] Runners who reduced their training from 81 km per week to 24 km per week suffered no loss in $\dot{V}O_2$ max, nor any significant changes in heart-rate response during submaximal running. They did, however, show an improvement of about 5% in leg power, calculated from a vertical jump test. Unfortunately, little information is available to demonstrate the influence of tapering on performance in team sports and in long-duration endurance events like cycling and marathon running. Before guidelines can be offered for athletes in these sports, research is needed to demonstrate that similar benefits can be generated by such periods of reduced training.

■ IN REVIEW . . . ■

1. Many athletes decrease their training intensity prior to a competition to avoid reductions in strength, power, and performance capacity that accompany high-intensity training. This practice is called tapering.
2. Muscle strength increases significantly during the tapering period.
3. Less training is needed to maintain previous gains than was originally needed to attain them, so tapering does not lead to a loss of conditioning.

Detraining

What happens to highly conditioned athletes who have fine-tuned their performance skills to a peak level but find that the competitive season and daily training have come to a sudden end? Most athletes in team sports

go into physical hibernation at this time. Many have been working 2 to 5 hr each day to perfect their skills and improve their physical condition and welcome the opportunity to completely relax, purposely avoiding any strenuous physical activity. But how does physical inactivity affect highly trained athletes?

Much of our knowledge about physical detraining, which is the cessation of regular physical training, comes from clinical research with patients who have been forced into inactivity because of injury or surgery. Athletes generally agree that suffering the pain of an injury is bad enough, but the situation is even worse when it forces them to stop training. Most fear that all they have gained through hard training will be lost during a period of inactivity. But recent studies reveal that a few days of rest or reduced training will not impair and might even enhance performance. Yet at some point, training reduction or complete inactivity will produce a decrement in physiological function and performance.

In the following sections, we will examine physiological responses to detraining. We will look at specific areas of concern to the athlete:

- Muscle strength and power
- Muscular endurance
- Speed, agility, and flexibility
- Cardiorespiratory endurance

Muscle Strength and Power

When a broken limb is immobilized in a rigid cast, changes begin immediately in both the bone and the surrounding muscles. Within only a few days, the cast that was applied tightly around the injured limb is loose. After several weeks, a large space separates the cast and the limb. Skeletal muscles undergo a substantial decrease in size, known as atrophy, when they remain inactive. This is accompanied by considerable loss of muscle strength and power. Total inactivity leads to rapid losses, but even prolonged periods of reduced activity lead to gradual losses that eventually can become quite significant.

In a similar fashion, research confirms that muscle strength and power are both reduced once the athlete stops training. But these changes are relatively small during the first few months. In one study, no strength loss was noted 4 weeks after completion of a 3-week resistance training program.[5] In another investigation, only 45% of the original strength gained from a 12-week training program had been lost when the subjects, who did no further training, were reevaluated 1 year later.

A study with collegiate swimmers revealed that even with up to 4 weeks of inactivity, terminating

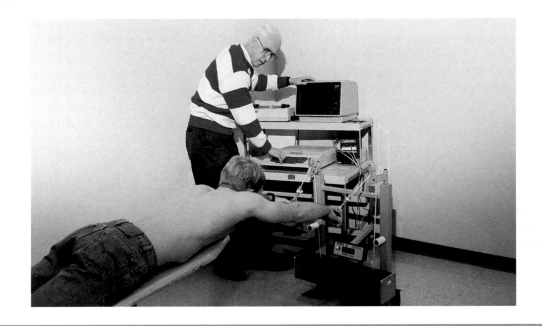

Figure 13.8   Measurements of arm strength and power using a Biokinetic Swim Bench.

training did not affect arm or shoulder strength. No strength changes were seen in these swimmers, whether they spent 4 weeks at complete rest or whether they reduced their training frequency to 1 or 3 sessions per week. But swimming power was reduced by 8% to 13.5% during the 4 weeks of reduced activity, whether the swimmers underwent complete rest or merely reduced training frequency.

Interestingly, this study's measurement techniques for strength and power differed in a significant respect. The strength of the swimmers was measured on land, using the semi-accommodating swim bench (see Figure 13.8), but their power was measured in the water, using tethered swimming, which allows the swimmers to use more natural actions (tethered swimming is discussed and illustrated in chapter 1).

The results of these measurements, depicted in Figure 13.9, suggest that the less-specific land measurements of muscle strength might not have accurately reflected the performance loss that the swimmers experienced. Although muscle strength might not have diminished during the 4 weeks of reduced training, the swimmers might have lost their ability to apply force during swimming, probably due to a loss of skill. As swimming coaches would say, the swimmers appeared to have lost their feel for the water.

The physiological mechanisms responsible for the loss of muscle strength as a consequence of either immobilization or inactivity are not clearly understood. Muscle atrophy causes a noticeable decrease in muscle mass and water content, which could partly account

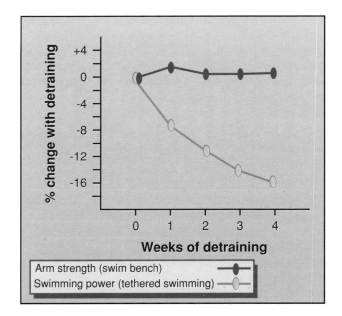

Figure 13.9   Percentages of change in arm strength and swimming power during 4 weeks of detraining. Arm strength was assessed from performance on a swim bench, and swimming power was assessed from performance of tethered swimming.

for a loss in maximal development of muscle fiber tension. When muscles aren't used, the frequency of their neurological stimulation is reduced and normal fiber recruitment is disrupted. Thus, part of the strength loss associated with detraining could result from an inability to activate some muscle fibers.

Research indicates that after training is terminated, an athlete can retain gained muscle strength and power for periods of up to 6 weeks. By instead continuing to train once every 10 to 14 days, athletes can usually maintain strength gains for much longer periods. Evidently, muscle requires minimal stimulation to retain the strength, power, and size gained during training.

This has extremely important implications for the injured athlete. The athlete can save much time and effort during rehabilitation by performing even a low level of exercise with the injured limb, starting in the first few days of recovery. Simple isometric actions are very effective for rehabilitation because their intensity can be graded and they don't require joint movement. Any program of rehabilitation, however, must be designed in cooperation with the supervising physician.

On the surface, all these findings seem to conflict with the observations noted earlier that periods of total inactivity, such as limb immobilization, cause sizeable losses in muscle strength, power, and mass. But apparently most individuals who either stop or decrease their training regimen get sufficient exercise through walking, stair climbing, pushing, pulling, and lifting to allow them to retain most of the strength they previously gained through strength training. With immobilization, though, virtually no activation occurs to stimulate the contractile processes. Strength and mobility are rapidly lost under such conditions.

Changes in Muscular Endurance

Muscular endurance performance decreases after only 2 weeks of inactivity. At this time, not enough evidence is available to determine whether this performance decrement results from changes in the muscle or from changes in cardiovascular capacity. In this section, we will examine muscle changes that are known to accompany detraining and which could cause a decrease in muscular endurance.

The localized muscle adaptations that occur during periods of inactivity are well documented, but knowledge of the exact role these changes play in the loss of muscular endurance still eludes us. We know from postsurgery cases that after a week or two of cast-immobilization, the activities of oxidative enzymes such as succinate dehydrogenase and cytochrome oxidase decrease by 40% to 60%. Data collected from swimmers, shown in Figure 13.10, indicate that the muscles' oxidative potential decreases much more rapidly than the subjects' maximal oxygen uptake with detraining. Although reduced oxidative

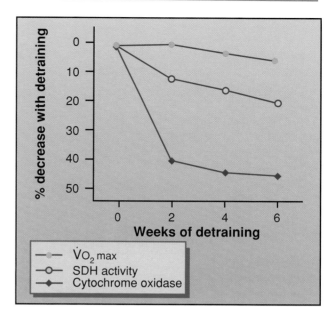

Figure 13.10   Percentages of decrease in $\dot{V}O_2$ max, muscle succinate dehydrogenase (SDH) activity, and cytochrome oxidase activity during 6 weeks of detraining.

enzyme activity would be expected to impair muscular endurance, more must be involved or $\dot{V}O_{2\ max}$ would decrease along with these enzyme activities.

In contrast, when athletes stop training, the activities of their muscles' glycolytic enzymes, such as phosphorylase and phosphofructokinase, change little, if at all, for at least 4 weeks. In fact, with up to 84 days of detraining, Coyle et al. observed no change in glycolytic enzyme activities, but a nearly 60% decrease in the activities of various oxidative enzymes.[8] This means that with detraining, the muscles' capacity for anaerobic performance is maintained longer than their capacity for aerobic performance. This might at least partly explain why performance times in sprint events are unaffected with a month or more of inactivity, but the ability to perform longer endurance events may decrease significantly with as little as 2 weeks of detraining.

One notable change in the muscle during detraining is a change in its glycogen content. Endurance-trained muscle tends to increase its glycogen storage. But 4 weeks of detraining has been shown to decrease muscle glycogen by 40%.[3] Figure 13.11 illustrates the drop in muscle glycogen accompanying 4 weeks of detraining in competitive collegiate swimmers and in untrained subjects. The untrained people showed no change in muscle glycogen content after 4 weeks of inactivity, but the swimmers' values decreased until they were about equal to those of the untrained people.

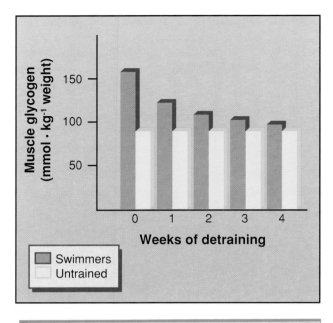

Figure 13.11 Changes in glycogen content of the deltoid muscle in competitive swimmers during 4 weeks of detraining. Note that muscle glycogen had nearly returned to the untrained level at the end of this period.

Table 13.1 Blood Lactate, pH, and Bicarbonate (HCO_3^-) After a Standard-Paced, 200-yd Front Crawl Swim in Eight Collegiate Swimmers Undergoing Detraining

Measurement	Weeks of detraining			
	0[a]	1[b]	2	4
Lactate ($mmol \cdot L^{-1}$)	4.2	6.3	6.8	9.7[c]
pH	7.259	7.237	7.236	7.183[c]
HCO_3^- ($mmol \cdot L^{-1}$)	21.1	19.5[c]	16.1[c]	16.3[c]
Swim time (s)	130.6	130.1	130.5	130.0

[a]The values at week 0 represent the measurements taken at the end of 5 months of training.

[b]The values at weeks 1, 2, and 4 are the results obtained after 1, 2, and 4 weeks of detraining, respectively.

[c]Denotes a significant difference from the value at the end of training or week 0.

detraining Lactate↑ pH↓ HCO₃-↓ time α

This indicates that the trained swimmers' improved capacity for muscle glycogen storage appears to be reversed during detraining.

Measurements of blood lactate and pH after a standard work bout have been used to assess the physiological changes that accompany training and detraining. For example, a group of collegiate swimmers were required to perform a standard-paced, 200-yd (183-m) swim at 90% of their seasonal best following 5 months of training, and then to repeat this test once a week for the following 4 weeks of detraining. The results are shown in Table 13.1. Blood lactate levels, taken immediately after this standard swim, changed very little during the first few weeks of inactivity. But at the end of the fourth week of detraining, the swimmers' acid-base balance was significantly disturbed. This reflected a significant rise in blood lactate levels and a significant drop in the levels of bicarbonate (a buffer). These findings support the theory that the muscles' oxidative and anaerobic energy systems change slowly and are probably unaffected by only a few days of rest. Only during periods of complete inactivity (immobilization) do such changes impair performance in the first week or two.

Muscle fiber composition does not appear to change during short periods of inactivity. But some clinical cases have reported dramatic changes in the percentage of slow-twitch and fast-twitch fibers, with a shift toward more FT fibers, in athletes who have undergone immobilization following surgery. However, these findings have not been replicated, so we cannot draw valid conclusions about the effects of detraining on muscle fiber composition.

Another structural change that has been proposed as a possible reason for the decrease in muscular endurance involves blood flow to the muscles. Some research suggests that the capillary supply in the muscles can decrease during detraining. This would impair oxygen delivery to the muscles, decreasing their oxidative potential. However, the findings on this are inconclusive.

Loss of Speed, Agility, and Flexibility

Training produces less improvement in speed and agility than it does in strength, power, muscular endurance, flexibility, and cardiovascular endurance. Consequently, losses of speed and agility that occur with inactivity are relatively small. Also, peak levels of both can be maintained with a limited amount of training. But this does not imply that the sprinter in track can get by with training only a few days a week. Success in actual competition relies on factors other than basic speed and agility, such as correct form, skill, and the ability to generate a strong finishing sprint. Many hours of practice are required during the week to tune performance to its optimal level, but most of this time is spent developing performance qualities other than speed and agility.

Flexibility, on the other hand, is lost rather quickly during inactivity, so it must be worked on throughout the year. Stretching exercises should be incorporated into both in-season and off-season training programs. But, during the off-season, many athletes tend to ignore flexibility training because it can be regained so rapidly. Although flexibility can be reestablished in little time, the athlete should maintain the desired flexibility level year-round. Reduced flexibility can increase athletes' susceptibility to serious injury.

Changes in Cardiorespiratory Endurance

The heart, like other muscles in the body, is strengthened by endurance training. Inactivity, on the other hand, can substantially decondition the heart and the cardiovascular system. The most dramatic examples of this are seen in studies conducted on subjects undergoing long periods of total bed rest—they weren't allowed to leave their beds, and physical activity was kept to an absolute minimum.[22] Cardiovascular function was assessed while the subjects performed at a constant rate of work both before and following a 21-day period of bed rest. The cardiovascular effects that accompanied bed rest included

- a considerable increase in submaximal heart rate,
- a 25% decrease in submaximal stroke volume,
- a 25% reduction in maximal cardiac output, and
- a 27% decrease in maximal oxygen consumption.

The reductions in cardiac output and $\dot{V}O_2 \text{ max}$ appear to result from a reduced stroke volume, which is probably due to a combined decrease in heart volume, total blood volume, plasma volume, and ventricular contractility.

Interestingly, the two most highly conditioned subjects in this study (the two who had the highest $\dot{V}O_2 \text{ max}$ values) experienced greater decrements in $\dot{V}O_2 \text{ max}$ than the three less-fit people, as shown in Figure 13.12. Furthermore, the untrained subjects regained their initial conditioning levels (before bed rest) in the first 10 days of reconditioning, but the well-trained subjects needed about 40 days for full recovery. This suggests that more highly trained individuals cannot afford long periods with little or no endurance training. The athlete who totally abstains from physical training at the completion of the season will experience great difficulty getting back into physical condition when the new season begins.

Recent studies have shown that impairment of cardiovascular function following a few weeks of detraining is largely due to a reduction in blood volume, which in turn diminishes the stroke volume of the heart.[7] Two to four weeks of reduced activity following months of training for cycling and running resulted in a 9% decrease in blood volume and a 12% decrease in both stroke volume and plasma volume. As a result, $\dot{V}O_2 \text{ max}$ dropped by 5.9%. After they were detrained, the subjects were infused with a dextran (sugar) solution to expand

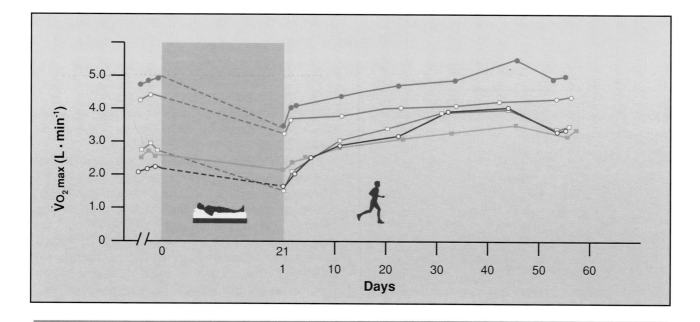

Figure 13.12 Changes in $\dot{V}O_2$ max with 20 days of bed rest. Adapted from Saltin et al. (1968).

their blood volume until it exceeded their trained level. As shown in Table 13.2, this improved cardiovascular function and $\dot{V}O_2$ max, though it proved of little benefit to endurance performance.

Studies have also observed changes in trained subjects' endurance performance during periods of inactivity. This reduction in cardiorespiratory endurance is much greater than the reductions of strength, power, and muscular endurance for the same period of inactivity. Drinkwater and Horvath studied seven female track athletes at the end of the competitive season and again 3 months after formal training ended.[9] During that 3-month period, the athletes participated in typical physical activities of their age group, including required physical education. At the end of the 3 months, $\dot{V}O_2$ max in the subjects had decreased an average of 15.5%. The new $\dot{V}O_2$ max levels were similar to those found in nonathletic girls of the same age.

So inactivity can significantly reduce $\dot{V}O_2$ max. How much activity is needed to prevent such considerable losses of physical conditioning? Studies show that physical conditioning can be maintained by training as few as three times per week, but less training leads to significant losses in the benefits of physical conditioning. A study by Brynteson and Sinning examined this issue.[2] Subjects exercised 5 days per week for 5 weeks to develop their initial training levels. They were then divided into four groups, exercising either one, two, three, or four times per week, to determine the minimal frequency needed to maintain the initial

training level. The researchers found that those who exercised at least three times per week were able to maintain their cardiovascular fitness levels, but the two groups that exercised only once or twice per week suffered significant losses in conditioning.

KEY POINT

Your body loses many of the benefits of training quickly if training is discontinued. Some minimal level of training is necessary to prevent these losses. Research indicates that at least three training sessions per week at an intensity of at least 70% of $\dot{V}O_2$ max are needed to maintain aerobic conditioning.

Although a decrease in training frequency and duration reduces aerobic capacity, the losses are only significant when frequency and duration are reduced by two thirds of the regular training load. However, training intensity apparently plays a more crucial role in maintaining aerobic power during periods of reduced training. Studies by Hickson et al. suggest that training intensity must be at least 70% of $\dot{V}O_2$ max to maintain the training-induced improvements in $\dot{V}O_2$ max.[11] In subjects who were previously trained for 10 weeks, as little as a one-third reduction in training intensity for 15 weeks produced a significant decrease in

- $\dot{V}O_2$ max,
- long-term (at 80% $\dot{V}O_2$ max until exhaustion) endurance, and
- cardiac size.

Short-term (4- to 8-min) endurance and body composition, however, were not changed by this one-third reduction in training intensity.

From these and other studies, it is apparent that cardiorespiratory endurance capacity is rapidly lost following the cessation of formal endurance training. Although complete bed rest provides the most dramatic decreases, even periods of light activity or formal endurance training frequency of only once or twice a week are not sufficient to prevent the loss of cardiovascular conditioning. Thus, an athlete must try to maintain his or her endurance capacity during the off-season, because once it is lost, regaining peak levels takes considerable time. Likewise, an injured athlete should get back into some modified form of endurance exercise as soon as possible to minimize the loss in cardiorespiratory endurance capacity.

Table 13.2 Effects of Detraining and Blood Volume Expansion

Parameter	Normal blood volume Trained	Normal blood volume Detrained	Expanded blood volume Detrained
Blood volume (ml)	5,177	4,692	5,412
Stroke volume[a] (ml)	166	146[b]	164
$\dot{V}O_2$ max (L · min^{-1})	4.42	4.16[b]	4.28
Exercise time to exhaustion (min)	9.13	8.44	8.06[c]

[a]Stroke volume measured during submaximal exercise.

[b]Denotes a significant difference from trained (normal blood volume) and detrained (expanded blood volume) values.

[c]Denotes a significant difference from the trained (normal blood volume) value.

Adapted from Coyle (1986).

IN REVIEW . . .

1. Detraining refers to the cessation of regular physical training. The effects of stopping training are quite minor compared to those that result from immobilization. In general, the greater the gains during training, the greater the losses during detraining simply because the well-trained person has more to lose than the untrained person.
2. Detraining causes muscle atrophy, which is accompanied by losses in muscle strength and power. However, muscles require only minimal stimulation to retain these qualities during periods of reduced activity.
3. Muscular endurance decreases after only 2 weeks of inactivity. Possible explanations for this are
   - decreased oxidative enzyme activities,
   - decreased muscle glycogen storage,
   - disturbance of the acid-base balance, and
   - decreased blood supply to the muscles.
4. Detraining losses in speed and agility are small, but flexibility is lost quickly. To avoid injury, athletes should engage in year-round flexibility training.
5. With detraining, losses of cardiorespiratory endurance are much greater than losses of muscle strength, power, and endurance.
6. To maintain cardiorespiratory endurance, training must be conducted at least three times per week, and training intensity should be at least 70% of the regular training intensity.

Cardiorespiratory greatest loss
maintain - 3x week at 70% vo₂max

Retraining

Recovery of conditioning after a period of inactivity, known as retraining, is affected by your fitness level and how long you were inactive. As mentioned earlier, the most highly trained individuals typically experience the greatest loss of conditioning from detraining. Because of this, these people also take considerably longer to regain their initial fitness levels than subjects who are less trained.

Two to three weeks of detraining have been shown to cause the following decrements in highly trained subjects:

- Decrease muscle oxidative enzyme activities by 13% to 24%
- Decrease performance time by about 25%
- Decrease $\dot{V}O_2$ max by about 4%

Following 15 days of retraining, only $\dot{V}O_2$ max had returned to its original trained level. Oxidative enzyme activities did not improve, and although performance time showed some improvement, it still remained 9% below the trained level. This suggests that even short periods of detraining significantly change physiological capacity in highly trained subjects, and that a longer period of retraining is necessary for these trained individuals to regain their conditioning.

As noted earlier, muscles that have been immobilized in a cast, whether for a few days or for many weeks, lose much of their strength, power, and endurance. After the cast is removed, most people can't begin activity immediately because they lack sufficient joint mobility. Regaining the range of joint motion is a relatively slow process, often taking several months for full recovery.

Several procedures have been proposed to speed the recovery of muscle function following immobilization. For example, when patients who had undergone surgical reconstruction of their anterior cruciate ligaments were given a cast that allowed some movement (20° to 60° range), full recovery of the knee's range of motion occurred in 4 weeks of retraining. But with an immovable cast, 16 weeks were needed to regain normal motion. The moveable cast resulted in minimal reduction of muscle fiber cross-sectional area and no reduction in oxidative enzyme activities.

Other studies have revealed effective ways to limit the reduction in muscle aerobic capacity following cast-immobilization. Compared to strength training alone, 20 to 60 min of daily cycling following cast removal leads to greater gains in muscle aerobic capacity and improved knee flexibility. Also, electrical stimulation of the muscles while they are immobilized prevents the usual decrease in their oxidative capacity and can also prevent muscle fiber atrophy.

IN REVIEW . . .

1. Retraining is the recovery of conditioning after a period of inactivity. It is affected by the person's fitness level and the duration and extent of the inactivity.
2. The time needed for retraining can be reduced in cases of immobilization if the cast used allows some range of movement.
3. Electrical stimulation of the muscles prevents the usual decrease in muscle oxidative capacity and can prevent muscle fiber atrophy.
4. The earlier an individual can resume active motion after immobilization or inactivity, the quicker the recovery of muscle function.

In Closing . . .

In this chapter we have examined how the quantity of training can affect your performance. We saw that too much training, either in the form of excessive training or overtraining, can actually impair your performance. Then we looked at the effects of too little training—detraining—either as a result of inactivity or, in the case of people recovering from an injury, immobilization. We saw that with detraining, many of the gains you achieved during regular training are quickly lost, especially your cardiovascular endurance. Finally, we briefly considered the process of retraining, during which you try to regain what you have lost through detraining.

Having dispelled the myth that more training always means better performance, in what other ways can athletes try to optimize their performance? In the next chapter, we turn our attention to the use of ergogenic aids.

Key Terms

detraining

excessive training

overtraining

overtraining syndrome

retraining

tapering

taper period

Study Questions

1. What are the causes of overtraining? How can it be identified? What is the suggested treatment for overtraining?
2. What physiological changes occur during the taper period that can be credited with improvements in performance?
3. What alterations occur in strength, power, and muscular endurance with physical detraining?
4. What changes take place in the muscle during periods of inactivity? During total muscle immobilization (casting)?
5. What alterations occur in speed, agility, and flexibility with physical detraining?
6. What changes occur in the cardiovascular system as one becomes deconditioned?
7. During periods of reduced training, what factors (frequency, intensity, or duration) must be stressed in order to prevent a decline in long-term endurance and aerobic capacity?
8. How can the negative effects of muscle immobilization be reduced?

References

1. Brahmi, Z., Thomas, J.E., Park, M., & Dowdeswell, I.R.G. (1985). The effect of acute exercise on natural killer cell activity of trained and sedentary subjects. *Journal of Clinical Immunology*, **5**, 321.

2. Brynteson, P., & Sinning, W.E. (1973). The effects of training frequencies on the retention of cardiovascular fitness. *Medicine and Science in Sports*, **5**, 29-33.

3. Costill, D.L., Fink, W.J., Hargreaves, M., King, D.S., Thomas, R., & Fielding, R. (1985). Metabolic characteristics of skeletal muscle during detraining from competitive swimming. *Medicine and Science in Sports and Exercise*, **17**, 339-343.

4. Costill, D.L., King, D.S., Thomas, R., & Hargreaves, M. (1985). Effects of reduced training on muscular power in swimmers. *Physician & Sports Medicine*, **13**(2), 94-101.

5. Costill, D.L., Maglischo, E., & Richardson, A. (1991). *Handbook of sports medicine: Swimming*. London: Blackwell Publishing.

6. Costill, D.L., Thomas, R., Roberger, R.A., Pascoe, D.D., Lambert, C.P., Barr, S.I., & Fink, W.J. (1991). Adaptations to swimming training: Influence of training volume. *Medicine and Science in Sports and Exercise*, **23**, 371-377.

7. Coyle, E.F., Hemmert, M.K., & Coggan, A.R. (1986). Effects of detraining on cardiovascular responses to exercise: Role of blood volume. *Journal of Applied Physiology*, **60**, 95-99.

8. Coyle, E.F., Martin, W.H. III, Sinacore, D.R., Joyner, M.J., Hagberg, J.M., & Holloszy, J.O. (1984). Time course of loss of adaptations after stopping prolonged intense endurance training. *Journal of Applied Physiology*, **57**, 1857-1864.

9. Drinkwater, B.L., & Horvath, S.M. (1972). Detraining effects in young women. *Medicine and Science in Sports*, **4**, 91-95.

10. Fitts, R.H., Costill, D.L., & Gardetto, P.R. (1989). Effect of swim-exercise training on human muscle fiber function. *Journal of Applied Physiology*, **66**, 465-475.

11. Hickson, R.C., Foster, C., Pollock, M.L., Galassi, T.M., & Rich, S. (1985). Reduced training intensities and loss of aerobic power, endurance, and cardiac growth. *Journal of Applied Physiology*, **58**, 492-499.

12. Houmard, J.A., Costill, D.L., Mitchell, J.B., Park, S.H., Fink, W.J., & Burns, J.M. (1990). Testosterone, cortisol, and creatine kinase levels in male distance runners during reduced training. *International Journal of Sports Medicine*, **11**, 41-45.

13. Houmard, J.A., Costill, D.L., Mitchell, J.B., Park, S.H., Hickner, R.C., & Roemmish, J.N. (1990). Reduced training maintains performance in distance runners. *International Journal of Sports Medicine*, **11**, 46-51.

14. Kirwan, J.P., Costill, D.L., Flynn, M.G., Mitchell, J.B., Fink, W.J., Neufer, P.D., & Houmard, J.A. (1988). Physiological responses to successive days of intense training in competitive swimmers. *Medicine and Science in Sports and Exercise*, **20**, 255-259.

15. Kirwan, J.P., Costill, D.L., Houmard, J.A., Mitchell, J.B., Flynn, M.G., & Fink, W.J. (1990). Changes in selected blood measures during repeated days of intense training and carbohydrate control. *International Journal of Sports Medicine*, **11**, 362-366.

16. Kuipers, H., & Keizer, H.A. (1988). Overtraining in elite athletes: Review and directions for the future. *Sports Medicine*, **6**, 79-92.

17. Mackinnon, L.T. (1989). Exercise and natural killer cells: What is the relationship? *Sports Medicine*, **7**, 141-149.

18. McCarthy, D.A., & Dale, M.M. (1988). The leucocytosis of exercise: A review and model. *Sports Medicine*, **6**, 333-363.

19. Morgan, W.P., Costill, D.L., Flynn, M.G., Raglin, J.S., & O'Conner, P.J. (1988). Mood disturbance following increased training in swimmers. *Medicine and Science in Sports and Exercise*, **20**, 408-414.

20. Mostardi, R., Gandee, R., & Campbell, T. (1975). Multiple daily training and improvement in aerobic power. *Medicine and Science in Sports*, **7**, 82.

21. Nilson, K., Schoene, R.B., Robertson, H.T., Escourrou, P., & Smith, N.J. (1981). The effect of iron repletion on exercise-induced lactate production in minimally iron deficient subjects. *Medicine and Science in Sports and Exercise*, **13**, 92.

22. Saltin, B., Blomqvist, G., Mitchell, J.H., Johnson, Jr., R.L., Wildenthal, K., & Chapman, C.B. (1968). Response to submaximal and maximal exercise after bed rest and training. *Circulation*, **38**(Suppl. 7).

23. Selye, H. (1956). *The stress of life*. New York: McGraw-Hill.

24. Sharp, R.L., Vitelli, C.A., Costill, D.L., & Thomas, R. (1984). Comparison between blood lactate and heart rate profiles during a season of competitive swim training. *Journal of Swimming Research*, **1**, 17-20.

25. Watt, E., Buskirk, E., & Plotnicki, B. (1973). A comparison of single versus multiple daily training regimens: Some physiological considerations. *Research Quarterly*, **44**, 119-123.

Selected Readings

Bompa, T.O. (1983). *Theory and methodology of training*. Dubuque: Kendall/Hunt.

Costill, D.L., Flynn, M.G., Kirwan, J.P., Houmard, J.A., Mitchell, J.B., Thomas, R., & Park, S.H. (1988). Effects of repeated days of intensified training on muscle glycogen and swimming performance. *Medicine and Science in Sports and Exercise*, **20**, 249-254.

Costill, D.L., Hinrichs, D., Fink, W.J., Hoopes, D. (1988). Muscle glycogen depletion during swimming interval training. *Journal of Swimming Research*, **4**(1), 15-18.

Fitzgerald, L. (1988). Exercise and the immune system. *Immunology Today*, **9**, 337-339.

Fry, R.W., Morton, A.R., & Keast, D. (1991). Overtraining in athletes: An update. *Sports Medicine*, **12**, 32-65.

Haggmark, T., Eriksson, E., & Jansson, E. (1986). Muscle fiber type changes in human skeletal muscle after injuries and immobilization. *Orthopedics*, **9**, 181-185.

Henriksson, J., & Reitman, J.S. (1977). Time course of changes in human skeletal muscle succinate dehydrogenase and cytochrome oxidase activities and maximal oxygen uptake with physical activity and inactivity. *Acta Physiologica Scandinavica*, **99**, 91-97.

Hickson, R.C., Kanakis, J.C., Moore, A.M., & Rich, S. (1981). Effects of frequency of training, reduced training and retraining on aerobic power and left ventricular responses. *Medicine and Science in Sports and Exercise*, **13**, 93.

Kirwan, J.P., Costill, D.L., Mitchell, J.B., Houmard, J.A., Flynn, M.G., Fink, W.J., & Beltz, J.D. (1988). Carbohydrate balance in competitive runners during successive days of intense training. *Journal of Applied Physiology*, **65**, 2601-2606.

Lehman, M., Foster., C., & Keul, J. (1993). Overtraining in endurance athletes: A brief review. *Medicine and Science in Sports and Exercise*, **25**(7), 854-862.

Morgan, W.P., Brown, D.R., Raglin, J.S., O'Connor, P.J., & Ellickson, K.A. (1987). Psychological monitoring of overtraining and staleness. *British Journal of Sportsmedicine*, **21**, 107-114.

Morse, L.J., Bryan, J.A., & Murle, J.P. (1972). Holy Cross football team hepatitis outbreak. *Journal of the American Medical Association*, **219**, 706-708.

Pate, R.R., Hughes, R.D., Chandler, J.V., & Ratliffe, J.L. (1978). Effects of arm training on retention of training effects derived from leg training. *Medicine and Science in Sports*, **10**, 71-74.

Sherman, W.M., Plyley, M.J., Pearson, D.R., Habansky, A.J., Vogelgesang, D.A., & Costill, D.L. (1983). Isokinetic rehabilitation after meniscectomy: A comparison of two methods of training. *Physician Sports Medicine*, **11**, 121-133.

Chapter 14

Ergogenic Aids and Performance

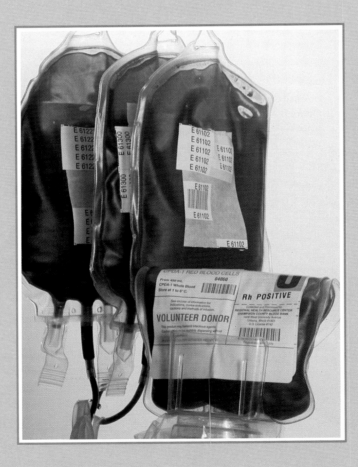

Chapter Overview

The skill levels of athletes in various sports improves from year to year. Athletic records reach new heights, and the margin between success and failure in the world of sport becomes smaller. Consequently, both coaches and athletes look for that slight edge that might assure victory. They might turn to ergogenic aids—substances or phenomena that enhance performance. Some of these aids can benefit performance, but others can have deadly consequences. In this chapter, we will examine various pharmacological, hormonal, and physiological agents that have been proposed to have ergogenic properties.

Chapter Outline

DIED of pneumonia following chemotherapy treatments for brain cancer, former NFL defensive end Lyle Alzado, 43, in Lake Oswego, Ore. Alzado, whose cancer was diagnosed in April 1991, believed he had contracted the disease through the use of anabolic steroids from 1969 to '91 and human growth hormone during his '90 comeback attempt. With the help of steroids, the 260-lb Alzado terrorized opponents during his 15 years (1971–85) with the Denver Broncos, the Cleveland Browns, and the Oakland Raiders. He led his teams in sacks three times, made All-Pro twice, played in two Super Bowls, and was voted Defensive Player of the Year in '77 and Comeback Player of the Year in '82. Though doctors say there is no proof that steroid or HGH use caused his cancer, the enfeebled Alzado said last August, "If what I've become doesn't scare you off steroids, nothing will."

—Reprinted from *Sports Illustrated*, May 25, 1992

In the never-ending quest for glory, athletes are often willing to try anything to improve their performance. For some, a special diet can be the deciding factor. Others might rely on stress reduction or hypnosis to alter their psychological states. Still others might try certain drugs or hormones.

Substances or phenomena that improve an athlete's performance are referred to as ergogenic aids. The variety of potential ergogenic aids is immense. Here are just a few examples:

- Weight lifters have taken anabolic steroids, hoping to increase muscle mass and strength.
- Distance runners have loaded up on carbohydrates a few days before competition to pack extra glycogen into their leg muscles.
- Hypnosis has been tried to help athletes through emotional or psychological problems.
- Even the cheers of the home crowd can place the home team at a distinct advantage.

The effects of proposed ergogenic substances are often shrouded in myth. Most athletes have received tips about ergogenic aids from a friend or coach and assume the information is accurate, but this is not always the case. Some athletes experiment with substances hoping for even a slight performance improvement regardless of possible harmful consequences. In the quest for performance perfection, a concern only with maximizing performance, coupled with a lack of knowledge about ergogenic substances, can prevent an athlete from making smart decisions.

The list of possible ergogenic aids is long, but the number that actually possess ergogenic properties is much shorter. In fact, some allegedly ergogenic substances or phenomena can actually impair performance. These are usually drugs, and Eichner has termed them ergolytic drugs.[19] Ironically and tragi-

cally, several ergolytic drugs have been promoted as ergogenic aids!

> ### KEY POINT
>
> **An ergogenic aid is any substance or phenomenon that enhances performance. An ergolytic substance is one that has a detrimental effect on performance. Some substances generally thought to be ergogenic are actually ergolytic.**

Table 14.1 provides a selected listing of substances, agents, and phenomena proposed to have ergogenic properties. These have been studied in sufficient depth to establish their efficacy. Many others have been proposed but not adequately researched. Table 14.2 lists proposed mechanisms of action by which ergogenic aids might work, along with examples.

This chapter focuses on pharmacological agents, hormones, and physiological agents. Nutritional supplements and substances will be addressed in chapter 15. Psychological phenomenon and mechanical factors are beyond the scope of this book, but have been reviewed in depth in Williams' book *Ergogenic Aids in Sport*.[44]

Researching Ergogenic Aids

Assume a professional superstar athlete consumes a particular substance several hours before game time and then has a successful performance. The athlete will likely attribute the success to this substance, even though there is no proof that ingesting the substance will ensure other athletes similar success.

Table 14.1 Proposed Ergogenic Aids

Category of aid	Proposed aid
Pharmacological agents	Alcohol
	Amphetamines
	Beta blockers
	Caffeine
	Cocaine and marijuana
	Diuretics
	Nicotine
Hormones	Anabolic steroids
	Human growth hormone
	Oral contraceptives
Physiological agents	Blood doping
	Erythropoietin
	Oxygen
	Warm-up and temperature variations
	Aspartic acid salts
	Bicarbonate loading
	Phosphate loading
Nutritional agents and substances	Carbohydrates
	Proteins
	Fats
	Vitamins and minerals
	Water and special beverages
Psychological phenomena	Hypnosis
	Covert rehearsal or mental practice
	Stress management
Mechanical factors	Clothing
	Equipment
	Environment—structures and surfaces

Table 14.2 Proposed Mechanism Through Which Ergogenic Aids Might Work

Proposed mechanism	Examples of various ergogenic aids
Act on muscle fibers	Anabolic steroids
	Growth hormone
	Protein
Act on heart and circulation	Alcohol
	Beta blockers
	Amphetamines
	Caffeine
	Cocaine and marijuana
Counteract CNS inhibition	Anabolic steroids
	Amphetamines
Counteract or delay onset or perception of fatigue	Amphetamines
	Aspartic acid salts
	Bicarbonate loading
	Phosphate loading
External mechanical factors	Clothing to reduce air or water resistance
	Playing surfaces such as tracks
	New equipment designs
	Shoes
Fuel supply for muscle and general muscle function	Carbohydrates
	Free fatty acids
	Vitamins and minerals
Increased oxygen delivery	Blood doping
	Phosphate loading
	Oxygen
Relaxation and stress reduction	Alcohol
	Beta-blocking drugs
	Hypnosis
	Stress management
Weight loss or weight gain	Diuretics
	Anabolic steroids
	Human growth hormone

Adapted from Fox et al. (1988).

Anyone can claim that a certain substance is ergogenic—and many substances have been so labeled strictly due to speculation—but before it can be legitimately classified as ergogenic, a substance must be proven to improve performance. Unfortunately, science, with its carefully controlled investigations, does not have all the answers. Still, scientific studies in this area are essential to differentiate between a true ergogenic response and a pseudoergogenic response, in which performance improves simply because the athlete expects improvement.

The Placebo Effect

The phenomenon by which your expectations of a substance determine your body's response to it is known as the placebo effect. This effect can seriously complicate the study of ergogenic qualities because researchers must be able to distinguish between the placebo effect and true responses to the substance being tested.

The placebo effect was clearly demonstrated in one of the earliest studies of anabolic steroids.[5] Fifteen male athletes who had been involved in heavy weight lifting for the previous 2 years volunteered for a weight-training experiment using anabolic steroids. They were told that those who made the greatest strength gains over a preliminary 4-month weight-training period would be selected for the second phase of the study, in which they would receive anabolic steroids.

Following the initial period, 8 of these 15 subjects were randomly selected to enter the treatment phase.

Only 6 of these subjects passed all medical screening tests and were allowed to continue to the treatment phase. This phase consisted of a 4-week period in which the subjects were told that they would receive 10 mg per day of Dianabol (an anabolic steroid), when, in fact, they received a placebo—an inactive substance typically provided in a form identical to the genuine drug.

Strength data were collected over the last 7 weeks of the pre-treatment period and over all 4 weeks of the treatment (placebo) period. Even though the subjects were experienced weight lifters, they continued to gain impressive amounts of strength during the pre-treatment period. However, strength gains while taking the placebo were substantially greater than during the pre-treatment period! As shown in Figure 14.1, the

What Does It Take to Get the Edge?

For some athletes, trying to get the competitive edge merely means following a comprehensive training program and a carefully controlled diet. But for others, ergogenic aids seem to be the answer. Some athletes might turn to a particular substance, yet others might try several substances at once in hopes of gaining the edge.

Melvin Williams, in the preface to his excellent book *Ergogenic Aids in Sport*, provides the following fictional example of the extremes to which some athletes will go.[44]

It was a special event, the tenth running of the New York City Marathon. Fred Lebow, initiator and director of the marathon, had national coverage on all three major television networks, and the Comsat Corporation arranged to have the race televised via satellite throughout the world. Lebow secured commitments from a variety of national corporations to guarantee a one million dollar prize to the winner.

Alberto Roe, the American record holder, had trained 8 to 10 hours per day over the past year in preparation for this event. He knew he was in peak condition and would shatter his current record. However, he also knew there would be serious challenges from the Japanese, Finns, East Germans, and New Zealanders. He was leaving nothing to chance.

In the past year, Alberto had trained at altitude for several months and had had three pints of blood removed and frozen. He had also used a new type of anabolic steroid that would maximize his red blood cell (RBCs) production and had consumed a special nutritional compound with iron, vitamin B_{12}, and folic acid to ensure optimal development of the RBCs.

During this time, the biomechanists working at Off Balance, the running gear company that sponsored Roe, had developed a polyethylene racing suit that would cut air resistance markedly at his racing speed and would permit an increase in heat dissipation. Moreover, they had developed a special racing shoe for him, weighing less than an ounce per pair and composed of a new elastomer that would double the rebounding force from the pavement.

During the last few days before the marathon, Roe began final preparations. The stored blood was infused into his veins and he initiated his carbohydrate-loading regimen with a new product designed to maximize the glycogen content in both the fast- and slow-twitch fibers. His personal sports psychologist was with him to help manage any stress at this crucial time that could disrupt his preparation for the race. He was given numerous posthypnotic suggestions to help him cruise through the race without fatigue, and he practiced the mental image of breaking the tape every hour.

About an hour before the race, Roe consumed a pint of water designed to maximize body water supplies for optimal temperature regulation. He also consumed a special amphetamine-caffeine mixture to provide an optimal anxiety level, carefully prescribed by his physician and sports psychologist. This mixture was also designed to optimize the free fatty acid levels in the blood in order to provide a glycogen-sparing effect. Every 2 miles during the race a handler would give him special fluid solutions and some concentrated oxygen through a specially designed breathing apparatus.[44]

Dr. Williams fails to provide the outcome of this race, but he paints an accurate picture of the extremes to which athletes, coaches, clinicians, and scientists go to gain a competitive edge. Some of the proposed aids in this example are still futuristic, but many have already been tried.

group improved an average of 10.2 kg (2%) during the 7-week pre-treatment period, but improved 45.1 kg (10%) during the 4-week treatment (placebo) period! This represents an average gain in strength of 1.5 kg per week during the pre-treatment period and 11.3 kg per week during the treatment period, indicating nearly a 10-fold increase in strength gains from the placebo alone! Furthermore, placebos are inexpensive, risk free, and legal for use in sport.

I [JHW] repeatedly witnessed the placebo effect while conducting a large series of studies investigating the effects of beta-blocking drugs on the ability to perform single bouts of exercise or to train aerobically. The Human Subjects Committee, a committee mandated by the federal government to oversee all research conducted with human subjects in the United States, requires that all human subjects receive a full disclosure of the risks associated with any experimental intervention so they can provide informed consent before participating. Before the start of each study, a cardiologist presented a comprehensive background on beta-blocking drugs to each subject, including the drugs' significance in treating various cardiovascular diseases and potential side effects associated with their use. I was amazed to note that over the course of 6 years of study, the most serious side effects almost always appeared in the subjects taking the placebo!

Thus, when evaluating a substance for possible ergogenic qualities, researchers must remember that witnessing an ergogenic effect does not necessarily prove that a substance is truly ergogenic. All studies of potential ergogenic substances must include a placebo group so researchers can compare responses resulting from the test substance with those resulting from a placebo.

> ### KEY POINT
>
> **Though the placebo effect has a psychological origin, the body's physical response to a placebo is not merely imagined—it is quite real. This clearly illustrates how effective our mental state can be in altering our physical state.**

Limitations of Research

To satisfy the scientific community, scientists often rely on laboratory techniques to evaluate the efficacy of any potential ergogenic aid. Often, however, scientific studies cannot provide absolutely clear answers to the questions under study. With elite athletes, success is defined in fractions of a second or tenths of an inch. Laboratory tests are often unable to detect such subtle differences in performance.

Scientists can be greatly limited by the accuracy of their equipment or techniques. All research methods have some margin of error. If the results fall within that margin of error, the researcher cannot be certain that the result is an effect of the substance being tested. The results might reflect limitations of the research methodology. Unfortunately, because of measurement error, individual differences, and the day-to-day variability of subjects' responses, a potential ergogenic aid must exert a major effect before scientific tests can prove that it is ergogenic.

The testing situation can also limit accuracy. Performance in a laboratory is considerably different than performance in the field where the athlete usually performs, so laboratory results won't always accurately reflect results found in the field. Yet an advantage of laboratory testing is that the environment can be carefully controlled, which isn't possible in the field, where several new variables—temperature, humidity, wind, and distractions—can affect the results. Thorough testing of a potential ergogenic aid should include both field and laboratory studies.

Realizing that science is limited in its ability to determine the efficacy of a substance, we can now examine some proposed ergogenic aids. We will consider substances in three classes:

1. Pharmacological agents
2. Hormonal agents
3. Physiological agents

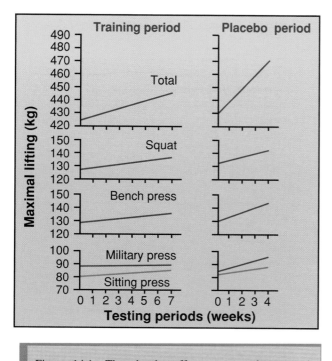

Figure 14.1   The placebo effect on muscular strength gains. Adapted from Ariel and Saville (1972).

Pharmacological Agents

Numerous pharmacological agents, or drugs, have been suggested as having ergogenic properties. The International Olympic Committee (IOC), the United States Olympic Committee (USOC), the International Amateur Athletic Federation (IAAF), and the National Collegiate Athletic Association (NCAA) all publish extensive lists of banned substances, most of which are pharmacological agents. Each athlete, coach, athletic trainer, and team physician must know which drugs are prescribed for and taken by the athlete, and they must check these drugs periodically against the listing of banned substances, because the list changes frequently. (The United States Olympic Committee has a drug education hotline that provides up-to-date information: 1-800-233-0393.) Athletes have been disqualified and have had to relinquish medals, ribbons, awards, and prizes after testing positive for a banned substance. In most cases, the medication had been used legitimately to treat a known medical condition.

We will review only drugs for which a research base has been established. Many other drugs have been touted as being ergogenic, but controlled studies must yet be conducted to determine if they are effective. The drugs we will discuss are

- alcohol,
- amphetamines,
- beta blockers,
- caffeine,
- cocaine,
- diuretics,
- marijuana, and
- nicotine.

Alcohol

Alcohol consumption is the number one drug problem in the United States today. Alcohol can be classified as a food or nutrient because it provides energy (7 $kcal \cdot g^{-1}$), but it can also be considered an antinutrient because it can interfere with the metabolism of other nutrients. Alcohol is also correctly classified as a drug because of its depressant effects on the central nervous system (CNS). However, psychologically, alcohol ingestion appears to result in a two-part response: an initial sensation of excitement, followed by depressive effects.[45]

Alcohol in Sports: The ACSM Position

Recently there has been considerable concern about increasing numbers of athletes becoming alcoholics as a result of their indiscriminate use of alcohol. This typically results from social drinking, not from using alcohol as an ergogenic aid. Most professional teams in all sports have now established alcohol and drug rehabilitation programs with professional groups to assist the treatment of athletes who admit to or who are identified as having a problem with substance abuse. The American College of Sports Medicine (ACSM) published the 1982 position statement, "The Use of Alcohol in Sports," which presents an excellent summary of the literature and general recommendations about alcohol use and abuse.[1] The ACSM concluded as follows:

1. The acute ingestion of alcohol can exert a deleterious effect upon a wide variety of psychomotor skills such as reaction time, hand-eye coordination, accuracy, balance, and complex coordination.

2. Acute ingestion of alcohol will not substantially influence metabolic or physiological functions essential to physical performance such as energy metabolism, maximal oxygen consumption, ($\dot{V}O_2$ max) heart rate, stroke volume, cardiac output, muscle blood flow, arteriovenous oxygen difference, or respiratory dynamics. Alcohol consumption may impair body temperature regulation during prolonged exercise in a cold environment.

3. Acute alcohol ingestion will not improve and may decrease strength, power, local muscular endurance, speed, and cardiovascular endurance.

4. Alcohol is the most abused drug in the United States and is a major contributing factor to accidents and their consequences. Also, it has been documented widely that prolonged excessive alcohol consumption can elicit pathological changes in the liver, heart, brain, and muscle, which can lead to disability and death.

5. Serious and continuing efforts should be made to educate athletes, coaches, health and physical educators, physicians, trainers, the sports media, and the general public regarding the effects of acute alcohol ingestion upon human physical performance and on the potential acute and chronic problems of excessive alcohol consumption.

Proposed Ergogenic Benefits

Some athletes use alcohol primarily for its psychological effects. It is thought to improve self-confidence and calm the nerves. Some athletes believe alcohol reduces inhibitions and makes them more alert.

Physiologically, many people view alcohol as a good carbohydrate source. It has also been touted as a means for reducing pain and muscle tremor. Its reputation for reducing tremor and anxiety made alcohol a potential ergogenic aid for shooting sports, but these sports have banned it.

Proven Effects

Unfortunately, little is known about the influence of varying amounts of alcohol on athletic performance. Although alcohol intoxication causes erratic and unpredictable performance, the influence of small amounts of alcohol just before or during a contest is not well understood.

In the absence of field studies of alcohol use during competition, laboratory studies have been conducted to observe the effects of small and moderate doses of alcohol on psychomotor skills such as

- simple reaction time,
- choice reaction time (person must choose the appropriate reaction),
- movement time,
- speed,
- sensorimotor coordination, and
- information processing.

Studies suggest that most psychomotor functions associated with sport performance are impaired by alcohol, not improved.[45] Although athletes can feel more alert and self-confident, their reaction time, coordination, movement, and thinking are all impaired. Small amounts of alcohol impair psychomotor skills, yet athletes are unaware of these changes and often believe that their performance has improved.

Well-controlled research studies also consistently support the conclusion that alcohol ingestion has no ergogenic effects on

- strength,
- power,
- speed,
- local muscular endurance, or
- cardiorespiratory endurance.

Risks of Alcohol Use

More important than its lack of ergogenic qualities, alcohol has many ergolytic features. Alcohol is a poor source of carbohydrates and, as mentioned earlier, is an antinutrient. Its depressant effects on the CNS dull pain sensation, but pain indicates injury, and physical activity while injured always carries a great risk of increasing the extent of injury. Although a reduction

in muscle tremor and anxiety might occur, the accompanying impairment of psychomotor skills offsets any advantage you might gain.

Alcohol suppresses the release of antidiuretic hormone (ADH), causing your body to excrete more water in the urine. This can, in turn, transiently decrease your blood pressure and cause dehydration (see Figure 14.2). This can have serious consequences during athletic performance, especially in hot environments. Alcohol also causes peripheral vasodilation (dilation of blood vessels in the skin). Loss of body heat through the blood vessels in your skin can trigger hypothermia in cold environments, because more heat is lost from your body than is desirable.

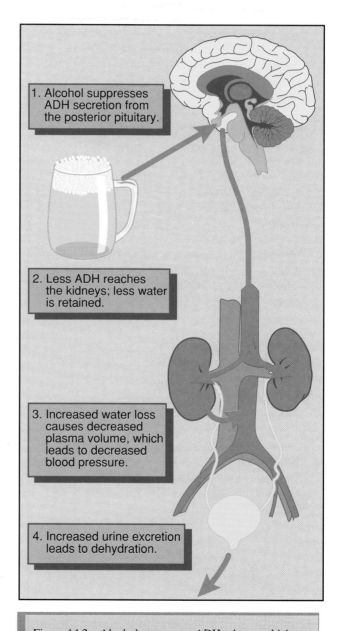

1. Alcohol suppresses ADH secretion from the posterior pituitary.

2. Less ADH reaches the kidneys; less water is retained.

3. Increased water loss causes decreased plasma volume, which leads to decreased blood pressure.

4. Increased urine excretion leads to dehydration.

Figure 14.2   Alcohol suppresses ADH release, which can lead to decreased blood pressure and dehydration, both of which impair performance.

■ IN REVIEW . . . ■

1. Alcohol consumption is the number one drug problem in the United States today. Alcohol is correctly classified as a drug because of its depressant effects on the CNS.
2. Alcohol is used by athletes primarily for its psychological effects. It is thought to improve self-confidence, calm nerves, reduce anxiety and inhibitions, increase mental alertness, and reduce pain and muscle tremor.
3. Most measures of psychomotor function are impaired by alcohol consumption, not improved, and no improvements in physiological function have been observed.
4. Alcohol use can negatively affect the athlete's health as well as performance.

Amphetamines

Amphetamine and its derivatives are CNS stimulants. They are also considered sympathomimetic amines, which means their activity mimics that of the sympathetic nervous system. They have been used as appetite suppressants in medically supervised weight-loss programs. During World War II, army troops used amphetamines to combat fatigue and to improve endurance. The drugs soon found their way into the athletic arena, where they were considered stimulants with possible ergogenic properties.

Proposed Ergogenic Benefits

Athletes have found amphetamines readily available even though they are prescription drugs. Amphetamines are used by athletes for many reasons. Psychologically, the drugs are thought to increase concentration and mental alertness. Their stimulating effect decreases mental fatigue. Athletes anticipate more energy and motivation and often feel more competitive when using amphetamines. The drugs also produce a state of euphoria, which is part of their attraction as so-called recreational drugs. Often athletes report a heightened sense of ability which they feel spurs them on to higher performance levels.

In terms of actual performance, amphetamines are thought to help athletes run faster, throw farther, jump higher, and delay the onset of total fatigue or exhaustion. Athletes who use these drugs expect virtually every aspect of performance to be enhanced.

Proven Effects

Generally, for any physiological, psychological, or performance variable that has been investigated, some studies show that amphetamines have no effect, others demonstrate an ergogenic effect, and still others indicate an ergolytic effect. As potent central nervous system stimulants, amphetamines do increase your state of arousal, which leads to a sense of increased energy, self-confidence, and faster decision making. People who take amphetamines experience

- decreased sense of fatigue,
- increased systolic and diastolic blood pressure,
- increased heart rate,
- redistribution of blood flow to skeletal muscles,
- elevation of blood glucose and free fatty acids, and
- increased muscle tension.[28]

Do these effects aid physical performance? Although studies are not in total agreement, the more recent studies, which have used better experimental designs and controls, show that amphetamines can enhance skills that are important in athletic performance, specifically

- speed,
- power,
- endurance,
- concentration, and
- fine motor coordination.[14,28,42]

The results of one of the better-controlled studies are presented in Table 14.3.[12] Subjects in this study received either a placebo or 15 mg per 70 kg of body weight of the amphetamine dexedrine, administered 2 hr before testing. Following amphetamine administration, significant increases were found in

- knee extension strength,
- acceleration,
- time to exhaustion during maximal treadmill testing,
- peak lactate response following the maximal treadmill test, and
- maximum heart rate.

Even though the time to exhaustion on the treadmill was increased, there were no differences in aerobic power.[12] The increased time to exhaustion likely reflects the subjects' psychological response to the drug, making them feel more energetic, delaying mental fatigue, and thus allowing them to work longer.

As mentioned previously, though, such laboratory tests might not accurately duplicate conditions encoun-

Table 14.3 Physical and Physiological Performance Changes With the Use of Amphetamines

Variable	Placebo	Drug	Mean difference	% difference
Elbow flexion strength (newtons)	681	724	43	6.3
Knee extension strength (newtons)	1,264	1,550	286	22.6[a]
Leg power (watts)	623	642	19	3.0
Peak speed (s per 10 yd)	1.11	1.11	0	0.0
Acceleration for 30-yard run (m · s⁻²)	2.89	3.00	0.11	3.8[a]
Aerobic power (L · min⁻¹)	3.96	3.97	0.01	0.3
Time to exhaustion (s)	427	446	19	4.4[a]
Peak lactate (mmol · L⁻¹)	13.3	14.4	1.1	8.3[a]
Maximum heart rate (beats · min⁻¹)	191	195	4	2.1[a]

[a]A statistically significant difference indicating a better performance while on amphetamines.

Adapted from Chandler and Blair (1980).

Table 14.4 The Acute and Chronic Side Effects of Amphetamines

Acute, mild	Acute, severe	Chronic
Restlessness	Confusion	Addiction
Dizziness	Assaultiveness	Weight loss
Tremor	Delirium	Psychosis
Irritability	Paranoia	Paranoid delusions
Insomnia	Hallucinations	Dyskinesias
Euphoria	Convulsions	Compulsive/
Uncontrolled	Cerebral hemorrhage	stereotypic/
movements	Angina/myocardial	repetitive
Headache	infarction	behavior
Palpitations	Circulatory collapse	Vasculitis
Anorexia		Neuropathy
Nausea		
Vomiting		

Adapted from Wadler and Hainline (1989).

Amphetamines can be psychologically addictive because of the euphoria and energized feelings they cause. But the drugs can also be physically addictive if taken regularly, and a person's tolerance to them builds with continued use, requiring increasingly larger doses over time to obtain the same effects. Amphetamines can also be toxic. Extreme nervousness, acute anxiety, aggressive behavior, and insomnia are frequently mentioned side effects of regular usage. Table 14.4 lists acute and chronic side effects of amphetamines.[42]

Beta Blockers

The sympathetic nervous system exerts its influence on bodily functions through adrenergic nerves—those that use norepinephrine as their neurotransmitter. Neural impulses traveling through these nerves trigger the release of norepinephrine, which crosses the synapses and binds to adrenergic receptors at the target cells. These adrenergic receptors are classified into two groups: alpha-adrenergic receptors and beta-adrenergic receptors.

Beta-adrenergic blockers, or beta blockers, are a class of drugs that block the beta-adrenergic receptors, preventing binding of the neurotransmitter. This greatly reduces the effects of stimulation by the sympathetic nervous system. Beta blockers are generally prescribed for the treatment of hypertension, angina pectoris, and certain cardiac arrhythmias. They are also prescribed as a preventative in the treatment of

tered in a field situation. Also, athletes might be consuming far greater doses of amphetamines than allowed in controlled research studies. Future studies must take this into account.

Risks of Amphetamine Use

Experience suggests that amphetamine use is inherently dangerous. Deaths have been attributed to excessive amphetamine usage. Because of the elevation of heart rate and blood pressure, amphetamine users place greater stress on their cardiovascular systems. The drugs can also trigger cardiac arrhythmias in some susceptible individuals. Also, rather than delaying the onset of fatigue, amphetamines likely delay the sensation of fatigue, enabling the athletes to push dangerously beyond normal limits to the point of circulatory failure. Deaths have occurred when athletes have pushed themselves far beyond the normal point of exhaustion.

in the treatment of migraine headaches, to reduce the symptoms of anxiety and stage fright, and for initial recovery from heart attacks.

Proposed Ergogenic Benefits

Because the sympathetic response gears the body up for physical activity (through the fight-or-flight mechanism), it is difficult to understand why athletes might turn to beta blockers as ergogenic aids. Beta blocker use in sport has been limited mostly to sports where anxiety and tremor could impair performance. When a person stands on a force platform (a highly sophisticated device that measures mechanical forces), measurable body movement is detected each time the heart beats. This movement is sufficient to affect a shooter's aim. Accuracy in shooting sports improves if the rifle or pistol can be shot or the arrow released between heartbeats. Beta blockers can slow a shooter's heart rate, allowing more time to stabilize the aim prior to shooting or releasing.

Beta blockers have also been postulated to enhance physiological adaptations to endurance training.[45] Research has shown that with chronic use of beta-blocking drugs the body increases its number of beta receptors. Apparently, the body responds to beta receptor blockage by increasing the number of beta receptors. It is theorized that endurance training while taking beta-blocking drugs would increase an athlete's number of beta receptors, allowing a greater sympathetic response after the drugs are discontinued.

Proven Effects

Beta blockers decrease the effects of sympathetic nervous system activity. This is well illustrated by the marked reduction in maximal heart rate with beta blocker administration. It is not unusual for a 20-year-old male athlete with a normal maximal heart rate of 190 beats per minute to have a maximal heart rate of only 130 beats per minute when taking beta-blocking drugs. Resting and submaximal heart rates are also reduced by these drugs. Several studies have confirmed improved scores, as a result of this heart-rate reduction, in shooting sports where subjects used beta blockers. Because of this, the IOC, the USOC, and the NCAA have banned the use of beta blockers for these sports.

The body contains two types of beta-adrenergic receptors: beta-1 and beta-2. Nonselective beta blockers affect both types of receptors, but beta-1 selective blockers primarily affect only the beta-1 receptors. Beta-1 receptors are located mainly in the heart, so a beta-1 selective blocker decreases the heart's rate and contractility. Beta-2 receptors are located in blood vessels, the lungs, the liver, skeletal muscle, and the intestines. Because they block both receptor types, nonselective beta blockers have greater overall effects than selective ones—they can affect blood flow, air

flow, and metabolism. If an athlete must take a beta-blocking drug for a medical condition, selective blockers are usually preferred because they have fewer negative effects on performance.

Laboratory studies have shown that beta-blocking drugs reduce

- maximal oxygen uptake, particularly in highly trained individuals;
- maximal ventilatory capacity, because air flow through the airways is reduced;
- submaximal and maximal heart rate;
- maximal cardiac output, because the stroke volume cannot increase enough to compensate for the reduced heart rate; and
- blood pressure, because cardiac output is reduced.[47]

Results of these laboratory studies have been confirmed by controlled studies during actual competition. In a study of long-distance runners, 10-km race times were greatly affected by beta-blocking drugs.[3] Under both control and placebo conditions, the runners averaged 35.8 min to complete the 10-km race. When using a nonselective beta blocker, the runners averaged 41.0 min (14.5% longer), but when using a selective beta-1 blocker, the runners averaged 39.2 min (9.5% longer).

Finally, beta-blocking drugs appear to have little influence on strength, power, and local muscular endurance (in activities that elicit fatigue in less than 2 min).[45] Thus, depending on the type of performance desired, beta blockers can be ergogenic (accuracy in shooting sports), ergolytic (decreased aerobic capacity), or without effect (strength, power, and local muscular endurance).

Risks of Beta Blocker Use

Most risks from beta blockers are associated with prolonged use, not isolated incidents of use as in athletics. Beta blockers can induce bronchospasm in people with asthma. They can cause cardiac failure in people who have underlying problems with cardiac function. In people with bradycardia, these drugs can lead to heart block. The decreased blood pressure they cause can result in lightheadedness. Some people with Type II diabetes can become hypoglycemic because beta blockers increase insulin secretion. These drugs, through their various effects, can cause pronounced fatigue, which can inhibit athletic performance and decrease motivation.

Caffeine

Caffeine, one of the most widely consumed drugs in the world, is found in coffee, tea, cocoa, soft drinks, and various other foods.[14] This drug is also common in several over-the-counter medications, often even in simple aspirin compounds. Caffeine is a central nervous system stimulant, and its effects are similar to those noted previously for amphetamines, though weaker. The caffeine contents of some common products are listed in Table 14.5.

Proposed Ergogenic Benefits

As with amphetamines, caffeine is generally touted as improving alertness, concentration, reaction time, and energy levels. People taking the drug often feel stronger and more competitive. They believe they can perform longer before the onset of fatigue and that if they are fatigued beforehand the fatigue is reduced.

Proven Effects

Because of its effects on the central nervous system, caffeine

- increases mental alertness,
- increases concentration,
- elevates mood,
- decreases fatigue and delays its onset,
- decreases reaction time,
- enhances catecholamine release,
- increases free-fatty-acid mobilization, and
- increases the use of muscle triglycerides.

In terms of ergogenic properties, caffeine was initially studied for potential effects that could benefit endurance activities. The first studies, conducted by Costill and his colleagues, demonstrated marked improvements in endurance performance in competitive cyclists who ingested a caffeinated beverage, compared to when they consumed a placebo beverage.[15,29] Caffeine increased endurance times in fixed-pace work bouts and decreased times in fixed-distance races.

Although several studies were unable to replicate these results, the most recent studies have demonstrated substantial ergogenic effects of caffeine ingestion in recreational cyclists and highly trained distance runners.[26,40] It is now generally concluded that caffeine does improve endurance performance, possibly through increased mobilization of free fatty acids, which leads to sparing of muscle glycogen for later use. But the actual mechanisms by which caffeine improves endurance performance might be more complex. It is now well documented that caffeine lowers your perception of effort at a given rate of work, potentially allowing you to perform at a higher rate of work for the same perceived effort. Cellular mechanisms are also presently being explored.[17]

Caffeine might also improve performance in sprint and strength types of activities.[4,13] Unfortunately, fewer studies have investigated this area, but caffeine might facilitate calcium exchange at the sarcoplasmic reticulum and increase the activity of the sodium-potassium pump, better maintaining the muscle membrane potential.

Risks of Caffeine Use

In people who are not accustomed to using caffeine, who are sensitive to it, or in anyone who consumes high doses, caffeine can produce nervousness, restlessness, insomnia, and tremors. Caffeine also acts as a diuretic, increasing an athlete's risk for dehydration and heat-related illness when performing in hot environments. It can disrupt normal sleep patterns, contributing to fatigue. Caffeine is also physically addictive—even for the daily coffee drinker. Abrupt discontinuation of caffeine intake can result in headache, fatigue, irritability, and gastrointestinal distress.

Cocaine

Little is known about the influence of the so-called recreational drugs, such as cocaine, on athletic performance. Cocaine acts as a central nervous system stimulant. Cocaine can also be characterized as a sympathomimetic drug, and its actions are very similar to those of amphetamines.

Cocaine blocks the reuptake of norepinephrine and dopamine (two major neurotransmitters) by the neurons after they are released. Recall that norepinephrine is released by sympathetic nerves, including those supplying the heart. Both norepinephrine and dopamine are used in the brain. By blocking their reuptake, cocaine potentiates these neurotransmitters' effects throughout the body.

Table 14.5   Caffeine Contents of Some Common Products[a]

Substance	Caffeine (mg)
Standard dose Prolamine	280
Standard dose Dexatrim, Dietac	200
Standard dose No Doz, Vivarin	100-200
6 oz automatic drip coffee	181
6 oz automatic perk coffee	125
Standard dose of some aspirin products (see labels)	30-128
6 oz hot tea (strong)	65-107
6 oz iced tea	70-75
6 oz instant coffee	54-75
12 oz cola beverages	32-65
12 oz Mountain Dew	54
12 oz Mello Yellow	51
8 oz chocolate milk	48
2 oz chocolate candy	45
1 oz baking chocolate	45

[a]Recommended caffeine intake is less than 250 mg per day.

Adapted from Tribole (1991).

IN REVIEW . . .

1. Amphetamines are CNS stimulants that increase mental alertness, elevate mood, decrease the sense of fatigue, and produce euphoria.
2. The most recent studies indicate that amphetamines can increase strength, acceleration, maximal lactate responses during exhaustive exercise, and time to exhaustion.
3. Amphetamines elevate both heart rate and blood pressure, and can trigger cardiac arrhythmias. Excessive use of these drugs has been blamed for some deaths, and the drugs can be both psychologically and physically addictive.
4. Beta blockers block beta-adrenergic receptors, preventing neurotransmitter binding.
5. Beta blockers slow the resting heart rate, which is a distinct advantage for shooters who try to release the arrow or squeeze the trigger between heartbeats to minimize the slight tremor associated with each beat. But these drugs impair endurance performance, reducing $\dot{V}O_2$ max in highly trained people because cardiac output is reduced (stroke volume cannot fully compensate for the reduced heart rate).
6. Beta blockers can cause bradycardia and even heart block, hypotension, bronchospasm, pronounced fatigue, and decreased motivation. Selective beta blockers have fewer side effects than nonselective blockers, and should usually be prescribed whenever an athlete must receive these drugs.
7. Caffeine, one of the most widely consumed drugs in the world, is also a CNS stimulant, and its effects are similar to those of amphetamine, but weaker.
8. Caffeine increases mental alertness and concentration, elevates mood, decreases fatigue and delays its onset, increases catecholamine release and mobilization of free fatty acids, and increases muscle use of free fatty acids to spare glycogen.
9. Caffeine can cause nervousness, restlessness, insomnia, tremors, and diuresis. Diuresis increases susceptibility to heat injury.

Proposed Ergogenic Benefits

Though cocaine use has become far too common in athletics, most is recreational use. But some athletes believe cocaine is an ergogenic aid. The drug creates an intense euphoria that is thought to increase self-confidence and motivation. Like amphetamines, cocaine masks both fatigue and pain, increases alertness, and makes the athlete feel energetic.

Proven Effects

Because of the dangers involved with cocaine use, few studies have been conducted on its ergogenic properties. Considering only the well-controlled studies, no evidence indicates that cocaine has any ergogenic properties, regardless of its similarities to amphetamine.

Risks of Cocaine Use

Athletes must recognize that even if athletic performance could benefit from cocaine, the risks associated with its use far outweigh any benefits. Several comprehensive reviews of the research literature conclude that tremendous health risks and no known performance benefits are associated with cocaine use.[11,14,33,42] Deaths of some prominent sports figures have been directly attributed to cocaine use.

Cocaine can induce psychological problems such as agitation, irritability, restlessness, and anxiety. It can cause insomnia and, with habitual use, can result in cocaine psychosis, in which the user hallucinates and can become paranoid.

Physiologically, repeated cocaine inhalation can inflame and ultimately destroy nasal tissues. More importantly, the drug increases norepinephrine's effects on the heart, which can cause serious, even fatal, arrhythmias. By drastically increasing the stimulation of the heart, cocaine puts a tremendous strain on even a healthy heart. Because these effects occur so rapidly, the heart is suddenly faced with this tremendous stress and can go into cardiac arrest. With the added stress of physical performance, the risk of death is greatly increased.

Cocaine is one of the most highly addictive drugs known, particularly in its purest form—crack, or rock cocaine. Now, with the deadly crack cocaine becoming increasingly available in virtually all communities, the cocaine problem in this country has become considerably more serious. Among athletes, cocaine use frequently starts as recreational use, but quickly becomes an addiction. Users experience intense cravings for the tremendous high cocaine provides. They turn to the drug more often and need higher doses to achieve the same high. Once they are hooked, cocaine becomes their obsession.

Diuretics

Diuretics affect the kidneys, increasing urine formation. Used appropriately, they rid the body of excess fluid and are frequently prescribed to control hypertension and reduce edema (water retention) associated with congestive heart failure or other conditions.

Proposed Ergogenic Benefits

Diuretics are generally used as ergogenic aids for weight control. For decades, diuretics have been used by some jockeys, wrestlers, and gymnasts to keep their weight down. More recently, they have been used by anorexics and bulimics for weight loss.[48]

Some athletes who are taking banned drugs have also turned to diuretics, but not to enhance their performance. Because diuretics increase fluid loss, these athletes hope that the extra fluid in their urine will dilute the concentration of banned drugs, thus decreasing the likelihood that the banned substances will be detected during drug testing. This, along with any means used to alter the urine in an effort to escape drug detection, is called masking.[42]

Proven Effects

Diuretics lead to significant weight loss, but no evidence suggests any other potentially ergogenic effects. In fact, several side effects make diuretics ergolytic. The fluid loss results primarily from losses in extracellular fluid, including plasma. For athletes, particularly those dependent on moderate to high levels of endurance, this reduction in plasma volume reduces maximal cardiac output, which in turn reduces aerobic capacity and impairs performance.

Risks of Diuretic Use

Diuretics also hinder thermoregulation. As internal body heat increases, more blood must be diverted to the skin so the heat can be lost to the environment. However, when blood plasma volume is diminished, as with diuretic use, more blood must be kept in the central regions to maintain central venous blood pressure and adequate blood supply and blood pressure to the vital organs. Thus less blood is available to be shunted to the skin and heat loss is impaired.

Electrolyte imbalance can also occur. Many of the diuretics cause fluid loss by assuring electrolyte loss. A diuretic called furosemide inhibits sodium reabsorption in the kidneys, thus allowing more of it to be excreted in the urine. Because fluid follows the sodium, more fluid will also be excreted. Electrolyte imbalances can occur with losses of either sodium or potassium. These imbalances can cause fatigue and muscle cramping. More serious imbalances can lead to exhaustion, cardiac arrhythmias, and even cardiac arrest. Deaths of some athletes have been attributed to electrolyte imbalances caused by diuretic use.

Marijuana

Marijuana is another so-called recreational drug. Like alcohol, it can elicit both stimulant and depressant effects.[45] It acts primarily on the central nervous system, but its mode of action is poorly understood.

Proposed Ergogenic Benefits

Marijuana has not been proposed as ergogenic. In fact, it generally is ergolytic.[19] However, use of this drug is quite common, especially among younger athletes, so it must be considered in terms of its effects on performance. Many who use marijuana seek the sense of euphoria and relaxation it produces. Like alcohol, it is often a means of escape or a way to reduce tension. Many youths deem its use appropriate merely because their peers are smoking it.

Proven Effects

Marijuana impairs performance of skills requiring

- hand-eye coordination,
- fast reaction time,
- motor coordination,
- tracking ability, and
- perceptual accuracy.[42]

Of major concern in athletes is the ''amotivational syndrome'' seen frequently in marijuana users. This is characterized by apathy, impaired judgment, loss of ambition, and an inability to carry out long-term plans.

Risks of Marijuana Use

Health risks of marijuana use are still under investigation. Personality changes are noted with just a few marijuana cigarettes. Short-term memory is impaired, which has led to concerns that marijuana might cause permanent brain damage. High intake of the drug can cause hallucinations and psychotic-like behavior.

Another concern with marijuana is how the drug is ingested. It is usually smoked, though it can be eaten. The serious health consequences associated with cigarette smoking are common knowledge. Do these same health problems arise from marijuana smoking? Are there other health problems resulting from the combustion of different chemicals in marijuana? These questions are still unanswered.

Nicotine

Athletes have used nicotine as a stimulant. The most familiar nicotine form is cigarettes, and fortunately fewer people now smoke. But among athletes the smokeless forms—chewing tobacco (chew), snuff (dip), and compressed tobacco (plug)—are still popular and their use appears to be increasing.

As with other recreational drugs, some athletes turn to nicotine for possible ergogenic effects, but many are addicted and use nicotine on a daily basis, so its effects carry over into their athletic performance.

Proposed Ergogenic Benefits

Nicotine is a stimulant. Some athletes believe it makes them more alert and better able to concentrate. Yet, paradoxically, the drug is also reported to have a calming effect, opposite that of a stimulant. For this reason, many athletes also use it to soothe jittery nerves.

Proven Effects

Nicotine has generally been found to be detrimental, or of little value, to athletic performance. In general, smokers have demonstrated lower $\dot{V}O_2$ max values than nonsmokers; such lower values are associated with increased carbon monoxide binding to hemoglobin, which reduces oxygen transport capacity. Nicotine from cigarettes or smokeless tobacco causes increased heart rate, blood pressure, and autonomic reactivity. Other changes noted after nicotine use include vasoconstriction, decreased peripheral circulation, increased secretion of antidiuretic hormone and catecholamines, and increased blood lipid levels, plasma glucose, glucagon, insulin, and cortisol. The effects on performance parameters have not been studied adequately to draw any conclusions.

Risks of Nicotine Use

Nicotine has serious long-term health effects. The drug is highly addictive, which is why so many people who first try tobacco with their peers find themselves years later with a serious habit that is difficult to break.

Many of nicotine's risks relate to the method of ingestion. Smokeless forms are known to cause cancers of the mouth, pharynx, and larynx, and smoking is linked to several cancers, most notably lung cancer. Smokers are often more susceptible to respiratory infections, because cigarette smoke paralyzes the cilia in the respiratory tract, which sweep particulate matter away from the lungs. When the cilia are paralyzed, this cleansing action is diminished or halted and particles can settle into the alveoli, blocking or damaging them. Smoking also can lead to emphysema. Smoking also leads to serious cardiovascular changes. It raises blood cholesterol levels and promotes atherosclerosis, which can directly lead to myocardial infarction or stroke. A smoker's risk of a heart attack is twice that of a nonsmoker, and smoking is the main risk factor for sudden cardiac death.

━━ IN REVIEW . . . ━━

1. Cocaine is a CNS stimulant. Although not generally considered ergogenic, some athletes associate the euphoria it creates with increased self-confidence and motivation. There is no evidence that cocaine is in any way ergogenic.
2. Cocaine is extremely addictive. It has tremendous potential for triggering major psychological disorders and has numerous undesirable physiological effects, most involving heart function, that can lead to death.
3. Diuretics affect the kidneys, increasing urine formation and excretion. They are often used by athletes for weight reduction or maintenance, and also by those trying to mask use of other drugs during drug testing.
4. Weight loss is the only proven ergogenic effect of diuretics, but this weight loss is primarily from the extracellular fluid compartment, including blood plasma. This leads to dehydration, which can impair thermoregulation and cause electrolyte imbalances.
5. Marijuana acts on the CNS and can elicit both stimulant and depressant effects.
6. Marijuana has not been proposed to have ergogenic qualities. It is in fact ergolytic. It impairs performance that requires hand-eye coordination, fast reaction time, motor coordination, tracking ability, and perceptual accuracy.
7. Marijuana use can lead to personality changes, short-term memory impairment, hallucinations, and psychotic-like behavior. When smoked, it might pose the same risks as cigarette smoking.
8. Nicotine is a stimulant, ingested either by smoking or in smokeless forms—chewing tobacco, snuff, and compressed tobacco. Some athletes believe nicotine makes them more alert and better able to concentrate, yet also more calm.
9. Nicotine is generally detrimental to performance. It causes several changes in cardiovascular, metabolic, respiratory, and hormonal function that can impair both submaximal and maximal performance.
10. Proven risks of nicotine use include various forms of cancer and cardiovascular disease.

Another effect is impaired circulation to the extremities. Smoking is the major factor contributing to peripheral vascular disease, in which the blood vessels to the extremities are constricted. The American Heart

KEY POINT

Many pharmacological agents don't have ergogenic properties, yet some athletes believe that they do. Several substances are banned not because they are ergogenic but because their use carries high risks. Such bans are intended to keep athletes from trying harmful substances with the erroneous notion that they will enhance performance, when in fact some of these substances can be lethal.

However, several drugs, both prescription or over-the-counter, possibly have ergogenic properties, such as ephedrine, which is common in cold and sinus medications. Many of these drugs are banned, which can cause disqualification of uninformed athletes who are merely trying to shake off some ailment, often following their doctors' advice. Before taking any drug for any reason, athletes should always check the banned substances lists if they plan to compete.

Association reports that this disease is found almost exclusively in smokers. This places athletes who smoke at a much higher risk of frostbite when performing in cold environments.

Hormonal Agents

The use of hormonal agents as ergogenic aids in competitive athletics began in the late 1940s or early 1950s. Anabolic steroids were the hormones most frequently used by athletes between the 1950s and the 1980s. During the last half of the 1980s, a new potential ergogenic aid emerged with the introduction of synthetic human growth hormone, and women began experimenting with oral contraceptives (birth control pills) to see if manipulating their menstrual cycles could facilitate athletic performance.

Although numerous scientific studies have been conducted on anabolic steroids and sport, little is known about the effects of human growth hormone and birth control pills on sport performance. Both anabolic steroids and human growth hormone are banned for all sports and the medical risks associated with their use are high. Medical risks are also associated with taking oral contraceptives, but their use in sport is unregulated at this time.

We now turn our attention to the three major hormone groups being used (or abused) by athletes today:

1. Anabolic steroids
2. Human growth hormone
3. Oral contraceptives

Anabolic Steroids

Androgenic-anabolic steroids, commonly referred to simply as anabolic steroids, are nearly identical to the male sex hormones (see chapter 6). The anabolic (building) properties of these steroid hormones accelerate growth by increasing the rate of bone maturation and increasing the development of muscle mass. For years, anabolic steroids have been given to youngsters with delayed growth patterns to normalize their growth curves. The development of synthetic steroids has allowed alteration of the natural chemical composition of these hormones to reduce their androgenic (masculinizing) properties and increase their anabolic effects on muscle.

Proposed Ergogenic Benefits

Theoretically, steroid administration will increase fat-free mass and strength. Consequently, an athlete who depends on muscle size, body size, or strength might be tempted to take steroids. Early claims that aerobic capacity improved with anabolic steroid use also caught the attention of endurance athletes. Anabolic steroids have also been postulated to facilitate recovery from exhaustive training bouts, allowing athletes to train hard on subsequent days. This potential benefit has stirred the interest of athletes from almost all sports. The potential for anabolic steroid use among athletes is very high, and this continues to be a major sports problem.

Proven Effects

The limitations of scientific research have been apparent in the study of effects of anabolic steroids. Results of early investigations were almost evenly divided. Many studies found no significant change in body size or physical performance attributable to taking steroids, yet many other studies found steroids to have considerable positive influence on increasing muscle mass and strength. One basic problem with almost all research conducted in this area to date is the inability to observe in the research laboratory the effects of the drug dosages being used in the athletic world. Some athletes are estimated to be taking five to ten times the recommended maximum daily dosage. Obviously, it would be unethical to design a study using dosages that exceed the recommended maximum. Fortunately, there is another option. Let's examine what the research does show about the effects of steroids on performance.

Muscle Mass and Strength. Researchers have been able to observe athletes who, on their own, are taking higher steroid doses. In one study, the effects of relatively high doses were observed in seven male weight lifters.[27] Two treatment periods, each lasting 6 weeks, were separated by a 6-week interval without treatment. Half of the subjects received a placebo during the first treatment period and the steroid during the second treatment period. The other half received the medications in reverse order—steroid first, then placebo. When the data from all subjects were analyzed, results showed that while on the steroid, the weight lifters had significant increases in

- body mass;
- potassium and nitrogen, indicating an increased fat-free mass;
- muscle size; and
- leg performance and strength.

These increases did not occur during the placebo period. Results of this study are summarized in Figure 14.3.

In a second study, body composition changes were observed in a professional bodybuilder and a competitive weight lifter.[22] Both were on self-prescribed high doses of steroids. The bodybuilder had been on the high dose for 140 days and the weight lifter for 125 days. Fat-free body mass increased an average of 19.2 kg, and fat mass decreased almost 10 kg.

Forbes plotted the results of a number of different studies using different dosages.[22] He concluded that only minimal increases of 1 to 2 kg in fat-free body mass occur with low doses of anabolic steroids. But with high doses, fat-free body mass increases markedly. His results show a threshold level for steroid doses, with only very high doses resulting in substantial increases in fat-free body mass.

In 1987, the American College of Sports Medicine published a revision of their 1977 position statement on the use of anabolic-androgenic steroids in sports.[2] They concluded that steroids in the presence of an adequate diet can increase total body mass, and often increase fat-free mass. Furthermore, they concluded that the normal gains in muscle strength associated with high-intensity exercise and proper diet can be increased by anabolic steroid use in some individuals. Several more recent reviews have reached the same conclusions.[34,42]

Cardiorespiratory Endurance. Several early studies reported increases in $\dot{V}O_2$ max with the use of anabolic steroids. These results were consistent with the known effects of steroid administration on increasing red blood cell production and total blood volume. However, in these studies $\dot{V}O_2$ max was estimated indirectly. In later, better-controlled studies, $\dot{V}O_2$ max was measured directly and anabolic steroids produced no benefit.

The American College of Sports Medicine's position statement concludes that anabolic steroids do not increase either aerobic power or the capacity for muscular exercise.[2] However, none of the studies investigating anabolic steroid use and improvement in aerobic capacity involved trained endurance athletes.

Recovery From Training. Finally, the theory that anabolic steroids facilitate recovery from high-intensity training is attractive. A major concern in training elite athletes

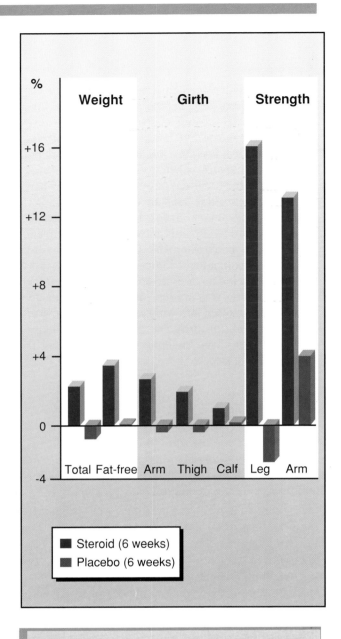

Figure 14.3 Percentage of changes in body size, body composition, and strength when using anabolic steroids and a placebo. Adapted from Hervey et al. (1981).

today is how to reduce the negative physiological and psychological effects associated with high-intensity training, enabling the athlete to continue to train at peak levels day after day. At this time, though, no available data about steroid use support this idea.

Risks of Anabolic Steroid Use

Although use of anabolic steroids can be beneficial for certain types of athletic performance, several major issues must be addressed. It is neither morally nor ethically right for athletes to use drugs to improve their chances in competition. Most athletes feel it is wrong for those they compete against to artificially improve their performance. Yet many of these same athletes feel compelled to use steroids in an effort to compete with the other athletes in their sport or event who are chronic steroid users. Fair competition is not possible if you are the only athlete in a particular competition who has remained steroid-free.

How widespread is this problem? Though in the past steroid use was a problem primarily in male-dominated sports, many women athletes are now taking steroids to increase their fat-free body mass, strength, and performance. Steroid use among athletes has also worked its way down to the high school and junior high school levels. Furthermore, steroid use among adolescent nonathletes who simply want to look good has also sharply increased.

At one time, it was estimated that 80% of all weight lifters, shot-putters, discus throwers, and javelin throwers of national caliber were using anabolic steroids, and this was considered by many to be a conservative number.

Although the pressures on the athlete are great, are the potential gains worth the possible risks associated with steroid use? These drugs are illegal and athletes risk being banned from their sports. More important, however, are the medical risks associated with steroid use, especially with the massive doses often used by athletes. Steroid use by people who are not physically mature can lead to early closure of the epiphyses of the long bones, so final stature can be reduced. Use of anabolic steroids suppresses the secretion of gonadotropic hormones, which control the development and function of the gonads (testes and ovaries). In males, decreased gonadotropin secretion can cause testicular atrophy, decreased secretion of testosterone, and a reduced sperm count. Decreased testosterone can lead to enlargement of the male breasts. In females, gonadotropins are required for ovulation and secretion of estrogens, so a decrease in these hormones disrupts those processes and menstruation. In addition, these hormonal disturbances in females can lead to masculiniza-

tion—breast regression, enlargement of the clitoris, deepening of the voice, and growth of facial hair.

Prostate gland enlargement in males is another possible side effect of steroid use. Liver damage from a form of chemical hepatitis brought on by steroid use has also been identified, and it can lead to liver tumors.

Cardiomyopathy (diseased heart muscle) has been reported in chronic steroid users. Scientists have found markedly depressed HDL-cholesterol levels—reductions of 75% or more—in athletes on even moderate steroid doses (see Figure 14.4). HDL-cholesterol has antiatherogenic properties, meaning it prevents the development of atherosclerosis. Low levels of it are associated with a high risk for both coronary artery disease and heart attack (see chapter 20).

Substantial personality changes have occurred with steroid use. The most notable change is a marked increase in aggressive behavior, or the "roid rage." Some teens have become extremely violent and have attributed these drastic mood changes to steroid use. Evidence also suggests drug dependency can result from steroid use. As a final point of great concern, neither scientists nor physicians know the potential long-term effects of chronic steroid use.

The American College of Sports Medicine's position statement and recent reviews provide more detail on the potential ergogenic effects and health risks associated with anabolic steroid use.[2,6,34,42,51] Most governing bodies of sports likely to be affected by anabolic

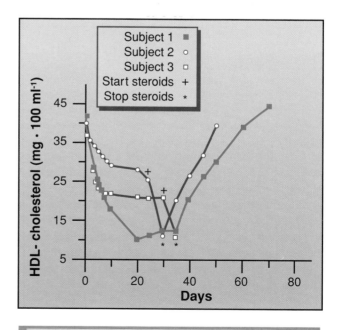

Figure 14.4   Changes in HDL-cholesterol levels as a result of using anabolic steroids. Adapted from Costill et al. (1984).

steroid use have developed educational materials for their athletes in hopes of preventing steroid use. Also, national governing bodies for most sports have instituted aggressive year-round testing programs in which athletes are randomly tested for steroid use.

▬ IN REVIEW . . . ▬

1. Anabolic steroids are more appropriately termed androgenic-anabolic steroids because in their natural state they include both androgenic (masculinizing) and anabolic (building) properties. Synthetic steroids have been designed to maximize the anabolic effects while minimizing androgenic effects.
2. Anabolic steroids have been proposed to increase muscle mass, strength, and endurance capacity, and to facilitate recovery from exhaustive training bouts.
3. Anabolic steroids can increase muscle mass and strength, but this effect is dose dependent. They do not increase endurance capacity and their ability to facilitate recovery from exhaustive exercise has not been proven.
4. Considerable risks are associated with use of anabolic steroids, including personality changes, "roid rage," testicular atrophy, reduced sperm count, breast enlargement in men and breast regression in women, prostate gland enlargement in men, masculinization in women, liver damage, and cardiovascular disease.

Human Growth Hormone

For years, the medical treatment for hypopituitary dwarfism has been administration of human growth hormone (hGH), a hormone secreted by the anterior pituitary gland. Prior to 1985, this hormone was obtained from cadaver pituitary extracts, and the supply was limited. Since the introduction of genetically engineered human growth hormone in the mid-1980s, availability is no longer an issue, although the cost is still high.

During the 1980s, realizing this hormone's numerous functions, athletes started investigating human growth hormone as a possible substitute for or complement to their use of anabolic steroids.

Proposed Ergogenic Benefits

Growth hormone (GH) has five functions of interest to athletes:

1. Stimulation of protein and nucleic acid synthesis in skeletal muscle

2. Stimulation of bone growth (elongation) if bones are not yet fused (important to young athletes)
3. Increase in lipolysis, leading to an increase in free fatty acids and an overall decrease in body fat
4. Increase in blood glucose levels
5. Enhancement of healing after musculoskeletal injuries

Athletes turned to this hormone thinking it would increase muscle development. Along with this comes an increase in fat-free mass. Often GH is used with anabolic steroids to maximize the anabolic effects. Some athletes, however, turn to GH instead of steroids because it is very difficult for drug testing to distinguish between synthetic growth hormone and the body's own natural supply of GH.

Proven Effects

Research on whether or not growth hormone aids healing is inconclusive at this time, but several studies have reported on other effects. One study involved healthy men, 61 to 81 years of age. Following a 6-month treatment period in which 12 men received GH 3 times a week, researchers found that

- fat-free body mass increased by 9%,
- fat mass decreased by 14%, and
- lumbar vertebral bone density increased by 2%.

A control group of 9 men showed no change in any of these measurements over the same period.[38]

In another study, young men were randomly assigned to one of two groups. Both underwent resistance training, but one group was given a placebo while the other received GH.[50] Following a 12-week training period, the GH group showed the greatest increases in

- fat-free body mass,
- total body water,
- whole-body protein synthesis rate, and
- whole-body protein balance (rate of synthesis − breakdown).

When looking at specific muscles, however, the two groups did not differ significantly. Muscle size, muscle strength, and the rate of muscle protein synthesis for the quadriceps were not any greater in the GH group than in the placebo group, indicating that resistance exercise alone resulted in similar increases in these areas, irrespective of GH use.

Some athletes also take other drugs and certain amino acid supplements to stimulate GH release from the pituitary. To date, little evidence suggests that this practice is effective.

Risks of Growth Hormone Use

As with steroids, potential medical risks are associated with growth hormone use. Acromegaly can result from taking GH after the bones have fused. This disorder results in bone thickening, which causes broadening of the hands, feet, and face; skin thickening; and soft tissue growth. Internal organs typically enlarge. Ultimately the victim suffers muscle and joint weakness and often heart disease. Cardiomyopathy is the most common cause of death with GH use. Glucose intolerance, diabetes, and hypertension can also result from GH use.

Oral Contraceptives

Oral contraceptives (birth control pills) contain synthetic versions of natural estrogens and progesterones. They function as contraceptives by preventing ovulation.

Proposed Ergogenic Benefits

Oral contraceptives have been proposed as potential ergogenic aids because they can control the athlete's menstrual cycle. Many women athletes find that their performance is unaffected by their menstrual cycle, but others notice a difference. Those who have cyclic fluctuations in their performance frequently suffer from premenstrual syndrome (PMS), experiencing emotional or physical symptoms, and often both, 3 to 5 days prior to menstruation. Many experience dysmenorrhea (difficult or painful menstruation).

Proven Effects

Shangold has stated that it is rarely advisable or necessary to manipulate an athlete's menstrual cycle to improve her performance.[39] However, she states that it might be appropriate to consider using oral contraceptives to regulate the cycle for special events of great importance in those few elite women athletes who perform better in the follicular (early cycle) phase than at other times. This can be accomplished by administering low-dose oral contraceptives continuously (not cyclically) for several months prior to the competitive event, continuing until 10 days before the competition. Withdrawal bleeding can be expected within 3 days of discontinuation. This assures the athlete of a predictable bleeding pattern and leaves her with low levels of both estrogen and progesterone at the time of the event. This approach is relatively safe.

Risks of Oral Contraceptive Use

Though the use of oral contraceptives is quite widespread, these drugs are not without medical risks. Some of the risks include

- nausea,
- weight gain,
- fatigue,
- hypertension,
- liver tumors,
- blood clots,
- stroke, and
- heart attack.

The risk of the last three is increased tremendously for women who also smoke.

IN REVIEW . . .

1. Human growth hormone stimulates synthesis of protein and nucleic acid in skeletal muscle, stimulates bone growth, increases lipolysis (thus decreasing body fat), increases blood glucose levels, and enhances healing of musculoskeletal injuries.
2. Growth hormone has not been studied extensively for its potential ergogenic effects. The limited research available supports its ability to increase fat-free mass and decrease fat mass, but GH might have little or no effect on increasing muscle mass and strength.
3. Risks associated with GH use include acromegaly, hypertrophy of internal organs, muscle and joint weakness, diabetes, hypertension, and heart disease.
4. Oral contraceptives have been proposed as ergogenic aids for women athletes due to their ability to regulate the menstrual cycle.
5. Little research at this time supports the use of oral contraceptives for ergogenic purposes, though the drugs may be beneficial for elite women athletes who suffer from PMS or dysmenorrhea.
6. Risks associated with oral contraceptives include nausea, weight gain, fatigue, hypertension, liver tumors, blood clots, stroke, and heart attack.

Physiological Agents

Many physiological agents have been proposed as ergogenic aids. The goal behind these is to improve the body's physiological response during exercise. With these agents, an athlete typically adds something that occurs naturally in the body to try to improve performance. The reasoning is that if natural levels of a substance are beneficial to performance, higher levels should be even better. Several physiological agents have been proven effective, but generally only under very specific conditions or for certain events or sports.

As with hormonal agents, many athletes consider use of these substances to be more ethical than use of pharmacological agents because these substances are naturally found in the body. They also often assume that because these substances are normally in the body, they must be safe at any level. Unfortunately, our bodies can be very unforgiving, and this assumption can be fatal.

We will look at only a few examples of physiological agents being used as ergogenic aids:

- Blood doping
- Erythropoietin
- Oxygen supplementation
- Aspartic acid
- Bicarbonate loading
- Phosphate loading

Blood Doping

Although altering blood composition in any way can be considered blood doping, the term has taken on a more specific meaning. Blood doping refers to any means by which a person's total volume of red blood cells is increased. This is often accomplished by transfusion of red blood cells, either previously donated by the individual (autologous transfusions) or from someone else with the same blood type (homologous transfusions).

Proposed Ergogenic Benefits

Knowing that oxygen is carried through the body bound to hemoglobin, it seems logical that increasing the number of red blood cells available to ferry the oxygen to the tissues could benefit performance. Increasing the number of oxygen carriers should increase your blood's oxygen-carrying capacity, allowing more oxygen to be delivered to your active tissues. If this happens, your aerobic endurance, and thus your performance, could be substantially increased. That is the premise underlying blood doping.

Proven Effects

Ekblom et al. created quite a stir in the sports world in the early 1970s.[21] In one of their studies, they withdrew between 800 and 1,200 ml of blood from their subjects, then reinfused the red blood cells into those subjects about 4 weeks later. Results showed a considerable improvement in $\dot{V}O_2$ max (9%) and treadmill performance time (23%). Over the next few years, several studies failed to confirm these original findings, but several others demonstrated an ergogenic effect.

Thus the research literature was divided on the effectiveness of blood doping until a major breakthrough occurred in 1980 as a result of a study by Buick et al.[9] Eleven highly trained distance runners were tested at different times during the study:

1. Before blood withdrawal
2. After allowing the body adequate time to reestablish normal red blood cell levels but before reinfusion of the removed blood
3. Following a sham reinfusion of 50 ml of saline (a placebo)
4. Following reinfusion of 900 ml of blood that had originally been withdrawn and preserved by freezing
5. After the elevated red blood cell levels had returned to normal

As shown in Figure 14.5, the researchers found a substantial increase in $\dot{V}O_2$ max and treadmill time following the reinfusion of the red blood cells (Group A), and no change following the sham reinfusion (Group B). This increase in $\dot{V}O_2$ max persisted for up to 16 weeks, but the increase in treadmill time decreased within the first 7 days.

Maximizing the Benefits. Why was the Buick et al. study a major breakthrough? Gledhill helped explain the controversy arising from the early studies.[23,24] Many early studies that found no improvement with blood doping had reinfused only small volumes of red blood cells, and the reinfusion was conducted within 3 to 4 weeks of the blood withdrawal. First, it appears that you must withdraw and reinfuse 900 ml or more of whole blood. Increases in $\dot{V}O_2$ max and performance are not as great when smaller volumes are used. In fact, some studies using smaller volumes failed to find any differences.

Second, it appears that you must wait for at least 5 to 6 weeks and possibly as long as 10 weeks before reinfusion. This is based on the time it takes your body to reestablish your blood's prewithdrawal hematocrit.

Finally, early studies refrigerated the withdrawn blood. Maximum storage time under refrigeration is approximately 5 weeks. Furthermore, when blood is refrigerated, approximately 40% of the red blood cells are destroyed or lost. Later studies have used frozen storage. Freezing allows an almost unlimited storage time, and only about 15% of the red blood cells are lost.

Gledhill concluded that blood doping results in significant improvements in $\dot{V}O_2$ max and endurance performance when done under optimal conditions:[23,24]

- A minimum of 900 ml of blood reinfusion
- A 5- to 6-week minimum interval between withdrawal and reinfusion
- Blood storage by freezing

He has also shown that these improvements are the direct result of the blood's increased hemoglobin content, not increased cardiac output due to an expanded plasma volume.

Blood Doping and Endurance. Does an increase in $\dot{V}O_2$ max and treadmill time as a result of blood doping translate into improved endurance performance? Sev-

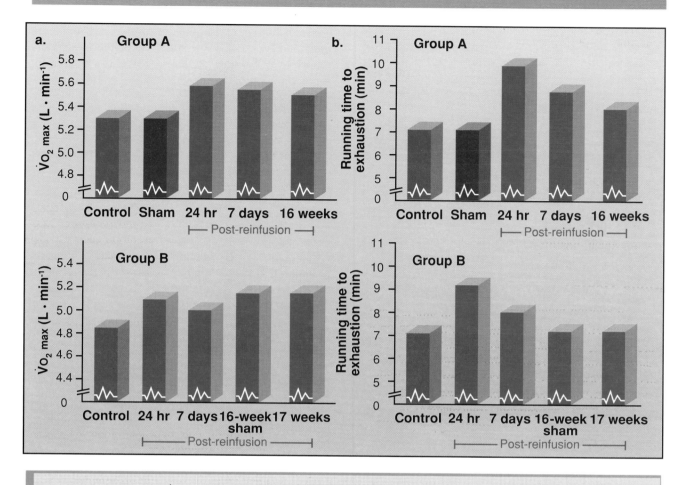

Figure 14.5   Changes in V̇o₂ max and running time to exhaustion following reinfusion of red blood cells. Adapted from Buick et al. (1980).

eral studies have addressed this issue. One study observed 5-mi (8-km) treadmill run times in a group of 12 experienced distance runners. Their times were checked before and after saline (placebo) infusion, and before and after blood infusion.[46] The 5-mi (8-km) run times on the treadmill were significantly faster following blood infusion, but this difference became significant only over the last 2.5 mi (4 km). The blood infusion trials were 33 s faster (3.7%) over the last 2.5 mi (4 km), and 51 s faster (2.7%) over the full 5.0 mi (8 km) compared to the placebo trials.

A second study, looking at 3-mi (4.8-km) run times in a group of six trained distance runners, reported a decrease of 23.7 s following blood doping. This decrease was significantly different from the runners' blind control trials.[25] Subsequent studies confirmed improvements in distance running and cross-country skiing performance with blood doping. Figure 14.6 illustrates the improvement in run time with blood doping for distances of up to 11 km.

Risks of Blood Doping

Although this procedure is relatively safe in the hands of competent physicians, it has inherent dangers. Adding more blood into the cardiovascular system can overload it, causing the blood to become too viscous, which could lead to clotting and possibly heart failure. With autologous blood transfusions, in which the recipient receives his or her own blood, mislabeling of the blood could occur. With homologous blood transfusions, in which blood is received from a matched donor, several other complications can occur. The reinfused blood could be mismatched. An allergic reaction could be triggered. The athlete may experience chills, fever, and nausea. The athlete also risks contraction of hepatitis or acquired immune deficiency syndrome (AIDS).

The potential risks of blood doping, even without considering the legal, moral, and ethical issues involved, outweigh any potential benefits.

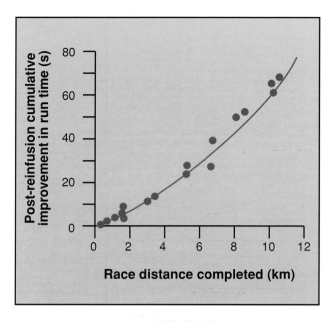

Figure 14.6 Improvements in running times for distances of up to 11 km following reinfusion of red blood cells from two units of freeze-preserved blood. Adapted from Spriet (1991).

Erythropoietin

Erythropoietin could easily be included in the preceding section on blood doping because it falls into that class, but the mechanism is somewhat different, so we'll examine it separately. Erythropoietin is a naturally occurring hormone produced by the kidneys. It stimulates red blood cell production. In fact, this hormone is responsible for the elevated red blood cell production seen when training at altitude—training in the presence of a lower partial pressure of oxygen stimulates erythropoietin release.

Human erythropoietin can now be cloned through genetic engineering, so it is widely available. This hormone increases the hematocrit substantially when administered to renal failure patients.

Proposed Ergogenic Benefits

Theoretically, if administered to athletes, human erythropoietin would have the same effects as the reinfusion of red blood cells. The goal of its use is to increase the red blood cell volume, thus increasing the blood's oxygen-carrying capacity.

Proven Effects

Erythropoietin's ability to increase oxygen capacity was demonstrated in 1991 when the first study was done of the effects of subcutaneous injections of low doses of human erythropoietin on maximal treadmill time and $\dot{V}O_2$ max. The study involved moderately trained to well-trained subjects.[20] Six weeks after erythropoietin administration,

- both hemoglobin concentration and hematocrit increased 10%,
- $\dot{V}O_2$ max increased 6% to 8%, and
- time to exhaustion on the treadmill increased 13% to 17%.

Seven of the 15 subjects had been through a previous study of red blood cell reinfusion, conducted 4 months earlier. Increases in $\dot{V}O_2$ max and treadmill time were almost identical in both studies, and these improvements were attributed directly to the increase in hemoglobin.

Risks of Erythropoietin Use

Serious consequences can arise from erythropoietin use. Some deaths among competitive cyclists, reported in the early 1990s, were alleged to be linked to erythropoietin use. This allegation has not been confirmed.

The outcome of erythropoietin use is less predictable than that of red blood cell reinfusion. Once the hormone has been put into the body, no one can predict how much red blood cell production will occur. This places the athlete at great risk of substantial increases in blood viscosity, which could lead to clotting or heart failure.

Oxygen Supplementation

You're watching the professional football game of the week on television. The star running back breaks loose for a 35-yd (32-m) touchdown run, struggles back to the bench, grabs a face mask, and starts breathing 100% oxygen to facilitate his recovery. How much does he gain by using oxygen supplementation instead of just breathing ordinary air?

Proposed Ergogenic Benefits

Obviously, the purpose of taking in oxygen is to increase the oxygen content of the blood, as with blood doping. Blood doping attempts to do this by increasing the oxygen-carrying capacity of the blood; oxygen supplementation tries to achieve this directly by providing more oxygen. By increasing the available oxygen, athletes hope to fend off fatigue for longer periods. This technique has also been suggested as a means to speed recovery between exercise bouts.

Proven Effects

Initial attempts to investigate the ergogenic properties of pure oxygen began in the early 1900s, but it was not until the 1932 Olympic Games that oxygen was considered a potential ergogenic aid for athletic performance. That year, Japanese swimmers won impressive victories, and many attributed their success to breathing pure oxygen before competing. However, it is unclear whether their success was due to their use of oxygen or to the fact that they were better athletes.

Of historical note, one of the first studies to observe the effects of breathing oxygen on performance was conducted by Sir Roger Bannister, a physician-scientist who is world renowned for his research in neurological disorders.[7] As an athlete, Dr. Bannister was the first person in the world to break the 4-minute-mile barrier!

Oxygen can be administered

- immediately prior to competition,
- during competition,
- during recovery from competition, or
- during any combination of these.

Oxygen breathing before exercise has a limited effect on performance of that exercise bout. The total amount of work or the rate of work (exercise intensity) can be increased by breathing oxygen if the bout is of short duration and occurs within a few seconds after breathing oxygen. During these short bouts, submaximal work can be performed at a lower pulse rate. However, no improvement occurs unless the exercise follows within seconds of breathing oxygen.

For exercise bouts exceeding 2 minutes or when more than 2 minutes lapse between oxygen breathing and actual performance, oxygen supplementation's influence is greatly diminished. This simply reflects the limits of the body's oxygen storage potential—extra oxygen dissipates rapidly; it is not stored.

When oxygen is administered during exercise, definite performance improvements occur. The total amount of work performed and the rate of work performed increase substantially. Likewise, submaximal work is performed more efficiently with lower physiological cost to the individual. Peak blood lactate levels are depressed following exhaustive exercise performed while breathing oxygen, even though considerably more work can be performed.

Studies have been unable to demonstrate any clear advantage to oxygen breathing during the recovery period. Recovery does not seem to be facilitated, nor does subsequent performance improve. In an unpublished study in our laboratory [JHW], subjects performed an exhaustive, all-out ride on a cycle ergometer for 60 s. They were then immediately switched to breathing a gas mixture of either pure oxygen or air for a 2-min recovery period. This was immediately followed by a second all-out 60-s ride. Neither the recovery during the 2-min interval between the exhaustive bouts, nor the total work accomplished in the

second bout, was facilitated by oxygen breathing. This is illustrated in Figure 14.7. A similar study with professional soccer players running on a treadmill also found no improvements in recovery or subsequent performance on the second exhaustive bout as a result of oxygen breathing.[49]

From a practical standpoint, oxygen administration prior to exercise would have little value because of the relatively short time that oxygen stores remain elevated. The nature of most sports doesn't allow an athlete to go immediately from oxygen breathing into competition. Regardless of the ergogenic effects of oxygen intake during performance, administration during exercise has limited value for obvious reasons: During which sports or events could you carry a cylinder of oxygen without significant restriction of movement?

The recovery period seems the only practical time to administer oxygen, but it would only be worthwhile if oxygen administration speeds the recovery process, allowing the athlete to re-enter the contest more fully recovered. However, such an effect has not been substantiated by research.

Risks of Oxygen Use

At this time, no known risks are associated with oxygen use. More research must be conducted to determine its safety. However, oxygen is flammable, so oxygen

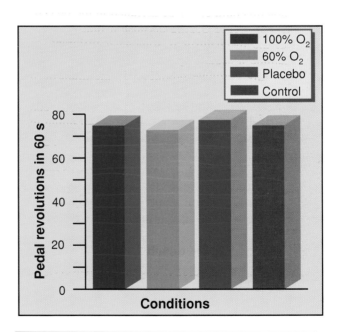

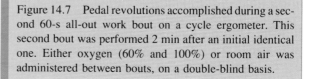

Figure 14.7 Pedal revolutions accomplished during a second 60-s all-out work bout on a cycle ergometer. This second bout was performed 2 min after an initial identical one. Either oxygen (60% and 100%) or room air was administered between bouts, on a double-blind basis.

equipment should never be near any heat source or flame, nor should it be allowed near anyone who is smoking.

IN REVIEW . . .

1. Blood doping refers to an artificial increase in a person's total volume of red blood cells. It has been proposed to improve endurance performance by increasing the blood's oxygen-carrying capacity.
2. Early studies produced conflicting results, but more recent work found major increases in maximal oxygen uptake, time to exhaustion, and actual performance in cross-country skiing and distance running.
3. Risks associated with blood doping include major complications such as blood clotting, heart failure, and administration of mislabeled blood and its potential consequences, such as transfusion reactions, transmission of hepatitis, and transmission of the virus that causes AIDS.
4. Erythropoietin is the naturally occurring hormone that stimulates red blood cell production. It has been proposed as an ergogenic aid with the premise that increasing the number of red blood cells would increase the blood's oxygen-carrying capacity.
5. Little research exists to substantiate this role for erythropoietin, but one study has demonstrated increased maximal oxygen consumption and increased time to exhaustion.
6. Because we cannot predict the magnitude of the body's response to erythropoietin administration, it is very dangerous. The hormone can lead to death if red blood cells are overproduced, because increased blood viscosity can cause clotting and heart failure.
7. Oxygen administration during exercise improves performance but is too cumbersome to be practical. Administration before or immediately after exercise has not been proven ergogenically effective.
8. There are no serious risks associated with brief (2- to 3-min) periods of oxygen breathing.

Aspartic Acid

Blood ammonia concentrations increase with increasing intensity and duration of exercise. These increases in blood ammonia have been associated with fatigue. Ammonia is toxic to our bodies. To decrease the toxic effects, excess ammonia is converted by the liver into a less harmful substance—urea. Aspartic acid is an amino acid involved in this conversion process in the liver.

Proposed Ergogenic Benefits

It has been hypothesized that administering aspartates (aspartic acid salts) might facilitate the clearing of ammonia from the blood, thereby delaying fatigue.

Proven Effects

Research on this topic is not conclusive. As an example, in one study eight healthy young male subjects exercised to exhaustion on a cycle ergometer. Each subject exercised at a constant rate of 75% of $\dot{V}O_2$ max and completed two trials: one with aspartates and one with a placebo.[35] Researchers found no significant difference in time to exhaustion between the two trials. Several years later, a second study used an almost identical experimental design but a slightly higher dose of aspartate. This study found significant differences in endurance times for the two groups.[43] At this time, it is impossible to draw any conclusions concerning aspartate's potential as an ergogenic aid. Well-controlled, systematic studies must be conducted, with varying doses of aspartates and varying intensities of exercise.

Risks of Aspartic Acid Use

At this time, no known risks are associated with the use of aspartic acid. However, insufficient data are available. More research must be conducted to determine its safety.

Bicarbonate Loading

Recall from chapter 9 that bicarbonates are an important part of the buffering system necessary to maintain the acid-base balance of body fluids. Scientists naturally began to investigate whether performance in highly anaerobic events, in which large amounts of lactic acid are formed, could be improved by enhancing the body's buffering capacity through elevation of the blood's bicarbonate concentrations.

Proposed Ergogenic Benefits

By ingesting agents that increase the bicarbonate concentrations in the blood plasma, such as sodium bicarbonate (baking soda), it is possible to increase blood pH, making the blood more alkaline. It was proposed that increasing plasma bicarbonate levels would provide additional buffering capacity, allowing higher concentrations of lactate in the blood. Theoretically, this could delay the onset of fatigue in short-term, all-out anaerobic work such as all-out sprinting.

Proven Effects

Oral intake of sodium bicarbonate elevates the plasma bicarbonate concentrations. However, this has little effect on the intracellular concentrations of bicarbonate in muscle. This was thought to limit the potential benefits of bicarbonate ingestion to anaerobic bouts of exercise lasting longer than 2 min because bouts less than 2 min would be too brief to allow much hydrogen ions (H^+, from the lactic acid) to diffuse out of the muscle fibers into the extracellular fluid where they could be buffered.

However, in 1990, Roth and Brooks described a cell membrane lactate transporter that operates in response to the pH gradient.[37] Increasing the extracellular buffering capacity by ingesting bicarbonate increases the extracellular pH, which, in turn, increases transport of lactate from the muscle fiber via this membrane transporter to the blood plasma and other extracellular fluids. This should allow improvement in anaerobic performances for events even briefer than 2 min.

Although the theory proposing bicarbonate ingestion as an ergogenic aid for anaerobic performance is sound, the research literature is, again, conflicting. However, Linderman and Fahey, in their review of the research literature, found several important patterns in the research that had been conducted that might explain these conflicts.[32] They concluded that bicarbonate ingestion had little or no effect on performances of less than 1 min or of more than 7 min, but for performances between 1 and 7 min, the ergogenic effects were evident. Furthermore, they found that the dose was important. Most studies that used a dose of 300 mg · kg^{-1} of body mass showed a benefit, whereas most studies of lower dosage showed little or no benefit. Thus, it appears that bicarbonate ingestion of 300 mg · kg^{-1} of body mass can enhance the performance of those all-out, maximal anaerobic activities of from 1 to 7 min duration.

An example of a study supporting these conclusions is illustrated in Figure 14.8. In this study, blood bicarbonate concentrations were artificially elevated by bicarbonate ingestion before and during five sprint-cycling bouts, each lasting 1 min (see Figure 14.8a).[16] Performance on the final trial improved by 42%! This elevation in blood bicarbonate levels reduced the concentration of free H^+ both during and after exercise (see Figure 14.8b), thereby elevating blood pH. The authors concluded that in addition to improving buffering capacity, the extra bicarbonate appeared to speed the removal of H^+ ions from the muscle fibers, thereby lessening the drop in intracellular pH. Six years later, in 1990, Roth and Brooks reported the presence of a

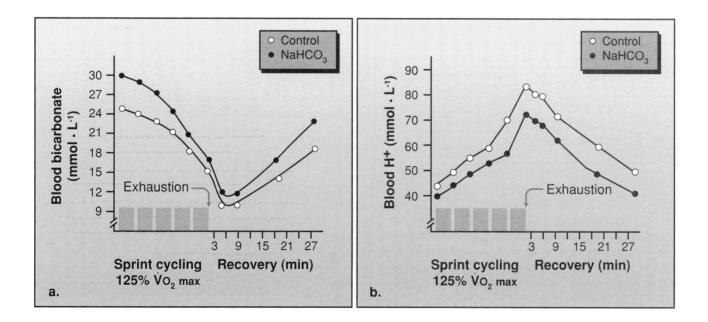

Figure 14.8   Concentrations of (a) blood bicarbonate (HCO_3^-) and (b) blood hydrogen ion (H^+) before, during, and after five sprint cycling bouts with and without ingestion of sodium bicarbonate ($NaHCO_3$). The fifth sprint was performed to exhaustion. The elevated blood HCO_3^- concentrations caused an elevation of blood H^+, less of a drop in blood pH, and faster recovery after the sprints. Adapted from Costill et al. (1984).

lactate transporter in the muscle cell membrane, as described earlier, which works precisely as Costill et al. had originally postulated.[16,37]

Risks of Bicarbonate Loading

Although sodium bicarbonate has long been used as a remedy for indigestion, many authors studying bicarbonate loading have reported severe gastrointestinal discomfort, including diarrhea, cramps, and bloating, when using high doses of bicarbonate. This can be prevented by ingesting as much water as desired, and by dividing the total bicarbonate dosage of at least $300 \text{ mg} \cdot \text{kg}^{-1}$ of body mass into five equal parts over a 1- to 2-hr period.[32] Also, several studies have found sodium citrate to have similar effects on buffering capacity and improved performance, but without gastrointestinal discomfort.[30,36]

Phosphate Loading

Since the early 1900s, scientists have been interested in the possibility of increasing the dietary consumption of phosphorus to improve cardiovascular and metabolic function during exercise. Several of the early studies suggested that phosphate loading, which involves ingestion of sodium phosphate as a dietary supplement, was an effective ergogenic aid.

Proposed Ergogenic Benefits

Phosphate loading has been proposed to have numerous potential benefits during exercise. These include elevation of extracellular and intracellular phosphate levels, which would increase the availability of phosphate for oxidative phosphorylation and phosphocreatine synthesis, thus improving your body's energy production capacity. It is also thought to enhance 2,3-diphosphoglycerate (2,3-DPG) synthesis in the red blood cells. This substance facilitates the release of oxygen from the red blood cells. This increase would shift the hemoglobin-oxygen dissociation curve to the right, permitting greater oxygen unloading in the active muscles.[42] Phosphate loading has also been proposed to improve the cardiovascular response to exercise, improve the body's buffering capacity, and consequently improve endurance capacity and performance.

Proven Ergogenic Benefits

Only a few studies have been conducted to determine the ergogenic benefits of phosphate loading. Unfortunately, the results are divided. Several studies show significant improvements in $\dot{V}O_2$ max and time to exhaustion.[10,31,41] However, several others show no effects.[8,18] There appear to be some potential benefits to phosphate loading, but additional research is needed to confirm this.

Risks of Phosphate Loading

At this time, no known risks are associated with phosphate loading. However, because insufficient research has been conducted to date, more studies are needed to determine its safety.

■—— IN REVIEW . . . ——■

1. Aspartic acid is an amino acid involved in the liver's conversion of ammonia to urea. Because excess ammonia is associated with fatigue, ingestion of aspartates has been postulated to reduce the ammonia that builds up during exercise, thus delaying fatigue.
2. Research on the effectiveness of aspartic acid as an ergogenic aid is insufficient and conflicting. More research is needed to determine its ergogenic potential and safety.
3. Bicarbonate is an important component of the body's buffering system, needed to maintain normal pH by neutralizing excess acid.
4. Bicarbonate loading is proposed to increase the blood's alkalinity, thus increasing the buffering capacity so that more lactate can be cleared. This would delay the onset of fatigue.
5. Bicarbonate ingestion of at least $300 \text{ mg} \cdot \text{kg}^{-1}$ body weight can delay fatigue and increase performance in all-out bouts of exercise lasting more than 1 min but less than 7 min.
6. Bicarbonate loading can cause gastrointestinal distress, including cramping, bloating, and diarrhea.
7. Ingestion of sodium phosphate has been postulated to improve general cardiovascular and metabolic functioning. During exercise, phosphate loading has been proposed to elevate phosphate levels throughout the body, which would increase the potential for oxidative phosphorylation and phosphocreatine synthesis, enhance oxygen release to the cells, improve cardiovascular response to exercise, improve the body's buffering capacity, and improve endurance capacity.
8. Little research at this time supports the use of phosphate loading as an ergogenic aid. Existing research is conflicting, and the risks of phosphate loading are largely unknown.

In Closing . . .

In this chapter, we reviewed some common substances and procedures thought to have ergogenic properties. All athletes must recognize the legal, ethical, moral, and medical consequences of using any ergogenic agent. The list of banned substances grows daily. Athletes using banned substances risk disqualification from a particular competition and they can be banned from competition in their sport for a year or more. In their quest for the perfect performance, athletes can easily get caught up in the hype surrounding various substances and the purported benefits they might bestow. Unfortunately, too many are blinded by ambition and do not consider the consequences of their actions until their career has been jeopardized or their health seriously impaired.

We have discussed the categories of pharmacological, hormonal, and physiological ergogenic aids. In the next chapter we turn our attention to nutritional ergogenic aids and the dietary needs of athletes.

Key Terms

alcohol
amphetamine
anabolic steroids
aspartic acid
beta blockers
bicarbonate loading
blood doping
caffeine
cocaine
diuretics
ergogenic
ergogenic aid
ergolytic

erythropoietin
hormonal agents
human growth hormone
marijuana
nicotine
oral contraceptives
oxygen supplementation
pharmacological agents
phosphate loading
physiological agents
placebo
placebo effect

Study Questions

1. What is the meaning of the term ergogenic aid? What is an ergolytic effect?
2. Why is it important to include control groups and placebos when studying the ergogenic properties of any substance or phenomenon?
3. How does the use of alcohol in moderate or large doses affect athletic performance?
4. What is presently known about the use of amphetamines in athletic competition? What are the potential risks of using amphetamines?
5. Under what circumstances might beta blockers be ergogenic aids? What are some of their ergolytic properties?
6. How might caffeine improve athletic performance?
7. What is known about cocaine and marijuana as ergogenic aids?
8. Are diuretics ergogenic? What are some risks associated with their use?
9. What are the effects of anabolic steroid use on athletic performance? What are some of the medical risks of steroid use?
10. What is known about human growth hormone as a potential ergogenic aid? What are the risks associated with its use?
11. How are oral contraceptives used as potential ergogenic aids?
12. What is blood doping? Does blood doping improve athletic performance?
13. How is erythropoietin theorized to benefit performance?
14. How beneficial is the breathing of oxygen prior to the start of competition, during competition, and during the recovery from competition?
15. What are the potential ergogenic properties of aspartates, bicarbonate, and phosphate?

References

1. American College of Sports Medicine Position Statement. (1982). The use of alcohol in sports. *Medicine and Science in Sports and Exercise*, **14**, ix-xi.

2. American College of Sports Medicine Position Statement. (1987). The use of anabolic-androgenic steroids in sports. *Medicine and Science in Sports and Exercise*, **19**, 534-539.

3. Anderson, R.L., Wilmore, J.H., Joyner, M.J., Freund, B.J., Hartzell, A.A., Todd, C.A., & Ewy, G.A. (1985). Effects of cardioselective and nonselective beta-adrenergic blockade on the performance of highly trained runners. *American Journal of Cardiology*, **55**, 149D-154D.

4. Anselme, F., Collomp, K., Mercier, B., Ahmaïdi, S., & Préfaut, C. (1992). Caffeine increases maximal anaerobic power and blood lactate concentration. *European Journal of Applied Physiology*, **65**, 188-191.

5. Ariel, G., & Saville, W. (1972). Anabolic steroids: The physiological effects of placebos. *Medicine and Science in Sports and Exercise*, **4**, 124-126.

6. Bahrke, M.S., Yesalis, C.E., & Wright, J.E. (1990). Psychological and behavioural effects of endogenous testosterone levels and anabolic-androgenic steroids among males: A review. *Sports Medicine*, **10**, 303-337.

7. Bannister, R.G., & Cunningham, D.J.C. (1954). The effects on the respiration and performance during exercise of adding oxygen to the inspired air. *Journal of Physiology*, **125**, 118-137.

8. Bredle, D.L., Stager, J.M., Brechue, W.F., & Farber, M.O. (1988). Phosphate supplementation, cardiovascular function, and exercise performance in humans. *Journal of Applied Physiology*, **65**, 1821-1826.

9. Buick, F.J., Gledhill, N., Froese, A.B., Spriet, L., & Meyers, E.C. (1980). Effect of induced erythrocythemia on aerobic work capacity. *Journal of Applied Physiology*, **48**, 636-642.

10. Cade, R., Conte, M., Zauner, C., Mars, D., Peterson, J., Lunne, D., Hommen, N., & Packer, D. (1984). Effects of phosphate loading on 2,3-diphosphoglycerate and maximal oxygen uptake. *Medicine and Science in Sports and Exercise*, **16**, 263-268.

11. Cantwell, J.D., & Rose, F.D. (1986). Cocaine and cardiovascular events. *The Physician and Sportsmedicine*, **14**(11), 77-88.

12. Chandler, J. V., & Blair, S.N. (1980). The effect of amphetamines on selected physiological components related to athletic success. *Medicine and Science in Sports and Exercise*, **12**, 65-69.

13. Collomp, K., Ahmaïdi, S., Chatard, J.C., Audran, M., & Préfaut, C. (1992). Benefits of caffeine ingestion on sprint performance in trained and untrained swimmers. *European Journal of Applied Physiology*, **64**, 377-380.

14. Conlee, R.K. (1991). Amphetamine, caffeine, and cocaine. In D.R. Lamb & M.H. Williams (Eds.), *Ergogenics—enhancement of performance in exercise and sport* (pp. 285-325). Dubuque, IA: Brown & Benchmark.

15. Costill, D.L., Dalsky, G.P., & Fink, W.J. (1978). Effects of caffeine ingestion on metabolism and exercise performance. *Medicine and Science in Sports*, **10**, 155-158.

16. Costill, D.L., Verstappen, F., Kuipers, H., Janssen, E., & Fink, W. (1984). Acid-base balance during repeated bouts of exercise: Influence of HCO_3. *International Journal of Sports Medicine*, **5**, 228-231.

17. Dodd, S.L., Herb, R.A., & Powers, S.K. (1993). Caffeine and exercise performance: An update. *Sports Medicine*, **15**, 14-23.

18. Duffy, D.J., & Conlee, R.K. (1986). Effects of phosphate loading on leg power and high intensity treadmill exercise. *Medicine and Science in Sports and Exercise*, **18**, 674-677.

19. Eichner, E.R. (1989). Ergolytic drugs. *Sports Science Exchange*, **2**(15), 1-4, Chicago: Gatorade Sports Science Institute.

20. Ekblom, B., & Berglund, B. (1991). Effect of erythropoietin administration on maximal aerobic power. *Scandinavian Journal of Medicine and Science in Sports*, **1**, 88-93.

21. Ekblom, B., Goldbarg, A.N., & Gullbring, B. (1972). Response to exercise after blood loss and reinfusion. *Journal of Applied Physiology*, **33**, 175-180.

22. Forbes, G.B. (1985). The effect of anabolic steroids on lean body mass: The dose response curve. *Metabolism*, **34**, 571-573.

23. Gledhill, N. (1982). Blood doping and related issues: A brief review. *Medicine and Science in Sports and Exercise*, **14**, 183-189.

24. Gledhill, N. (1985). The influence of altered blood volume and oxygen transport capacity on aerobic performance. *Exercise and Sport Sciences Reviews*, **13**, 75-93.

25. Goforth, H.W., Jr., Campbell, N.L., Hodgdon, J.A., & Sucec, A.A. (1982). Hematologic parameters of trained distance runners following induced erythrocythemia. *Medicine and Science in Sports and Exercise*, **14**, 174 (abstract).

26. Graham, T.E., & Spriet, L.L. (1991). Performance and metabolic responses to a high caffeine dose during prolonged exercise. *Journal of Applied Physiology*, **71**, 2292-2298.

27. Hervey, G.R., Knibbs, A.V., Burkinshaw, L., Morgan, D.B., Jones, P.R.M., Chettle, D.R., & Vartsky, D. (1981). Effects of methandienone on the performance and body composition of men undergoing athletic training. *Clinical Science*, **60**, 457-461.

28. Ivy, J.L. (1983). Amphetamines. In M.H. Williams (Ed.), *Ergogenic aids in sport* (pp. 101-127). Champaign, IL: Human Kinetics.

29. Ivy, J.L., Costill, D.L., Fink, W.J., & Lower, R.W. (1979). Influence of caffeine and carbohydrate feedings on endurance performance. *Medicine and Science in Sports*, **11**, 6-11.

30. Kowalchuk, J.M., Maltais, S.A., Yamaji, K., & Hughson, R.L. (1989). The effect of citrate loading on exercise performance, acid-base balance and metabolism. *European Journal of Applied Physiology*, **58**, 858-864.

31. Kreider, R.B., Miller, G.W., Williams, M.H., Somma, C.T., & Nasser, T.A. (1990). Effects of phosphate loading on oxygen uptake, ventilatory anaerobic threshold, and run performance. *Medicine and Science in Sports and Exercise*, **22**, 250-256.

32. Linderman, J., & Fahey, T.D. (1991). Sodium bicarbonate ingestion and exercise performance: An update. *Sports Medicine*, **11**, 71-77.

33. Lombardo, J.A. (1986). Stimulants and athletic performance: Cocaine and nicotine. *Physician and Sportsmedicine*, **14**(12), 85-91.

34. Lombardo, J.A., Hickson, R.C., & Lamb, D.R. (1991). Anabolic/androgenic steroids and growth hormone. In D.R. Lamb & M.H. Williams (Eds.), *Ergogenics—enhancement of performance in exercise and*

sport (pp. 249-278). Dubuque, IA: Brown & Benchmark.

35. Maughan, R.J., & Sadler, D.J.M. (1983). The effects of oral administration of salts of aspartic acid on the metabolic response to prolonged exhausting exercise in man. *International Journal of Sports Medicine*, **4**, 119-123.

36. McNaughton, L.R. (1990). Sodium citrate and anaerobic performance: Implications of dosage. *European Journal of Applied Physiology*, **61**, 392-397.

37. Roth, D.A., & Brooks, G.A. Lactate transport is mediated by a membrane-bound carrier in rat skeletal muscle sarcolemmal vesicles. *Archives of Biochemistry and Biophysics*, **279**, 377-385.

38. Rudman, D., Feller, A.G., Nagraj, H.S., Gergans, G.A., Lalitha, P.Y., Goldberg, A.F., Schlenker, R.A., Cohn, L., Rudman, I.W., & Mattson, D.E. (1990). Effects of human growth hormone in men over 60 years old. *New England Journal of Medicine*, **323**, 1-6.

39. Shangold, M.M. (1988). Gynecologic concerns in exercise and training. In M. Shangold & G. Mirkin (Eds.), *Women and exercise: Physiology and sports medicine* (pp. 186-194). Philadelphia: F.A. Davis.

40. Spriet, L.L., MacLean, D.A., Dyck, D.J., Hultman, E., Cederblad, G., & Graham, T.E. (1992). Caffeine ingestion and muscle metabolism during prolonged exercise in humans. *American Journal of Physiology*, **262**, E891-E898.

41. Stewart, I., McNaughton, L., Davies, P., & Tristram, S. (1990). Phosphate loading and the effects on $\dot{V}O_2$ max in trained cyclists. *Research Quarterly for Exercise and Sport*, **61**, 80-84.

42. Wadler, G.I., & Hainline, B. (1989). *Drugs and the athlete*. Philadelphia: F.A. Davis.

43. Wesson, M., McNaughton, L., Davies, P., & Tristram, S. (1988). Effects of oral administration of aspartic acid salts on the endurance capacity of trained athletes. *Research Quarterly for Exercise and Sport*, **59**, 234-239.

44. Williams, M.H. (Ed.) (1983). *Ergogenic aids in sport*. Champaign, IL: Human Kinetics Publishers.

45. Williams, M.H. (1991). Alcohol, marijuana, and beta blockers. In D.R. Lamb & M.H. Williams (Eds.), *Ergogenics—enhancement of performance in exercise and sport* (pp. 331-369). Dubuque, IA: Brown & Benchmark.

46. Williams, M.H., Wesseldine, S., Somma, T., & Schuster, R. (1981). The effect of induced erythrocythemia upon 5-mile treadmill run time. *Medicine and Science in Sports and Exercise*, **13**, 169-175.

47. Wilmore, J.H. (1988). Exercise testing, training, and beta-adrenergic blockade. *Physician and Sportsmedicine*, **16**(12), 45-52.

48. Wilmore, J.H. (1991). Eating and weight disorders in the female athlete. *International Journal of Sports Nutrition*, **1**, 104-117.

49. Winter, F.D., Snell, P.G., & Stray-Gundersen, J. (1989). Effects of 100% oxygen on performance of professional soccer players. *Journal of the American Medical Association*, **262**, 227-229.

50. Yarasheski, K.E., Campbell, J.A., Smith, K., Rennie, M.J., Holloszy, J.O., & Bier, D.M. (1992). Effect of growth hormone and resistance exercise on muscle growth in young men. *American Journal of Physiology*, **262**, E261-E267.

51. Yesalis, C.E., Wright, J.E., and Bahrke, M.S. (1989). Epidemiological and policy issues in the measurement of the long term health effects of anabolic-androgenic steroids. *Sports Medicine*, **8**, 129-138.

Selected Readings

Catlin, D., Wright, J., Pope, H., Jr., & Liggett, M. (1993). Assessing the threat of anabolic steroids. *The Physician and Sportsmedicine*, **21**(8), 37-44.

Clarkson, P.M. (1993). Nutritional ergogenic aids: Caffeine. *International Journal of Sport Nutrition*, **3**, 103-111.

Heigenhauser, G.J.F., & Jones, N.L. (1991). Bicarbonate loading. In D.R. Lamb & M.H. Williams (Eds.), *Ergogenics—enhancement of performance in exercise and sport* (pp. 183-207). Dubuque, IA: Brown & Benchmark.

Lamb, D.R., & Williams, M.H. (Ed.) (1991). *Ergogenics—enhancement of performance in exercise and sport*. Dubuque, IA: Brown & Benchmark.

Morgan, W.P. (Ed.) (1972). *Ergogenic aids and muscular performance*. New York: Academic Press.

Rogol, A.D. (1989). Growth hormone: Physiology, therapeutic use, and potential for abuse. *Exercise and Sport Sciences Reviews*, **17**, 353-377.

Spriet, L.L. (1991). Blood doping and oxygen transport. In D.R. Lamb & M.H. Williams (Eds.), *Ergogenics—enhancement of performance in exercise and sport* (pp. 213-242). Dubuque, IA: Brown & Benchmark.

Wright, J.E. (1981). Anabolic steroids and athletics. *Exercise and Sport Sciences Reviews*, **8**, 149-202.

Yarasheski, K.E., Zachwieja, J.J., Angelopoulos, T.J., & Bier, D.M. (1993). Short-term growth hormone treatment does not increase muscle protein synthesis in experienced weight lifters. *Journal of Applied Physiology*, **74**(6), 3073-3076.

Chapter 15

Nutrition and Nutritional Ergogenics

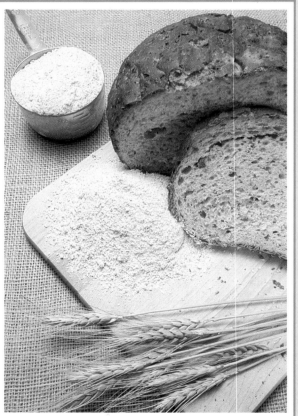

© John & Diane Harper/Photo Network

Chapter Overview

The intense effort and energy expenditure of sports training and competition places unusual demands on the diet of athletes. In fact, athletes in some sports, such as swimming and distance running, can have trouble balancing their energy intake to the caloric demands of training. For these reasons, the major dietary concern of many athletes is the amount of food they consume, rather than what they eat. Yet, in their quest for success, most athletes have at some time searched for a magic food that will produce a winning performance. As we saw in the previous chapter, any substance with such performance-enhancing properties is said to be ergogenic. Unfortunately, diet manipulations are typically based on testimonials from more successful performers, poorly designed research studies, invalid commercial advertising claims, and misinterpretation of nutritional research. Few areas of exercise science are more fraught with fads than the field of sport nutrition. Too often this leads to the use of unfounded nutritional practices.

In this chapter, we will examine the substances we ingest and their importance beyond their role in bioenergetics. We will focus on the optimal composition of the diet and the special dietary needs of the athlete. And we will carefully examine how nutrition can affect performance, focusing on the potential ergogenic properties of various nutrients and dispelling many myths.

In 1970 we [DLC] conducted a study in an effort to determine why athletes who train or compete intensely on repeated days gradually become chronically fatigued. Trained marathon runners were asked to run on a treadmill for 2 hr on 3 successive days at a pace equivalent to their best marathon performance. During this period they ate a normal mixed diet containing 50% of calories from carbohydrate, 35% from fat, and 15% from protein. On the average, the runners covered about 32 km (20 mi) in the 2 hr, becoming more and more fatigued with each succeeding day. By the third day, none of the runners could maintain the pace of the previous days, and all had to terminate the run before completing the 2-hr effort. Why did they become chronically fatigued? Muscle biopsy data revealed that their glycogen levels were extremely low, suggesting that the diet was inadequate to meet the energy needed for exercise. Could the runners' diet have been changed to prevent this fuel deficit? In the following discussion we will focus on the role of nutrition for training and optimal performance.

Optimal physical performance requires a careful dietary balance of the essential nutrients. The United States government (The National Research Council, Subcommittee on the Tenth Edition of the Recommended Dietary Allowances) has established standards for optimal nutrient intake that are termed Recommended (Daily) Dietary Allowances, abbreviated RDA. The RDA of a substance is an estimate of an intake adequate to maintain good health. RDA values are guidelines to help people of average activity levels gauge their diets.

However, the nutritional needs of very active athletes can exceed the RDAs considerably. Individual caloric needs are quite variable, depending on the athlete's size, gender, and sport choice. Some athletes have been reported to need as many as 12,000 kcal per day! Also, some competitive sports require adherence to rigid weight standards. Athletes who participate in these sports must closely monitor their weight and thus their caloric intake. Too often this leads to nutritional abuses, dehydration, and serious health risks. In addition, the dietary tactics used by some athletes to achieve excessive weight loss are of increasing concern because of the potential association with eating disorders, such as anorexia nervosa and bulimia nervosa.

A person's diet should contain a relative balance of carbohydrate, fat, and protein. Of the total calories consumed, the recommended balance for most people is

- carbohydrate, 55% to 60%;
- fat, no more than 30% (less than 10% saturated); and
- protein, 10% to 15%.

Although all foods can ultimately be broken down to carbohydrate, fat, or protein, these nutrients are not all that the body needs. Let's look at the classes of nutrients.

The Six Nutrient Classes

The energy from the foods we eat is essential to our ability to sustain physical activity, but we rely on foods for much more than energy. Food can be categorized into six classes of nutrients, each with specific functions in the body:

1. Carbohydrate
2. Fat (lipid)
3. Protein
4. Vitamins
5. Minerals
6. Water

In the following discussion, we will examine the physiological importance to the athlete of each of these classes.

Carbohydrate

A carbohydrate (CHO) is classified as either monosaccharide, disaccharide, or polysaccharide. Monosaccharides are the simple one-unit sugars (such as glucose, fructose, and galactose) that cannot be reduced to a simpler form. Disaccharides (such as sucrose, maltose, and lactose) are composed of two monosaccharides. For example, sucrose (table sugar) consists of glucose and fructose. Polysaccharides contain more than two monosaccharides. Common polysaccharides include starch and glycogen, both composed completely of glucose units. Larger polysaccharides, for example, starches, are commonly referred to as complex carbohydrates. All carbohydrates must be broken down to monosaccharides before the body can use them.

Carbohydrate serves many functions in the body:

- It is a major energy source, particularly during high-intensity exercise.
- Its presence regulates fat and protein metabolism.
- The nervous system relies exclusively on it for energy.
- Muscle and liver glycogen are synthesized from it.

Major sources of carbohydrate include grains, fruits, vegetables, milk, and concentrated sweets. Refined sugar, syrup, and cornstarch are nearly pure carbohydrates. Many concentrated sweets such as candy, honey, jellies, molasses, and soft drinks contain few if any other nutrients.

Carbohydrate Consumption and Glycogen Storage

Your body stores excess carbohydrate, primarily in your muscles and liver, as glycogen. Because of this, your carbohydrate consumption directly influences your muscle glycogen storage and your ability to train and compete in endurance events. As shown in Figure 15.1, athletes who train intensely and eat a low-carbohydrate diet (40% of total calories) often experience a day-to-day decrease in muscle glycogen. When these athletes consume a high-carbohydrate diet (70% of total calories), their muscle glycogen levels recover

almost completely within 22 hr of the training bouts. In addition, athletes perceive training as easier when their muscle glycogen is maintained throughout a workout.

Early studies demonstrated that when men eat a diet containing a normal amount of carbohydrate (about 55% of total calories ingested) their muscles store about 100 mmol of glycogen per kg of muscle. One study showed that diets containing less than 15% carbohydrate lead to storage of only 53 mmol · kg^{-1}, but rich carbohydrate diets (60% to 70% CHO) lead to storage of 205 mmol · kg^{-1}. When subjects exercised to exhaustion at 75% of their maximal oxygen uptake, their exercise times were proportional to the amount of muscle glycogen stored before the test, as shown in Figure 15.2.

More recent studies have shown that glycogen storage replacement is not simply determined by carbohydrate intake. Exercise with an eccentric (muscle lengthening) component, such as running and weight

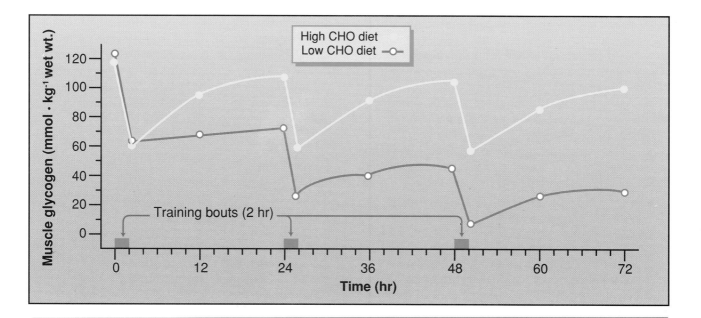

Figure 15.1   The influence of dietary carbohydrates on muscle glycogen stores during repeated days of training. Adapted from Costill and Miller (1980).

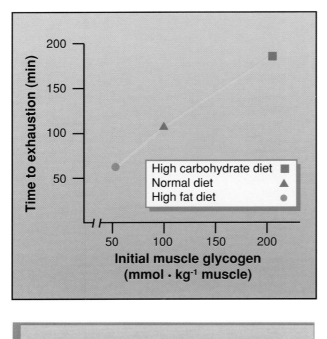

Figure 15.2   The relationship between muscle glycogen content and exercise time to exhaustion.

lifting, can induce some muscle damage and impair glycogen resynthesis. In these situations, muscle glycogen levels can appear quite normal during the first 6 to 12 hr after exercise, but glycogen resynthesis slows or stops completely as muscle repair begins.

The precise cause for this response is unknown, but conditions in the muscle could inhibit muscle glucose uptake and glycogen storage. For example, within 12 to 24 hr after intense eccentric exercise, damaged muscle fibers are infiltrated with inflammatory cells (leukocytes, macrophages, etc.) that remove cellular debris resulting from damage to the cells' membranes. This repair process can require a significant amount of the blood glucose, reducing the amount of glucose available for resynthesizing muscle glycogen. In addition, some evidence suggests that eccentrically exercised muscle is less sensitive to insulin, which would limit muscle fiber uptake of glucose. Perhaps future studies will more fully explain why eccentric-type activities delay glycogen storage. But for now we can only observe that glycogen recovery from various forms of exercise can differ and that this should be considered for optimal training and competition.

When athletes eat only as much food as hunger dictates, they often fail to consume enough carbohydrate to compensate for the amount used during training or competition. This imbalance between glycogen use and carbohydrate intake might explain, in part, why some athletes become chronically fatigued and

need 48 hr or more to restore normal muscle glycogen levels. Athletes who train exhaustively on successive days require a diet rich in carbohydrate to reduce the heavy, tired feeling associated with muscle glycogen depletion.

Carbohydrate Type

Simple carbohydrates (sugars), properly called monosaccharides, such as glucose or fructose, are absorbed from the digestive system quickly. Because of this, ingestion of simple carbohydrates causes hyperglycemia, meaning the blood glucose level is elevated. Insulin then helps move the glucose from the blood into the cells. This overloads the cells' energy-producing systems, so the excess carbohydrate is converted to fat. This can, in turn, elevate the blood concentration of triglycerides and cholesterol (both are fat derivatives), which is associated with a higher risk of heart disease. Complex carbohydrates, such as starch, require more time for complete breakdown, so they produce a slower and smaller rise in blood glucose. Because of this, complex carbohydrates have less impact on blood lipid levels.

These effects of carbohydrate on blood lipid levels were observed in relatively inactive subjects. But in endurance athletes, most carbohydrate consumed is used for glycogen storage. Their blood lipid levels change very little with carbohydrate ingestion, because training depletes their glycogen reserves and this, in turn, triggers increased glycogen synthesis.

With all of this information, we might expect that altering the relative amounts of simple and complex carbohydrates in an athlete's diet would affect the rate and quantity of glycogen formation. Tests of this theory, however, are inconclusive. Because of conflicting reports, any potential benefits from the preferential use of either simple or complex carbohydrates for muscle glycogen replacement are unclear.

Ergogenic Properties of Carbohydrate

As noted earlier, muscle glycogen provides a major resource for energy during exercise. Because muscle glycogen depletion has been shown to be a major cause of fatigue and ultimate exhaustion in events lasting more than an hour, efforts to load the muscle with extra glycogen before starting the exercise have been considered ergogenic for performance. Early studies demonstrated that men who ate a carbohydrate-rich diet for 3 days stored nearly twice their normal amounts of muscle glycogen.[1] When asked to exercise to exhaustion at 75% $\dot{V}O_{2\,max}$, their exercise times significantly increased. This practice, called glycogen loading, is widely used by distance runners, cyclists, and other athletes who must perform exercise for several hours. We will discuss this practice in greater detail later in this chapter.

Blood glucose levels become low (hypoglycemia) during exhaustive long-distance running and cycling, and this might contribute to fatigue. Several studies have shown that subjects' performances improve when they are given carbohydrate feedings during exercise lasting 1 to 4 hr.[13] Comparisons of subjects when they received carbohydrate feedings and when they received placebos revealed no performance differences during the early phase of the exercise, but during the final stage of the experiments, performance was greatly improved with carbohydrate feedings, as shown in Figure 15.3.

Although we don't fully understand how carbohydrate feedings improve performance, most scientists believe that maintaining blood glucose near normal levels allows the muscles to obtain more energy from blood glucose. Carbohydrate feedings during exercise do not spare muscle glycogen use, but may help to maintain glycogen reserves. Endurance performance (more than 1 hr) can be enhanced when carbohydrate is consumed within 5 min before the exercise begins, more than 2 hr before exercise (such as during the precompetition meal), and at frequent intervals during the activity.

An athlete should not ingest carbohydrate foods during the period 15 to 45 min before exercise because it could cause hypoglycemia shortly after the exercise begins, which could lead to early exhaustion by depriving the muscle of one of its energy sources. As shown in Figure 15.4, carbohydrate ingested during that period stimulates insulin secretion, causing an elevation of insulin when the activity begins. In response, glucose uptake by the muscles reaches an abnormally high rate, leading to hypoglycemia. Not everyone experiences this reaction, but sufficient evidence indicates that carbohydrate should be avoided in the period 15 to 45 min before exercise.

Why don't carbohydrate feedings during exercise produce the same hypoglycemic effects observed with pre-exercise feedings? Sugar feedings during exercise result in smaller increases in both blood glucose and insulin, lessening the threat of an overreaction that leads to a sudden drop in blood glucose. This finer control on blood glucose during exercise might be caused by increased muscle fiber permeability that decreases the need for insulin, or insulin binding sites may be altered during muscular activity. Regardless of the cause, carbohydrate intake during exercise appears to supplement the carbohydrate supply needed for muscular activity.

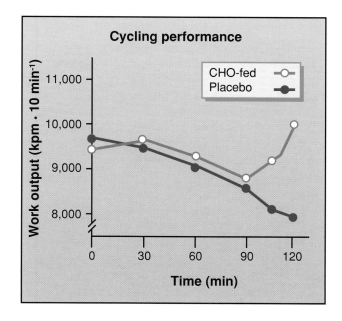

Figure 15.3 The influence of carbohydrate and placebo feedings on 2-hr cycling performance. Note the increase in work output from 90 min to 120 min with carbohydrate feedings.

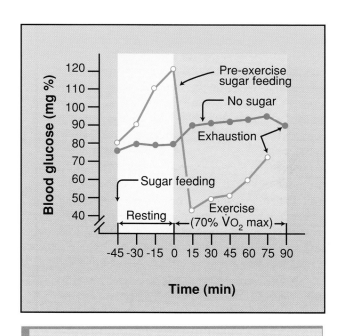

Figure 15.4 The effects of pre-exercise carbohydrate feedings on blood glucose levels during exercise. Note the drop in blood glucose to hypoglycemic levels with sugar feeding 45 min prior to exercise. Adapted from Costill et al. (1977).

Fat

Fat, also termed lipid, is a class of organic compounds with limited water solubility. It exists in the body in many forms, such as triglycerides, free fatty acids (FFA), phospholipids, and sterols. The body stores most fat as triglycerides, composed of three molecules of fatty acids and one molecule of glycerol. Triglycerides are our most concentrated source of energy.

Dietary fat, especially cholesterol and triglycerides, has a major role in cardiovascular disease (chapter 20), and excessive fat intake has also been linked to other diseases such as cancer. But, in spite of the negative publicity, fat serves many vital functions in the body:

- It is an essential component of cell membranes and nerve fibers.
- It is a primary energy source, providing up to 70% of our total energy in the resting state.
- Vital organs are supported and cushioned by it.
- All steroid hormones in the body are produced from cholesterol.
- Fat-soluble vitamins gain entry into and are transported through the body via fat.
- Body heat is preserved by the insulating subcutaneous fat layer.

The most basic unit of fat is the fatty acid, which is the part used for energy production. Fatty acids occur in two forms: saturated and unsaturated. Unsaturated fats contain one (monounsaturated) or more (polyunsaturated) double bonds between carbon atoms, and each double bond takes the place of two hydrogen atoms. A saturated fatty acid possesses no double bonds, so it has the maximum amount of hydrogen bound to the carbons. Excessive saturated fat consumption is a risk factor for numerous diseases.

Fats derived from animal sources generally contain more saturated fatty acids than fats derived from plants. Also, fats that are more highly saturated tend to be solids at room temperature, whereas less-saturated fats tend to be liquids. The tropical oils are notable exceptions: Palm, palm kernel, and coconut oil are plant-derived fats that are liquids at room temperature, but they are very high in saturated fat. And, although many vegetable oils are low in saturated fats, they are often used in foods as hydrogenated shortening. The process of hydrogenation adds hydrogen to the fat, increasing its saturation. Saturated fat contents of some common fats are shown in Figure 15.5.

Fat Consumption

Fat can enhance food's palatability by absorbing and retaining flavors and by affecting the food's texture. For this reason, it is quite common in our diets. Americans typically consume between 35% to 45% of their

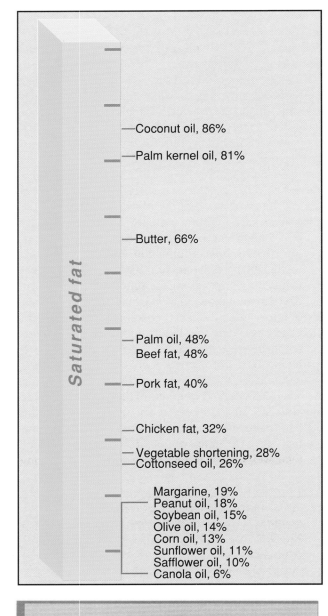

Figure 15.5   Percentages of saturated fat in some common fats and oils. Data from Tribole (1992).

total caloric intake as fat. This percentage has increased significantly since the early 1900s. Most nutritionists recommend that fat consumption should not exceed 30% of total calories consumed. Guidelines accompanying the USDA's new food guide pyramid advise us to limit saturated fats to less than 10% of total caloric intake.

Ergogenic Properties of Fat

For the athlete, fat is especially important as an energy source. Muscle and liver glycogen stores in the body are limited, so the use of fat (free fatty acids, or FFA) for energy production can delay exhaustion. Clearly, any change that allows the body to use more fat would

Calculating the Fat Content of Foods

We're told that reading labels on our foods is important so that we can make wise nutrition choices, but these labels are often confusing. This is especially true with fat content. The fat content of a food can be calculated in terms of

- the weight of the fat,
- its percentage of the food's total weight,
- the kilocalories it provides, or
- its percentage of the total calories.

We are advised to restrict our fat intake to less than 30% of our total calories, but food labels don't always give this information. With some simple math, you can do your own calculations. Table 15.1 compares 1-cup servings of four types of milk. The first column shows the weight of the serving and the second shows what percentage of the milk's weight is water. The third column indicates the total number of kilocalories per serving (recall that in human nutrition, the capitalized Calorie is actually a kilocalorie).

The last four columns are measurements of fat content. First we see the actual weight of the fat; for example, 1 c of whole milk contains 8.15 g of fat. The next column gives the percentage of the total weight that is fat. This shows us that whole milk is only 3.3% fat. That sounds great, because we are trying to keep fat consumption down to less than 30%, but 3.3% is the percentage of the total *weight*, not of the total *calories*.

Recall from chapter 5 that 1 g of fat contains 9 kcal of energy. Multiply the 8.15 g by 9 kcal · g^{-1} and you find that fat accounts for 73.4 kcal in 1 c of whole milk. Now comes the final calculation: what percent of the total calories is this? Simply dividing the kcal of fat by the total kcal in the milk (73.4 / 150) reveals that 48.9% of the total kcal in whole milk is from fat. This far exceeds our target of less than 30%!

Perhaps math is not your strong point, especially when walking the aisles at the grocery store and reading tiny print on confusing food labels. An easier method can be used to calculate the total percentage of calories from fat. Most foods list both the total (kilo)calories per serving and the grams of fat per serving. To keep your fat intake below 30% of your total calories, select foods that have no more than 3 g of fat per 100 (kilo)calories, because

3 g of fat per 100 kcal × 9 kcal · g^{-1} of fat
= 27 kcal of fat per 100 kcal
= 27% total kcal from fat

Table 15.1 Calculating the Fat Content of Foods

Food type	Weight (g)	H$_2$O (% wt)	Energy (kcal)	Fat (g)	Fat (% wt)	Fat (kcal)	Fat (% kcal)
Whole milk (8 oz)	244	88	150	8.15	3.3	73.4	48.9
2% low fat milk (8 oz)	244	89	121	4.78	2.0	43.0	35.6
1% low fat milk (8 oz)	244	90	102	2.54	1.0	22.9	22.4
Skim milk (8 oz)	245	91	86	0.44	0.2	4.0	4.6

KEY POINT

Fat constitutes 35% to 45% of the total calories consumed in the typical American diet. This is well above the recommended maximum of 30% or less, which many feel is essential for good health, disease prevention, and optimal athletic performance.

be an advantage, particularly for endurance performance. In fact, one adaptation that occurs in response to endurance training is an increased ability to use fat as an energy source. Unfortunately, merely eating fat does not stimulate the muscles to burn fat. Instead, eating fatty foods only tends to elevate plasma triglycerides, which must then be broken down before the free fatty acids can be used for energy production. To increase the use of fat, the FFA levels in the blood, not the triglyceride levels, must be increased.

Dietary attempts to elevate plasma FFA have been relatively unsuccessful. Some foods that contain the stimulant caffeine promote fat use and improve performance in prolonged, exhaustive exercise when they are consumed an hour before exercise. But many people have negative reactions to caffeine and show no performance improvements. Despite the potential performance advantages offered by ingesting caffeine (chapter 14), its ethical use is questionable because it can confer an unnatural advantage. Though international governing bodies, such as the International Olympic Committee, have attempted to ban the use of caffeine, policing its use is difficult and impractical.

Protein

Protein is a class of nitrogen-containing compounds formed by amino acids. Protein serves numerous functions in our bodies:

- It is the major structural component of the cell.
- It is used for growth, repair, and maintenance of body tissues.
- Hemoglobin, enzymes, and many hormones are produced from it.
- Normal blood osmotic pressure is maintained by proteins in the plasma.
- Antibodies for disease protection are formed from it.
- Energy can be produced from it.

Twenty amino acids have been identified as necessary for human growth and metabolism (Table 15.2). Of these, eleven or twelve are termed nonessential amino acids, meaning that our bodies synthesize them so we don't rely on dietary intake for their supply. The remaining eight or nine are termed essential amino acids because we cannot synthesize them, thus they are an essential part of our daily diets. Absence of one of these essential amino acids from the diet precludes formation of any proteins that contain that amino acid, and thus any tissue requiring those proteins cannot be maintained.

A dietary protein source that contains all of the essential amino acids is called a complete protein. Meat, fish, poultry, eggs, and milk are examples. The proteins in vegetables and grains are called incomplete proteins because they do not supply all of the essential amino acids. This concept is important for people on vegetarian diets (discussed later in this chapter).

Protein Consumption

Protein accounts for approximately 5% to 15% of the total calories consumed per day in the United States. Many experts believe this is two to three times the actual amount needed. The RDAs for protein are shown in Table 15.3. The RDA depends on individual body weight and composition. Males typically require more protein than females because males weigh more and have greater muscle mass. In general, though, an allowance of 0.8 g per kg of body weight is considered appropriate for adults.

Ergogenic Properties of Protein

Should athletes who are training for strength and muscle bulk increase their protein intake? Amino acids are the body's building blocks, so protein is essential for the growth and development of body tissues. For many years, protein supplementation was believed essential for athletes. In fact, muscle was once thought to consume itself as fuel for its own actions, so protein supplementation was considered necessary to prevent muscle wasting. Now we know that little protein is consumed as fuel for muscular work. When available, fat and carbohydrate are preferentially selected as energy sources.

Does protein supplementation enhance performance? Horstman has concluded that the average diet in the Western culture adequately meets the protein needs of the athlete.[17] In theory, protein needs for heavy physical training or work should be met, even when energy expenditure exceeds 5,000 kcal per day, if the proportion of protein in the total energy (kcal) consumed is maintained. But are these needs met in reality? Subjects who consume a protein supplement have shown significant strength gain, but similar results are achieved when they receive a placebo.

Studies with college men revealed that those who engaged in a month of weight training and followed diets containing either 0.8 g or 2.4 g of protein per kg of body weight each day retained more protein than a

Table 15.2 The Essential and Nonessential Amino Acids

Essential	Nonessential
Isoleucine	Alanine
Leucine	Arginine
Lysine	Asparagine
Methionine	Aspartic acid
Phenylalanine	Cysteine
Threonine	Glutamic acid
Tryptophan	Glutamine
Valine	Glycine
Histidine (children)[a]	Proline
	Serine
	Tyrosine

[a]Histidine is not synthesized in young children, so it is an essential amino acid for that age group, but not for adults.

Table 15.3 Protein Requirements for Male and Female Teens and Adults

Males	Recommended Dietary Allowance[a] (g)	Females	Recommended Dietary Allowance[a] (g)
Teen	45	Teen	46
Adult	58-63	Adult	44-50

[a]Recommended Dietary Allowance (RDA) is based on 1989 standards set by the National Research Council.

group of men who followed the same diet but did not train.[21] Nitrogen excretion in urine, an indicator of protein use, decreased significantly in the training group. The weight-trained men retained enough protein for a 2-kg increase in fat-free body mass. Comparing the need for protein and the gains in fat-free body mass suggested that the intake of only 0.8 g of protein per kg of body weight per day might have been low. Instead, the higher intake of 2.4 g might have better met the subjects' protein needs. In another study, two groups of men consumed different amounts of protein (1.4 g and 2.8 g per kg of body weight per day) during a prolonged period of intense physical training.[8] Only the group on the high protein diet significantly increased fat-free body mass.

During the early stages and heavy periods of training, some endurance athletes may need as much as 1.6 g of protein per kg of body weight each day.[20] This is more than the RDA for adults. For strength training, research findings are still unclear, though most researchers agree that an intake of 0.9 g per kg of body weight per day might be adequate for those who are simply maintaining their muscle mass.

Thus, at the present time, little scientific support exists to justify the extremely high-protein diets consumed by many athletes. In fact, some health risks might be associated with excessive protein intake because it places greater demands on the kidneys to excrete the unused amino acids. A diet containing 12% to 15% of calories from protein should be adequate for most athletes unless their total energy intake is deficient.

Vitamins

Vitamins are a group of unrelated organic compounds that perform specific functions to promote growth and to maintain health. We need them in relatively small quantities, but without them we could not utilize the other nutrients we ingest. Vitamins act primarily as catalysts in chemical reactions. They are essential for energy release, for tissue building, and for metabolic regulation. Vitamins can be classified into one of two major categories: fat soluble or water soluble. The fat-soluble vitamins, A, D, E, and K, are absorbed from the digestive tract along with and bound to lipids (fats). These vitamins are stored in the body, so excessive intake can cause toxic accumulations. The B-complex vitamins and vitamin C are water soluble. They are absorbed from the digestive tract along with water. Any excess of these vitamins is excreted, mostly in the urine, but vitamin toxicity has been reported with some of these. Table 15.4 lists the various vitamins, as well as the RDA, good dietary sources, major functions, and symptoms of deficiencies and toxicities for each.

▬ IN REVIEW . . . ▬

1. Carbohydrates are sugars and starches. They exist in the body as monosaccharides, disaccharides, and polysaccharides. All carbohydrates must be broken down into monosaccharides before the body can use them as a fuel.
2. Muscle glycogen loading by eating a diet rich in carbohydrate offers major ergogenic benefits to performance.
3. Fats, or lipids, exist in the body as triglycerides, free fatty acids, phospholipids, and sterols. They are stored primarily as triglycerides, which are our bodies' most concentrated energy source. A triglyceride molecule can be broken down into one glycerol and three fatty acid molecules. Only the free fatty acids are used by the body for energy production.
4. Although fat is a major energy source, dietary attempts to elevate free fatty acids have been only partially successful. Caffeine can promote the use of fat and improve prolonged exhaustive exercise, but its use is regulated by many governing bodies.
5. The smallest unit of protein is an amino acid. All proteins must be broken down to amino acids before the body can use them. Only the nonessential amino acids can be synthesized in our bodies. The essential amino acids must be attained through our diets. Protein is not a primary energy source in our bodies, but it can be used for energy production.
6. The RDA for protein may be a bit low for athletes involved in intense resistance training or for endurance athletes during early or heavy periods of training. However, extremely high-protein diets offer no benefits and could damage the kidneys.

Most vitamins have some function important to the athlete. For example:

- Vitamin A is crucial for normal growth and development because it plays an integral role in bone development.
- Vitamin D is essential for intestinal absorption of calcium and phosphorus, and thus for bone development and strength. By regulating calcium absorption, this vitamin also has a key role in neuromuscular function.
- Vitamin K is an intermediate in the electron transport chain, making it important for oxidative phosphorylation.

Of all the vitamins, though, only the B-complex vitamins and vitamins C and E have been extensively

Table 15.4 Vitamin Requirements for Adult Men and Women

Vitamin	Fat (F) or water (W) soluble	Source	Function	Symptoms of deficiency	Recommended Dietary Allowance[a]
A (retinol)	F	From provitamin carotene found in yellow and green vegetables; preformed in liver, egg yolk, butter, and milk	Necessary for rhodopsin synthesis, normal health of epithelial cells, and bone and tooth growth	Rhodopsin deficiency, night blindness, retarded growth, skin disorders, and increased infection risk	800 µg in females 1,000 µg in males
B₁ (thiamine)	W	Yeast, grains, and milk	Involved in carbohydrate and amino acid metabolism; necessary for growth	Beriberi—muscle weakness (including cardiac muscle), neuritis, and paralysis	1.1 mg in females 1.5 mg in males
B₂ (riboflavin)	W	Green vegetables, liver, wheat germ, milk, and eggs	Component of flavin adenine dinucleotide (FAD); involved in citric acid cycle	Eye disorders and skin cracking, especially at corners of the mouth	1.3 mg in females 1.7 mg in males
Pantothenic acid (part of B₂ complex)	W	Liver, yeast, green vegetables, grains, and intestinal bacteria	Constituent of coenzyme A, glucose production from lipids and amino acids, and steroid hormone synthesis	Neuromuscular dysfunction and fatigue	4-7 mg
B₃ (niacin)	W	Fish, liver, red meat, yeast, grains, peas, beans, and nuts	Component of nicotinamide adenine dinucleotide (NAD); involved in glycolysis and citric acid cycle	Pellagra—diarrhea, dermatitis, and mental disturbance	15 mg in females 19 mg in males
B₆ (pyridoxine)	W	Fish, liver, yeast, tomatoes, and intestinal bacteria	Involved in amino acid metabolism	Dermatitis, retarded growth, and nausea	1.6 mg in females 2.0 mg in males
Folic acid	W	Liver, green leafy vegetables, and intestinal bacteria	Nucleic acid synthesis; hematopoiesis	Macrocytic anemia (enlarged red blood cells)	180 µg in females 200 µg in males
B₁₂ (cyanocobalamin)	W	Liver, red meat, milk, and eggs	Necessary for erythrocyte production; some nucleic acid and amino acid metabolism	Pernicious anemia and nervous system disorders	2.0 µg
C (ascorbic acid)	W	Citrus fruit, tomatoes, and green vegetables	Collagen synthesis; general protein metabolism	Scurvy—defective bone formation and poor wound healing	60 mg
D (cholecalciferol, ergosterol)	F	Fish liver oil, enriched milk, and eggs; pro-vitamin D converted by sunlight to cholecalciferol in the skin	Promotes calcium and phosphorus use, normal growth, and bone and teeth formation	Rickets—poorly developed, weak bones; osteomalacia; bone reabsorption	10 µg

(continued)

Table 15.4 *(continued)*

E (alpha-tocopherol)	F	Wheat germ, cotton-seed, palm, and rice oils; grain, liver, and lettuce	Prevents catabolism of certain fatty acids; may prevent miscarriage	Muscular dystrophy and sterility	8 mg in females 10 mg in males
H (biotin), often considered part of the B-vitamin group	W	Liver, yeast, eggs, and intestinal bacteria	Fatty acid and purine synthesis; movement of pyruvic acid into citric acid cycle	Mental and muscle dysfunction, fatigue, and nausea	Unknown. 0.3 to 1.0 mg recommended
K (phylloquinone)	F	Alfalfa, liver, spinach, vegetable oils, cabbage, and intestinal bacteria	Required for synthesis of a number of clotting factors	Excessive bleeding due to retarded blood clotting	65-80 µg

[a]Recommended Dietary Allowance (RDA) is based on 1989 standards set by the National Research Council.

investigated for their potential to facilitate athletic performance. In the following sections we will briefly consider each of these.

B-Complex Vitamins

The B-complex vitamins were once thought to be a single vitamin. Now more than a dozen B-complex vitamins have been identified. These vitamins' essential roles in cellular metabolism cannot be overemphasized. Among their diverse functions, they serve as cofactors in various enzyme systems involved in the oxidation of food and the production of energy. Consider just a few examples. Vitamin B_1 (thiamin) is needed for the conversion of pyruvic acid to acetyl CoA. Vitamin B_2 (riboflavin) becomes FAD, which acts as a hydrogen acceptor during oxidation. Vitamin B_3 (niacin) is a component of NADP, a coenzyme in glycolysis. Vitamin B_{12} has a role in amino acid metabolism and is also needed for the production of red blood cells, which transport oxygen for oxidation. The B-complex vitamins have such a close inter-relationship that a deficiency in one can impair utilization of the others. Symptoms of deficiencies vary with the vitamins involved.

Several studies have shown that supplementation of one or more of the B-complex vitamins facilitates performance. However, most researchers agree that this is only true if the individual being studied suffers a preexisting B-complex deficiency.[3,6] Creating a deficiency in one or more of the B-complex vitamins usually impairs performance, but this is reversed when the deficiency is corrected with supplementation. No compelling evidence supports advocating supplementation when there is no deficiency.

Vitamin C

Vitamin C (ascorbic acid) is common in our foods but deficiencies can occur, such as in people who smoke, use oral contraceptives, have surgery, or run a fever. This vitamin is important for the formation and maintenance of collagen, a crucial protein found in connective tissue, so it is essential for healthy bones, ligaments, and blood vessels. Vitamin C also functions in

- the metabolism of amino acids;
- synthesis of some hormones, such as the catecholamines (epinephrine and norepinephrine) and the anti-inflammatory corticoids; and
- promoting iron absorption from the intestines.

Many people also believe vitamin C assists healing, combats fever and infection, and prevents or cures the common cold. Though evidence to date is inconclusive, the role of vitamin C in the fight against disease is an area of major interest.

Vitamin C supplementation has produced equivocal findings in the research conducted to date. However, those who have reviewed this area generally agree that, even with the increased requirements of training, vitamin C supplementation will not improve performance when no deficiency exists.

Vitamin E

Vitamin E is stored in muscle and fat. This vitamin's functions are not well established. It is known to enhance the activity of vitamins A and C by preventing their oxidation. Indeed, the most important role of vitamin E is its action as an antioxidant. It disarms free radicals (highly reactive molecules) that could otherwise severely damage cells, disrupting metabolic processes. This process also prevents lung damage from many of the pollutants that we inhale. Vitamin E has received considerable media attention over the years as a potential miracle vitamin that might prevent or alleviate a number of medical conditions, such as rheumatic fever, muscular dystrophy, coronary artery disease, sterility, menstrual disorders, and spontaneous abortions. Such claims generally lack supporting scientific evidence; however, recent reports suggest that people who take more than 400 mg of vitamin E per day are at less risk of coronary artery disease.

A large segment of the athletic population likely consumes large supplementary doses of vitamin E. It is postulated to benefit performance through its relationship with oxygen use and energy supply. However, reviews have generally concluded that vitamin E supplementation does not improve athletic performance.

Minerals

A number of inorganic substances known as minerals are essential for normal cellular functions. Minerals account for approximately 4% of your body weight. Some are present in high concentrations in your skeleton and teeth, but minerals are also found throughout your body, in and around every cell, dissolved in your body's fluids. They can be present either as ions or combined with various organic compounds. Mineral compounds that can dissociate into ions in the body are called electrolytes.

By definition, macrominerals are those of which your body needs more than 100 milligrams per day. Microminerals, or trace elements, are those needed in smaller amounts. Table 15.5 provides a list of the seventeen essential minerals, their major functions, symptoms of deficiencies and excesses, and their recommended daily allowances.

Unlike vitamins, mineral intake is less likely to be supplemented by the athletic population. Far less concern has been shown by athletes for their mineral status, possibly because far fewer ergogenic qualities have been ascribed to specific minerals. Of the minerals, calcium and iron have been most frequently investigated.

Calcium

Calcium is the most abundant mineral in your body, constituting approximately 40% of its mineral content. Calcium is well known for its importance in building and maintaining healthy bones, and that is where most of it is stored. But it is also essential for nerve impulse transmission. Calcium plays major roles in enzyme activation and regulation of cell membrane permeability, both important for metabolism. And this mineral is also essential for normal muscle function: Recall from chapter 2 that calcium is stored in the sarcoplasmic reticulum of muscles and released when the muscle fibers are stimulated. It is required for formation of the actin-myosin–cross-bridges that cause the fibers to contract.

Sufficient calcium intake is critical to our health. If we do not consume enough, calcium will be removed from its storage sites in the body, especially the bones.

This condition is called osteopenia. It weakens the bones and can lead to osteoporosis, a common problem in postmenopausal women. Unfortunately, few studies have been conducted on calcium supplementation; these suggest that supplementation is of no value in the presence of an adequate (RDA) dietary intake of calcium.

Phosphorus

Phosphorus is closely linked to calcium. It constitutes approximately 22% of your body's total mineral content. About 80% of this phosphorus is combined with calcium (calcium phosphate), providing strength and rigidity to the bones. Phosphorus is an essential part of metabolism, cell membrane structure, and the buffering system (to maintain constant blood pH). As we saw in chapter 5, phosphorus plays a major role in bioenergetics—it is an essential component of ATP.

Iron

Iron—a micromineral—is present in the body in relatively small amounts (35 to 50 mg per kg of body weight). It plays a crucial role in oxygen transportation—iron is required for the formation of both hemoglobin and myoglobin. Hemoglobin, located in the red blood cells, binds with oxygen in the lungs and then transports it to the body tissues via the blood. Myoglobin, found in muscle, combines with oxygen and stores it until needed.

Iron deficiency is prevalent throughout the world. By some estimates, as much as 25% of the world's population is iron deficient. The major problem associated with this condition is iron-deficiency anemia, in which hemoglobin levels are reduced, decreasing the blood's oxygen-carrying capacity. This causes fatigue, headaches, and other symptoms. Iron deficiency is a more common problem in women than in men because both menstruation and pregnancy cause iron losses that must be replenished. This problem is compounded by the fact that women generally consume less food, and thus less iron, than men.

Iron has received much attention in the research literature. Women are considered anemic only when their hemoglobin content is below 11 g per 100 ml of blood. But in the United States, 22% of all women between the ages of 17 and 44 are thought to be iron deficient despite having normal hemoglobin values. Studies generally suggest that 22% to 25% of female athletes and 10% of male athletes are iron deficient. But these numbers may be conservative—Risser et al. found that 31% of a group of varsity women athletes at two major United States universities were iron deficient.[23]

When iron supplements are given to those who are iron deficient, performance measures, particularly aerobic capacity, are typically improved. However,

Table 15.5 Mineral Requirements for Adult Men and Women

Mineral	Function	Symptoms of deficiency	Recommended Dietary Allowance[a]
Calcium	Bone and teeth formation, blood clotting, muscle activity, and nerve function	Spontaneous nerve discharge and tetany	1,200 mg
Chlorine	Blood acid-base balance; hydrochloric acid production in stomach	Acid-base imbalance	Not established
Chromium	Associated with enzymes in glucose metabolism	Unknown	50-200 µg
Cobalt	Component of vitamin B_{12}; erythrocyte production	Anemia	Not established
Copper	Hemoglobin and melanin production; electron-transport system	Anemia and loss of energy	1.5-3.0 mg
Fluoride	Provides extra strength in teeth; prevents dental caries	No real pathology	1.5-4.0 mg
Iodine	Thyroid hormone production; maintenance of normal metabolic rate	Decrease of normal metabolism	150 µg
Iron	Component of hemoglobin; ATP production in electron-transport system	Anemia, decreased oxygen transport, and energy loss	10 mg in males 15 mg in females
Magnesium	Coenzyme constituent; bone formation; muscle and nerve function	Increased nervous system irritability, vasodilation, and arrhythmias	280 mg in females 350 mg in males
Manganese	Hemoglobin synthesis; growth; activation of several enzymes	Tremors and convulsions	2.5-5.0 mg
Molybdenum	Enzyme component	Unknown	75-250 µg
Phosphorus	Bone and teeth formation; important in energy transfer (ATP); component of nucleic acids	Loss of energy and cellular function	1,200 mg
Potassium	Muscle and nerve function	Muscle weakness, abnormal electrocardiogram, and alkaline urine	Not established
Selenium	Component of many enzymes	Unknown	55 µg in females 70 µg in males
Sodium	Osmotic pressure regulation; nerve and muscle function	Nausea, vomiting, exhaustion, and dizziness	Not established; probably about 2,500 mg
Sulfur	Component of hormones, several vitamins, and proteins	Unknown	Not established
Zinc	Component of several enzymes; carbon dioxide transport and metabolism; necessary for protein metabolism	Deficient carbon dioxide transport and deficient protein metabolism	12 mg in females 15 mg in males

[a]Recommended Dietary Allowance (RDA) is based on 1989 standards set by the National Research Council.

supplementation of iron in those who are not deficient appears to have no benefit.

Sodium, Potassium, and Chloride

Sodium, potassium, and chloride are distributed throughout all body fluids and tissues. Sodium and chloride are primarily found in the fluid outside of your cells and in your blood plasma, but potassium is located mainly in your cells. This selective distribution of these three minerals establishes the electrical charge separation found across neuron and muscle cell membranes. Thus these minerals enable neural impulses to control muscle activity (chapter 3). In addition, they are responsible for maintaining the body's water balance and distribution, normal osmotic equilibrium, acid-base balance (pH), and normal cardiac rhythm.

Western diets are replete with sodium, so dietary deficiency is unlikely. However, minerals are lost with sweating, so any condition causing excessive sweating, such as extreme exertion or exercise in a hot environment, can deplete these minerals. When discussing mineral imbalances, we often focus on deficiencies. However, many of these minerals also have negative effects when taken in excess. In fact, excess potassium can cause heart failure! Individual needs vary, but megadosing is never advisable.

IN REVIEW . . .

1. Vitamins perform numerous functions in our bodies and are essential for normal growth and development. Many are involved in metabolic processes, such as those leading to energy production.
2. Vitamins A, D, E, and K are fat soluble. These can accumulate to toxic levels in the body. Vitamins C and B-complex are water soluble. Excesses of these are excreted, so toxicity is rarely a problem. Several of the B-complex vitamins are involved in the processes of energy production.
3. Macrominerals are minerals of which we require more than 100 mg per day. Microminerals (trace elements) are those of which we require smaller amounts.
4. Minerals are required for numerous physiological processes, such as muscle contraction, oxygen transport, fluid balance, and bioenergetics. Minerals can dissociate into ions, which can participate in numerous chemical reactions. Because minerals can produce ions, they are also called electrolytes.
5. Vitamins and minerals do not appear to have any ergogenic value. Taking them in amounts greater than the RDA will not improve performance.

Water

Seldom is water thought of as a nutrient because it has no caloric value. Yet its importance in maintaining life is second only to oxygen's. Water constitutes about 60% of a typical young male's (or 50% of a young female's) total body weight. It has been estimated that

---

KEY POINT

A water loss of 9% to 12% of a person's total body weight can lead to death.

---

we can survive losses of up to 40% of our body weight in fat, carbohydrate, and protein. But a water loss of 9% to 12% of body weight can be fatal.

The body's fluid compartments are illustrated in Figure 15.6. Approximately 60% to 65% of the water in our bodies is contained in our cells and is referred to as intracellular fluid. The remainder is outside the cells, referred to as the extracellular fluid. This includes the interstitial fluid surrounding the cells, the blood plasma, lymph, and some other fluids.

With respect to exercise, water plays several critical roles. For example:

- Red blood cells carry oxygen to your active muscles via the blood plasma, which is primarily water.
- Nutrients such as glucose, fatty acids, and amino acids are transported to your muscles by blood plasma.
- CO_2 and other metabolic wastes leave the cells and then enter the blood plasma to be cleared from your body.
- Hormones that regulate metabolism and muscular activity during exercise are transported by the blood plasma to their targets.
- Body fluids contain buffering agents to maintain proper pH when lactate is being formed.
- Water facilitates the dissipation of body heat that is generated during exercise.
- Blood plasma volume is a major determinant of blood pressure, and thus cardiovascular function.

In the next sections, we will more closely examine the role of water in exercise and performance.

IN REVIEW . . .

1. Water is our most important nutrient. We would die much more quickly if deprived of water than we would if deprived of any other nutrient.
2. Water is found in the intracellular compartment (inside the cells) and the extracellular compartment (outside the cells). Extracellular fluids include blood plasma, lymph, interstitial fluid, and other body fluids.
3. Among its most important functions, water provides transportation between and delivery to the body's different tissues, regulates body temperature, and maintains blood pressure for proper cardiovascular function.

Water and Electrolyte Balance

For optimal performance, the body's water and electrolyte contents should remain relatively constant. Unfor-

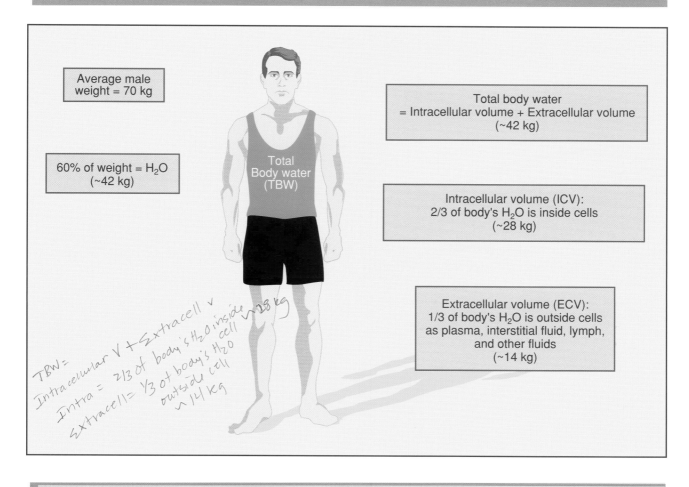

Figure 15.6   The body's fluid compartments.

tunately, this doesn't always happen during exercise. In the next sections, we will examine the balance between water and electrolytes, how exercise affects it, and the impact on performance when this balance is disrupted.

Water Balance at Rest

Under normal resting conditions, our body water content is relatively constant: Our water intake equals our water output. About 60% of our daily water intake is obtained from the fluids we drink and about 30% is from the foods we consume. The remaining 10% is produced in our cells during metabolism (recall from chapter 5 that water is a by-product of oxidative phosphorylation). Metabolic water production varies from 150 to 250 ml per day depending on the rate of energy expenditure—higher metabolic rates produce more water. The total daily water intake from all sources averages about 33 ml per kg of body weight per day. For a 70-kg (154-lb) person, that would be 2.31 L per day.

Water output, or water loss, occurs from four sources:

1. Evaporation from the skin
2. Evaporation from the respiratory tract
3. Excretion from the kidneys
4. Excretion from the large intestine

Human skin is permeable to water. Water diffuses to the skin's surface where it evaporates into the environment. In addition, the gases we breathe are constantly being humidified by water as they pass through our respiratory tracts. These two types of water loss (from the skin and respiration) occur without our sensing them. Thus, they are termed insensible water losses. Under cool, resting conditions, these losses account for about 30% of daily water loss.

The majority of water loss—60% when at rest—occurs from our kidneys, which excrete water and waste products as urine. Under resting conditions, the kidneys excrete about 50 to 60 ml of water per hour. Another 5% of the water is lost by sweating (though this is often considered along with insensible water loss), and the remaining 5% is excreted from the large intestine in the feces. The sources of water intake and water output at rest are depicted in Figure 15.7.

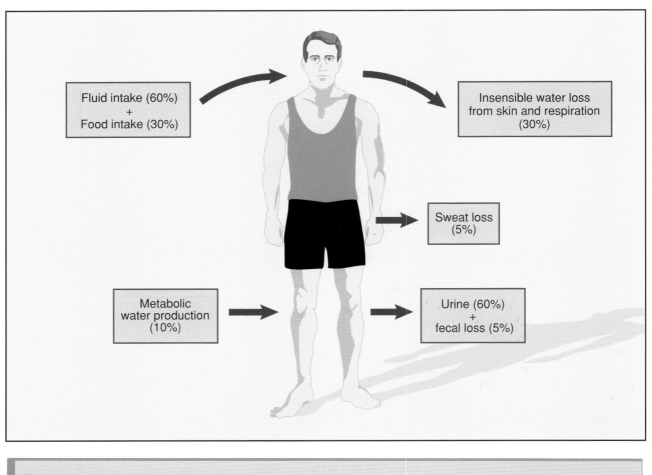

Figure 15.7   Sources of body water gains and losses at rest.

Water Balance During Exercise

Water loss is accelerated during exercise. Your body's ability to lose the heat generated during exercise depends primarily on the formation and evaporation of sweat, as seen in Table 15.6. As your body's temperature rises, sweating increases in an effort to prevent overheating. But at the same time, more water is produced during exercise because of increased oxidative metabolism. Unfortunately, the amount produced even during the most intense effort has only a small impact on the dehydration resulting from heavy sweating. During an hour of intense effort, for example, a 70-kg person might metabolize about 245 g of carbohydrate. This would produce about 146 ml of water. During that same period, however, sweat losses could exceed 1,500 ml, approximately 10 times more than generated metabolically. Nevertheless, the water produced during oxidative metabolism helps minimize, if only to a small degree, the dehydration that occurs during exercise.

During a marathon race, a runner's muscles can produce nearly 500 ml of water over 2 to 3 hr.

Table 15.6   Comparison of Water Loss From the Body at Rest in a Cool Environment and During Prolonged Exhaustive Exercise

Source of loss	Resting		Prolonged exercise	
	ml • hr⁻¹	% total	ml • hr⁻¹	% total
Insensible loss				
Skin	14.6	15	15	1.1
Respiration	14.6	15	100	7.5
Sweating	4.2	5	1200	90.6
Urine	58.3	60	10	0.8
Feces	4.2	5	—	0
Total	95.9 ml • hr⁻¹		1325 ml • hr⁻¹	

In general, the amount of sweat produced during exercise is determined by

- environmental temperature,
- body size, and
- metabolic rate.

These three factors influence the body's heat storage and temperature. Heat is transferred from warmer areas to cooler ones, so heat loss from the body is impaired with high environmental temperatures. Body size is important because large individuals generally need more energy to do a given task, so they usually have higher metabolic rates, producing more heat. But they also have more surface area (skin), which allows more sweat formation and evaporation.

As exercise intensity increases, so does the metabolic rate. This increases body heat production which, in turn, increases sweating. To conserve water during exercise, blood flow to the kidneys decreases in an attempt to prevent dehydration, but, like the increase in metabolic water production, this too may be insufficient. Under extreme exercise and environmental heat stress, sweating and respiratory evaporation can cause rapid losses of as much as 2 to 3 L of water per hour. (Chapter 11 contains additional information about body water losses during exercise in warm environments.)

During an event such as the marathon, sweating and water loss from respiration may reduce body water content by 6% to 10%, despite efforts to drink fluids.

Dehydration and Exercise Performance

Even minimal changes in your body's water content can impair endurance performance. Without adequate fluid replacement, a subject's exercise tolerance shows a pronounced decrease during long-term activity because of water loss through sweating. Studies have shown that dehydrated people are intolerant of prolonged exercise and heat stress.[1,7] Distance runners, for example, are forced to slow their pace by about 2% for each percent of body weight lost by dehydration. A runner capable of running 10,000 m in 35 min when normally hydrated will be slowed by 2 min 48 s (8% of normal time) when dehydrated by 4%.

The impact of dehydration on the cardiovascular and thermoregulatory systems is quite predictable. Fluid loss decreases plasma volume. This decreases blood pressure which, in turn, reduces blood flow to

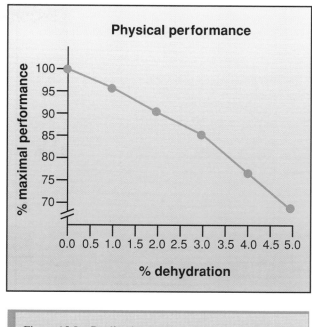

Figure 15.8   Decline in exercise performance with dehydration. Adapted from Saltin and Costill (1988).

the muscles and skin. In an effort to overcome this, heart rate increases. Because less blood reaches the skin, heat dissipation is hindered and the body retains more heat. Thus, when a person is dehydrated by more than 2% of body weight, both heart rate and body temperature are elevated during exercise. If the loss reaches 4% or 5% of body weight, the capacity for prolonged aerobic effort declines by 20% to 30%, as shown in Figure 15.8.

However, the effects of dehydration on performance in shorter, less aerobic events are less dramatic. In exercise bouts lasting only a few seconds, in which ATP is generated primarily via the ATP-PCr and glycolytic systems, performance seems to be unaffected. Although research findings are mixed, most researchers agree that dehydration has a minimal effect on performance in short, explosive, highly anaerobic events (like weight lifting). Wrestlers commonly dehydrate to get a weight advantage during competition. Most rehydrate prior to competition and experience only small decrements in performance. The effects of dehydration on exercise performance are shown in Table 15.7.

Thus far we have examined only the effects of dehydration on performance. In addition to the body water lost during endurance events, many nutrients, especially minerals, escape with sweat. In the following discussion, we will examine the effects of heavy

Table 15.7 The Influence of Dehydration (Hypohydration) on Selected Physiological Parameters and Performance

Measurement	Dehydration
Physiological parameters	
Strength	Unchanged
Sprint running	Unchanged
Reaction time	Small increase
Endurance	Decreased
Submaximal exercise performance	
Heart rate	Increased
Oxygen uptake	Unchanged
Body temperature	Increased
Blood lactate	Increased
Maximal exercise performance	
$\dot{V}O_2$ max	Decreased
Heart rate	Unchanged
Blood lactate	Increased

sweating, not only on water balance, but also on the electrolyte composition of body tissues.

Electrolyte Balance During Exercise

As mentioned earlier, normal body function depends on a balance between water and electrolytes. We have discussed the effects of water loss on performance.

IN REVIEW . . .

1. Water balance depends on electrolyte balance, and vice versa.
2. At rest, water intake equals water output. Water intake includes water ingested from foods and fluids, and from metabolic water, a by-product of metabolic processes. The majority of water output at rest is generated by the kidneys, but water is also lost across the skin, from the respiratory tract, and in the feces.
3. During exercise, metabolic water production increases as the metabolic rate increases.
4. Water loss during exercise increases because, as heat in the body increases, more water is lost in sweat. Sweat becomes the primary avenue for water loss during exercise. In fact, the kidneys decrease their excretion in an effort to prevent dehydration.
5. When dehydration exceeds 2% of body weight, prolonged physical performance is notably impaired. Also in response to dehydration, heart rate and body temperature increase.

Now we can turn our attention to the effects of the other component of this delicate balance: electrolytes. When large amounts of water are lost from the body, such as during exercise, the balance between water and electrolytes can quickly be disrupted. In the next sections, we will examine the effects of exercise on electrolyte balance. Our focus will be on the two major routes for electrolyte loss: sweating and urine production.

Electrolyte Loss in Sweat

Human sweat is a filtrate of blood plasma, so it contains many substances found there, including sodium, chloride, potassium, magnesium, and calcium. Although sweat tastes salty, it contains far fewer minerals than the plasma and other body fluids. In fact it is 99% water.

Sodium and chloride are the predominant ions in sweat and blood. As seen in Table 15.8, the concentrations of sodium and chloride in sweat are roughly one third those found in plasma and five times those found in muscle. Each of these three fluids' osmolality, which is the ratio of solutes (such as electrolytes) to fluid, is also shown. Sweat's electrolyte concentration can vary considerably between individuals. It is strongly influenced by

- rate of sweating,
- state of training, and
- state of heat acclimatization.

At the elevated rates of sweating reported during endurance events, sweat contains large amounts of sodium and chloride but little potassium, calcium, and magnesium. One study examined the effects of a sweat loss of nearly 4.1 kg (9 lbs), which represented a 5.8% reduction in body weight.

Based on estimates of the athlete's total body electrolyte content, such losses would lower the body's sodium and chloride content by only about 5% to 7%. Total body levels of potassium and magnesium, two ions principally confined to the inside of the cells,

Table 15.8 Electrolyte Concentrations and Osmolality in Sweat, Plasma, and Muscle of Men Following 2 hr of Exercise in the Heat

Site	Electrolytes (mEq · L⁻¹)				Osmolality
	Na⁺	Cl⁻	K⁺	Mg⁺⁺	(mOsm · L⁻¹)
Sweat	40–60	30–50	4–6	1.5–5	80–185
Plasma	140	101	4	1.5	295
Muscle	9	6	162	31	295

would decrease by about 1%. These losses probably have no measurable effect on an athlete's performance.

As electrolytes are lost in sweat, the remaining ions are redistributed among the body tissues. Consider potassium. It diffuses from active muscle fibers as they contract, entering the extracellular fluid. The increase this causes in extracellular potassium levels does not equal the amount of K^+ that is released from active muscles because potassium is being taken up by inactive muscles and other tissues while the active muscles are losing it. During recovery, intracellular potassium levels normalize quickly. Some researchers suggest that these muscle potassium disturbances during exercise might contribute to fatigue by altering the membrane potentials of neurons and muscle fibers, making it more difficult to transmit impulses.

Electrolyte Loss in Urine

In addition to clearing wastes from the blood and regulating water levels, the kidneys also regulate the body's electrolyte content. Urine production is the other major source of electrolyte loss. At rest, electrolytes are excreted in the urine as necessary to maintain homeostatic levels, and this is the primary route for electrolyte loss. But as your body's water loss increases during exercise, your urine production rate decreases considerably in an effort to conserve water (the mechanisms involved were discussed in chapter 6). Consequently, with very little urine being produced, electrolyte loss by this avenue is minimized.

The kidneys play another role in electrolyte management. If, for example, a person eats 250 mEq of salt (NaCl) the kidneys will normally excrete 250 mEq of these electrolytes to keep their body content constant. Heavy sweating and dehydration, however, trigger the release of the hormone aldosterone from the adrenal gland. This hormone stimulates renal reabsorption of sodium. Consequently, the body retains more sodium than usual during the hours and days after a prolonged exercise bout. This elevates the body's sodium content, increasing the osmolality of the extracellular fluids.

This increased sodium content triggers thirst, which compels the person to consume more water, which is then retained in the extracellular compartment. The increased water consumption reestablishes normal osmolality in the extracellular fluids but leaves these fluids expanded, which dilutes the other substances present there. This expansion of the extracellular fluids has no negative effects and is temporary. Fluid levels return to normal within 48 to 72 hr after the exercise.

IN REVIEW ...

1. The loss of large amounts of water can disrupt electrolyte balance, though electrolytes are rather dilute in sweat, which is 99% water.
2. Electrolyte loss during exercise occurs primarily along with water loss from sweating. Sodium and chloride are the most abundant electrolytes in sweat.
3. At rest, excessive electrolytes are excreted in the urine by the kidneys. But urine production declines tremendously during exercise, so little electrolyte loss occurs by this route.
4. Dehydration causes the hormone aldosterone to promote renal retention of Na^+ and Cl^-, raising their concentrations in the blood. This triggers thirst in an effort to make us consume more fluid to replace what has been lost.

Replacement of Body Fluid Losses

Your body loses more water than electrolytes when you are sweating heavily. This raises the osmotic pressure in your body fluids, because your electrolytes become more concentrated. Because of this, your need to replace body water is greater than your need for electrolytes, because only by replenishing your water content can the electrolytes return to normal concentrations. But how does your body know when this is necessary?

Thirst

When you feel thirsty, you drink. The thirst sensation is regulated by your hypothalamus. It triggers thirst when the plasma's osmotic pressure is increased. Unfortunately, your body's thirst mechanism doesn't precisely gauge your state of dehydration. You don't sense thirst until well after dehydration begins. Even when you are dehydrated, you might desire fluids only at intermittent intervals.

The control of thirst is not fully understood. When permitted to drink water as their thirst dictates, people can require 24 to 48 hr to completely replace water lost through heavy sweating. In contrast, dogs and burros can drink up to 10% of their total body weight within the first few minutes after exercise or heat exposure, replacing all lost water. Because of our sluggish drive to replace body water and in order to prevent chronic dehydration, we are advised to drink more fluid than our thirst indicates. Because of the increased water loss during exercise, it is imperative that athletes' water intakes are sufficient to meet their bodies' needs, and it is essential that they rehydrate during and after an exercise bout.

Benefits of Fluids During Exercise

Drinking fluids during prolonged exercise, especially during hot weather, has obvious benefits. Water intake will minimize

- dehydration,
- body temperature increases, and
- cardiovascular stress.

As seen in Figure 15.9, when subjects became dehydrated during several hours of treadmill running in the heat (40 °C) without fluid replacement, their heart rates increased steadily throughout the exercise. When they were deprived of fluids, the subjects became exhausted and couldn't complete the 6-hr exercise. Ingesting amounts of either water or a saline solution equal to their weight losses prevented dehydration and kept their heart rates lower. Even warm fluids (near body temperature) provide some protection against overheating, but cold fluids enhance body cooling because some of the deep body heat is used to warm cold drinks to body temperature.

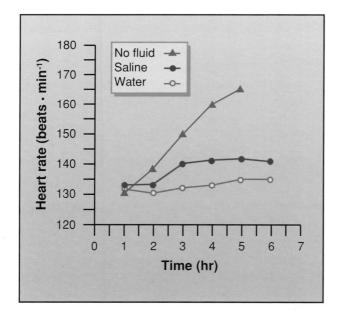

Figure 15.9   Effects of prolonged exercise in the heat on heart rate when subjects receive no fluid, a saline solution, and water.

Hyponatremia

Fluid replacement is beneficial, but can too much of a good thing be bad? In the last few years, several cases of hyponatremia have been reported in endurance athletes. From a clinical point of view, hyponatremia is defined as a blood sodium concentration below the normal range of 136 to 143 mmol $\cdot$ L^{-1}. Symptoms of hyponatremia appear in stages: weakness, disorientation, seizures, and coma if the condition is not reversed. How likely is hyponatremia to occur?

The processes that regulate fluid volumes and electrolyte concentrations are highly effective, so consuming enough water to dilute plasma electrolytes is difficult under normal circumstances. Marathoners who lose 3 to 5 L of sweat and drink 2 to 3 L of water maintain normal plasma concentrations of sodium, chloride, and potassium. Distance runners who run 25 to 40 km per day in warm weather and do not salt their food don't develop electrolyte deficiencies. And normal electrolyte levels were maintained even when subjects consumed only 30% as much potassium as they normally would while losing 3 to 4 L of sweat daily for 8 consecutive days.[9]

Some research has suggested that during ultramarathon running (more than 42 km, or 26.2 mi), athletes can experience hyponatremia. A case study of two runners who collapsed after an ultramarathon race (160 km, or 100 mi) in 1983 revealed that their blood sodium concentration had decreased from a normal value of 140 mEq $\cdot$ L^{-1} to values of 123 and 118 mEq $\cdot$ L^{-1}.[15] One of the runners experienced a grand mal seizure; the other became disoriented and confused. Examining the runners' fluid intakes and estimating their sodium intakes during the run suggested that they diluted their sodium contents by consuming fluids that contained too little sodium. A study by Barr et al., however, showed that when subjects consumed more than 7 L (about 2 gal) of plain water during 6 hr of exercise in the heat, their plasma sodium concentration decreased only negligibly, by about 3.9 mmol $\cdot$ L^{-1}.[2]

The ideal situation would be to replace water at the exact rate that it is being lost, or to add sodium to the ingested fluid to prevent hyponatremia. The problem with the latter approach is that sports drinks that contain no more than 25 mmol Na$^+$ $\cdot$ L^{-1} are apparently too weak to prevent sodium dilution, but stronger concentrations cannot be tolerated. The precise causes of the observed cases of exercise hyponatremia remain unclear. Only a small number of cases have been reported. Thus it is probably inappropriate to form conclusions from this information to design a fluid replacement regimen for people who must exercise for long periods in the heat.

■ IN REVIEW . . . ■

1. Our need to replace lost body fluid is greater than our need to replace lost electrolytes.
2. Our thirst mechanism does not exactly match our hydration state, so we should consume more fluid than we are aware that we need.
3. Water intake during prolonged exercise reduces the risk of dehydration and optimizes our bodies' cardiovascular and thermoregulatory functions.
4. In some cases, drinking too much fluid with too little sodium has led to hyponatremia (low plasma levels of sodium), which can cause confusion, disorientation, and even seizures.

The Athlete's Diet

Athletes place considerable demands on their bodies every day they train and compete. Their bodies must be as finely tuned as possible. This, by necessity, must include optimal nutrition. Too often, athletes spend considerable time and effort perfecting skills and attaining top physical condition while ignoring proper nutrition and sleep. Performance deterioration can often be traced to poor nutrition.

Unfortunately, we know very little about the eating habits of athletes. To gain insight into their practices, a group of highly trained distance runners' diets were recorded during a period of training and during the three days before a marathon. The results are shown in Table 15.9. The 22 runners (11 men, 11 women) had running experience ranging from recreational to international-level competition. The findings revealed little dietary difference between elite and average runners. Diet did not appear to determine success or failure among these performers. Although specific diet items varied, when food was analyzed for percentage of fat, protein, and carbohydrate, or for vitamin and mineral content, the overall differences were small.

Interestingly, the runners came very close to meeting the RDAs. These runners ate diets containing 50% carbohydrate, 36% fat, and 14% protein. We might at first consider the carbohydrate intake of these runners to be low, knowing the need for a high carbohydrate diet when training for distance running. But these runners actually ate more than enough carbohydrate to meet the energy needs of training. Their total calorie intake was nearly 50% higher than expected for nontraining people of similar size (about 65.8 kg, or 145 lb), so their total carbohydrate intake was well above average.

Table 15.9 A Comparison of the 22 Runners' Diets With the Recommended Daily Allowance (RDA).

Diet composition	Runners' average	RDA
Calories (kcal · day⁻¹)	3,012	(2,000)
Carbohydrate (g)	375	(250)
Protein (g)	112	(70)
Saturated fats (g)	42	(26)
Unsaturated fats (g)	64	(54)
Total fat (g)	122	(66-100)
Cholesterol (mg)	377	(300)
Fiber (g)	7	(3-6)
Vitamin A (IU)	10,814	5000
Vitamin B1 (mg)	1.9	1.5
Vitamin B2 (mg)	2.5	1.7
Vitamin B6 (mg)	2.2	2.0
Vitamin B12 (µg)	3.8	2.0
Folic acid (µg)	230	200
Niacin (mg)	27.3	19.0
Pantothenic acid (mg)	5.3	4-7
Vitamin C (mg)	205	60
Vitamin E (mg)	5.2	10
Iron (mg)	25	15
Potassium (g)	4.3	—[a]
Calcium (mg)	1,300	1,200
Magnesium (mg)	400	350
Phosphorus (mg)	200	800-1,200
Sodium (g)	2,600	(2,500)[b]

Note. Figures shown in parentheses represent estimates of the average values in the American diet, which may or may not be healthy. Even where the figure is low, as with folic acid and vitamin E, that does not necessarily suggest a deficiency since the RDA is somewhat arbitrary with a large safety factor.

[a]RDA is not established.

[b]RDA is not established. This is an estimate.

Most of the runners studied did not use vitamin supplements, contrary to some recent surveys about the habits of runners. Still, these runners consumed adequate amounts of most vitamins and minerals to at least equal the RDA. Unless a runner's vitamin intake falls well below the RDA for an extended period of time, no effects on performance are expected. Though diets rich in simple carbohydrates tend to be deficient in some of the B-complex vitamins, only two runners consumed too little vitamin B₁₂. Participants also obtained ample dietary fiber, another item associated with good health.

In the last 3 days before a marathon, the subjects changed both their training and their eating habits. They reduced their daily distance from an average of 13.7 km (8.5 mi) to 3.7 km (2.3 mi). In an attempt to load their muscles with glycogen, the runners increased their daily caloric intake from 3,012 kcal during training to a premarathon average of 3,730 kcal.

Several athletes ate more than 5,000 kcal a day, nearly twice their rate of caloric expenditure during that period, but such overeating might theoretically hurt their performances. During this period, the marathoners had reduced their running distance, so they were burning only about 2,526 kcal per day while eating 3,730 kcal per day. The daily surplus of 1,204 kcal over 3 days could result in storage of an extra pound (0.45 kg) of unnecessary and unproductive fat (1 lb of fat contains 3,500 kcal). For performance, however, eating a bit too much food, principally carbohydrates, is probably better than risking not being fully loaded with muscle and liver glycogen at the time of competition.

These results are from only one study of highly trained distance runners. They are not meant to reflect the typical diet of all athletes. Athletes in different sports might eat differently.

The Vegetarian Diet

In an effort to eat a healthy diet and to increase their carbohydrate intake, many athletes have adopted vegetarianism. Vegans are strict vegetarians who eat only food from plant sources. Lactovegetarians also consume dairy products. Ovovegetarians add eggs to their plant food diets, and lacto-ovovegetarians eat plant foods, dairy products, and eggs.

Can athletes survive on a vegetarian diet? The answer is a qualified yes. Athletes who are strict vegans must be very careful in the selection of the plant foods they eat to provide a good balance of the essential amino acids and adequate sources of vitamin A, riboflavin, vitamin B_{12}, vitamin D, calcium, iron, and sufficient calories. Some professional athletes have noted significant deterioration in athletic performance after switching to strict vegetarian diets. The problem is usually traced to unwise selection of foods. Including milk and eggs in the diet decreases the risk of nutritional deficiencies. Anyone contemplating switching to a vegetarian diet should either read authoritative material on the subject written by qualified nutritionists or consult a registered dietician.

The Precompetition Meal

For years, athletes have received the traditional steak dinner several hours before competition. This practice might have originated from the early belief that muscle consumes itself to fuel its own activity, and that steak would provide the necessary protein to counteract this loss. But we now know that steak is probably the worst food an athlete could eat prior to competing. Steak contains a high percentage of fat, which requires several hours for full digestion; during competition, the digestive system would compete with the muscles for the available blood supply. Also, nervous tension is typically high before a big competition, so even the choicest steak cannot truly be enjoyed at this time. The steak would be more satisfying, and less likely to disturb performance, if the athlete eats it either the night before or after the competition. But if steak is out, what should the athlete eat before competing?

Although the meal ingested a few hours before competition might contribute little to muscle glycogen stores, it can insure a normal blood glucose level and prevent hunger. This meal should contain only about 200 to 500 kcal and consist mostly of carbohydrate foods that are easily digested. Foods such as cereal, juice, and toast are digested rather quickly and won't leave the athlete feeling full during competition. In general, this meal should be consumed at least two hours prior to competition. The rates at which food is digested and nutrients are absorbed into the body are quite individualized, so timing the precompetition meal might depend on prior experience.

A liquid precompetition meal might be less likely to result in nervous indigestion, nausea, vomiting, and abdominal cramps. Such feedings are commercially available and generally have been found useful both before and between events. As with any precompetition feeding, however, they should be avoided in the final hour before competition. Finding time to feed athletes is often difficult when they must perform in multiple preliminary and final events. Under these circumstances, a liquid feeding that is low in fat and high in carbohydrate might be the only solution.

Glycogen Loading

In the preceding discussion we have established that different diets can markedly influence muscle glycogen stores and that endurance performance depends largely on these stores. The theory is that the greater the amount of glycogen stored, the better the potential endurance performance, because fatigue will be delayed. Thus an athlete's goal is to begin an exercise bout or competition with as much stored glycogen as possible.

Based on muscle biopsy studies conducted in the mid-1960s, Åstrand proposed a plan to help runners store the maximum amount of glycogen.[1] This process is known as glycogen loading. According to Åstrand's regimen, athletes should prepare for competition by completing an exhaustive training bout 7 days before the event. For the following 3 days, they should eat fat and protein almost exclusively to deprive the muscles of carbohydrate, which, in turn, increases the activity of glycogen synthase, an enzyme responsible for glycogen synthesis. Athletes should then eat a carbohydrate-rich diet for the remaining days. Because glycogen synthase activity is increased, increased carbohydrate intake results in greater muscle glycogen storage. Training intensity and volume during this 6-day period should be markedly reduced to prevent additional muscle glycogen depletion, thus maximizing liver and muscle glycogen reserves.

This regimen has been shown to elevate muscle glycogen stores to twice the normal level, but it is somewhat impractical for most highly trained competitors. During the 3 days of low carbohydrate intake, athletes generally find training difficult. They are also often irritable and unable to perform mental tasks and typically show signs of low blood sugar, such as muscle weakness and disorientation. In addition, the exhaustive depletion bouts of exercise performed 7 days before the competition have little training value and can impair glycogen storage rather than enhance it. This depletion exercise also exposes athletes to possible injury or overtraining.

Considering these limitations, many propose that the depletion run and the low carbohydrate aspects of Åstrand's regimen should be eliminated. Instead, the athlete should simply reduce training intensity a week before competition and eat a normal mixed diet containing 55% of the calories from carbohydrate until three days before the competition. For these days, training should be reduced to a daily warm-up of 10 to 15 min of activity, accompanied by a carbohydrate-rich diet. Following this plan, as seen in Figure 15.10, glycogen will be elevated to about 200 mmol per kg of muscle, the same level attained with Åstrand's regimen, and the athlete will be better rested for competition.

Diet is also important in preparing the liver for the demands of endurance exercise. Liver glycogen stores decrease rapidly when a person is deprived of carbohydrates for only 24 hr, even when at rest. With only 1 hr of strenuous exercise, liver glycogen decreases by 55%. Thus, hard training combined with a low carbohydrate diet can empty the liver glycogen stores. A single carbohydrate meal, however, quickly restores liver glycogen to normal. Clearly, a carbohydrate-rich diet in the days preceding competition will maximize the liver glycogen reserve and minimize the risk of hypoglycemia during the event.

Water is stored in the body at a rate of about 2.6 g of water for each gram of glycogen. Consequently, the increase or decrease in muscle and liver glycogen generally produces a change in body weight of from

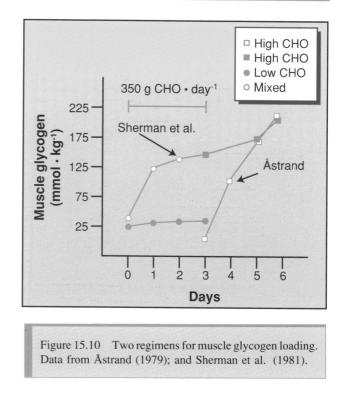

Figure 15.10   Two regimens for muscle glycogen loading. Data from Åstrand (1979); and Sherman et al. (1981).

1 to 3 lb (0.45 to 1.36 kg). Some scientists have proposed that muscle and liver glycogen stores can be monitored by recording the athlete's early morning weight immediately after rising, after emptying the bladder, and before eating breakfast. A sudden drop in weight might reflect a failure to replace glycogen, a deficit in body water, or both.

Athletes who must train or compete in exhaustive events on successive days should replace muscle and liver glycogen stores as rapidly as possible. Although liver glycogen can be totally depleted after 2 hr of exercise at 70% $\dot{V}_{O_2 max}$, it is replenished within a few hours when a rich carbohydrate meal is consumed. Muscle glycogen resynthesis, on the other hand, is a slower process, taking several days to return to normal after an exhaustive exercise bout like the marathon (see Figure 15.11).[4,24] Studies in the late 1980s revealed that muscle glycogen resynthesis was most rapid when individuals were fed at least 50 g (about 0.7 g per kg of body weight) of glucose every 2 hr after the exercise.[5,19] Feeding subjects more than this amount did not appear to accelerate the replacement of muscle glycogen. During the first 2 hr after exercise, the rate of muscle glycogen resynthesis is 7% to 8% per hr (7 to 8 mmol per kg of muscle per hr), which is somewhat faster than the normal rate of 5% to 6% per hr.[18] Thus, an athlete recovering from an exhaustive endurance event should ingest sufficient carbohydrate as soon after exercise as is practical.

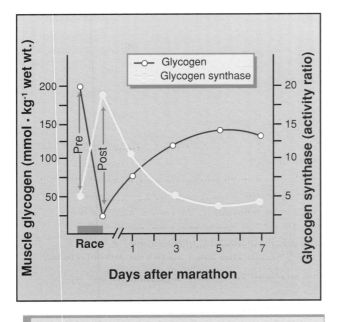

Figure 15.11 Muscle glycogen resynthesis is a slow process, requiring several days to restore normal muscle glycogen storage following exhaustive exercise.

Table 15.10 Effects of Solution Composition on the Rate of Gastric Emptying

Solute characteristic	Effect on the rate of emptying
Volume of the solution	Increases with larger volumes
Caloric content	Decreases as the caloric density increases
Osmolality	Decreases with hyperosmolar solutions
Temperature	Cooler fluids empty faster than warm solutions
pH	Decreased emptying with more acid solutions

Gastrointestinal Function During Exercise

Before solutions can be absorbed into the blood, they must pass through the stomach and into the small intestine, where digestion is completed and nutrients are absorbed into the blood. In this section, we will examine gastrointestinal function during exercise and what impact this has on designing the optimal sports drink. How does the gastrointestinal system handle an ingested solution during exercise?

Gastric Emptying

While ingested food is in the stomach, it is mixed with gastric secretions that contain digestive enzymes to break the food down into smaller subunits, hydrochloric acid that activates some enzymes and kills bacteria, and numerous electrolytes. These secretions are important to proper digestion of the ingested food and absorption of the nutrients it contains. Once the food is mixed with these secretions, it empties from the stomach into the small intestine (the duodenum).

Although neural and hormonal regulation of gastric emptying are not fully understood, we know that a wide variety of stimuli affect the rate at which a solution passes through the stomach. As shown in Table 15.10, these stimuli include

- the volume of ingested food,
- the caloric content of the ingested food,
- the composition and osmolality of the gastric contents,
- the temperature of the ingested food, and
- the pH of the ingested food.

Aside from these factors, limited data suggest that caffeine, emotional distress, diurnal (daily cycle) variations, environmental conditions, and phase of the menstrual cycle might also influence gastric emptying.[10]

But what about exercise? We mentioned earlier that feedings of carbohydrate solutions during endurance exercise can benefit performance, but how is the rate of gastric emptying affected by exercise? Let's examine the impact of various exercise components.

Exercise Intensity

Gastric emptying slows significantly during intense exercise (above 70% to 80% $\dot{V}O_{2\,max}$). As early as 1833, Beaumont noted that severe fatiguing exercise retards digestion. Nearly a century later, researchers reported that even moderate exercise (running 2 to 3 mi, or 3.2 to 4.8 km) after a light meal slowed gastric emptying and reduced gastric secretion in young men.

In contrast, less intense activity, such as walking, actually increased the gastric emptying rate and did not reduce gastric secretion. This has been confirmed by recent studies. In addition, Beaumont found that gastric emptying is more rapid when walking and talking with a friend than when walking alone, demonstrating that psychological factors are also important. What conclusions can be drawn from all this?

Most studies have shown that intense exercise reduces the gastric emptying rate. But for less intense exercise, maintained below 70% to 80% of the subject's $\dot{V}O_{2\,max}$, the gastric emptying rate does not differ from that when the subject is at rest.[11,22] Thus, the physiological mechanisms regulating gastric emptying at rest and during light- to moderate-intensity activity are assumed to be similar. The cause of the differences in emptying rate that have been noted with less-intense exercise might be related to the specific type of exercise (which we will discuss later in this chapter).

The intensity of exercise needed to impair gastric emptying also can vary with the subjects' level of fitness. In one subject, merely walking quickly slowed gastric emptying. Yet in another subject who trained regularly, running 2 mi (3.2 km) had no effect on gastric function. Thus the more fit the individual, the less impact exercise has on gastric function, because at the same rate of work a more-fit person exercises at a lower percentage of $\dot{V}O_{2\,max}$ than a less-fit person.

Exercise Duration

To determine the effects of exercise duration on the rate of gastric emptying, a series of studies examined this rate at four points during 2 hr of cycling.[11] Despite the fatiguing effects of the exercise, no change in the gastric emptying rate occurred throughout the activity. As a consequence of these studies, data on gastric emptying measured at rest are assumed to apply during prolonged activities (less than 2 hr). These activities are generally performed at intensities below 80% $\dot{V}O_{2\,max}$, so the gastric emptying rate is not affected.

Mode of Exercise

Now we have examined the effects of exercise intensity and duration on gastric function, but not all types of exercise cause the same effects. For example, water and carbohydrate solutions have been shown to empty 38% faster during moderate treadmill exercise than when subjects remained inactive after the feeding.[22] Submaximal cycling might also increase the gastric emptying rate, though recent investigations of this have presented conflicting results.[10]

To compare the influence of various exercise modes, the gastric emptying rates for carbohydrate solutions were studied during 20 and 120 min of rest, cycling, and running.[10] Emptying was consistently faster during the running trials than during the cycling trials, and 20 min of either form of exercise induced faster gastric emptying than 20 min of rest. But the emptying rate for 120 min of cycling was not significantly different than when at rest. In a separate study, no difference in gastric emptying rates occurred during cycling and resting bouts lasting from 15 to 120 min.

Thus the influence of cycling on gastric emptying is not clear. However, moderately intense running or walking does appear to facilitate gastric emptying. Anecdotal evidence suggests that cross-country skiing might also accelerate gastric emptying, but little information is available concerning the influence of other modes of activity.[10] At best, we can conclude that different modes of exercise can affect gastric emptying rates differently.

Intestinal Absorption of Nutrients

When ingesting carbohydrate feedings during endurance exercise, intestinal absorption is somewhat delayed because most carbohydrate solutions are held in the stomach for a short time as the stomach attempts to dilute the solution by mixing it with gastric secretions. For this reason, the first traces of any sugar solution do not appear in the blood for 5 to 7 min after consumption. This delay allows the stomach to deliver fluids that can be rapidly absorbed to the small intestine.

Digestion is completed in the small intestine, then nutrients are absorbed from the intestinal wall into the blood to meet the body's needs. This process directly affects the maintenance of fluid and fuel homeostasis during exercise. Not all products of digestion are absorbed at the same rate or via the same mechanisms. In the following discussion, we'll summarize the major factors governing absorption in the intestine.

About 9 L of fluid are presented to the intestines each day:[16]

- 2 L from ingested fluid
- 1.5 L from saliva
- 5.5 L from gastrointestinal secretions

Of this amount, approximately 60% is absorbed from the duodenum and jejunum, 20% from the ileum, and 15% from the large intestine. The remainder stays in the large intestine and is excreted with the feces.

How does exercise affect intestinal absorption? Most physiologists agree that moderate to intense exercise reduces blood flow to the gut. Because substances must be absorbed from the intestinal wall into the blood, reductions in blood flow suggest less opportunity for absorption. However, Fordtran and Saltin found that exercise at 75% of $\dot{V}O_{2\,max}$ did not impair intestinal absorption of fluid containing carbohydrate and sodium chloride.[14] This led to the conclusion that, under most exercise situations, intestinal blood flow and normal peristaltic action do not play major roles in altering absorption.

During highly intense effort, however, such as in long-distance running and triathlon competitions, the relatively high incidence of gastrointestinal distress suggests that some serious alterations in intestinal function might occur. Abdominal cramps, for example, can indicate interruptions in oxygen (and hence blood) supply.

Diarrhea associated with endurance exercise (such as marathon running) appears to be of a psychogenic or emotional nature. The anxiety or emotional stimulation associated with competition may speed the passage of materials through the intestines, reducing the amount of time for water absorption. This exercise-induced diarrhea is caused by excessive stimulation of the parasympathetic nervous system. This stimulates both intestinal motility and mucus secretion in the distal colon. These two factors prevent normal absorption of water from the feces, leading to diarrhea. Some cases of gastrointestinal bleeding have also been noted. These might indicate ischemic (oxygen deprivation) injury to the intestinal lining.

A variety of factors might affect intestinal absorption during exercise, such as the mode of exercise, environmental temperature, and the formulation of ingested solutions. Some studies have shown that during exercise the absorption rate is reduced for water, Na+, K+, and Cl-. However, most studies have concluded that exercise does not influence intestinal absorption.[14,16]

Designing Sports Drinks

We mentioned earlier that ingesting carbohydrate solutions during exercise can benefit performance by ensuring adequate fuel for energy production and adequate fluid for rehydration. Now that we have discussed the nutrient needs of athletes and how exercise affects gastrointestinal function, we can consider what types of feedings are best during exercise. As we have seen, adequate carbohydrate intake is essential for maintaining athletes' energy levels. For this reason, the sports drink industry has focused on carbohydrate solutions. Let's examine some of the factors that must be considered when designing sports drinks to maximize performance.

Carbohydrate Type

Although the body relies on it for energy production, is glucose the best sugar to include in sports drinks? Other sugar molecules may empty from the stomach faster than glucose. For example, earlier studies with solutions of maltodextrin (complex chains of glucose) showed that a 5 g per 100 ml solution emptied from the stomach faster than a glucose solution of similar concentration. However, subsequent research has not supported this finding, leading most investigators to conclude that the rates of gastric emptying for these two carbohydrate forms differ little, if any. But fructose might leave the stomach faster than other carbohy-

drates. Fructose at concentrations below 200 mmol · L⁻¹, when given alone, caused little or no slowing of gastric emptying. Some other forms of sugar, such as sucrose, maltose, galactose, and lactose, might even inhibit gastric emptying. So, along with concentration, the type of carbohydrate in the solution is important. Most commercial sports drinks contain mixtures of glucose, sucrose, fructose, high fructose corn syrup, and maltodextrins.

Carbohydrate Concentration

In general, carbohydrate solutions empty more slowly from the stomach than either water or a weak sodium chloride (salt) solution.[11,12,14] Research suggests that a solution's caloric content, a reflection of its concentration, might be a major determinant of how quickly it empties from the stomach and is absorbed in the intestine. Rich solutions remain in the stomach longer than either water or weak solutions. As illustrated in Figure 15.12, increasing the glucose concentration of a drink drastically reduces the gastric emptying rate. For example, 400 ml of a weak glucose solution (139 mmol · L⁻¹) is almost completely emptied from the stomach in 20 min, but emptying a similar volume of a strong glucose solution (834 mmol · L⁻¹) can require nearly two hours.

However, when even a small amount of a strong glucose drink leaves the stomach it can contain more

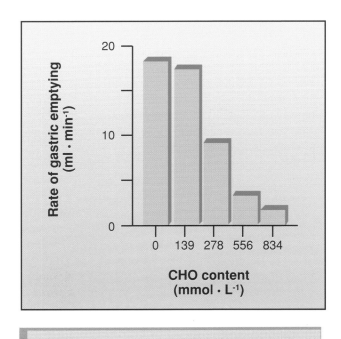

Figure 15.12 The relationship between a solution's carbohydrate concentration and the rate of gastric emptying.

sugar than a larger amount of a weaker solution simply because of its higher concentration. Table 15.11 shows that despite their slower rates of gastric emptying, strong sugar solutions deliver more glucose (in kcal) per minute to the intestine than weak ones.

Results of early studies suggested that sports drinks should have less than 2.5 g of sugar per 100 ml of water to speed their passage through the stomach. Unfortunately, such a small amount of carbohydrate contributes little to energy reserves. Even if you drank 200 ml (about 7 oz) of such a drink every 15 min during a long run, you would take in only 20 g of carbohydrate per hour. Recent studies suggest that to improve performance, athletes should consume at least 50 g of sugar per hour.

Most sports drinks on the market contain only about 6 to 8 g of sugar per 100 ml. An endurance athlete would need to drink about 625 to 833 ml of these drinks every hour to get enough carbohydrates to do any good. Most people can drink only about 270 to 450 ml (9 to 15 oz) per hour during exercise. Thus, only drinks containing at least 11 g of carbohydrate per 100 ml would be of any value. The sports drinks currently on the market fall far short of this. Besides, such a rich mixture might be delayed in the stomach, might draw water from the stomach's lining, and can cause an uncomfortable feeling of fullness.

Rehydration With Sports Drinks

Just adding fluid to the body during exercise lessens the risk of serious dehydration. But some research indicates that adding glucose to rehydrative beverages, aside from supplying an energy source, might also stimulate both water and sodium absorption. Recall that when sodium is retained, it causes more water to be retained. Furthermore, some exercise physiologists believe that Na^+ is required for glucose transport.

These beliefs are used to justify adding sodium to sports drinks, but the interactions of glucose and sodium are still unconfirmed. Studies on the topic have examined intestinal content through a tube that bypasses the stomach. Thus these studies ignore the normal gastric contributions of sodium and other ions to the ingested solutions, so the addition of sodium to sports drinks remains controversial. Still other people have suggested that the addition of amino acids to a glucose and electrolyte solution will enhance its absorption, but, again, this remains unconfirmed.

What Works Best

Athletes will not drink solutions that taste bad. Unfortunately, we all have different taste preferences. To further confound the issue, what tastes good before and after a long, hot bout of exercise will not necessarily taste good during the event. A recent study tested the taste preferences of runners and cyclists during 60 min of exercise. Most of the 50 subjects chose a drink with a light flavor and no strong aftertaste. For this criterion, nearly all of the commercial sports drinks failed.

So what should the athlete drink during training and competition? Under the extreme stress of hot weather, water is the primary need. Although a good case can be made for plain water, most agree that definite nutritional benefits can be gained by adding carbohydrate to the solution. The inclusion of 4 to 8 g of carbohydrate per 100 ml should not compromise the delivery of water to the body tissues. Consuming 100 to 150 ml of solution every 10 or 15 min should reduce the risk of dehydration and hyperthermia and provide an energy supplement. In events lasting less than an hour, the need for fluids is very small because dehydration is not very significant in these events and the body's carbohydrate stores are sufficient to sustain the activity for this period.

Clearly, how to design the best drink for rehydration is still debatable. In light of the commercial competition surrounding sports drinks, the debate over the

Table 15.11 Composition of Water and Glucose Solutions Before and 20 min After Ingestion

Variables	Water		5 g glucose per 100 ml		10 g glucose per 100 ml	
	Before	Residue	Before	Residue	Before	Residue
Osmolality (mOsm $\cdot$ L^{-1})	23	87	266	245	532	434
Sodium (mEq $\cdot$ L^{-1})	0.7	7.9	1.5	18.6	1.9	14.5
Potassium (mEq $\cdot$ L^{-1})	0.1	4.11	0.11	5.21	0.10	3.63
Glucose (g per 100 ml)	0.0	0.0	5.0	3.3	10.0	6.5
pH	4.76	2.05	3.50	2.29	3.46	2.40
Gastric secretion[a] (ml)	—	32	—	52	—	65

[a]Gastric secretion denotes the volume of secretion calculated to be present in the residue.

ideal exercise drink will probably continue for some time.

IN REVIEW . . .

1. The composition of ingested materials can be significantly altered while in the stomach by the addition of electrolytes and water.
2. The volume of stomach contents is one of the strongest regulators of the gastric emptying rate. Larger volumes of ingestate trigger neural receptors in the walls of the stomach and duodenum. This stimulation causes the emptying rate to increase.
3. The type and concentration of the ingestate also affects gastric emptying. Strong carbohydrate solutions empty more slowly than weaker ones, but because of their concentrations these stronger solutions can still deliver more glucose to the intestines than faster-emptying but weaker solutions. Fat is a strong inhibitor of gastric emptying.
4. Intense exercise slows gastric emptying significantly, but lighter exercise can actually increase the rate. Psychological factors also seem to be involved.
5. Even though intense exercise decreases blood flow to the intestines, absorption does not seem to be hindered. But cramping and other symptoms during high-intensity exercise indicate that some disturbance of intestinal function occurs.
6. Various ideas have been proposed about which solution would be best absorbed from the gastrointestinal tract. Plain water is good; adding carbohydrate is probably even better. But to date no ideal solution has been identified.

In Closing . . .

In this chapter we have examined the nutritional needs of the athlete, considering the importance of the six nutrient classes to exercise and athletic performance. We also discussed several ways in which athletes try to use nutritional supplementation for ergogenic purposes. We dispelled the myth of the value of the precompetition steak dinner and explored the effectiveness of commercial sports drinks. Now that we have a thorough knowledge of the importance of a balanced diet, we will turn our attention to another aspect of the athlete's diet. In the next chapter we will consider the effects of body weight on athletic performance.

Key Terms

dehydration
electrolytes
essential amino acids
extracellular fluid
gastric emptying
glycogen loading
hyponatremia
intestinal absorption

intracellular fluid
macrominerals
microminerals (trace
   elements)
nonessential amino acids
osmolality
thirst mechanism
vitamins

Study Questions

1. What are the six categories of nutrients?
2. What role does dietary fat play in endurance performance?
3. What is an appropriate protein allowance for a normally active adult male? Female?
4. Discuss the value of using protein supplements to enhance performance in strength and endurance events.
5. Which vitamins are most likely to be deficient in the athlete's diet?
6. How does dehydration affect exercise performance? What effect does dehydration have on exercise heart rate and body temperature?
7. How does the body regulate electrolyte balance during acute exercise and chronic exercise?
8. Describe the preferred precompetition meal.
9. Describe the methods used to maximize muscle glycogen storage (glycogen loading).
10. Describe the proper dietary regimen to glycogen load the muscle prior to an exhaustive event lasting 3 to 4 hours.
11. Discuss the value of consuming carbohydrate during and after endurance exercise.
12. List the factors that regulate the rate of gastric emptying. Which of these appear to have the greatest impact on gastric emptying during exercise?
13. What characteristics/components should the ideal sports drink have?
14. What foods can be considered as ergogenic aids to performance? In which events will the athlete benefit from consuming these foods?

References

1. Åstrand, P.-O. (1979). Nutrition and physical performance. In M. Rechcigl (Ed.), *Nutrition and the world food problem*. S. Karger: Basel.

2. Barr, S.I., Costill, D.L., Fink, W.J., & Thomas, R. (1991). Effect of increased training volume on blood lipids and lipoproteins in male collegiate swimmers.

Medicine and Science in Sports and Exercise, **23**, 795-800.

3. Belko, A.Z. (1987). Vitamins and exercise—an update. *Medicine and Science in Sports and Exercise*, **19**, S191-S196.

4. Blom, P., Costill, D.L., & Vollestad, N.K. (1987). Exhaustive running: Inappropriate as a stimulus of muscle glycogen super-compensation. *Medicine and Science in Sports and Exercise*, **19**, 398-403.

5. Blom, P., Vollestad, N.K., & Costill, D.L. (1986). Factors affecting changes in muscle glycogen concentration during and after prolonged exercise. *Acta Physiologica Scandinavica*, **128**(Suppl. 556), 67-74.

6. Bruce, R., Ekblom, B., & Nilsson, I. (1985). The effect of vitamin and mineral supplements and health foods on physical endurance and performance. *Proceeding of the Nutrition Society*, **44**, 283-295.

7. Claremont, A.D., Costill, D.L., Fink, W., & VanHandel, P. (1976). Heat tolerance following diuretic-induced dehydration. *Medicine and Science in Sports and Exercise*, **8**, 239-243.

8. Consolazio, C.F., Johnson, H.L., Nelson, R.A., Dramise, J.G., & Skala, J.H. (1975). Protein metabolism during intensive physical training in the young adult. *American Journal of Clinical Nutrition*, **28**, 29-35.

9. Costill, D.L. (1977). Sweating: Its composition and effect of body fluids. *Annals of the New York Academy of Science*, **301**, 160-174.

10. Costill, D.L. (1990). Gastric emptying of fluids during exercise. In C. Gisolfi and D. Lamb (Eds.) *Perspectives in exercise science and sports medicine: Vol. 3. Fluid homeostasis during exercise* (pp. 97-127). Indianapolis: Benchmark Press.

11. Costill, D.L., & Saltin, B. (1974). Factors limiting gastric emptying during rest and exercise. *Journal of Applied Physiology*, **37**, 679-683.

12. Coyle, E.F., Costill, D.L., Fink, W.J., & Hoopes, D.G. (1978). Gastric emptying rates for selected athletic drinks. *Research Quarterly*, **49**, 119-124.

13. Coyle, E.F., Hagberg, J.M., Hurley, B.F., Martin, W.H., Ehsani, A.A., & Holloszy, J.O. (1983). Carbohydrate feeding during prolonged strenuous exercise can delay fatigue. *Journal of Applied Physiology*, **55**, 230-235.

14. Fordtran, J.S., & Saltin, B. (1967). Gastric emptying and intestinal absorption during prolonged severe exercise. *Journal of Applied Physiology*, **23**, 331-335.

15. Frizzell, R.T., Lang, G.H., Lowance, D.C., & Lathan, S.R. (1986). Hyponatremia and ultramarathon running. *Journal of the American Medical Association*, **255**, 772-774.

16. Gisolfi, C.V., Summers, R.W., & Schedl, H.P. (1990). Intestinal absorption of fluids during rest and exercise. In *Perspectives in exercise science and sports medicine: Vol. 3. Fluid homeostasis during exercise*. Indianapolis: Benchmark Press.

17. Horstman, D.H. (1972). Nutrition. In W.P. Morgan (Ed.), *Ergogenic aids and muscular performance* (pp. 343-365). New York: Academic Press.

18. Ivy, J.L., Katz, A.L., Cutler, C.L., Sherman, W.M., & Coyle, E.F. (1988). Muscle glycogen synthesis after exercise: Effect of time of carbohydrate ingestion. *Journal of Applied Physiology*, **64**, 1480-1485.

19. Ivy, J.L., Lee, M.C., Brozinick, Jr., J.T., & Reed, M.J. (1988). Muscle glycogen storage after different amounts of carbohydrate ingestion. *Journal of Applied Physiology*, **65**, 2018-2023.

20. Lemon, P.W.R., & Proctor, D.N. (1991). Protein intake and athletic performance. *Sports Medicine*, **12**, 313-325.

21. Marable, N.L., Hickson, J.F., Korslund, M.K., Herbert, W.G., Desjardins, R.F., & Thye, F.W. (1979). Urinary nitrogen excretion as influenced by a muscle-building exercise program and protein intake variation. *Nutrition Reports International*, **19**, 795-805.

22. Neufer, P.D., Costill, D.L., Fink, W.J., Kirwan, J.P., Fielding, R.A., & Flynn, M.G. (1986). Effects of exercise and carbohydrate composition on gastric emptying. *Medicine and Science in Sports and Exercise*, **18**, 658-662.

23. Risser, W.L., Lee, E.J., Poindexter, H.B.W., West, M.S., Pivarnik, J.M., Risser, J.M.H., & Hickson, J.F. (1988). Iron deficiency in female athletes: Its prevalence and impact on performance. *Medicine and Science in Sports and Exercise*, **20**, 116-121.

24. Sherman, W.M., Costill, D.L., Fink, W.J., Hagerman, F.C., Armstrong, L.E., & Murray, T.F. (1983). Effect of a 42.2-km footrace and subsequent rest or exercise on muscle glycogen and enzymes. *Journal of Applied Physiology*, **55**, 1219-1224.

Selected Readings

Åstrand, P.-O. (1967). Diet and athletic performance. *Federation Proceedings*, **26**, 1772-1777.

Beaumont, W. (1833). *Experiments and observations on the gastric juice and the physiology of digestion*. New York: Dover Publishing.

Bergstrom, J. (1962). Muscle electrolytes in man: Determined by neutron activation analysis in needle biopsy specimens. A study on normal subjects, kidney patients, and patients with chronic diarrhea. *Scandinavian Journal of Clinical Laboratory Investigation*, **14**(Suppl. 68).

Bergstrom, J., Hermansen, L., Hultman, E., & Saltin, B. (1967). Diet, muscle glycogen and physical performance. *Acta Physiologica Scandinavica*, **71**, 140-150.

Bergstrom, J., & Hultman, E. (1967). A study of the glycogen metabolism during exercise in man. *Scandinavian Journal of Clinical Laboratory Investigation*, **19**, 218-228.

Brooks, G.A. (1987). Amino acid and protein metabolism during exercise and recovery. *Medicine and Science in Sports and Exercise*, **19**, S150-S156.

Brouns, F., & Beckers, E. (1993). Is the gut an athletic organ? *Sports Medicine*, **15**, 242-257.

Burke, L.M., & Read, R.S.D. (1993). Dietary supplements in sport. *Sports Medicine*, **15**(1), 43-65.

Christensen, E.H., & Hansen, O. III. (1939). Arbeitsfahigkeit and Ernahrung. *Scandinavian Archives of Physiology*, **81**, 160-171.

Clement, D.B., & Asmundson, R.C. (1982). Nutritional intake and hematological parameters in endurance runners. *Physician and Sportsmedicine*, **10**, 37-43.

Coggan, A.R., & Coyle, E.F. (1987). Reversal of fatigue during prolonged exercise by carbohydrate infusion or ingestion. *Journal of Applied Physiology*, **63**, 2388-2395.

Coggan, A.R., & Swanson, S.C. (1992). Nutritional manipulations before and during endurance exercise: Effects on performance. *Medicine and Science in Sports and Exercise*, **24**, S331-S335.

Costill, D.L. (1988). Carbohydrates for exercise: Dietary demands for optimal performance. *International Journal of Sports Medicine*, **9**, 1-18.

Costill, D.L., Bennett, A., Branam, G., & Eddy, D. (1973). Glucose ingestion at rest and during prolonged exercise. *Journal of Applied Physiology*, **34**, 764-769.

Costill, D.L., Cote, R., & Fink, W. (1982). Dietary potassium and heavy exercise: Effects on muscle water and electrolytes. *American Journal of Clinical Nutrition*, **36**, 266-275.

Costill, D.L., Dalsky, G.P., & Fink, W.J. (1978). Effects of caffeine ingestion on metabolism and exercise performance. *Medicine and Science in Sports*, **10**, 155-158.

Costill, D.L., & Miller, J.M. (1980). Nutrition for endurance sport: Carbohydrate and fluid balance. *International Journal of Sports Medicine*, **1**, 2-14.

Coyle, E.F. (1991). Timing and method of increased carbohydrate intake to cope with heavy training, competition, and recovery. *Journal of Sports Sciences*, **9**, 29-52.

Coyle, E.F., Coggan, A.R., Hemmert, M.K., & Ivy, J.L. (1986). Muscle glycogen utilization during prolonged strenuous exercise when fed carbohydrates. *Journal of Applied Physiology*, **61**, 165-172.

Foster, C., Costill, D.L., & Fink, W.J. (1979). Effects of pre-exercise feedings on endurance performance. *Medicine and Science in Sports*, **11**, 1-5.

Gontzea, I., Sutzescu, P., & Dumitrache, S. (1974). The influence of muscular activity on nitrogen balance and on the need of man for proteins. *Nutrition Reports International*, **10**, 35-43.

Havel, R.J., Pernow, B., & Jones, N.L. (1966). Uptake and release of free fatty acids and other metabolism in the legs of exercising man. *Journal of Applied Physiology*, **23**, 90-96.

Haymes, E.M. (1983). Proteins, vitamins, and iron. In M.H. Williams (Ed.), *Ergogenic aids in sport* (pp. 27-55). Champaign, IL: Human Kinetics.

Hermansen, L., Hultman, E., & Saltin, B. (1967). Muscle glycogen during prolonged severe exercise. *Acta Physiologica Scandinavica*, **71**, 129-139.

Hiller, W.D.B., O'Toole, M.L., Fortess, E.E., Laird, R.H., Imbert, P.C., & Sisk, T.D. (1987). Medical and physiological considerations in triathlons. *American Journal of Sports Medicine*, **15**, 164-167.

Howald, H., & Segesser, B. (1975). Ascorbic acid and athletic performance. *Annals of the New York Academy of Science*, **258**, 458-464.

Hultman, E. (1967). Studies on muscle metabolism of glycogen an active phosphate in man with special reference to exercise and diet. *Scandinavian Journal of Clinical Laboratory Investigation*, **19** (Suppl. 94).

Hunt, J.N., & Knox, M.T. (1969). Regulation of gastric emptying. In *Handbook of physiology: Vol. IV. Alimentary canal* (pp. 1917-1935). Washington D.C.: American Physiological Society.

Karlsson, J., & Saltin, B. (1971). Diet, muscle glycogen, and endurance performance. *Journal of Applied Physiology*, **31**, 203-206.

Kozlowski, S., & Saltin, B. (1964). Effect of sweat loss on body fluids. *Journal of Applied Physiology*, **19**, 1119-1124.

Lentner, C. (Ed.) (1981). *Geigy scientific tables: Vol. 1. Units of measurement, body fluids, composition of the body, nutrition* (pp. 232-234). Geneva, Switzerland: Ciba-Geigy.

McDonald, R., & Keen, C.L. (1988). Iron, zinc and magnesium nutrition and athletic performance. *Sports Medicine*, **5**, 171-184.

Minaim, H., & McCallum, R.W. (1984). The physiology and pathophysiology of gastric emptying in humans. *Gastroenterology*, **86**, 1592-1610.

Mitchell, J.B., Costill, D.L., Houmard, J.A., Fink, W.J., Pascoe, D.D., & Pearson, D.R. (1989). Influence of carbohydrate dosage on exercise performance and glycogen metabolism. *Journal of Applied Physiology*, **67**, 1843-1949.

Mitchell, J.B., Costill, D.L., Houmard, J.A., Flynn, M.G., Fink, W.J., & Beltz, J.D. (1988). Effects of carbohydrate ingestion on gastric emptying and exercise performance. *Medicine and Science in Sports and Exercise*, **20**, 110-115.

Nielsen, B., Sjogaard, G., Ugelvig, J., Knudsen, B., & Dohlmann, B. (1986). Fluid balance in exercise dehydration and rehydration with different glucose-electrolyte drinks. *European Journal of Applied Physiology*, **55**, 318-325.

Noakes, T.D., Goodwin, N., Rayner, B.L., Branker, T., & Taylor, R. (1985). Water intoxication: A possible complication during endurance exercise. *Medicine and Science in Sports and Exercise*, **17**, 370-375.

Noakes, T.D., Norman, R.J., Buck, R.H., Godlonton, J., Stevenson, K., & Pittaway, D. (1990). The incidence of hyponatremia during prolonged ultraendurance exercise. *Medicine and Science in Sports and Exercise*, **22**, 165-170.

Owen, M.D., Kregel, K.C., Wall, P.T., & Gisolfi, C.V. (1985). Effects of carbohydrate ingestion on thermoregulation, gastric emptying and plasma volume during exercise in the heat. *Medicine and Science in Sports and Exercise*, **17**, 185. (Abstract)

Pate, R.R. (1983). Sports anemia: A review of the current research literature. *Physician Sportsmedicine*, **11**, 115-131.

Piehl, K. (1974). Time course for refilling of glycogen stores in human muscle fibres following exercise-induced glycogen depletion. *Acta Physiologica Scandinavica*, **90**, 297-302.

Rennie, M.J., & Holloszy, J.O. (1977). Inhibition of glucose uptake and glycogenolysis by availability of oleate in well-oxygenated perfused skeletal muscle. *Biochemistry Journal*, **168**, 161-170.

Saltin, B. (1964). Aerobic and anaerobic work capacity after dehydration. *Journal of Applied Physiology*, **19**, 1114-1118.

Saltin, B. & Hermansen, L. (1967). Glycogen stores and prolonged severe exercise. In G. Blix (Ed.), *Nutrition and physical activity* (pp. 32-46). Uppsala: Almqvist & Wiksells.

Sherman, W.M. (1992). Recovery from endurance exercise. *Medicine and Science in Sports and Exercise*, **24**, S336-S339.

Sherman, W.M., Costill, D.L., Fink, W.J., Armstrong, L.E., & Hagerman, F.C. (1983). The marathon: Recovery from acute biochemical alterations. *Biochemistry of Exercise*, **13**, 312-317.

Sherman, W.M., Costill, D.L., Fink, W.J., & Miller, J.M. (1981). Effects of exercise-diet manipulation on muscle glycogen and its subsequent utilization during performance. *International Journal of Sports Medicine*, **2**, 1-15.

Smith, N.J., & Worthington-Roberts, B. (1989). *Food for sport*. Palo Alto, CA: Bull Publishing.

Tarnopolsky, M.A., MacDougall, J.D., & Atkinson, S.A. (1988). Influence of protein intake and training status on nitrogen balance and lean body mass. *Journal of Applied Physiology*, **64**, 187-193.

Van Handel, P. (1983). Caffeine. In M.H. Williams (Ed.), *Ergogenic aids in sport* (pp. 128-163). Champaign, IL: Human Kinetics.

Vellar, O.D. (1968). Studies on sweat losses of nutrients. I. Iron content of whole body sweat and its association with other sweat constituents, serum iron levels, hematological indices, body surface area and sweat rate. *Scandinavian Journal of Clinical Laboratory Investigation*, **1**, 157-167.

Weight, L.M., Noakes, T.D., Labadarios, D., Graves, J., Jacobs, P., & Berman, P.A. (1988). Vitamin and mineral status of trained athletes including the effects of supplementation. *American Journal of Clinical Nutrition*, **47**, 186-191.

Chapter 16

Optimal Body Weight for Performance

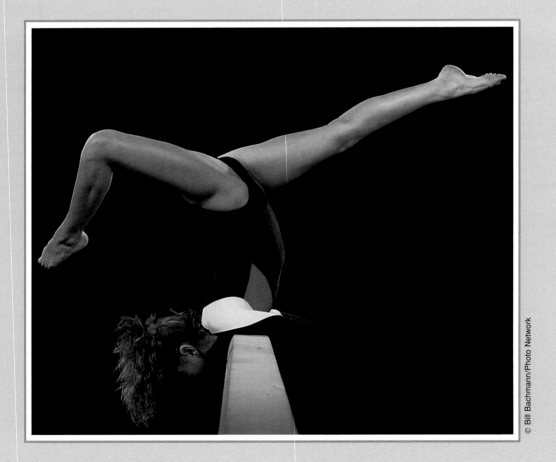

Chapter Overview

An athlete's body size, build, and composition play major roles in determining athletic success. Of primary concern is the athlete's fat mass and fat-free mass. The ideal body type varies with each sport. The endurance runner strives for leanness, minimizing the load that must be carried during a distance run, but the sumo wrestler tries hard to maximize his weight, because the tradition of his sport dictates that "bigger is better." Athletes of various weights can participate successfully in some sports, such as football, depending on the position they play. Yet other sports, such as wrestling, set rigid weight standards for participants that often force athletes to shed large amounts of weight in a short time. Many turn to crash diets, fasting, or the current fad diet, too often with little or no regard to the overall effects this has on health or performance.

In this chapter, we will focus on body composition and how it affects physical performance. We will discuss the significance of both fat-free mass and relative body fat, then put these into perspective by looking at the ideal ranges found in elite performers. We will explore the use of weight standards and the medical problems that are common when athletes use unrealistic methods to try to make weight. Finally, we will examine the proper way to plan weight loss so that a goal weight can be met and maintained without impairing performance.

Chapter Outline

A former major league baseball player made minimum salary during his first few years in the majors. Early preseason polls projected his team to finish the season at the bottom of its division, but the team ended up in the World Series. This player became one of the best at his position in the National League during that season, and once the World Series was over he asked management for a substantial salary increase ($75,000 in the mid-1970s). Management agreed to his salary demands contingent on his loss of 25 lb (11 kg)! The player refused to lose the weight, so the parties were deadlocked.

The team physician suggested sending the player to a major university for an accurate body composition assessment, and both parties agreed. A hydrostatic weighing was performed, and the results showed that the player had less than 6% body fat, with only a total of 11 lb (5 kg) of fat! Because 3% to 4% body fat is necessary for survival, this player had only 4 to 5 lb (about 2 kg) of fat to lose, and that loss wasn't advised because he was already at the lower level recommended for wrestlers, who are known for their rapid weight-loss techniques. Management was satisfied; this player received his salary increase and he did not have to lose weight.

In this case, the athlete's weight was well above the weight range for his height and he had a peculiar gait—a gait commonly referred to as a waddle. The combination of being overweight by the standard height-weight charts and having a waddle led management to demand the 25-lb (11-kg) weight loss. Had the athlete agreed to management's demand, he would have likely destroyed his career as a professional athlete. How many athletes have been faced with a similar situation? How many gave in?

Coaches and athletes today are acutely aware of the importance of achieving and maintaining optimal body weight for peak performance in sports. Appropriate size, build, and body composition are critical to success in almost all athletic endeavors. Compare the specific performance requirements of the 5-ft, 100-lb (152-cm, 45-kg) Olympic gymnast and those of the 6-ft, 9-in.; 325-lb (206-cm, 147-kg) defensive lineman in professional football. Body shape, size, and composition are largely predetermined by the genes inherited from one's parents. But this doesn't mean athletes should dismiss these components of their physical profile, feeling that nothing can be done to change or improve them. Although size and body build can be altered only slightly, body composition can change substantially with diet and exercise. Resistance training can substantially increase muscle mass, and a sound diet combined with vigorous exercise can significantly decrease body fat. Such changes can be of major importance to achieving optimal athletic performance.

Body Build, Body Size, and Body Composition

What are the differences between body build, body size, and body composition? Body build refers to morphology, or the form and structure of the body. Most scientific systems for classifying body build have identified three major components:

1. Muscularity
2. Linearity
3. Fatness

Each athlete's build is a unique combination of these three components. Athletes in certain sports usually exhibit a predominance of one component over the other two. The bodybuilder primarily exhibits muscularity, the 7-ft, 2-in. (218-cm) basketball center who weighs only 180 lb (82 kg) exhibits linearity, and the sumo wrestler exhibits fatness. Most athletes are more balanced between muscularity and linearity, but muscularity tends to dominate in male athletes.[5]

Body size refers to the height and mass (weight) of an individual. Body size is often categorized as short or tall, large or small, heavy or light. Distinctions between these categories can vary depending on the specific performance requirements, so body size must be considered relative to the specific sport, the athlete's position, or the type of event. For example, among males a height of 6 ft, 3 in. (190.5 cm) would be short for a professional basketball player, but tall for a long-distance runner. Similarly, in professional football a weight of 230 lb (104 kg) would be heavy for a quarterback, just right for a linebacker, but light for a defensive end.

Body composition refers to the body's chemical composition. Figure 16.1 illustrates four models of body composition. The first two divide the body into its various chemical and anatomical components; the last two simplify body composition into two components. The major difference between these last two models is the terminology of lean body mass and fat-free mass. Behnke originally proposed the concept of lean body mass, defined to include fat-free mass and essential fat—the amount of fat necessary for survival.[8] Although this model is conceptually sound, it presents measurement problems: It isn't possible to differentiate between essential and nonessential fat. Consequently, most scientists have adopted the two-component model that includes fat mass and fat-free mass, which is the model used in this book. Fat mass is often discussed in terms of relative body fat, which is the percentage of the total body mass that is composed of fat. Fat-free mass simply refers to all body tissue that is not fat.

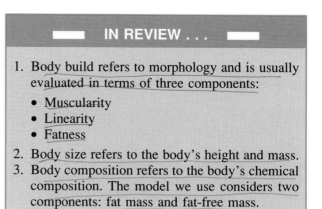

IN REVIEW . . .

1. Body build refers to morphology and is usually evaluated in terms of three components:
   - Muscularity
   - Linearity
   - Fatness
2. Body size refers to the body's height and mass.
3. Body composition refers to the body's chemical composition. The model we use considers two components: fat mass and fat-free mass.

Assessing Body Composition

Assessment of body composition provides additional information, beyond the basic measures of height and weight, to both the coach and the athlete. As an example, if the center fielder of a major league baseball team is 6 ft, 3 in. (190.5 cm) tall and weighs 200 lb (91 kg), is he at his ideal playing weight? Knowing that 10 lb (about 5 kg) out of a total weight of 200 lb (91 kg) is fat weight and that the remaining 190 lb (86 kg) is fat-free weight provides considerably more insight than weight alone. In this example, only 5% of his body weight is fat, which is about as low as any athlete should go. Armed with this knowledge,

KEY POINT

The fat-free mass, formerly referred to as the lean body mass, is composed of all of the body's nonfat tissue, including bone, muscle, organs, and connective tissue.

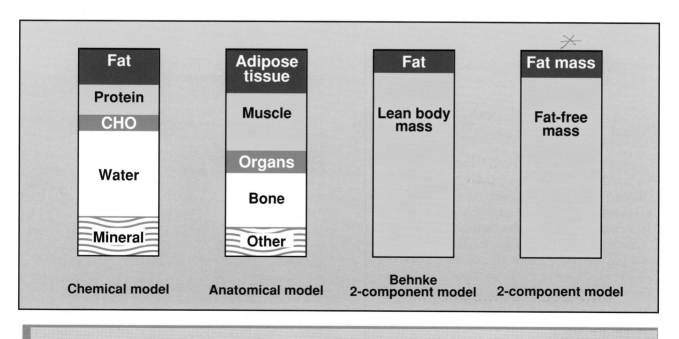

Figure 16.1   Four models of body composition. Adapted from Wilmore (1992).

both athlete and coach realize that this athlete's body composition is ideal. They should not be concerned with weight loss, even though standard height-weight charts indicate that the athlete is overweight. However, another baseball player of the same weight (200 lb, or 91 kg) who has 50 lb (23 kg) of fat would be 25% fat. This would constitute a serious weight problem—he would be overfat. In most sports, the higher the percent body fat, the poorer the performance. An accurate assessment of the athlete's body composition provides valuable insight into what weight allows optimal performance.

Appropriate goal weights for competition cannot be established simply by considering an athlete's present weight. An athlete can be overweight by the standard height-weight tables yet have a normal or below-normal body fat content. Likewise, an athlete can be within the acceptable weight range for his or her height but be overfat. Standard height-weight tables do not provide accurate estimates of what athletes should weigh because they do not take body composition into account.

This was established in Welham and Behnke's classic 1942 study relating body composition to athletics. They studied the body compositions of a group of professional football players.[21] Of these 25 professional athletes, 17 had been classified as physically unqualified for military duty or for first-class insurance because of their weight. But of these 17 "overweight" players, 11 were found to have very low levels of body fat. Their overweight condition was the result of excess fat-free mass, not fat mass. The average relative body fat for these athletes was only 9.3%. This demonstrates that knowing the composition of an athlete's weight is more important than relying on standard height-weight tables. But how do you determine an athlete's body composition?

KEY POINT

Although total body size and weight are important for most athletes, an athlete's body composition is generally of greater concern. Being *overweight* is usually not a problem, but being *overfat* typically has a negative impact on athletic performance. Standard height-weight tables do not provide accurate estimates of what an athlete should weigh because they do not take into account the composition of the weight. An athlete can be overweight according to these tables, yet have very little body fat.

Densitometry

Densitometry involves measuring the density of the athlete's body. Density (D) is defined as mass divided by volume:

$$D_{body} = mass_{body} \div volume_{body}$$

The mass of the body is the athlete's scale weight. Body volume can be obtained by several different techniques, but the most common is hydrostatic weighing, in which the athlete is weighed while totally immersed in water. The difference between the athlete's scale weight and underwater weight, when corrected for the density of water, equals the body's volume. This volume must be further corrected to account for air trapped in the body. The amount of air trapped in the gastrointestinal tract is difficult to measure, but fortunately it is a small volume (about 100 ml) and is usually ignored. The gas trapped in the lungs, however, must be measured because its volume is generally large, averaging 1,500 ml in young adult males and 1,200 ml in young adult females, depending on size.

Figure 16.2 illustrates the hydrostatic weighing technique used for two professional football players of identical height and weight but substantially different body compositions. Table 16.1 shows the calculations of their body composition, demonstrating that Dave is nearly twice as fat as Jack. For both of these athletes to reach a relative body fat value of 10%, Jack would have to lose less than 1 lb (about 0.5 kg), but Dave would need to lose nearly 20 lb (8.7 kg).

Table 16.1 Comparison of the Underwater Weighing Values, Body Composition Determinations, and Goal Weight Calculations in Two Professional Football Players of the Same Height and Weight

Variable	Jack	Dave
Height	188 cm (74 in.)	188 cm (74 in.)
Weight	93 kg (205 lb)	93 kg (205 lb)
Underwater weight	6.5 kg	5.0 kg
Volume	86.5 L	88.0 L
Density	1.075 g • ml⁻¹	1.057 g • ml⁻¹
Relative fat	10.5%	18.4%
Fat weight	9.7 kg (21.4 lb)	17.1 kg (37.7 lb)
Fat-free weight	83.3 kg (183.6 lb)	75.9 kg (167.3 lb)
Goal weight at 10% fat	92.6 kg (204.2 lb)	84.3 kg (185.9 lb)
Weight loss to achieve goal weight	0.4 kg (0.8 lb)	8.7 kg (19.1 lb)

Note. volume = weight − underwater weight
density = weight ÷ volume

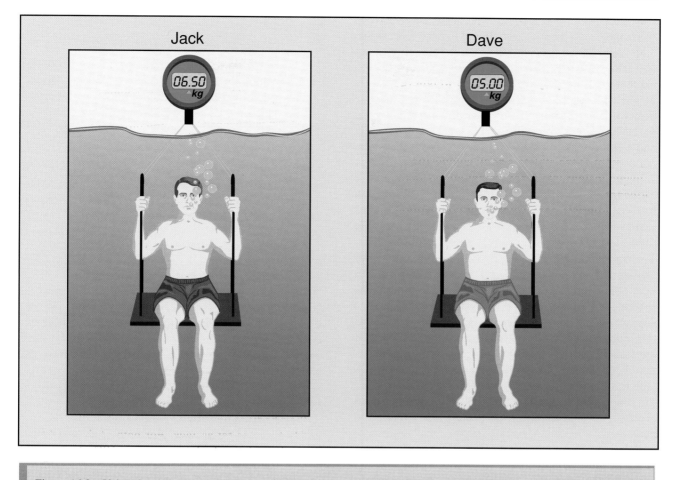

Figure 16.2   Using the underwater weighing technique on two professional football players of the same weight but different body compositions.

Densitometry has long been the technique of choice for assessing body composition. New techniques are typically compared against densitometry to determine their accuracy. However, densitometry has its limitations. If body weight, underwater weight, and lung volume during underwater weighing are measured correctly, the resulting body density value is accurate. Densitometry's major weakness is in the conversion of body density to an estimate of relative body fat.[12]

Accurate estimates of the densities of fat mass and fat-free mass are required when using the two-component model of body composition. The equation most often used to convert body density to an estimate of relative body fat is the standard equation of Siri:

$$\% \text{ body fat} = (495 \div D_{body}) - 450$$

This equation assumes that the densities of the fat mass and the fat-free mass are relatively constant in all people. Indeed, the density of fat at different sites is very consistent in the same individual, and relatively consistent between people. The value generally used is $0.9007 \text{ g} \cdot \text{cm}^{-3}$. But determining the density of the fat-free mass (D_{FFM}), which the equation of Siri assumes is 1.100, is more problematic. To determine this density, we must make two assumptions:

1. The density of each tissue comprising the fat-free mass is known and remains constant.
2. Each tissue type represents a constant proportion of the fat-free mass (for example, we assume that bone always represents 17% of the fat-free mass).

Exceptions to either of these assumptions cause error when converting body density to relative body fat, and this error can be substantial. Unfortunately, the density of the fat-free mass varies considerably between people.

This point is illustrated by considering the data from three athletes, shown in Table 16.2.[22] If Edna, Vicki, and Susan each had the same total body density of 1.060, using the standard equation of Siri we would estimate that the relative body fat for each woman is 17.0%. However, this equation would be appropriate only for Edna, because she is the only one with a D_{FFM} of 1.100. If new equations were developed for Vicki and Susan, using their correct fat-free mass densities, Vicki's relative body fat would be 21.8% (her D_{FFM} is 1.115) and Susan's would be 11.5% (her D_{FFM} is 1.085). Thus, for the same body density, which is all that can be measured, the true relative body fat in these athletes varied from 11.5% to 21.8%. Although this example seems to exaggerate the point, the point itself is valid.

As just mentioned, the density of a mature, fully grown person's fat-free mass is generally assumed to be $1.100 \text{ g} \cdot \text{cm}^{-3}$. Due primarily to known differences in bone mass and total body water, evidence now supports using lower values for children, females, and the elderly and higher values for people of African ancestry.[10,16] In our example, Vicki is a mature African-American athlete and Susan is an 11-year-old white athlete. The D_{FFM} values obtained from the sum of the proportional densities for Vicki (1.115) and Susan (1.085) are almost identical to the values that have been established for African-American and adolescent populations. Research is progressing in this area. Population-specific equations are now available for select populations, improving the accuracy of converting body density to relative body-fat values.[10]

Other Laboratory Techniques

Many other laboratory techniques are available for assessing body composition. These include radiography, magnetic resonance imaging, hydrometry (for measuring total body water), photon absorptiometry, total body electrical conductivity, and dual-energy x-ray absorptiometry. Most of these techniques are complex and require expensive equipment. None of them are likely to be used for assessing athletic populations, so we will not discuss them. These techniques have been extensively reviewed by others.[3,11]

> **KEY POINT**
>
> Inaccuracies in densitometry largely reflect the variation in the density of the fat-free mass from one individual to another. Density of fat-free mass is affected by age, gender, and race.

Field Techniques

Several field techniques are also available for assessing body composition. These techniques are more accessible than laboratory techniques because the equipment is less costly and cumbersome, so they can be used more easily by the coach, the trainer, or even the athlete.

Skinfold Fat Thickness

The most widely applied field technique involves measuring the skinfold fat thickness (see Figure 16.3) at one or more sites and using the values obtained to estimate body density, relative body fat, or fat-free mass. It is generally recommended that the sum of the measurements from three or more skinfold sites be used in a quadratic equation to estimate body density.[14] A quadratic equation more accurately describes the relationship between the sum of skinfold measurements and body density than a linear equation does. With linear equations the density of a lean person is underestimated, which causes overestimation of body fat. The difference between the quadratic and linear regression lines are demonstrated in Figure 16.4. Skinfold fat thickness measurements using quadratic equa-

Table 16.2 Differences in the Density of the Fat-Free Mass (D_{FFM}) in Three Female Athletes

Body tissue	Edna D_t	%	D_p	Vicki D_t	%	D_p	Susan D_t	%	D_p
Muscle	1.065	46	0.490	1.065	41	0.437	1.065	46	0.490
Bone	1.350	17	0.229	1.350	22	0.297	1.260	17	0.214
Remainder	1.030	37	0.381	1.030	37	0.381	1.030	37	0.381
D_{FFM}			1.100			1.115			1.085

Note. D_t = density of the tissue; % = percent contribution of this tissue to the total fat-free mass; D_p = proportional density of the tissue ($D_t \cdot \% / 100$); D_{FFM} = density of the fat-free mass, which is the sum of the proportional densities.

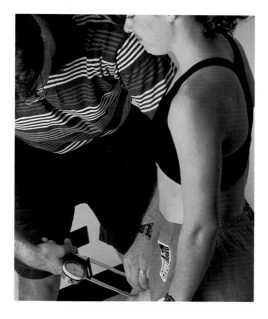

Figure 16.3   Measuring skinfold fat thickness.

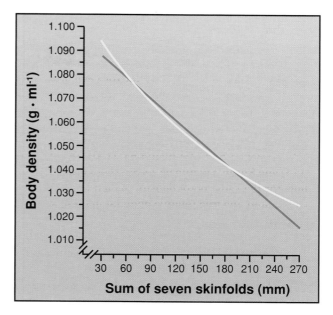

Figure 16.4   The curvilinear relationship between the sum of seven skinfold fat thickness measurements and body density. The two lines represent the quadratic (curvilinear line) regression and the linear (straight line) regression. Adapted from Jackson and Pollock (1978).

tions provide reasonably accurate estimates of total body fat or relative fat, with correlations ranging from 0.90 to 0.96.

KEY POINT

Laboratory techniques such as densitometry and radiography provide reasonable estimates of true body composition—relative body fat, fat mass, and fat-free mass. Multiple skinfold fat thickness measurements used in an equation appropriate for the population being assessed also provide a good estimate of body composition.

Bioelectric Impedance

Two other field techniques were introduced during the 1980s. Measuring bioelectric impedance is a simple procedure that takes just 5 minutes to perform. Four electrodes are attached to the body at the ankle, the foot, the wrist, and the back of the hand, as shown in Figure 16.5. An undetectable current is passed through the distal electrodes (hand and foot). The proximal electrodes (wrist and ankle) receive the current flow. Electrical conduction through the tissues between the electrodes depends on the water and electrolyte distribution in that tissue. Fat-free mass contains almost all of the body water and the conducting electrolytes. As a result, conductivity is much greater in the fat-free

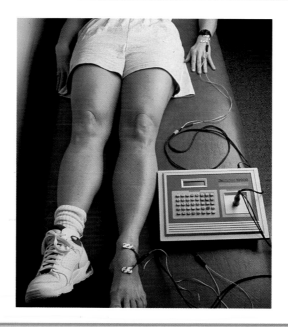

Figure 16.5   The bioelectric impedance technique for assessing relative body fat.

mass than in the fat mass. In other words, the electrical current moves more easily and more quickly through the fat-free mass. The fat mass has a much greater impedance, meaning that it is much more difficult for the current to flow through the fat mass. Thus the amount of current flow through the tissues reflects the relative amount of fat contained in that tissue.

With the bioelectric impedance technique, measurement of the impedance, the conductivity, or both are transformed into estimates of relative body fat. Estimates of relative body fat based on bioelectric impedance highly correlate with body fat measurements obtained through hydrostatic weighing (r = about 0.90 to 0.94). However, the relative body fat in lean athletic populations tends to be overestimated with bioelectric impedance due to the nature of the equations that are used. More sport-specific equations are being developed.

Infrared Interactance

Infrared interactance is a procedure that is based on the principles of light absorption and reflection using near-infrared spectroscopy. A probe is placed on the skin above the site to be measured. The probe emits electromagnetic radiation through a central bundle of optic fibers. Optic fibers on the periphery of the same probe absorb the energy reflected back from the tissues, and that energy is then passed on to a spectrophotometer for measurement. The amount of energy that is reflected back reflects the composition of the tissue directly under

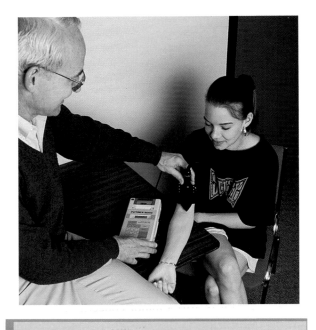

Figure 16.6   The Futrex infrared technique for assessing relative body fat.

the probe to a depth of several inches. This technique is quite accurate when multiple sites are assessed. A commercial model of the apparatus is now available that uses only a single site, the biceps, as depicted in Figure 16.6. This procedure seems promising, but the studies conducted to date are insufficient to determine its validity for athletic populations.

Body Composition and Sports Performance

Many athletes believe that they must be big to be good in their sport, because size has traditionally been associated with performance quality: The bigger the athlete, the better the performance. But big does not always mean better. In the following sections, we consider how performance can be affected by body composition.

Fat-Free Mass

Rather than being concerned with total body size or weight, most athletes should be concerned specifically with fat-free mass. Maximizing fat-free mass is desirable for athletes involved in activities that require strength, power, and muscular endurance. But increased fat-free mass is likely to be undesirable for the endurance athlete, such as a distance runner, who must move his or her total body mass horizontally

---

IN REVIEW . . .

1. Knowing a person's body composition is more valuable for predicting performance potential than knowing merely height and weight.
2. Densitometry is the method of choice for assessing body composition and has long been considered the most accurate, though it does carry certain risks of error. It involves measuring the density of the athlete's body by dividing his or her body mass by body volume, which is typically determined by hydrostatic weighing. Body composition can be calculated, though there is some margin of error.
3. The density of the fat-free mass is generally assumed to be 1.100 g · cm^{-3} for a fully mature person, but lower values are suggested for children, females, and the elderly and higher values for people of African ancestry.
4. Field techniques for assessing body composition include measuring skinfold fat thickness, bioelectric impedance, and infrared interactance. These techniques are less costly and more accessible for the athlete and the coach than are the laboratory techniques.

for extended periods. A higher fat-free mass is an additional load that must be carried and might impair the athlete's performance. This might also be true for the high jumper, long jumper, triple jumper, and pole-vaulter who must maximize either their vertical or horizontal distances or both. Additional weight, even though it is active fat-free mass, can decrease rather than facilitate performance in these athletes.

Eventually, techniques will be available to allow extensive evaluations of athletes not only to estimate their fat mass and fat-free mass but also their potential for increasing their fat-free mass. This would allow athletes to design training programs that would develop their fat-free mass to this projected maximum while maintaining their fat mass at relatively low levels.

Relative Body Fat

Relative body fat is also a major concern of athletes. Adding additional fat to the body just to increase the athlete's weight and overall size is generally detrimental to performance. Many studies have shown that the higher the percentage of body fat, the poorer the person's performance. This is true of all activities in which the body weight must be moved through space, such as in sprinting and long jumping (it is less important for more stationary activities, such as archery and shooting). In general, leaner athletes perform better.

One study determined the relationship between weight, body fat, and performance in young men.[15] Results clearly indicated that degree of fatness, not total body weight, had the greatest influence on the performance of four fitness and athletic ability tests, shown in Table 16.3. Other studies have clearly shown that body fatness is associated with poorer performance on tests of

- speed,
- endurance,
- balance and agility, and
- jumping ability.

Endurance athletes try to minimize their fat stores because excess weight is proven to impair their performance. Both absolute fat and relative body fat can profoundly influence running performance in highly trained distance runners. Less fat generally leads to better performance. Male runners normally have much less relative body fat than female runners, which is thought to be one of the most important reasons for the differences in running performance between elite men and women distance runners.[23] This was confirmed in a study of men and women runners who when matched by their 15-mi road race times did not differ in relative body fat.[13]

In another study, male and female runners performed both submaximal and maximal runs on the treadmill and an all out 12-min run.[6] Each male runner performed his tests under normal conditions and also while carrying external weight added to the trunk to simulate the relative body fat of the female runner to whom he had been matched (see Figure 16.7). With the added weight, the metabolic cost of submaximal exercise was increased and maximal oxygen uptake was reduced. Furthermore, the large performance differences noted between the males and females in all three unweighted tests were reduced considerably when the males ran with the added weight.

Heavyweight weight lifters might be exceptions to the general rule that less fat is better. These athletes add large amounts of fat weight just prior to competi-

> **KEY POINT**
>
> Excessive body fat is associated with decreased athletic performance in activities where the body mass must be moved through space. Speed, endurance, balance and agility, and jumping ability are all negatively affected by a high level of fatness.

Table 16.3 The Effect of Relative Body Fat on Selected Performance Tests

| Performance test | Level of fatness (% body fat) | | |
	Low (<10%)	Moderate (10-15%)	High (>15%)
75-yd dash (s)	9.8	10.1	10.7
220-yd dash (s)	29.3	31.6	35.0
Standing long jump (ft)[a]	23.8	22.7	20.2
Sit-ups in 2 min	43.4	41.6	36.2

Note. The men in this study were classified into one of three levels of fatness: Low, Moderate, and High.

[a]Sum of three trials.

Adapted from Riendeau et al. (1958).

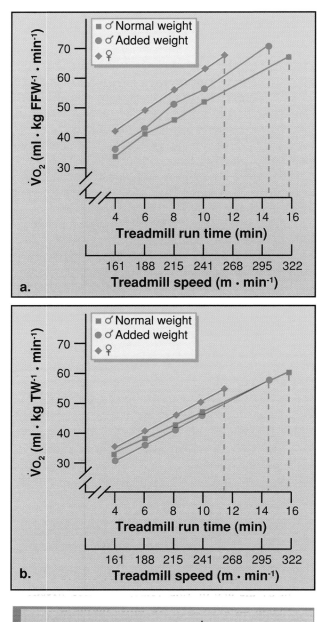

Figure 16.7 Gender differences in V̇o₂, expressed relative to fat-free mass (FFM) and total weight (TW), decrease when male runners have external weight added around their trunks. The dashed lines indicate V̇o₂ max.

Performance in swimming also seems to be an exception to this general rule. In one study, the relationship between body fatness and swimming performance was determined in 284 competitive female swimmers, ages 12 to 17 years.[19] Examining their best times in their best events and in the 100-yd freestyle revealed that swim performance was unrelated to relative body fat and only slightly related to fat-free mass. Body fat might provide some advantage to the swimmer because it improves buoyancy, which can reduce body drag in the water and reduce the metabolic cost of staying on the surface of the water.

■■■ IN REVIEW . . . ■■■

1. The ideal body composition varies with different sports, but in general the less fat mass, the greater the performance.
2. Maximizing fat-free mass is desirable for athletes in sports that require strength, power, and muscular endurance but can be a hindrance to endurance athletes who must be able to move their total body mass for extended periods.
3. The degree of fatness has more influence on performance than does total body weight. In general, the greater the relative body fat, the poorer the performance. Possible exceptions to this include heavyweight weight lifters, sumo wrestlers, and swimmers.

Weight Standards

Coaches and athletes alike are always looking for that winning edge. Once a coach or an athlete hits on something that works and performances improve, the word quickly spreads. The widespread use of anabolic steroids is a classic example. What started out in the late 1940s and early 1950s as experimentation among a small number of bodybuilders and weight lifters has spread throughout the world of sport to where the majority of the elite athletes in certain sports are habitual steroid users. A similar phenomenon has accompanied the emphasis on leanness in athletes.

The elite athlete has long been esteemed for representing the most desirable physical and physiological characteristics for performance in a sport or activity. Theoretically, the elite athlete's genetic foundation and years of intense training have combined to provide the ultimate athletic profile for that sport. These elite athletes set the standards toward which others aspire.

In the 1970s, we [JHW] had the opportunity to test many of the United States' elite women track and

tion with the premise that the additional weight will lower their center of gravity and give them a greater mechanical advantage in lifting. Research has not yet confirmed the value of this additional fat weight. The sumo wrestler is another notable exception to the theory that overall size is not the major determinant of athletic success. In this sport, the larger individual has a decided advantage, but even so, the wrestler with the higher fat-free mass should have the best overall success.

field athletes.[23] In addition to treadmill testing, each athlete underwent a body composition assessment. The results of these assessments are presented in Figure 16.8. Looking just at the distance runners, many of the best were below 12% body fat. The two top distance runners had only about 6% fat. One of these had won six consecutive international cross-country championships, and the other held what was then the best time in the world for the marathon. From these results, we could be tempted to suggest that any girl or woman distance runner should have between 6% and 12% relative body fat if she has world-class aspirations. However, one of the best distance runners in the United States at that time, who was within 2 years of taking over the top spot, had a relative body fat of 17%. Furthermore, one of the women in this study had a relative body fat of 37%, and she set the best time in the world for the 50-mi run within 6 months of her evaluation! More than likely, neither of these women would have gained an advantage if they had been forced to drop their weight to achieve 12% body fat or lower.

Body weight has been a general concern in several sports for many years. Over the past 10 to 15 years, this concern has become more widespread, and most sports have now adopted weight standards designed to ensure that athletes have the optimal body size and composition for maximum performance. Unfortunately, this is not always the result.

Inappropriate Use of Weight Standards

Weight standards have been seriously abused. Coaches have seen that athletes' performances generally improve as body weight decreases. This has led some coaches to adopt the philosophy that if small weight losses improve performance a little, then major weight losses should improve it even more. Not only coaches are guilty of making this assumption—athletes and their parents also are drawn into this way of thinking. As an example, a university athlete, considered one of the best in the United States in her sport, had dieted and exercised down to such a low body weight that her relative body fat was less than 5%. If anyone who joined the team appeared to be leaner, she would work even harder to reduce her weight and fat content. This woman's athletic performance began to deteriorate, and she started to develop injuries that never seemed to heal. She was eventually diagnosed with anorexia nervosa (chapter 19) and underwent professional treatment. But her career as an elite athlete is over.

Making Weight: Risks With Severe Weight Loss

Male athletes are not immune to problems associated with excessive weight loss and disordered eating. The medical and scientific communities have been concerned over problems in male athletes associated with making weight. The major concern has centered around the sport of wrestling. In 1986, a survey was conducted that involved 63 collegiate wrestlers representing 15 teams at the Eastern Intercollegiate Wrestling Association Championships.[20] These wrestlers began wrestling at an average age of 10.9 years. They started cutting weight by the age of 13.5 years, and these wrestlers lost weight an average of 15 times during a normal season. The average for the most weight lost at any one time was 15.8 lb (7.2 kg). For this specific championship meet, the average weight loss for these wrestlers was 9.7 lb (4.4 kg) in less than 3 days. Wrestlers typically make weight by combining food restriction, fluid deprivation, thermal dehydration, and increased activity. The influence of these practices on performance and physiological function is outlined in Table 16.4. The potential health hazards of such practices led the American College of Sports Medicine to publish the 1976 position statement "Weight Loss in Wrestlers."[1]

Many schools, districts, or state-level organizations organize sports other than wrestling on the basis of size, with weight as the predominant factor. Often the athlete attempts to achieve the lowest possible weight to gain an advantage over opponents. In so

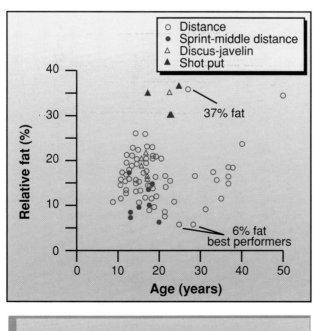

Figure 16.8   Relative body fat in elite female track and field athletes. Data from Wilmore et al. (1977).

Table 16.4 The Effects of the Single and Combined Influences of Food Restriction, Fluid Deprivation, and Thermal Dehydration on Selected Parameters

Parameters	Effects
Performance factors	
Aerobic power	Decreased
Muscular strength	No change
Muscular endurance	Decreased
Muscular power	Unknown
Speed of movement	Unknown
Run time to exhaustion	Decreased
Work performed	Decreased
Physiological factors	
Cardiac output	Decreased
Blood volume	Decreased
Plasma volume	Decreased
Heart rate	Increased
Stroke volume	Decreased
Core temperature	Increased
Sweat rate	Decreased
Muscle water	Decreased
Muscle electrolytes	Decreased

Adapted from Tipton and Oppliger (1984).

doing, many athletes have jeopardized their health. In the following sections, we examine a few of the consequences of severe weight loss in athletes.

Dehydration

Fasting or very low calorie diets lead to large amounts of weight loss, primarily through dehydration. Athletes trying to make weight might exercise in rubberized sweat suits, sit in steam and sauna baths, chew on towels to lose saliva, and keep their fluid intake to a minimum. Such severe water losses compromise kidney and cardiovascular function and are potentially dangerous. Weight losses of 2% to 4% of the athlete's weight through dehydration can impair performance. The consequences of dehydrative weight loss, discussed in chapter 15, include

- decreased blood volume and blood pressure,
- decreased submaximal and maximal stroke volume and maximal cardiac output,
- decreased blood flow to and through the kidneys, and
- impaired thermoregulation.

Chronic Fatigue

Pushing body weight too low can have major repercussions. When weight drops below a certain optimal level, the athlete is likely to experience performance decrements and an increased incidence of illness and injury. The performance decrements can be due to many factors, including chronic fatigue that often accompanies major weight losses. The causes of this fatigue have not been established, but there are several likely possibilities.

The symptoms of an athlete who is chronically underweight (below optimal competitive weight) mimic those seen with overtraining (chapter 13). Both neural and hormonal components are involved in the phenomenon of overtraining. In most cases, the sympathetic nervous system appears to be inhibited and the parasympathetic system dominates. In addition, the hypothalamus does not function normally. These alterations lead to a cascade of symptoms that include chronic fatigue.[2,9]

This chronic fatigue could also be due to substrate depletion. Energy for almost all athletic activities is derived predominantly from carbohydrate. Carbohydrate also represents the smallest source of stored energy. The combined carbohydrate storage pools in muscle, liver, and extracellular fluid account for approximately 2,000 kcal of stored energy. When athletes are training hard and are not eating an adequate diet (when they are deficient either in total calories or in total carbohydrate calories), their carbohydrate energy stores become depleted. Most importantly to the athlete, liver and muscle glycogen levels decrease, which in turn reduces blood glucose levels. The combined effect of these decreases can be chronic fatigue and considerable declines in performance.[18] In addition, under these conditions the body also uses its protein stores as an energy substrate for exercise. This can, over time, gradually deplete muscle protein.[4]

Eating Disorders

The constant attention given to achieving and maintaining a prescribed weight goal, particularly if the weight goal is inappropriate, can lead to disordered eating. A high proportion of athletes, particularly females, have disordered eating. This term can simply refer to restricting food intake to levels that are below energy expenditure, but disordered eating can also involve pathological behaviors, such as self-induced vomiting and laxative abuse, to control body weight. Disordered eating can lead to clinical eating disorders, such as anorexia nervosa or bulimia nervosa. These disorders have become prevalent among female athletes. Each has strict criteria for diagnosis that set them apart from disordered eating in general.

Obtaining accurate estimates of the prevalence of eating disorders is difficult, if not impossible, particularly in athletic populations. However, a significant number of indicators suggest a high prevalence in select athletic populations. Over 90% of people with eating disorders are women. Among athletes, those in appearance sports (such as gymnastics, figure skating, diving, and dancing) and in endurance sports (such as running and swimming) seem at greatest risk. On certain teams, such as in these appearance and endurance sports, the prevalence of eating disorders might approach or even exceed 50% at the elite or world-class level. Athletes and coaches must realize the importance of the potential link between weight standards and eating disorders. The issue of eating disorders in athletes is a major focus of chapter 19.

Furthermore, a female athlete who is prone to disordered eating is open to a triad of disorders that are likely interrelated: anorexia nervosa or bulimia nervosa, menstrual dysfunction, and bone mineral disorders. This is now referred to as the female athlete triad.

KEY POINT

Eating disorders appear to be prevalent among elite female athletes. It is important to establish weight standards that maximize performance but minimize the risk of initiating an eating disorder.

Menstrual Dysfunction

Menstrual dysfunction, or abnormal menstruation, is widely recognized in female athletes, but its pathophysiology is not well understood. High prevalences of oligomenorrhea (infrequent or scant menstrual flow), amenorrhea (cessation of menstrual flow), and delayed menarche (first period) have been associated with sports that emphasize low body weight or low body fat. The combination of caloric restriction and a vegetarian diet is common among women endurance athletes. Substantial weight loss induced by either or both of these is associated with a shortened luteal phase and menstrual dysfunction.[17]

A strong link exists between anorexia nervosa and menstrual dysfunction. In fact, amenorrhea is one of the strict criteria necessary for the diagnosis of anorexia nervosa in females. A similar relationship has not yet been established with bulimia (see chapter 19), but an increasing number of athletes are found to be both bulimic and amenorrheic.

Bone Mineral Disorders

Bone mineral disorders are recognized as a potentially serious consequence of menstrual dysfunction.[7] The link between the two was first reported in 1984. Now a number of scientists are researching the relationship between athletic-induced amenorrhea and low bone mineral content or density. Past studies suggest that bone density increases with the resumption of normal menses (menstruation), but more recent observations suggest that the amount of bone that is regained might be limited and that bone density might remain well below normal even with reestablishment of normal menstrual function.[7] The long-term consequences of chronically low bone densities in an athletic population have not yet been established.

Establishing Appropriate Weight Standards

The potential for abuse of weight standards is clearly established. If standards are not set appropriately, athletes could be pushed well below optimal body weight. Thus it is critically important to properly set weight standards.

Body weight standards should be based on an athlete's body composition. Once body composition has been determined, the amount of fat-free mass is used to estimate what the athlete should weigh at a specific relative body fat. Consider an example in which the goal is to get a 160-lb (72.5-kg) woman swimmer with 25% body fat down to 18% body fat, as shown in Table 16.5. We know that her goal weight will be composed of 18% fat and 82% fat-free mass. So to estimate her goal weight at 18% body fat, we divide her fat-free mass by 82%, which is the fraction of her goal weight that is to be represented by her fat-free mass. This calculation (120 lb, or 54.4 kg, divided by 0.82) gives us a goal weight of 146 lb (66.3 kg), so this woman needs to lose 14 lb (6.4 kg).

Thus, the establishment of weight standards should translate into the establishment of standards of relative body fat for each sport. With this in mind, what is the recommended relative body fat for an elite athlete in any given sport? For each sport an optimal value or range of values for relative body fat should be established outside of which the athlete's performance is likely impaired. And, because fat distribution shows definite gender differences, the weight standards should be gender-specific. Representative ranges for

Table 16.5 Computing a Goal Weight for Performance in a Female Swimmer

Weight	160 lb
Relative fat	25%
Fat weight	40 lb (160 lb × 0.25)
Fat-free weight	120 lb (160 lb − 40 lb fat weight)
Goal % fat	18% (= 82% fat-free)
Goal weight	146 lb (= 120 lb / 0.82)
Weight loss goal	14 lb

males and females in various sports are presented in Table 16.6. In most cases, these values are representative of the elite athletes in those sports.

However, these values might not be appropriate for all athletes who engage in a specific activity. The existing techniques for measuring body composition include inherent errors, as we discussed earlier. Even with the better laboratory techniques, measurement of body density can introduce a 1% to 3% error, and an even greater error is associated with converting that

density to relative body fat. In addition, we must understand the concept of individual variability. Not every male distance runner will have his best performance at 6% body fat. Some will improve performance with slightly lower values. Others won't be able to get down to such low relative fat values, or they will find that their performance starts to decline at the suggested values. For these reasons, a range of values should be set for males and females in specific activities, recognizing individual variability, methodological error, and gender differences.

KEY POINT

It is important to establish realistic weight standards for athletes. This is generally best accomplished by using a range of relative fat values that are considered acceptable on the basis of the sport, age, and gender.

Table 16.6 Ranges of Relative Body Fat Values for Men and Women Athletes in Various Sports

Sport	% fat	
	Men	Women
Baseball/softball	8-14	12-18
Basketball	6-12	10-16
Body building	5-8	6-12
Canoe/kayak	6-12	10-16
Cycling	5-11	8-15
Fencing	8-12	10-16
Football	6-18	—
Golf	10-16	12-20
Gymnastics	5-12	8-16
Horse racing	6-12	10-16
Ice/field hockey	8-16	12-18
Orienteering	5-12	8-16
Pentathlon	—	8-15
Racquetball	6-14	10-18
Rowing	6-14	8-16
Rugby	6-16	—
Skating	5-12	8-16
Skiing	7-15	10-18
Ski jumping	7-15	10-18
Soccer	6-14	10-18
Swimming	6-12	10-18
Synchronized swimming	—	10-18
Tennis	6-14	10-20
Track and field		
Running events	5-12	8-15
Field events	8-18	12-20
Triathlon	5-12	8-15
Volleyball	7-15	10-18
Weight lifting	5-12	10-18
Wrestling	5-16	—

IN REVIEW . . .

1. Many sports enforce weight standards, with the goal of ensuring that the athletes are of optimal body size for participation. Unfortunately, athletes often turn to questionable, ineffective, or even dangerous methods of weight loss to reach their goal weight.
2. Severe weight loss in athletes can cause potential health problems, such as dehydration, chronic fatigue, disordered eating, menstrual dysfunction, and bone mineral disorders.
3. The chronic fatigue symptoms that often accompany severe weight loss mimic those of overtraining. This fatigue can also be caused by substrate depletion.
4. Body weight standards should be based on body composition. Thus these standards should emphasize relative body fat rather than total body mass.
5. For each sport, a range of values should be established, recognizing the importance of individual variation, methodological error, and gender differences.

Achieving Optimal Weight

Many athletes discover that they are considerably above their assigned playing weight with only a few weeks remaining before they report to training camp. Consider a 25-year-old professional football player who realizes his weight is 20 lb (9 kg) above his playing weight in the previous season. He must lose this excess weight by the start of the preseason training camp, a mere 4 weeks away. Failure will cost him a fine of $500 per day for each pound over his assigned weight. Exercise alone is of little value because he would need 9 to 12 months to lose this much weight through that means. Will this athlete accomplish his goal?

Crash Dieting

Our football player must lose 5 lb (about 2 kg) per week for the next 4 weeks, so he decides to embark on a crash diet, selecting whatever diet is in vogue, knowing that a person can lose 6 to 8 lb (about 3 kg) per week with such diets. He is not unique. Many athletes find themselves overweight and out of shape because of overeating and reduced activity during the off-season, and they typically wait until the last few weeks before their reporting dates to attack the problem. In our example, the football player might be able to shed 20 lb in 4 weeks with his crash diet. But much of this weight loss would be from body water and very little from stored fat. Several studies have reported that substantial weight losses occur with very low calorie diets (500 kcal per day or less), but of the weight lost, more than 60% comes from the body's fat-free tissue and less than 40% from fat depots.

Although much of our football player's weight is lost from water stores, a substantial amount of protein is lost as well. Also, most crash diets are based on a major reduction in carbohydrate intake. This reduced intake is insufficient to supply the body's needs for carbohydrate, and as a result the body's carbohydrate stores become depleted. Because water storage accompanies carbohydrate storage, the water stores are also reduced as the carbohydrate stores diminish. With every gram of carbohydrate used by the body, approximately 3 g of water are lost. The total body glycogen content is about 800 g, so depletion of the stored glycogen would result in a loss of approximately 2,400 g of water—slightly more than 5 lb (about 2.4 kg).

In addition, the body relies more heavily on free fatty acids for energy as its carbohydrate stores are depleted. As a result, ketone bodies, a by-product of fatty acid metabolism, accumulate in the blood causing a condition known as ketosis. This condition further increases water loss. Much of this water loss occurs during the first week of the diet.

Figure 16.9 illustrates these changes in body water, fat, protein, and carbohydrate during a period of 30 days of fasting. Carbohydrate depletion occurs within about 3 days. Protein content drops significantly in the same time period. The body's water content drops abruptly during the first 3 days. The rate of fat loss, though it drops somewhat in the second and third day, remains relatively unchanged for the remainder of the fasting period.

It is impossible for most people to lose more than 4 lb (about 2 kg) of fat per week, even under conditions of total fasting. This can be easily demonstrated. A pound of fat (adipose tissue) has the caloric equivalent of 3,500 kcal, so a deficit of 3,500 kcal is needed to lose 1 lb (0.45 kg) of fat. The resting metabolic rate

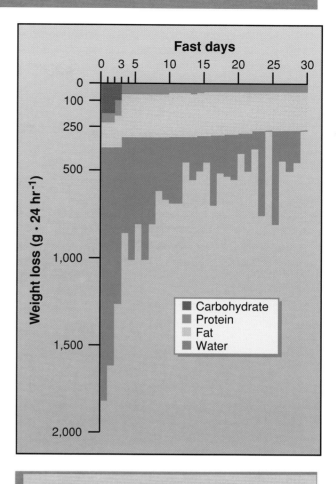

Figure 16.9 The composition of weight lost with 30 days of fasting.

of the professional football player in our previous example would be approximately 2,500 kcal per day. So if he fasted, he would have a 2,500 kcal deficit per day. The most he could lose each day would be about 0.7 lb (0.3 kg) (2,500 kcal per day divided by 3,500 kcal per lb, or 7,716 kcal per kg, of fat). However, research indicates that the total body metabolism is reduced by 20% to 25% during fasting. A 20% reduction in this athlete's resting metabolic rate would lower his total deficit to only 2,000 kcal per day, which would result in a maximum weight loss of only about 0.6 lb (about 0.3 kg) of fat per day. In 1 week of total fasting, this would result in a loss of only 4 lb (about 2 kg)! By increasing his activity level, our football player could increase this predicted rate of fat weight loss. But he would find it impossible to train very hard with no food intake and an almost total depletion of his glycogen stores. Also, few people can tolerate the discomfort associated with prolonged periods of fasting. The rapid weight losses experienced with crash diets are quickly regained, probably because when a balanced diet is substituted for the low-calorie, low-carbohydrate diet, the water that was lost is quickly regained as the carbohydrate stores are replenished.

Optimal Weight Loss

The sensible approach to reducing body fat stores is to combine moderate dietary restriction with increased exercise. Appetite is delicately balanced with the body's actual caloric needs. If you reduce your dietary intake by a mere 100 kcal each day (one slice of buttered bread), for example, you will lose 10 lb (about 4.5 kg) in 1 year, assuming that your activity level remains constant. But if you add to this an additional modest loss of 0.25 lb to 0.5 lb (0.1 kg to 0.2 kg) per week due to increased activity (such as a 3-day per week jogging program), your total weight loss would be 23 to 36 lb (about 10 to 16 kg) in a single year, and most of this weight loss would be from stored body fat!

When athletes exceed the upper end of the weight range for their sport, they should work toward achieving the upper end goal weight slowly, losing no more than 1 to 2 lb (less than 1 kg) per week. Losing more weight than that per week leads to losses in fat-free mass, which is usually not the desired outcome. When the upper limit of the range is reached, further weight loss should be undertaken only with close supervision of the coach, athletic trainer, or team physician. This weight loss should be achieved at an even slower rate: less than 1 lb (less than 0.5 kg) per week to assure that performance is not negatively affected. The rate of this loss should be reduced still more if performance is affected or if medical symptoms are noted.

Decreasing an athlete's caloric intake by 200 to 500 kcal per day will allow weight losses of about 1 lb (about 0.5 kg) per week, particularly if combined with a sound exercise program. This is a realistic goal, and such losses add up to a substantial weight loss over time. When trying to reduce weight, total daily calories should be consumed over at least three meals per day. Many athletes make the mistake of eating only one or two meals per day, skipping breakfast, lunch, or both, then consuming a large dinner. Research in animals has shown that, given the same number of total calories, the animals that eat their daily food ration in one or two meals gain more weight than those that nibble their ration throughout the day.

The purpose of weight-loss programs is to lose body fat, not fat-free mass. Because of this, the combination of diet and exercise is the preferred approach. Combining increased activity with caloric reduction prevents any significant loss of fat-free mass. In fact, body composition can be significantly altered with physical training. Chronic exercise can increase fat-free mass and decrease fat mass. The magnitude of these changes varies with the type of exercise used for training. Resistance training promotes gains in fat-free mass, and both resistance and endurance training promote loss of fat mass. To lose weight, athletes should combine a moderate resistance and endurance training program with modest caloric restriction.

As a final point, a balanced diet is, of course, essential to ensure that the athlete receives all necessary vitamins and minerals. Vitamin supplementation

KEY POINT

Athletes who are above their weight standard should lose weight gradually, not more than 1 to 2 lbs (about 1 kg) per week to preserve their fat-free mass. This should be accomplished by integrating a good diet containing 200 to 500 kcal less than their daily energy expenditure, with a reasonable increase in resistance and endurance activities.

IN REVIEW . . .

1. When severe (very low calorie) diets are followed, much of the weight loss that occurs is from water, not fat.
2. Most severe diets limit carbohydrate intake, causing carbohydrate stores to be depleted. Water is lost along with the carbohydrates, exacerbating the problem of dehydration. Also, the increased reliance on free fatty acids can lead to ketosis, which further enhances water loss.
3. The combination of diet and exercise is the preferred approach to optimal weight loss.
4. Athletes should lose no more than 1 to 2 lb (about 0.5 to 1.0 kg) per week until reaching the upper end of the desired weight range. After that, weight loss should be less than 1 lb (less than 0.45 kg) per week until goal weight is reached. More rapid weight losses result in loss of fat-free mass. Weight loss at this rate can be accomplished by a reduction in dietary intake of 200 to 500 kcal per day, especially when combined with a sound exercise program.
5. For fat loss, moderate resistance and endurance training is most effective. Resistance training also promotes gains in fat-free mass.

might or might not be necessary—results of research thus far are in conflict. But if the nutritional adequacy of the diet is at all questionable, a simple multivitamin that meets the RDA for that person is suggested.

In Closing . . .

With this chapter, we conclude our discussion on optimizing performance. We have discussed the effects of different amounts and types of training. We examined the use of ergogenic aids, their proposed benefits and effectiveness, and their health risks. We explored the importance of nutrition in keeping the athlete's body fueled and ready for maximal performance, and the use of diet manipulation to enhance performance. Finally, in this chapter, we discussed the importance of body composition, the way in which fat-free mass and relative body fat affect performance, and the best method for athletes to lose weight (body fat) to optimize their body composition for their chosen activity.

In the next part, we shift our focus away from athletes in general to the unique characteristics of special populations in sport. We will begin our discussion in chapter 17 as we examine special considerations for the young athlete.

Key Terms

bioelectric impedance	fat mass
body build	hydrostatic weighing
body composition	infrared interactance
body size	morphology
densitometry	relative body fat
fat-free mass	skinfold fat thickness

Study Questions

1. Differentiate between body build, body size, and body composition.
2. What tissues of the body constitute the fat-free mass?
3. What is densitometry? How is it used to assess the body composition of the athlete? What is the major weakness of densitometry with respect to its accuracy?
4. What are several field techniques for estimating body composition? What are their strengths and weaknesses?
5. What is the relationship of relative leanness and fatness to performance in sport?
6. What is more important to sports performance, body fat or body weight? Why?
7. What guidelines should be used to determine the athlete's goal weight?
8. What are potential problems associated with a fixation on body weight that is too low?
9. Why should the athlete avoid crash diets?
10. What is the lowest weight an athlete should be allowed to attain?
11. How much weight should an overweight athlete lose per week in order to maximize fat loss and minimize fat-free mass loss?

References

1. American College of Sports Medicine. (1976). Weight loss in wrestlers. *Medicine and Science in Sports and Exercise*, **8**, 11-13.

2. Barron, J.L., Noakes, T.D., Levy, W., Smith, C., & Millar, R.P. (1985). Hypothalamic dysfunction in overtrained athletes. *Journal of Clinical Endocrinology and Metabolism*, **60**, 803-806.

3. Brodie, D.A. (1988). Techniques for measurement of body composition (Parts I and II). *Sports Medicine*, **5**, 11-40, 74-98.

4. Butterfield, G. (1991). Amino acids and high protein diets. In D.R. Lamb & M.H. Williams (Eds.), *Ergogenics—enhancement of performance in exercise and sport* (pp. 1-27). Dubuque, IA: Brown & Benchmark.

5. Carter, J.E.L., Aubry, S.P., & Sleet, D.A. (1982). Somatotypes of Montreal Olympic athletes. In J.E.L. Carter (Ed.), *Physical structure of Olympic athletes* (pp. 53-80). New York: Karger.

6. Cureton, K.J., & Sparling, P.B. (1980). Distance running performance and metabolic responses to running in men and women with excess weight experimentally equated. *Medicine and Science in Sports and Exercise*, **12**, 288-294.

7. Drinkwater, B.L., Bruemner, B., & Chesnut, C.H. (1990). Menstrual history as a determinant of current bone density in young athletes. *Journal of the American Medical Association*, **263**, 545-548.

8. Grande, F., & Keys, A. (1980). Body weight, body composition and calorie status. In R.S. Goodhart & M.E. Shils (Eds.), *Modern nutrition in health and disease* (6th ed.) (p. 16). Philadelphia: Lea & Febiger.

9. Kuipers, H., & Keizer, H.A. (1988). Overtraining in elite athletes: Review and directions for the future. *Sports Medicine*, **6**, 79-92.

10. Lohman, T.G. (1986). Applicability of body composition techniques and constants for children and

youths. *Exercise and Sport Sciences Reviews*, **14**, 325-357.

11. Lukaski, H.C. (1987). Methods for the assessment of human body composition: Traditional and new. *American Journal of Clinical Nutrition*, **46**, 537-556.

12. Martin, A.D., & Drinkwater, D.T. (1991). Variability in the measures of body fat: Assumptions or technique? *Sports Medicine*, **11**, 277-288.

13. Pate, R.R., Barnes, C., & Miller, W. (1985). A physiological comparison of performance-matched female and male distance runners. *Research Quarterly for Exercise and Sport*, **56**, 245-250.

14. Pollock, M.L., & Jackson, A.S. (1984). Research progress in validation of clinical methods of assessing body composition. *Medicine and Science in Sports and Exercise*, **16**, 606-613.

15. Riendeau, R.P., Welch, B.E., Crisp, C.E., Crowley, L.V., Griffin, P.E., & Brockett, J.E. (1958). Relationships of body fat to motor fitness test scores. *Research Quarterly*, **29**, 200-203.

16. Schutte, J.E., Townsend, E.J., Hugg, J., Shoup, R.F., Malina, R.M., & Blomqvist, C.G. (1984). Density of lean body mass is greater in blacks than in whites. *Journal of Applied Physiology*, **56**, 1647-1649.

17. Shangold, M., Rebar, R.W., Wentz, A.C., & Schiff, I. (1990). Evaluation and management of menstrual dysfunction in athletes. *Journal of the American Medical Association*, **263**, 1665-1669.

18. Sherman, W.M. (1991). Carbohydrate feedings before and after exercise. In D.R. Lamb & M.H. Williams (Eds.), *Ergogenics—enhancement of performance in exercise and sport* (pp. 87-117). Dubuque, IA: Brown & Benchmark.

19. Stager, J.M., & Cordain, L. (1984). Relationship of body composition to swimming performance in female swimmers. *Journal of Swimming Research*, **1**, 21-26.

20. Steen, S.N., & Brownell, K.D. (1990). Patterns of weight loss and regain in wrestlers: Has the tradition changed? *Medicine and Science in Sports and Exercise*, **22**, 762-768.

21. Welham, W.C., & Behnke, A.R. (1942). The specific gravity of healthy men. *Journal of the American Medical Association*, **118**, 498-501.

22. Wilmore, J.H. (1992). Body weight and body composition. In K.D. Brownell, J. Rodin, & J.H. Wilmore, (Eds.), *Eating, body weight, and performance in athletes: Disorders of modern society* (pp. 77-93). Philadelphia: Lea & Febiger.

23. Wilmore, J.H., Brown, C.H., & Davis, J.A. (1977). Body physique and composition of the female distance runner. *Annals of the New York Academy of Sciences*, **301**, 764-776.

Selected Readings

Behnke, A.R., & Wilmore, J.H. (1974). *Evaluation and regulation of body build and composition.* Englewood Cliffs, N.J.: Prentice-Hall.

Brownell, K.D., Rodin, J., & Wilmore, J.H. (Eds.) (1992). *Eating, body weight, and performance in athletes: Disorders of modern society.* Philadelphia: Lea & Febiger.

Brownell, K.D., Steen, S.N., & Wilmore, J.H. (1987). Weight regulation practices in athletes: Analysis of metabolic and health effects. *Medicine and Science in Sports and Exercise*, **19**, 546-556.

Horswill, C.A. (1992). When wrestlers slim to win: What's a safe minimum weight? *The Physician and Sports Medicine*, **20**(9), 91-101.

Katch, F.I., & McArdle, W.D. (1988). *Nutrition, weight control, and exercise* (3rd ed.). Philadelphia: Lea & Febiger.

Lehman, M., Foster, C., & Keul, J. (1993). Overtraining in endurance athletes: A brief review. *Medicine and Science in Sports and Exercise*, **25**(7), 854-862.

Rosen, L.W., McKeag, D.B., Hough, D.O., & Curley, V. (1986). Pathogenic weight control behavior in female athletes. *The Physician and Sportsmedicine*, **14**(1), 79-86.

Sinning, W.E. (1985). Body composition and athletic performance. In D.H. Clarke & H.M. Eckert (Eds.), *Limits of human performance*. Champaign, IL: Human Kinetics.

Thornton, J.S. (1990). Feast or famine: Eating disorders in athletes. *Physician and Sportsmedicine*, **18**(4), 116-122.

Wilmore, J.H. (1983). Body composition in sport and exercise: Directions for future research. *Medicine and Science in Sports and Exercise*, **15**, 21-31.

Wilmore, J.H. (1992). Body weight standards and athletic performance. In K.D. Brownell, J. Rodin, & J.H. Wilmore, (Eds.), *Eating, body weight, and performance in athletes: Disorders of modern society*. Philadelphia: Lea & Febiger.

Special Populations in Sport and Exercise

From the previous parts of this book, we have gained a good understanding of the general principles of exercise and sport physiology. Now, in Part F, we turn our attention to how these principles are specifically applied to special populations. In chapter 17, Growth, Development, and the Young Athlete, we examine the processes of human growth and development and how different stages affect a young athlete's physiological capacity. We will also consider how these stages of growth and development might alter our strategies for training a young athlete for competition. In chapter 18, Aging and the Older Athlete, we will discuss how sport performance changes as we age, asking to what extent this change is due to physiological aging and how much of it might be due to an increasingly sedentary lifestyle. We will discover the important role that training can play in minimizing the loss of performance capacity and physical conditioning that accompanies the aging process. In chapter 19, Gender Issues and the Female Athlete, we will examine potential differences between women's and men's physiological responses to exercise and training and to what extent these differences are biological. We will also focus on issues specific to female athletes, including menstrual function, pregnancy, and osteoporosis, and we will discuss the high prevalence of eating disorders in this population.

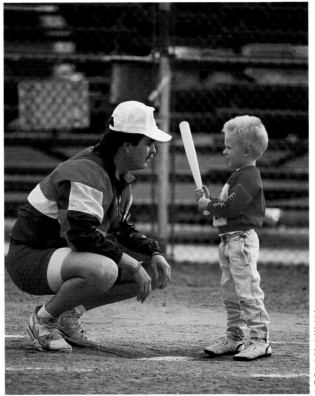

© F-Stock/Mark W. Lisk

Chapter 17
Growth, Development, and the Young Athlete

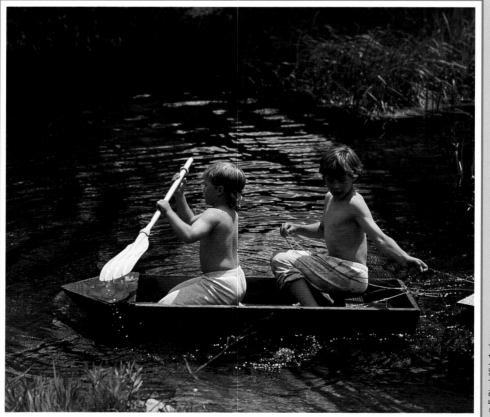

© F-Stock/Kirk Anderson

Chapter Overview

Competition in youth sports has grown considerably over the last several decades and is now a major part of the world of sport. Boys compete in Little League baseball and Pop Warner football, girls compete in Bobby Sox and Little League softball, and both participate in minibike racing, soccer, swimming, track and field, and long-distance running. With this growing interest in age-group competition, many questions have been raised. Is competition physically or psychologically harmful for the preadolescent? Should preadolescents be allowed to compete in such activities as long-distance running or strength training?

We will address these and similar questions in this chapter. We will begin by considering the processes of growth and development, then we will examine how these processes affect performance. Finally, we will discuss the training of young athletes.

Chapter Outline

In 1984, at age 16, Bulgarian weight lifter Naim Suleimanov lifted 170 kg (375 lb) from the floor to full arms' length overhead. He was able to perform this incredible feat at a body weight of only 123 lb (56 kg)! In other words, he was able to lift more than three times his body weight, something that no one else had ever been able to do. He was considered at the time to be the best competitive weight lifter in the world.

Growth, development, and maturation are terms that can be used to describe changes starting at conception and continuing through adulthood that occur in the body. Growth refers to an increase in the size of the body or any of its parts. Development refers to differentiation along specialized lines of function, so it reflects the functional changes that occur with growth. Finally, maturation refers to the process of taking on the adult form and becoming fully functional, and is defined by the system or function being considered. For example, skeletal maturity refers to having a fully developed skeletal system in which all bones have completed normal growth and ossification, whereas sexual maturity refers to having a fully functional reproductive system. The state of a child's or adolescent's maturity can be defined by

- chronological age,
- skeletal age, and
- stage of sexual maturation.

With the increasing popularity of youth sport and an emphasis on increasing children's physical fitness, we must understand the physiological bases for growth and development. Children and adolescents must not be regarded as mere miniature versions of adults. They are unique at each stage in their development. The growth and development of their bones, muscles, nerves, and organs largely dictate their physiological and performance capacities. As children increase in size, so do almost all of their functional capacities. This is true of motor ability, strength, and aerobic and anaerobic capacity. In the following sections, we will examine age-related changes in a child's physical abilities.

Growth and Development of the Tissues

To understand the physical capabilities of children and the potential impact that sport activity can have on young athletes, we must first consider the physical state of their bodies. In this section, we address issues related to the growth and development of selected body tissues.

Height and Weight

Specialists in the field of growth and development have spent considerable time analyzing the changes in height and weight that accompany growth. These two variables are most useful when we examine their rates of change. Change in height is assessed in terms of centimeters per year, and change in weight in terms of kilograms per year. Figure 17.1a shows that height increases rapidly during the first 2 years of life. In fact, the child reaches about 50% of adult height by age 2. After this, height increases at a progressively slower rate throughout childhood; thus there is a decline in the rate of its change. Just prior to puberty, the rate of change in height increases markedly, followed by an exponential decrease in the height growth rate until full height is attained at a mean age of about 16.5 years in girls and 18.0 years in boys. The peak rate of growth in height occurs at approximately 12.0 years in girls and 14.0 years in boys. Figure 17.1b reveals the same overall trend for the rate of change in weight. As with height, the peak rate of growth in body weight occurs at approximately 12.0 years in girls, but in boys this rate peaks at 14.5 years—slightly later than height.

KEY POINT

Girls mature physiologically about 2 to 2.5 years earlier than boys do.

Bone

Bones, joints, cartilage, and ligaments form the body's structural support. Bones provide points of attachment for the muscles, protect delicate tissues, act as reservoirs for calcium and phosphorus, and some are in-

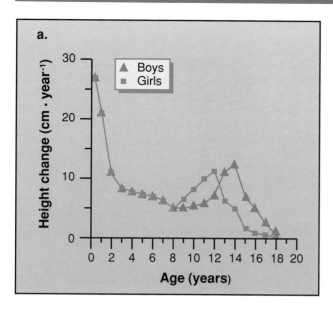

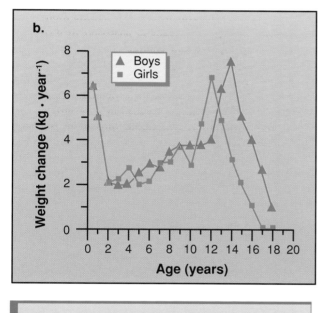

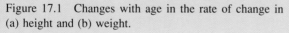

Figure 17.1   Changes with age in the rate of change in (a) height and (b) weight.

The Ossification Process

The general contour of the cartilage during embryonic development resembles the future shape of the mature bone. The central shaft of a long bone is referred to as the diaphysis, and each end of a long bone is an epiphysis. Ossification, through which cartilage is transformed into bone, begins at the diaphysis, as shown in Figure 17.2. The cartilage that will be transformed is covered by a fibrous membrane, the perichondrium. Ossification is initiated when this membrane is penetrated by blood vessels. Once the perichondrium is vascularized, it is called the periosteum, and the chondrocytes (cartilage-forming cells) in it become osteoblasts (bone-forming cells). Osteoblasts secrete substances that form a ring or collar of bone around the diaphysis. At the same time, the cartilage cells in the central area of the diaphysis undergo a series of complex changes, which eventually result in calcification of the bone. This area of bone formation is then known as the primary ossification center. The cartilage continues to grow in length and thickness, and the periosteal development and bone formation from the primary ossification center continue toward the epiphyses.

At birth, each of our long bones has a bony diaphysis and two cartilaginous epiphyses. Shortly after birth, secondary ossification centers arise in the epiphyses. With the establishment of these secondary centers, the epiphyses begin to ossify. Bone formation then occurs in the diaphysis and the epiphyses, leaving a plate of cartilage between the diaphysis and each epiphysis that is known as the epiphyseal, or growth, plate. These epiphyseal plates allow our bones to elongate as we grow. Cartilage growth continues on the epiphyseal border of these plates as cartilage is replaced on the diaphyseal border, so the growth plates remain approximately the same thickness.

Ossification is completed and bone growth ceases when the cartilage cells cease to grow and the epiphyseal plates are replaced by bone. This fuses the diaphysis with each epiphysis, and bone lengthening is then no longer possible. In the tibia (shin bone) of males ossification is completed in the distal epiphysis (ankle) by the average age of 17 years and in the proximal epiphysis (knee) by the average age of 20 years, although actual age varies considerably. In females, this fusion process is completed approximately 2 to 3 years earlier. The average ages at which the different bones in our bodies complete ossification differs widely, but bones typically begin to fuse in the preteens, and all are fused by the early twenties. On the average, girls achieve full bone maturity several years before boys.

The structure of mature long bones is complex. Bone is a living tissue that requires essential nutrients,

volved in blood cell formation. Early in fetal development the bones begin to develop from cartilage. Some flat bones, such as those of the skull, develop from fibrous membranes. The vast majority of bones instead develop from hyaline cartilage. During fetal development, as well as during the initial 14 to 22 years of life, membranes and cartilage are transformed into bone through the process of ossification, or bone formation. In this text, we are mostly concerned with the long bones of the body, so we will focus on their development.

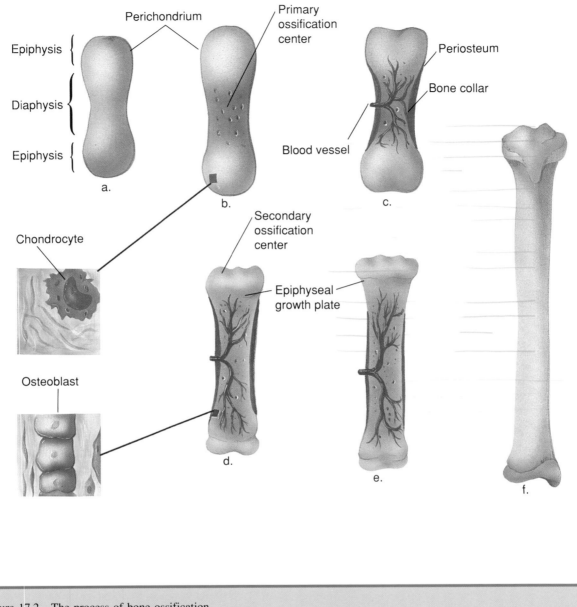

Figure 17.2   The process of bone ossification.

so it receives a rich blood supply. Bone consists of cells distributed throughout a matrix or lattice-type arrangement, and it is dense and hard due to deposits of lime salts, mainly calcium phosphate and calcium carbonate. For this reason, calcium is an essential nutrient, particularly during periods of bone growth and in the latter years of life when bone tends to become brittle due to aging. Bones also store calcium. When our blood calcium level is high, excess calcium can be deposited in our bones for storage, and when cal-

cium levels are too low, bone is resorbed, or broken down, to release calcium into the blood. And when injury occurs or when extra stress is placed on a bone, more calcium is deposited. Thus, throughout life, our bones are constantly changing.

Exercise is essential for proper bone growth. Although exercise has little or no influence on bone lengthening, it does increase bone width and bone density by depositing more mineral in the bone matrix, which increases the bone's strength.

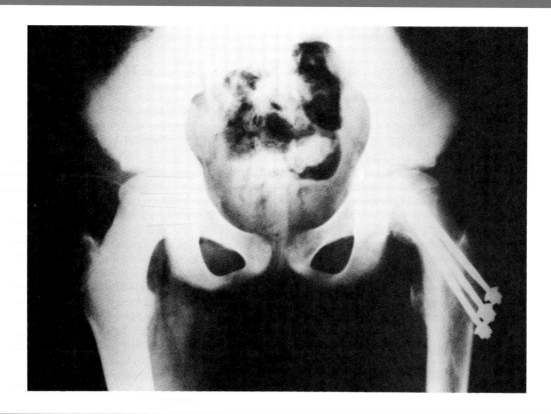

Figure 17.3   An x-ray of a slipped epiphysis at the head of the femur in an 8-year-old girl injured while playing competitive soccer, showing the three pins that were placed in the head of the femur to secure the epiphysis to the diaphysis.

■■■ KEY POINT ■■■

Exercise, along with an adequate diet, is essential for proper bone growth. Exercise affects primarily bone width, density, and strength but has little or no effect on length.

Bone Injuries Affecting Growth

In this chapter we must understand how injury of immature bones can affect bone growth and development. The greatest concern is the potential for injury at the epiphyseal plate. Fractures there can disturb the bone's blood (nutrient) supply and disrupt the growth process. Disruption of the growth of the femur, as an example, leads to different lengths of the two legs, the injured leg being much shorter. Fortunately, such injuries are rare and seldom occur in sports. In a study of 31 epiphyseal injuries, only 23% were sport induced. The remainder resulted from falls and vehicular accidents.[13] Figure 17.3 illustrates a slipped epiphysis of the head of the femur in an 8-year-old girl. The epiphysis of her femur was displaced, or had slipped, from its correct alignment with the diaphysis. The injury occurred during a championship soccer match, and her symptoms were initially diagnosed as a groin pull.

Traumatic epiphysitis (inflammation of the epiphysis) is a type of epiphyseal injury that occurs in young athletes. One form of this is "Little Leaguer's elbow," a condition that results from repetitive strains to the medial epicondylar epiphysis of the humerus (inner aspect of the elbow). Twelve-year-old boys can throw a baseball up to 80 mph (129 kph). This causes a sudden pull on the epiphysis that anchors the tendons of the involved muscles, and can even result in its separation (Figure 17.4). Short of a total separation, the stress of repetitive throwing can produce an inflammatory response—epiphysitis.

In Adams' widely publicized study published in 1965, x-ray examination revealed epiphysitis in all 80 pitchers in a group of 162 young boys.[1] Only a small percentage of the nonpitchers and of the control group of nonplayers exhibited this condition. But subsequent

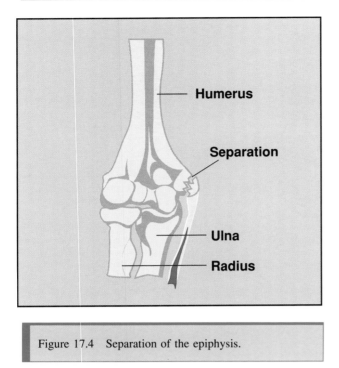

Figure 17.4   Separation of the epiphysis.

studies have not confirmed this initial study, reporting instead much lower percentages of epiphysitis in both pitchers and nonpitchers.

Another study reviewed 1,338 consecutive athletic injuries seen by four orthopedists in a major sports medicine practice. Of all of these injuries, 28% occurred in youths ages 15 years and younger.[14] Only 6% of the total injuries in those 15 years old and younger involved the epiphysis. The study also concluded that epiphyseal injuries do not always result in crippling or permanent trauma and that early recognition is important.

Of all youth sports, competitive baseball is of greatest concern because of its potential for serious epiphyseal injuries resulting primarily from the pitching motion. Some youth leagues have replaced the pitcher with a parent or coach, a pitching machine, or a batting tee from which the ball is hit. This is a sensible approach until the youngster reaches an age at which pitching is not so likely to cause injury. Tennis (tennis elbow) and swimming (swimmer's shoulder) are two other sports that share an increased risk of epiphyseal injury. Pop Warner football and other competitive activities have good records with regard to bone injuries. Although the potential for injury in football is generally considered high, the players' small size, player matching by size, and good protective equipment apparently provide a safe environment for young football players. Inappropriate equipment or a mismatch of players by size and ability increases the risk of injury.

IN REVIEW . . .

1. Growth in height is very rapid during the first 2 years of life, with a child reaching 50% of adult stature by age 2. After that, the rate is slower throughout childhood until a marked increase occurs near puberty.
2. The peak rate of height growth occurs at age 12.0 in girls and age 14.0 in boys. Full height is typically attained at age 16.5 in girls and age 18.0 in boys.
3. Growth in weight follows the same trend as height. The peak rate of weight increase occurs at age 12.0 in girls and at age 14.5 in boys.
4. Bones are formed through ossification, which spreads from primary (diaphysis) and secondary (epiphysis) ossification centers.
5. Injury at the epiphysis could cause early termination of growth.
6. Competitive baseball, especially the pitching motion, carries the highest risk of epiphyseal injury. Tennis and swimming also carry higher risks for young athletes.

Muscle

From birth through adolescence, the body's muscle mass steadily increases, along with the youngster's weight gain. In males, the total muscle mass increases from 25% of body weight at birth to 40% or more in the adult. Much of this gain occurs when the muscle development rate peaks at puberty. This corresponds to a sudden, almost 10-fold increase in testosterone production. Girls don't experience such rapid acceleration of muscle growth at puberty, but their muscle mass does continue to increase, although much more slowly than boys'. This rate difference is largely attributed to hormonal differences at puberty (see chapter 19).

Increases in muscle mass with age appear to result primarily from hypertrophy (increase in size) of existing fibers, with little or no hyperplasia (increase in fiber number). This hypertrophy results from increases in the myofilaments and myofibrils. Increases in muscle length as young bones elongate result from increases in the number of sarcomeres (they are added at the junction of the muscle and the tendon) and from increases in the length of existing sarcomeres. Muscle mass peaks when females reach 16 to 20 years of age and males reach 18 to 25 years, unless it is increased further through exercise, diet, or both.

KEY POINT

The increase in muscle mass with growth and development is accomplished primarily by hypertrophy of individual muscle fibers through increases in their myofilaments and myofibrils. Muscle length increases through the addition of sarcomeres and by increases in the length of existing sarcomeres.

Fat

Fat cells form and fat deposition starts in these cells early in fetal development, and this process continues indefinitely thereafter. Each fat cell can increase in size at any age from birth to death. Early studies investigating fat cell and fat mass development suggested that the number of fat cells became fixed early in life. This led many scientists to believe that maintaining a low total body fat content during this early period of development would minimize the total number of fat cells that develop, greatly reducing the likelihood of obesity as an adult. But more recent evidence suggests that the number of fat cells can continue to increase throughout life.[4] The most recent evidence suggests that as fat is added to the body, existing fat cells continue to fill with fat to a certain critical volume. Once these cells are filled to this point, new fat cells are formed. In light of this evidence, it is important to maintain good dietary and exercise habits throughout life!

KEY POINT

Fat storage occurs through increasing the size of existing fat cells and by increasing the number of fat cells. It appears that existing fat cells, as they become full, signal the need for the development of new fat cells.

The amount of fat that accumulates with growth and aging depends on

- your diet,
- your exercise habits, and
- heredity.

Heredity is unchangeable, but both diet and exercise can be altered to either increase or decrease your fat stores.

At birth, 10% to 12% of total body weight is fat. At physical maturity, the fat content reaches approximately 15% of total body weight for males and approximately 25% for females. This gender difference, like that seen in muscle growth, is primarily due to hormonal differences. When girls reach puberty, their estrogen levels increase, which promotes the deposition of body fat. The trend of body fat increasing with age is shown in Figure 17.5, which illustrates the relationship between subcutaneous fat (measured at the triceps and subscapular sites) and age for both males and females. The amount of subcutaneous fat is representative of total body fat. Figure 17.6 illustrates the changes in both fat mass and fat-free mass for both males and females for ages 8 to 28 years. It is important to realize that both fat and fat-free mass increase during this time period, so an increase in absolute fat does not necessarily mean a person is increasing relative fat.

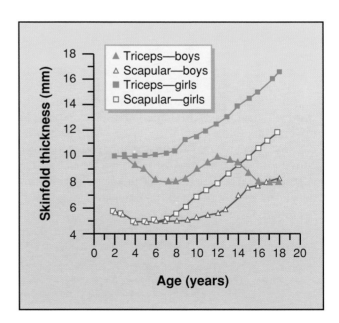

Figure 17.5 Changes in skinfold fat thickness at the triceps brachii and scapular sites in boys and girls from age 2 years to 18 years. Data from the NHANES-I, National Center for Health Statistics.

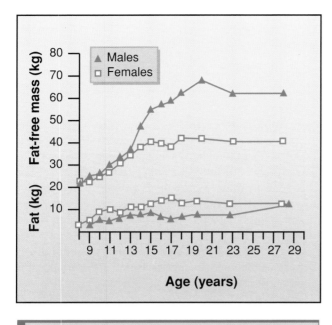

Figure 17.6 Changes in fat mass and fat-free mass for females and males from ages 8 to 28. Data from Forbes (1972).

The Nervous System

As children grow, they develop better balance, agility, and coordination as their nervous systems develop. Myelination of the nerve fibers must be completed before fast reactions and skilled movement can occur, because conduction of an impulse along a nerve fiber is considerably slower if myelination is absent or incomplete (chapter 3). Myelination of the cerebral cortex occurs most rapidly during childhood, but continues well beyond puberty. Although practicing an activity or skill can improve performance to a certain extent, the full development of that activity or skill is dependent on full maturation (and myelination) of the nervous system.

Physical Performance in Young Athletes

The function of almost all physiological systems improves until full maturity is reached or shortly before. After that, function plateaus for a period of time before starting to decline with advancing age. In this section, we focus on some of the changes in the young athlete that accompany growth and development. We will focus on

- motor ability,
- strength,

IN REVIEW . . .

1. Muscle mass increases steadily along with weight gain from birth through adolescence.
2. In males, the rate of muscle mass increase peaks at puberty, when testosterone production increases dramatically. Girls do not experience this sharp increase in muscle mass.
3. Muscle-mass increases in boys and girls result primarily from fiber hypertrophy with little or no hyperplasia.
4. Muscle mass peaks in girls between ages 16 and 20, and in boys between ages 18 and 25, though it can be increased more through diet and exercise.
5. Fat cells can increase in size and number throughout life.
6. The amount of fat accumulation depends on diet, exercise habits, and heredity.
7. At physical maturity, the body's fat content averages 15% in males and 25% in females. The differences are caused primarily by higher testosterone levels in males and higher estrogen levels in females.
8. Balance, agility, and coordination improve as children's nervous systems develop.
9. Myelination of nerve fibers must be completed before fast reactions and skilled movements are fully developed because myelination speeds the transmission of electrical impulses.

- pulmonary function,
- cardiovascular function,
- aerobic capacity,
- running economy,
- anaerobic capacity, and
- thermal stress.

Motor Ability

As shown in Figure 17.7, the motor ability of boys and girls generally increases with age for the first 18 years, although girls tend to plateau at about the age of puberty for most items tested. These improvements result primarily from development of the neuromuscular and endocrine systems and secondarily from the children's increased activity.

The plateau observed in the girls at puberty is likely explained by two factors. As mentioned earlier, the increase in estrogen levels at puberty or in the estrogen:testosterone ratio leads to increased fat deposition. Performance tends to decrease as fat increases. Probably of greater importance, though, is that around puberty many girls assume a much more sedentary lifestyle than boys. This is largely a matter of social

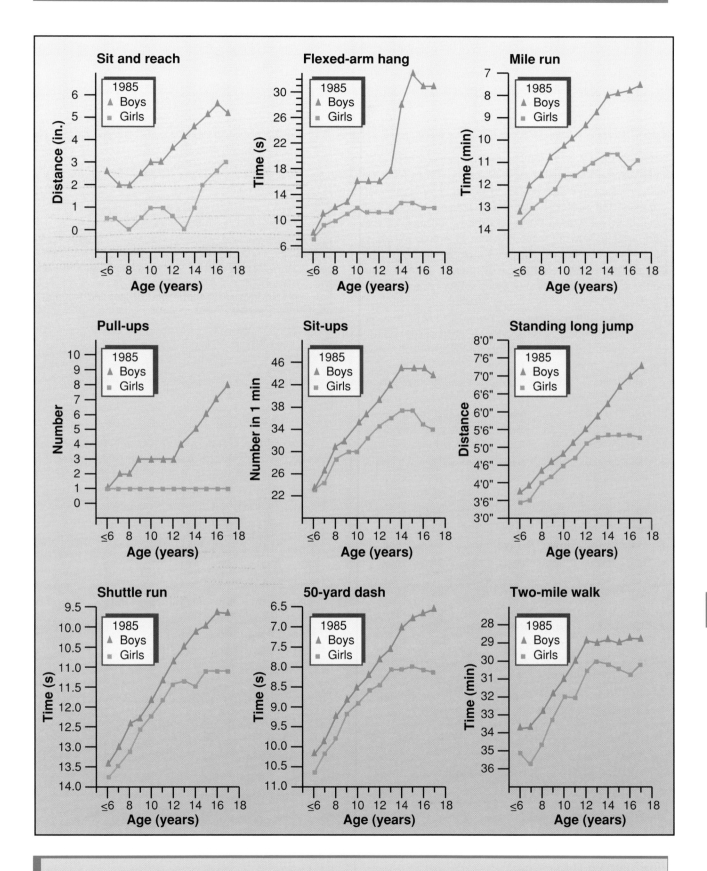

Figure 17.7   Changes in motor ability from the ages of 6 years to 17 years. Data from the President's Council on Physical Fitness and Sports (1985).

conditioning, as boys are encouraged to be more active and athletic than girls. As these girls become less active, their motor abilities tend to plateau. This trend might change because more opportunities for sport and activity are now available for girls.

Strength

Strength improves as muscle mass increases with age. Peak strength is usually attained by age 20 in females and between age 20 and 30 in males. The hormonal changes that accompany puberty lead to marked increases in strength in pubescent males, because of the increased muscle mass noted before. Brooks and Fahey have also observed that the extent of the development and the performance capacity of muscle is dependent on the relative maturation of the nervous system.[5] High levels of strength, power, and skill are impossible if the child has not reached neural maturity. Myelination of many motor nerves is incomplete until sexual maturity, so the neural control of muscle function is limited before that time.

Figure 17.8 illustrates changes in leg strength in a group of boys from the Medford Boys' Growth Study. The boys were followed longitudinally from age 7 to age 18.[6] The rate of strength gain increases noticeably around the age of 12, the typical age for onset of puberty. Similar longitudinal data for girls are not available. Cross-sectional data, however, indicate that girls experience a more gradual increase in strength and do not exhibit a marked change in their rate of strength gain with puberty.

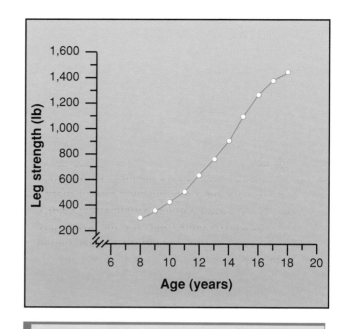

Figure 17.8 Gains with age in leg strength of young boys followed longitudinally over 12 years. Note the increase in the slope of the curve from 12 to 16 years of age. Data from Clarke (1971).

The changes in these volumes and flow rates are matched by the changes in the highest ventilation that can be achieved during exhaustive exercise, which is referred to as the maximal expiratory ventilation ($\dot{V}_{E\,max}$), or maximal minute ventilation. $\dot{V}_{E\,max}$ increases with age to the point of physical maturity, then decreases with aging. For example, cross-sectional data show that $\dot{V}_{E\,max}$ averages about 40 L · min^{-1} for 4- to 6-year-old boys and increases to 110 to 140 L · min^{-1} at full maturity. Girls follow the same general pattern, but their absolute values remain considerably lower, primarily due to their smaller size. These changes are associated with the growth of the pulmonary system, which parallels the general growth patterns of children.

Cardiovascular Function

Cardiovascular function undergoes numerous changes as the child grows and ages. Let's consider some of these changes during submaximal and maximal exercise.

Submaximal Exercise

Blood pressure while at rest and during submaximal levels of exercise is lower in the child than in the adult but progressively increases to adult values during the late teen years. Blood pressure is also directly related to body size: Larger people generally have higher blood pressures. In children, blood flow to active muscles

---

IN REVIEW . . .

1. Motor ability generally increases for the first 18 years of life, although in girls it tends to plateau around puberty. This plateau is probably due to increased estrogen levels, which promote greater fat deposition, as well as girls' typical assumption of a more sedentary lifestyle.
2. Strength improves as muscle mass increases with age.
3. Gains in strength also depend on neural maturation, because neuromuscular control is limited until myelination has been completed, usually around sexual maturity.

Pulmonary Function

Lung function changes markedly with age. All lung volumes increase until growth is completed. Peak flow rates follow the same pattern.

during exercise can be greater than in adults, because children have less peripheral resistance.

Recall that cardiac output is the product of heart rate and stroke volume. A child's smaller heart size and total blood volume result in a lower stroke volume, both at rest and during exercise, than in an adult. In an attempt to compensate for this, the child's heart rate response to a given rate of submaximal work (such as on a cycle ergometer) is higher than an adult's. As the child ages, heart size and blood volume increase along with body size. Consequently, stroke volume also increases for the same absolute rate of work.

However, a child's higher submaximal heart rate cannot completely compensate for the lower stroke volume. Because of this, the child's cardiac output is also somewhat lower than the adult's for the same absolute rate of work. To maintain adequate oxygen uptake during these submaximal levels of work, the child's arterial-venous oxygen difference (a-$\bar{v}O_2$ diff) is increased to further compensate for the lower stroke volume. The increase in a-$\bar{v}O_2$ diff is most likely due to increased blood flow to the active muscles—a greater percentage of the cardiac output goes to the active muscles.

These submaximal relationships are illustrated in Figure 17.9. In each case, the response of an 8-year-old boy is compared to that of a fully mature man.

Maximal Exercise

Maximum heart rate (HR max) is higher in young children but decreases linearly as they age. Young children under age 10 frequently have maximum heart rates exceeding 210 beats per minute, whereas the average 20 year old has a maximum heart rate of approximately 195 beats per minute. Results of cross-sectional studies suggest that maximum heart rate decreases by slightly less than one beat per year. Longitudinal studies, however, suggest that maximum heart rate decreases only 0.5 beats per minute per year. Longitudinal studies, in which the same people are followed over time, generally provide more accurate estimates of the true changes.

During maximal levels of exercise, as also seen with submaximal exercise, the child's smaller heart

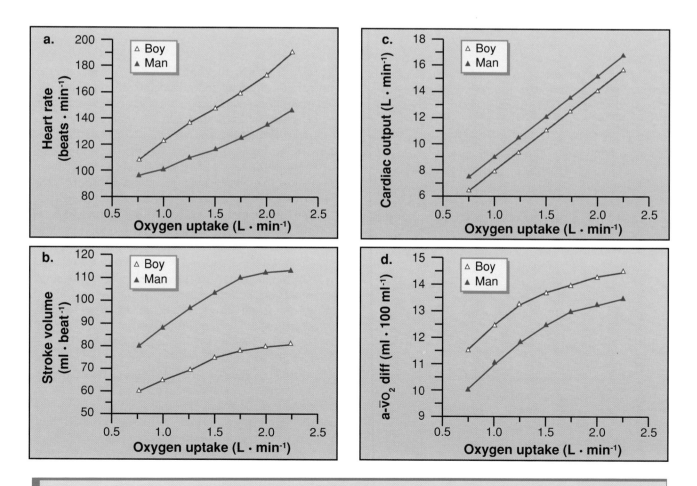

Figure 17.9   Submaximal (a) heart rate, (b) stroke volume, (c) cardiac output, and (d) arterial-venous oxygen difference in an 8-yr old boy and a fully mature man at fixed rates of oxygen uptake. Data from Bar-Or (1983).

and blood volume limit the maximal stroke volume that can be achieved. And again the elevated maximum heart rate cannot fully compensate for this, leaving the child with a lower maximal cardiac output than the adult. This limits the child's performance at high absolute rates of work (for example, pedaling at 100 W on a cycle ergometer) because the child's capacity for oxygen delivery is less than an adult's. However, for high relative rates of work in which the child is responsible for moving only his or her body mass, this lower maximal cardiac output is not as serious a limitation. In running, for example, a 25-kg (55-lb) child requires (in direct proportion to body size) considerably less

---

KEY POINT

Heart size is directly related to body size, so children have smaller hearts than adults have. As a result of this and a smaller blood volume, the child has a smaller stroke volume capacity. The higher maximum heart rate in the child can only partially compensate for this lower stroke volume capacity, and thus maximal cardiac output is lower than that of an equally trained adult.

IN REVIEW . . .

1. All lung volumes increase until physical maturity.
2. Until physical maturity, maximal ventilatory capacity and maximal expiratory ventilation increase in direct proportion to the increase in body size during exhaustive exercise.
3. Blood pressure is directly related to body size—it is lower in children than adults but increases to adult levels in the late teen years.
4. During both submaximal and maximal exercise, the child's smaller heart and blood volume result in a lower stroke volume than in adults. In partial compensation, the child's heart rate is higher than an adult's.
5. Even with increased heart rate, a child's cardiac output remains less than an adult's. In submaximal exercise, an increase in the a-$\bar{v}O_2$ diff ensures adequate oxygen delivery to the active muscles. But at maximal work rates oxygen delivery limits performance in activities other than those in which the child merely needs to move his or her body mass.

oxygen than a 90-kg (200-lb) man would require, yet the oxygen consumption rate per kilogram of body weight is about the same for both.

Aerobic Capacity

The purpose of the basic pulmonary and cardiovascular adaptations that occur in response to varying levels of exercise (rates of work) is to accommodate the exercising muscles' need for oxygen. Thus, increases in pulmonary and cardiovascular function that accompany growth suggest that aerobic capacity ($\dot{V}O_2$ max) similarly increases. In 1938, Robinson demonstrated this phenomenon in a cross-sectional sample of boys and men ranging in age from 6 to 91 years.[19] He found that $\dot{V}O_2$ max peaks between ages 17 and 21, then decreases linearly with age. Other studies have subsequently confirmed these observations. Studies of girls and women have shown essentially the same trend, although in females the decrease begins at a much younger age, generally age 12 to 15 (refer to chapter 19), probably due to an earlier assumption of a sedentary lifestyle. The changes in $\dot{V}O_2$ max with age, expressed in L · min^{-1}, are illustrated in Figure 17.10a.

Expressing $\dot{V}O_2$ max relative to body weight (ml · kg^{-1} · min^{-1}) provides a considerably different picture, as shown in Figure 17.10b. Values change little in boys from age 6 to young adulthood. For girls, however, little change occurs from age 6 to 13, but after age 13, aerobic capacities show a gradual decrease. Although these observations are of general interest, they might not accurately reflect the development of the cardiorespiratory system as children grow and their physical activity levels change. Several questions have been raised about the validity of using body weight to account for changes in the size of the cardiorespiratory and metabolic systems, such as when dividing absolute values by body weight, for example, $\dot{V}O_2$ per kg.

First, although $\dot{V}O_2$ max values expressed relative to body weight remain relatively stable or decline with age, endurance performance steadily improves. The average 14-year-old boy can run the mile (1.6 km) almost twice as fast as the average 5-year-old boy, yet their $\dot{V}O_2$ max values expressed relative to body weight are similar.[21] Second, although the increases in $\dot{V}O_2$ max that accompany endurance training in children are relatively small compared to adults, the performance increases in these children are relatively large. Body weight might not be the most appropriate variable to use in scaling $\dot{V}O_2$ max values for differences in body size in a young, growing child. The relationships between $\dot{V}O_2$ max, body dimensions, and system functions during growth are extraordinarily complex.[22]

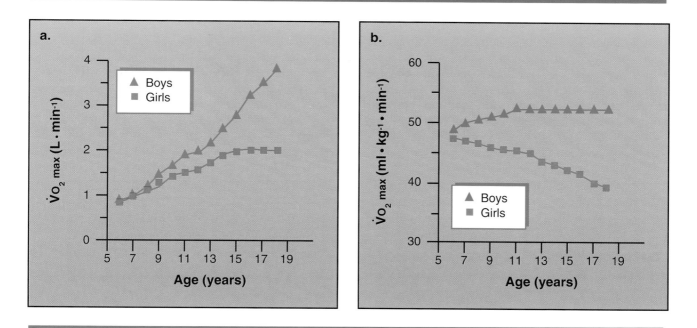

Figure 17.10 Changes in maximal oxygen uptake with age. Values are expressed in (a) $L \cdot min^{-1}$ and (b) relative to body weight, in $ml \cdot kg^{-1} \cdot min^{-1}$.

IN REVIEW . . .

1. As pulmonary and cardiovascular function improve with continued development, so does aerobic capacity.
2. $\dot{V}O_{2\,max}$, expressed in $L \cdot min^{-1}$, peaks between ages 17 and 21 years in males and between 12 and 15 years in females, after which it steadily decreases.
3. When $\dot{V}O_{2\,max}$ is expressed relative to body weight, it plateaus in males from age 6 to 25 years, but begins its decline at about age 13 in girls. However, expressing $\dot{V}O_{2\,max}$ relative to body weight might not provide an accurate estimate of aerobic capacity. Such $\dot{V}O_{2\,max}$ values do not reflect the significant gains in endurance performance capacity that are noted with both maturation and training.
4. The child's lower $\dot{V}O_{2\,max}$ value ($L \cdot min^{-1}$) limits endurance performance unless body weight is the major resistance to movement, such as in distance running.
5. When expressed relative to body weight, a child's $\dot{V}O_{2\,max}$ is similar to an adult's, yet in activities such as distance running a child's performance is far inferior to adult performance because of differences in economy of effort.

KEY POINT

Aerobic capacity ($\dot{V}O_{2\,max}$), when expressed in $L \cdot min^{-1}$, is lower in children than in adults at similar levels of training. This is due primarily to the child's lower maximal cardiac output capacity. When $\dot{V}O_{2\,max}$ values are expressed to reflect the differences in body size between children and adults, there is little or no difference in aerobic capacity.

Running Economy

How do growth-related changes in aerobic capacity affect a child's performance? For any activity that requires a fixed rate of work, such as cycling on an ergometer, the child's lower $\dot{V}O_{2\,max}$ limits endurance performance. But as noted earlier, for activities where body weight is the major resistance to movement, such as distance running, children should not be at a disadvantage because their $\dot{V}O_{2\,max}$ values expressed relative to body weight are already at or near adult values.

Yet the child cannot maintain as fast a running pace as the adult because of basic differences in economy of effort. At a given speed on a treadmill, the child will have a substantially higher submaximal oxygen consumption when expressed relative to body weight than the adult. Even if the child's lactate threshold occurred at the same relative oxygen consumption as the adult (at the same percentage of their respective $\dot{V}O_{2\,max}$ values), the child would be running at a much slower pace. Also, as children age, their legs lengthen, their muscles become stronger, and their running skills improve. Running economy increases and this improves their distance running pace even if the children are not training and if their $\dot{V}O_{2\,max}$ values don't increase.[7,12]

Rowland has hypothesized that the following factors, which change with growth and development, explain at least in part the lower running economy in children and its improvement with maturation:[21]

- Stride frequency
- Gait mechanics
- Musculotendinous elastic energy storage
- Surface-area-to-body-mass ratio
- Changes in body composition
- Thermal responses to exercise
- Substrate utilization
- Anaerobic capacity
- Ventilatory efficiency

Of these factors, thus far only stride frequency has been proven to be important (based on studies with youths ages 8 to 20 years). It is also possible that scaling oxygen consumption to body weight is inappropriate during growth and development, as discussed in the previous section.

Anaerobic Capacity

Children have a limited ability to perform anaerobic-type activities. This is demonstrated in several ways. Children cannot achieve adult concentrations of lactate in either muscle or blood for maximal and supramaximal rates of exercise, which indicates a lower glycolytic capacity. The lower lactate levels might reflect a lower concentration of phosphofructokinase, the key rate-limiting enzyme of glycolysis. However, lactate threshold, when expressed as a percentage of $\dot{V}O_{2\,max}$, does not appear to be a limiting factor in children because children's lactate thresholds are similar, if not somewhat higher, than those of similarly trained adults.

Children cannot achieve high respiratory exchange ratios during maximal or exhaustive exercise.

KEY POINT

Anaerobic capacity is lower in children than adults, which simply might reflect the lower concentration in children of the key rate-limiting enzyme phosphofructokinase.

Maximal respiratory exchange ratios in children are seldom above 1.10, and are sometimes below 1.00, but adult ratios are usually more than 1.10 and often greater than 1.15. This indicates that less CO_2 is produced in children for the same oxygen consumption, which in turn indicates less buffering of lactate.

Anaerobic mean and peak power output, as determined by the Wingate anaerobic power test (a 30-s–all-out maximal effort on a cycle ergometer) are also lower in the child than in the adult. Figure 17.11 illustrates this for 306 males who performed the Wingate test with both arms and legs.[10] Mean power output is the average power output for the entire 30-s test. Peak power output is the highest power output obtained during any 5-s interval during the test. Results indicate that anaerobic power increases with growth and development, even when the values are expressed relative to body weight (watts · kg^{-1}).

Bar-Or has summarized the development of both the aerobic and anaerobic characteristics in boys and girls from ages 9 through 16, using 18 years of age as the criterion for 100% of the adult value.[2] The changes with age are shown in Figure 17.12. Aerobic power is represented by the child's $\dot{V}O_{2\,max}$, whereas anaerobic power is represented by the child's performance on the Margaria step-running test (a field test). Maximum energy expenditure per kilogram represents the maximum energy-generating capacities of the aerobic and anaerobic systems, scaled to body weight (kg) to account for body size differences with growth.

IN REVIEW . . .

1. The child's ability to perform anaerobic activities is limited. A child has a lower glycolytic capacity, possibly because of a limited amount of phosphofructokinase.
2. Children cannot attain high respiratory exchange ratios during maximal or exhaustive exercise, suggesting less lactate production.
3. Anaerobic mean and peak power outputs are lower in children than in adults.

Thermal Stress

Laboratory experiments suggest that children are more susceptible to heat- and cold-induced illness or injury than adults are. But the number of reported cases of thermal illness or injury have not supported this theory. A major concern is the child's apparently lower capacity when exercising in the heat to dissipate heat through evaporation. Children appear to rely much more on convection and radiation, which are enhanced through greater peripheral vasodilation.[3] A child's lower capac-

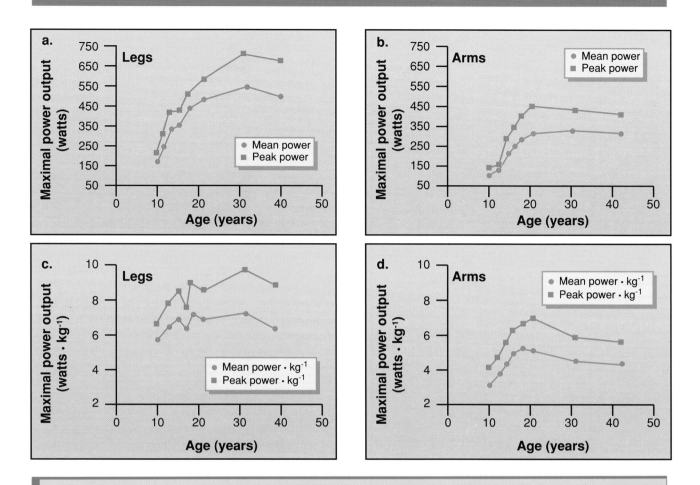

Figure 17.11   Mean and peak anaerobic power changes with age, expressed in (a and b) absolute values (watts) and (c and d) relative to body weight (watts · kg^{-1}). Adapted from Inbar and Bar-Or (1986).

ity for evaporative heat loss is largely the result of a decreased sweating rate. Individual sweat glands in children form sweat more slowly than those in adults and are less sensitive to increases in the body's core temperature than those in adults. Although young boys can acclimatize to exercise in the heat, their rate of acclimatization is slower than that of adults. Acclimatization data are not available on girls.

Only a few studies have focussed on children exercising in the cold. From the limited information available, children appear to have greater conductive heat loss than adults, due to a larger surface-area-to-mass ratio. This should place them at higher risk for hypothermia.

For both heat and cold stress, few studies have been conducted on children, and conclusions from the studies have sometimes been contradictory. More research is needed in this area to determine the risks faced by children who exercise in the heat and cold. In the meantime, a conservative approach is advisable. Children should be considered at an increased risk compared to adults.[3]

IN REVIEW . . .

1. Laboratory studies indicate that children are more susceptible to injury or illness from thermal stress, but the number of reported cases does not support this.
2. Children are capable of less evaporative heat loss than adults because children sweat less (less sweat is produced by each active sweat gland).
3. Young boys acclimatize to heat more slowly than adults do. Data on this topic are not available for girls.
4. Children appear to have greater conductive heat loss than adults, which should place children at greater risk for hypothermia in cold environments.
5. Until more is known about children's susceptibility to thermal stress, a conservative approach should be used for children who exercise in temperature extremes.

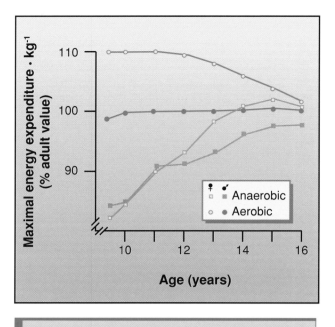

Figure 17.12 Development of aerobic and anaerobic characteristics in boys and girls ages 9 to 16 years. Values are expressed as a percentage of adult values. Adapted from Bar-Or (1983).

Training the Young Athlete

We have seen that, indeed, children are not just miniature adults. The young athlete is physiologically unique from the adult and must be considered differently. But does this mean that special consideration must be given to the young athlete when developing individualized programs of training? Training can improve the strength, aerobic capacity, and anaerobic capacity of the young athlete. Generally, the youngster will adapt well to the same type of training routine used by the mature athlete. But training programs for children and adolescents should be designed specifically for each age group, keeping in mind the developmental factors associated with that age. In this section, we address the issues of most concern for young athletes who are involved in

- resistance (strength) training,
- aerobic training, and
- anaerobic training.

Resistance (Strength) Training

For many years, the use of resistance training to increase muscular strength and endurance in prepubescent and adolescent boys and girls was highly controversial. Boys and girls were discouraged from using free weights for fear that they might injure themselves and prematurely stop the growth process. Furthermore, many scientists speculated that resistance training would have little or no effect on the muscles of prepubescent boys because their levels of circulating androgens were still low.

Studies on animals suggest that heavy-resistance exercise can lead to stronger, broader, and more compact bones. But these studies have not contributed much to our understanding of the benefits or risks associated with this form of activity because it is nearly impossible to load these animals to the same extent as youngsters can be loaded. Fortunately, several studies have been conducted in which both prepubescent and adolescent children have participated in resistance training. From these studies, Kraemer and Fleck have concluded that the risk of injury is very low. In fact, resistance training might offer some protection against injury, for example, by strengthening the muscles that cross a joint. Still, a conservative approach is recommended in prescribing resistance exercise for children, particularly preadolescents.[11]

Several studies conducted in the mid-1980s demonstrated that prepubescent boys and girls can participate safely in resistance training and they can gain substantial strength. In one study, prepubescent boys and girls took part in a 9-week progressive resistance training program.[24] They exercised 25 to 30 minutes per day, 3 days each week. Their mean strength increase was 42.9%, compared to a 9.5% increase in a nontraining control group. In a second study, 16 prepubescent males between ages 6 and 11 participated in a 14-week strength training program using isokinetic techniques with hydraulic resistance, while another 10 boys served as nontraining controls.[25] Isokinetic strength increased between 18% and 37% in the training group, but little or no change was observed in the control group. The authors felt that only one reported injury was related to the strength-training routine. The injured boy missed only three training sessions. Interestingly, an additional six subjects reported injuries from activities of normal daily living, independent of the strength-training program. None of the subjects demonstrated any damage to the epiphyses, bones, or muscles as a result of strength training.

In a final study, 33 prepubescent, pubescent, and postpubescent males underwent a 9-week resistance training program. All three groups had significant strength gains.[17] Researchers hypothesized that the pubescent group would experience the greatest strength gains because testosterone levels increase dramatically during this period, but this was not the case. In fact, the prepubescent group made greater gains than the pubescent group in several of the strength tests.

How are these increases in strength accomplished? The mechanisms allowing strength changes in children are similar to those for adults, with one minor exception: Prepubescent strength gains are accomplished largely without any changes in muscle size.[23] A comprehensive study of the mechanisms responsible for strength increases in prepubescent boys concluded that the likely determinants of the strength gains achieved are[18]

- improved motor skill coordination,
- increased motor unit activation, and
- other undetermined neurological adaptations.

Strength gains in the adolescent result primarily from neural adaptations and increases in both muscle size and specific tension. Kraemer and Fleck have provided a model that integrates various developmental factors that affect a person's potential for muscle strength adaptations with resistance training.[11] This model is illustrated in Figure 17.13. In this model, strength is influenced by the amount of fat-free mass, testosterone concentrations, the extent of nervous system development, and the differentiation of FT and ST muscle fibers. As previously mentioned, the early gains in strength up through puberty are largely the result of changes in neuromuscular patterns.

For actual training programs, resistance training for children should be prescribed in much the same way as is done for adults. Specific guidelines (Table

17.1) were established at a workshop in 1985 by a group representing eight different professional organizations: the American Orthopaedic Society for Sports Medicine, the American Academy of Pediatrics, the American College of Sports Medicine, the National Athletic Trainers Association, the National Strength and Conditioning Association, the President's Council on Physical Fitness and Sports, the U.S. Olympic Committee, and the Society of Pediatric Orthopaedics. Also, Kraemer and Fleck have established basic guidelines for the progression of resistance exercise in children, which are included in Table 17.2.[11] Further information on resistance training program designs for children is available.[9,11,23] Any youth resistance training program must be carefully supervised by competent instructors who have been trained specifically to work with children. Furthermore, resistance training should be only one part of a more comprehensive fitness program for this age group. In the next section we consider the value of aerobic and anaerobic training.

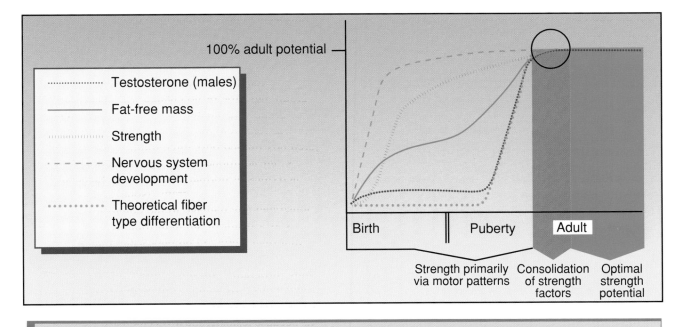

Figure 17.13   A theoretical interactive model that integrates various developmental factors that are related to the potential for muscle strength adaptations with training. Adapted from Kraemer and Fleck (1993).

Table 17.1 Strength Training Recommendations for Prepubescent Children

Equipment
1. Strength-training equipment should be of appropriate design to accommodate the size and degree of maturity of the prepubescent.
2. It should be cost-effective.
3. It should be safe, free of defects, and inspected frequently.
4. It should be located in an uncrowded area free of obstructions with adequate lighting and ventilation.

Program considerations
1. A preparticipation physical exam is mandatory.
2. The child must have the emotional maturity to accept coaching and instruction.
3. There must be adequate supervision by coaches who are knowledgeable about strength training and the special problems of prepubescents.
4. Strength training should be a part of an overall comprehensive program designed to increase motor skills and level of fitness.
5. Strength training should be preceded by a warm-up period and followed by a cool-down.
6. Emphasis should be on dynamic concentric contractions.
7. All exercises should be carried through a full range of motion.
8. Competition is prohibited.
9. No maximum lift should ever be attempted.

Prescribed program
1. Training is recommended two or three times a week for 20- to 30-min periods.
2. No resistance should be applied until proper form is demonstrated. Six to fifteen repetitions equal one set; one to three sets per exercise should be done.
3. Weight or resistance is increased in 1- to 3-lb increments after the prepubescent does 15 repetitions in good form.

Table 17.2 Basic Guidelines for Resistance Exercise Progression in Children

Age (years)	Considerations
7 or younger	Introduce child to basic exercises with little or no weight; develop the concept of a training session; teach exercise techniques; progress from body weight calisthenics, partner exercises, and lightly resisted exercises; keep volume low.
8-10	Gradually increase the number of exercises; practice exercise technique in all lifts; start gradual progressive loading of exercises; keep exercises simple; gradually increase training volume; carefully monitor toleration to the exercise stress.
11-13	Teach all basic exercise techniques; continue progressive loading of each exercise; emphasize exercise techniques; introduce more advanced exercises with little or no resistance.
14-15	Progress to more advanced youth programs in resistance exercise; add sport-specific components; emphasize exercise techniques; increase volume.
16 or older	Move child to entry-level adult programs after all background knowledge has been mastered and a basic level of training experience has been gained.

Note. If a child of any age begins a program with no previous experience, start the child at previous levels and move him or her to more advanced levels as exercise toleration, skill, amount of training time, and understanding permit.

Reprinted from Kraemer and Fleck (1992).

Aerobic and Anaerobic Training

Do prepubescent boys and girls benefit from aerobic training to improve their cardiorespiratory systems? This has also been a highly controversial area because several early studies indicated that training prepubescent children did not change their $\dot{V}O_{2\ max}$ values.[20] Interestingly, even without significant increases in $\dot{V}O_{2\ max}$, the running performance of the children studied did improve substantially. They could run a fixed distance faster following the training program. More recent studies have found small increases in aerobic capacity with training in prepubescent children, but these increases are less than would be expected for adolescents or adults. More

substantial changes in $\dot{V}O_{2\ max}$ appear to occur once children have reached puberty. The reasons for these findings are not well defined at this time. Because stroke volume appears to be the major limitation to aerobic performance in this age group, it is quite possible that further increases in aerobic capacity depend on heart growth.

Anaerobic training appears to improve children's anaerobic capacity. Following training, children have[2,8]

- increased resting levels of phosphocreatine, ATP, and glycogen;
- increased phosphofructokinase activity; and
- increased maximal blood lactate levels.

Ventilatory threshold, a noninvasive marker of lactate threshold, has also been reported to increase with endurance training in 10- to 14-year-old boys.[15]

Growth and Maturation

Many people have wondered what effect physical training might have on growth and maturation. In a comprehensive review of this area, Malina has made some interesting and relevant observations.[16] Regular training has no apparent effect on growth in height. It does, however, affect weight and body composition. Generally, regular training results in

- decreased total body fat,
- increased fat-free mass, and
- increased total body mass.

However, the gains in fat-free mass are generally limited to boys.

As for maturation, the age at which peak height velocity occurs is generally not affected by regular training, nor is the rate of skeletal maturation. But the data concerning the influence of regular training on indices of sexual maturation are not at all clear. Although some data suggest that menarche (the initial onset of menstruation) is delayed in highly trained girls, these data are confounded by a number of factors that weren't controlled for in the analysis. Malina concludes his review with the following statement: ''Responses of the developing individual to the physical activity of regular training are probably not sufficient to alter genotypically programmed growth and maturation processes. Thus, training has no apparent effect on stature and on maturation as ordinarily assessed in growth studies.''[16]

In Closing . . .

In this chapter, we have discussed children and young athletes. We have seen how, as their body systems grow and develop, children gain more control of movements. We have seen how their developing systems can sometimes limit performance capacities and how training can improve children's performances.

We have seen that, in general, the ability to perform increases as children approach physical maturity. But as we move beyond the point of physical maturity, our physiological functioning begins to decline. Having considered the developmental process, we are now ready to consider the aging process. How is performance affected as we move beyond our physiological prime? This will be our focus in the next chapter as we turn our attention to aging and the older athlete.

IN REVIEW . . .

1. Animal studies suggest that resistance training can lead to stronger, broader, more compact bones.
2. The risk of injury from resistance training in young athletes is relatively low and the programs they should follow are much like those of adults.
3. Strength gains achieved from resistance training in preadolescents result primarily from

   - improved motor skill coordination,
   - increased motor unit activation, and
   - other neurological adaptations.

   Unlike in adults, preadolescents who resistance train experience little change in muscle size.
4. Aerobic training in preadolescents does not alter $\dot{V}O_2$ max as much as would be expected for the training stimulus, possibly because $\dot{V}O_2$ max is dependent on heart size. But endurance performance does improve with aerobic training.
5. A child's anaerobic capacity is increased with anaerobic training.
6. Regular training typically results in

   - decreased total body fat,
   - increased fat-free mass, and
   - increased total body mass.

7. In general, growth and maturation rates and processes are probably not altered significantly by training.

Key Terms

development	maturation
diaphysis	myelination
epiphyseal plate	ossification
epiphysis	physical maturity
growth	puberty

Study Questions

1. What is the major concern when a bone that has not reached full growth breaks?
2. At what ages does fat-free body mass reach its peak rate of growth in males and in females?
3. What typical changes occur in fat cells with growth and development?
4. How does pulmonary function change with growth?
5. What changes occur in stroke volume for a fixed rate of work as the child grows? What factors explain these changes?
6. What changes occur in cardiac output for a fixed rate of work as the child grows? What factors explain these changes?

7. What changes occur in submaximal and maximal heart rate as the child grows?

8. Why does absolute aerobic or cardiorespiratory endurance capacity increase from age 6 to age 20?

9. How does the child differ from the adult with respect to thermoregulation?

10. How dangerous is resistance training in children? What advice would you give to these youngsters if they wanted to improve their strength? Can they improve strength, and if so, how does this occur?

11. What happens to aerobic capacity as the prepubescent child trains aerobically?

12. What happens to anaerobic capacity as the prepubescent child trains anaerobically?

13. How does physical activity and regular training affect the growth and maturation processes?

References

1. Adams, J. E. (1965). Injury to the throwing arm. *California Medicine*, **102**, 127-132.

2. Bar-Or, O. (1983). *Pediatric sports medicine for the practitioner: From physiologic principles to clinical applications*. New York: Springer-Verlag.

3. Bar-Or, O. (1989). Temperature regulation during exercise in children and adolescents. In C.V. Gisolfi & D.R. Lamb (Eds.), *Perspectives in exercise science and sports medicine: Youth, exercise and sport* (pp. 335-362). Carmel, IN: Benchmark Press.

4. Bjorntorp, P. (1986). Fat cells and obesity. In K.D. Brownell & J.P. Foreyt (Eds.), *Handbook of eating disorders: Physiology, psychology, and treatment of obesity, anorexia, and bulimia*. New York: Basic Books.

5. Brooks, G.A., & Fahey, T.D. (1984). *Exercise physiology: Human bioenergetics and its applications*. New York: Wiley.

6. Clarke, H.H. (1971). *Physical and motor tests in the Medford Boys' Growth Study*. Englewood Cliffs, NJ: Prentice-Hall.

7. Daniels, J., Oldridge, N., Nagle, F., & White, B. (1978). Differences and changes in $\dot{V}O_2$ among young runners 10 to 18 years of age. *Medicine and Science in Sports and Exercise*, **10**, 200-203.

8. Eriksson, B.O. (1972). Physical training, oxygen supply and muscle metabolism in 11–13-year old boys. *Acta Physiologica Scandinavica*, Suppl. 384.

9. Fleck, S.J., & Kraemer, W.J. (1987). *Designing resistance training programs*. Champaign, IL: Human Kinetics.

10. Inbar, O., & Bar-Or, O. (1986). Anaerobic characteristics in male children and adolescents. *Medicine and Science in Sports and Exercise*, **18**, 264-269.

11. Kraemer, W.J., & Fleck, S.J. (1993). *Strength training for young athletes*. Champaign, IL: Human Kinetics.

12. Krahenbuhl, G.S., Morgan, D.W., & Pangrazi, R.P. (1989). Longitudinal changes in distance-running performance of young males. *International Journal of Sports Medicine*, **10**, 92-96.

13. Larson, R.L. (1974). Physical activity and the growth and development of bone and joint structures. In G.L. Rarick (Ed.), *Physical activity: Human growth and development* (pp. 32-59). New York: Academic Press.

14. Larson, R.L., & McMahan, R.O. (1966). The epiphyses and the childhood athlete. *Journal of American Medical Association*, **196**, 607-612.

15. Mahon, A.D., & Vaccaro, P. (1989). Ventilatory threshold and $\dot{V}O_{2\,max}$ changes in children following endurance training. *Medicine and Science in Sports and Exercise*, **21**, 425-431.

16. Malina, R.M. (1989). Growth and maturation: Normal variation and effect of training. In C.V. Gisolfi & D.R. Lamb (Eds.), *Perspectives in exercise science and sports medicine: Youth, exercise and sport* (pp. 223-265). Carmel, IN: Benchmark Press.

17. Pfeiffer, R.D., & Francis, R.S. (1986). Effects of strength training on muscle development in prepubescent, pubescent, and postpubescent males. *Physician and Sportsmedicine*, **14**(9), 134-143.

18. Ramsay, J.A., Blimkie, C.J.R., Smith, K., Garner, S., MacDougall, J.D., & Sale, D.G. (1990). Strength training effects in prepubescent boys. *Medicine and Science in Sports and Exercise*, **22**, 605-614.

19. Robinson, S. (1938). Experimental studies of physical fitness in relation to age. *Arbeitsphysiologie*, **10**, 251-323.

20. Rowland, T.W. (1985). Aerobic response to endurance training in prepubescent children: A critical analysis. *Medicine and Science in Sports and Exercise*, **17**, 493-497.

21. Rowland, T.W. (1989). Oxygen uptake and endurance fitness in children: A developmental perspective. *Pediatric Exercise Science*, **1**, 313-328.

22. Rowland, T.W. (1991). ''Normalizing'' maximal oxygen uptake, or the search for the holy grail (per kg). *Pediatric Exercise Science*, **3**, 95-102.

23. Sale, D.G. (1989). Strength training in children. In C.V. Gisolfi & D.R. Lamb (Eds.), *Perspectives in*

exercise science and sports medicine: Youth, exercise and sport (pp. 165-216). Carmel, IN: Benchmark Press.

24. Sewall, L., & Micheli, L.J. (1986). Strength training for children. *The Journal of Pediatric Orthopaedia Strabismus*, **6**, 143-146.

25. Weltman, A., Janney, C., Rians, C.B., Strand, K., Berg, B., Tippitt, S., Wise, J., Cahill, B.R., & Katch, F.I. (1986). The effects of hydraulic resistance strength training in pre-pubertal males. *Medicine and Science in Sports and Exercise*, **18**, 629-638.

Selected Readings

Albinson, J.G., & Andrew, G.M. (1976). *Child in sport and physical activity*. Baltimore: University Park Press.

Åstrand, I. (1967). *Aerobic work capacity: Its relation to age, sex, and other factors* (Monograph No. 15). New York: American Heart Association.

Berg, K., & Eriksson, B.O. (Eds) (1980). *Children and exercise IX*. Baltimore: University Park Press.

Binkhorst, R.A., Kemper, H.C.G., & Saris, W.H.M. (Eds.) (1985). *Children and exercise XI*. Champaign, IL: Human Kinetics.

Blimkie, C.J.R. (1993). Resistance training during pre-adolescence: Issues and controversies. *Sports Medicine*, **16**, 389-407.

Boileau, R.A. (Ed.) (1984). *Advances in pediatric sport sciences: Vol. 1*. Champaign, IL: Human Kinetics.

Cronk, C.E., & Roche, A.F. (1982). Race and sex-specific reference data for triceps and subscapular skin folds and weight/stature². *American Journal of Clinical Nutrition*, **35**, 347-354.

Ekblom, B. (1969). Effect of physical training in adolescent boys. *Journal of Applied Physiology*, **27**, 350-355.

Forbes, G.B. Growth of the lean body mass during childhood and adolescence. *Journal of Pediatrics*, **64**, 822-827.

Gisolfi, C.V., & Lamb, D.R. (Eds.) (1989). *Perspectives in exercise science and sports medicine: Youth, exercise and sport*. Carmel, IN: Benchmark Press.

Krahenbuhl, G.S., Skinner, J.S., & Kohrt, W.M. (1985). Developmental aspects of maximal aerobic power in children. *Exercise and Sports Sciences Reviews*, **13**, 503-538.

Malina, R.M. (Ed.) (1988). *Young athletes: Biological, psychological, and educational perspectives*. Champaign, IL: Human Kinetics.

Malina, R.M., & Bouchard, C. (1991). *Growth, maturation, and physical activity*. Champaign, IL: Human Kinetics.

Oseid, S., & Carlsen, K.-H. (Eds.) (1989). *Children and exercise XIII*. Champaign, IL: Human Kinetics.

Rowland, T.W. (1990). Developmental aspects of physiological function relating to aerobic exercise in children. *Sports Medicine*, **10**, 255-266.

Rowland, T.W. (1990). *Exercise and children's health*. Champaign, IL: Human Kinetics.

Rutenfranz, J., Mocellin, R., & Klimt, F. (Eds.) (1986). *Children and exercise XII*. Champaign, IL: Human Kinetics.

Shephard, R.J. (1992). Effectiveness of training programmes for prepubescent children. *Sports Medicine*, **13**, 194-213.

Stull, G.A., & Eckert, H.M. (Eds.) (1986). *Effects of physical activity on children*. Champaign, IL: Human Kinetics.

Vaccaro, P., & Mahon, A. (1987). Cardiorespiratory responses to endurance training in children. *Sports Medicine*, **4**, 352-363.

Washington, R.L. (1989). Anaerobic threshold in children. *Pediatric Exercise Science*, **1**, 244-256.

Weltman, A. (1989) Weight training in prepubertal children: Physiologic benefit and potential damage. In O. Bar-Or (Ed.), *Advances in pediatric exercise sciences* (pp. 101-129). Champaign, IL: Human Kinetics.

Zanconato, S., Buchthal, S., Barstow, T.J., & Cooper, D.M. (1993). P-magnetic resonance spectroscopy of leg muscle metabolism during exercise in children and adults. *Journal of Applied Physiology*, **74**, 2214-2218.

Zauner, C.W., Maksud, M.G., & Melichna, J. (1989). Physiological considerations in training young athletes. *Sports Medicine*, **8**, 15-31.

Zwiren, L.D. (1989). Anaerobic and aerobic capacities of children. *Pediatric Exercise Science*, **1**, 31-44.

Chapter 18
Aging and the Older Athlete

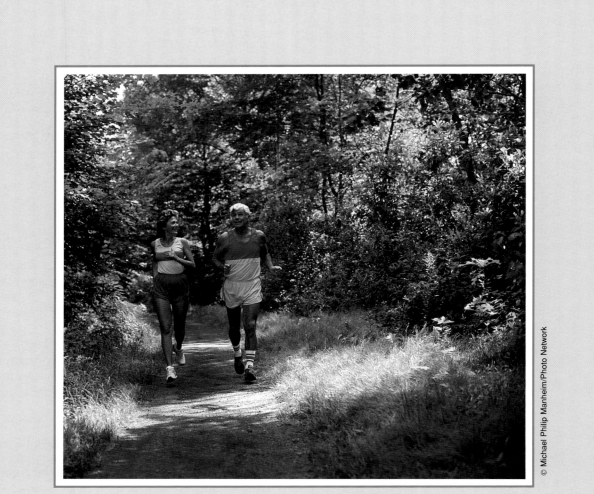

© Michael Philip Manheim/Photo Network

Chapter Overview

The number of adult men and women participating in competitive sports has increased dramatically over the past 20 years. Although many of these older competitors, often termed Masters athletes, engage in competition for recreation and fitness, others train with the same enthusiasm and intensity as young Olympians. Opportunities are now available for older adult athletes to compete in a wide variety of activities, including marathon running and weight lifting. The success and the standards of performance set by these Masters athletes are exceptional and often beyond comprehension. However, although these older athletes exhibit strength and endurance capacities that are far greater than those of untrained people of similar age, even the most highly trained older person experiences a decline in performance after the fourth or fifth decade of life.

What physiological changes occur during aging that affect exercise tolerance? Does intense physical activity pose any health risks in aging athletes? How trainable are middle-aged and older adults? We will attempt to answer these questions in this chapter. We begin by examining sports performance in older adults, then we consider age-related changes in cardiorespiratory endurance, muscle strength, tolerance of environmental stress, and body composition—and how these changes can affect performance. Finally, we consider how training can improve the older athlete's performance.

Few athletes continue to compete into middle and old age. One exception was the classic case of Clarence DeMar, who won his seventh Boston Marathon at age 42, placed 7th at age 50, and was 78th in a field of 153 runners at the age of 65. In all, he ran more than 1,000 distance races, including more than 100 marathons between 1909 and 1957, a period when it was not popular to exercise or engage in competition as an adult. His performances at the Boston Marathon alone spanned 48 years, from age 20 to 68. DeMar's last race in 1957, at age 68, was 15 km, which he ran despite advanced intestinal cancer and a colostomy. His best time for the Boston Marathon was 02:29:42 at age 36. Thereafter, his time gradually slowed to 03:58:37 at age 66.

$\bigvee$oluntary participation in strenuous physical activity on a regular basis is an unusual pattern of behavior that is not observed in most aging animals. Studies have shown that humans and lower animal forms tend to decrease their physical activity as they grow older. As shown in Figure 18.1, rats that were allowed to exercise freely ran an average of 28 to 29 mi (about 46 km) per week in the early months of life, but covered only 2 to 4 mi (about 3 to 6 km) per week during their final months.[14] In this regard, humans and rats have much in common.

In modern societies, the level of voluntary physical activity begins to decline soon after people reach adult maturity. In many ways we try to eliminate all forms of stress from our lives, including muscular effort. Technology has made virtually every aspect of life less physically demanding. Thus, older men and women who choose to participate in competitive sports or to train exhaustively do not follow natural human behavior patterns. Why do some older individuals choose to remain physically active when the natural tendency is to become sedentary? The psychological factors that motivate these older athletes, or Masters athletes, to compete are not clearly defined, but these athletes' goals probably do not differ substantially from those of their younger counterparts.

Considering the importance of exercise for maintaining muscle and cardiorespiratory health, it is not surprising that adult inactivity can lead to deterioration of one's capacity and tolerance for strenuous effort. Because of this, distinguishing between the effects of aging and those of reduced activity is difficult when studying lifelong changes in physiological function and physical performance. How does aging affect sport performance?

Sport Performance

Records in running, swimming, cycling, and weight lifting suggest that we are in our physical prime during our late 20s or early 30s. Using a cross-sectional approach, comparing these records with national and world records for Masters athletes in these events allows us to examine the effects aging has on the best performers. Unfortunately, we have little longitudinal information about the effects of aging on performance, because few studies have enabled us to follow physical performance in selected individuals over the span of their athletic careers. In the following sections, we will consider how aging affects certain types of physical performance.

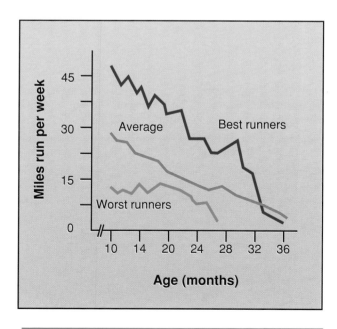

Figure 18.1 Voluntary running activity in rats throughout life. Adapted from Holloszy et al., (1985).

Running Performance

Running performance decreases with age, and the rate of this decline appears to be independent of distance.

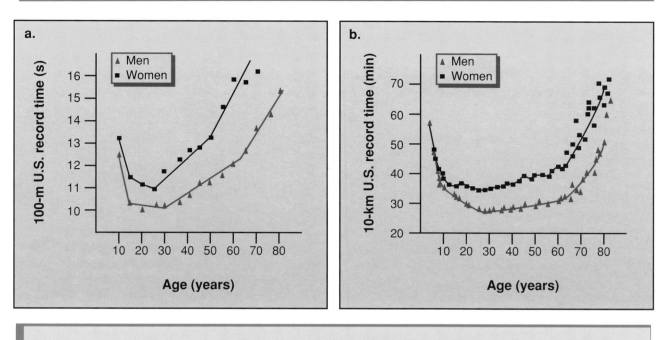

Figure 18.2   Change with age in men's and women's records for 100-m and 10-km runs. Adapted from Costill (1986).

Performance records for both 100-m and 10-km runs decrease by about 1% per year from age 25 to age 60, as shown in Figure 18.2. Beyond age 60, the records for men slow by nearly 2% per year. A sprint-running test of 560 women between ages 30 and 70 revealed a steady decrease in maximal running velocity of 8.5% per decade.[23] The patterns of change are about the same in both sprint- and endurance-running performances.

Swimming Performance

Swimming performance is affected by the aging process in much the same manner as running. As noted in Figure 18.3, average velocities for record performances in the 100-m front crawl decrease by about 1% per year for both men and women from age 25 to age 75. Because success in this sport depends on skill, as well as on strength and endurance, some Masters swimmers have achieved their personal best performances at 45 to 50 years of age. As an example, the data in Table 18.1 illustrate a male swimmer's best performances at age 20 and at age 50. Despite a 30-year lapse in swimming training, this swimmer was able to achieve his best performances when he resumed training at age 50. Although the precise reasons for these improvements are unknown, we can logically assume that they are the combined result of improvements in swimming technique, training methods, and swimming facilities, with little decrease in physiological capacity.

Cycling Performance

As with other strength and endurance sports, record-setting cycling performances are generally achieved in the age range of 25 to 35. Male and female cyclists' records (based on 40-km races) drop at about the same rate with age, an average of 20 s (approximately 0.6%)

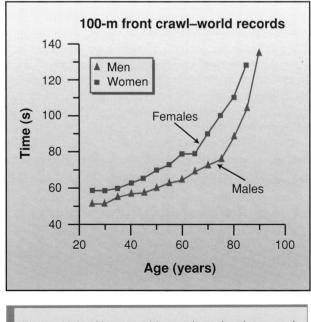

Figure 18.3   Changes with age in swimming records among Masters-level competitors.

Table 18.1 Swimming Performances at Age 20 and 50 Years for a Male Masters Swimmer

Distance (m)	Best performance (s)		Improvement %
	20 years	50 years	
50	27.2	26.5	2.6
100	62.7	60.3	3.8
200	147.8	137.7	6.8
400	318.8	288.9	9.4
1,500	1,403.0	1,227.0	12.5

Note. The best freestyle swimming (front crawl stroke) times were achieved at age 50, despite the fact that the swimmer was an accomplished collegiate swimmer at age 18 to 21 years. It is also interesting to mention that this swimmer trained by swimming about 1,500 meters per day at the age of 20 yr and 2,500 meters per day at age 50 yr.

Data from Ball State University, Human Performance Laboratory.

per year. The U.S. national cycling records for 20 km show a similar pattern for both men and women. For this distance, speed decreases by about 12 s (approximately 0.7%) per year from age 20 to nearly age 65.

Weight Lifting

In general, maximum muscle strength is achieved between the ages of 25 and 35. Beyond that age range, as noted in Figure 18.4, men's records for the sum of four power lifts decline at a steady rate of about 12.1 kg (approximately 1.8%) per year. Of course, as with other measurements of human performance, individual strength performances vary considerably. Some individuals, for example, exhibit greater strength at age 60 than people half their age.

Thus, most athletic performance declines at a steady rate during middle and advanced ages. This results from decrements in both muscular and cardiovascular endurance and strength. In the following discussion, we will turn our attention to the underlying physiological causes of these changes.

█ KEY POINT █

As we age, peak performances in both endurance and strength events decrease by about 1% to 2% per year, starting between ages 20 and 35.

Changes in Cardiorespiratory Endurance With Aging

To a large extent, endurance performance changes that accompany aging can be attributed to decrements in both central and peripheral circulation. Measurements

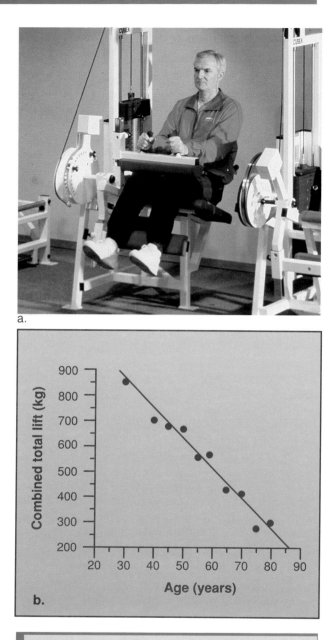

a.

b.

Figure 18.4 (a) An older athlete performing resistance training. (b) Changes in U.S. National Masters powerlifting records with age among male weight lifters. The values reported are combined totals for the squat, bench press, and deadlift.

of cardiac output and limb blood flow are not easily performed, so early studies of the effects of aging on the physiology of endurance exercise examined maximal oxygen uptake ($\dot{V}O_2$ max), which correlates well with cardiac output. More recently, efforts have been made to determine cardiac output and oxygen exchange in the leg muscles of exercising older subjects. Unfortunately, the number of such studies is limited. Consequently, our explanation of the decline in endurance performance among older men and

Table 18.2 Changes in $\dot{V}_{O_2 \, max}$ Among Normally Active Men

Age (years)	$\dot{V}_{O_2 \, max}$ (ml · kg^{-1} · min^{-1})	% change from 25 years
25	47.7	0
35	43.1	-9.6
45	39.5	-17.2
52	38.4	-19.5
63	34.5	-27.7
75	25.5	-46.5

women will, for the most part, be limited to the changes in maximal oxygen uptake (aerobic capacity).

Studies of Normally Active People

The first studies of aging and physical fitness were performed by Sid Robinson in the late 1930s.[25] He demonstrated that maximal oxygen uptake in normally active men declined steadily from age 25 to age 75 (Table 18.2). His cross-sectional data suggested that aerobic capacity declines an average of about 1% per year (10% per decade). This is the same rate of decline seen in endurance running, swimming, and cycling performances. More recently, a review of 11 cross-sectional studies, most involving men under age 70, examined the rate of decline in $\dot{V}_{O_2 \, max}$ with aging.[5] These studies indicated that the average rate of decrease in $\dot{V}_{O_2 \, max}$ for these men was about 0.8% to 1.1% per year.

Unfortunately, few longitudinal studies have been conducted in this area. Studies that have reexamined normally active men at various stages of their lives reveal a wide range of decline for aerobic capacity.[3,8,21] At least part of these variations can be attributed to the different activity levels and initial ages of the subjects. Nevertheless, the rate of decline in $\dot{V}_{O_2 \, max}$ is generally agreed to be approximately 10% per decade (−0.4 ml · kg^{-1} · min^{-1} per year) in relatively sedentary men.

It has been shown that, on the average, women demonstrate a lower rate of $\dot{V}_{O_2 \, max}$ decline than men during aging, approximately 0.2 to 0.5 ml · kg^{-1} · min^{-1} per year.[5] However, some studies suggest that there are no differences between men and women with regard to the decrease in aerobic capacity with age.[6,31] For example, a longitudinal study of 35 Swedish women revealed that, after 21 years, the women's $\dot{V}_{O_2 \, max}$ values had decreased by an average of 0.44 ml · kg^{-1} · min^{-1} per year, a rate that does not differ significantly from that reported for men. In fact, when calculated in terms of fat-free mass, $\dot{V}_{O_2 \, max}$ shows little gender difference with aging.

When comparing $\dot{V}_{O_2 \, max}$ values in men and women, comparisons per unit of body weight might not be accurate. Humans generally gain body weight during aging, and this tends to falsely lower $\dot{V}_{O_2 \, max}$ values, exaggerating the effects of aging. In addition, comparisons of such $\dot{V}_{O_2 \, max}$ values do not take into consideration the individuals' initial $\dot{V}_{O_2 \, max}$ values. For example, a decrease of 0.5 ml · kg^{-1} · min^{-1} per year would have more impact on a person who had an initial $\dot{V}_{O_2 \, max}$ of only 30 ml · kg^{-1} · min^{-1} than it would on someone with an initial value of 50 ml · kg^{-1} · min^{-1}. For these reasons, we should compare groups of people in terms of the percentage of change in their $\dot{V}_{O_2 \, max}$ values. This calculation is derived as follows:

$$\% \text{ change} = \frac{\text{final } \dot{V}_{O_2 \, max} - \text{initial } \dot{V}_{O_2 \, max}}{\text{initial } \dot{V}_{O_2 \, max}} \times 100$$

When percentage of change in $\dot{V}_{O_2 \, max}$ during aging is compared for men and women, both show a decline of about 1% per year. This decline is caused primarily by a reduction in maximum heart rate and stroke volume. These reductions decrease cardiac output, which limits oxygen transport to the muscles.

KEY POINT

$\dot{V}_{O_2 \, max}$ decreases by about 10% per decade with aging, starting in the late teens for women and in the mid-20s for men. This decrease is largely associated with a decrease in cardiorespiratory endurance activity.

Studies of Older Athletes

Sport physiology is a relatively new field—few laboratories were working in this field during the first half of this century. As a result, few longitudinal studies have been conducted on aging in athletes. The sparse data published about older athletes is typically limited to periods of 10 to 16 years. Pollock et al., for example, studied 24 older track athletes (ages 50 to 82) to evaluate the relationship between age and training over a 10-year period.[24] During that period, only 11 of the athletes remained highly competitive. The other 13 participants quit competing and reduced their training intensity. Those who continued to compete maintained their $\dot{V}O_2$ max values, but those who quit and reduced their training showed a significant decrease in $\dot{V}O_2$ max over the 10-year period. However, other changes were the same in both groups:

- Maximum heart rate decreased by about 7 beats per minute.
- Body weight decreased slightly from an average of 70.0 kg to 68.9 kg.
- Body fat increased significantly, from about 13.1% to 15.1%.

So even though both groups showed signs of aging, aging alone might not necessarily decrease aerobic capacity. When the intensity and volume of training are kept at a high level, $\dot{V}O_2$ max remains unchanged.

KEY POINT

For those older endurance athletes who maintain a high-intensity training program and continue high-level competition, $\dot{V}O_2$ max declines very little, if at all, at least over a period of from 10 to 15 years.

Figure 18.5 illustrates the changes in $\dot{V}O_2$ max among groups of untrained men, joggers, and highly trained runners. Although endurance training appears to offer a substantial aerobic advantage, aging seems to induce a similar decrease in $\dot{V}O_2$ max during middle age. Some caution must be used in drawing conclusions from these findings because the older runners and joggers probably didn't train with the same intensity and duration as the younger athletes. At least part of the decline in aerobic endurance with age might be related to the intensity and quantity of training performed.

Recently, highly competitive Masters distance runners were reexamined in a 25-year–follow-up study [DLC, unpublished]. These men were initially tested at 18 to 25 years of age. During the interval between testing sessions, the runners trained at about the same relative intensity as they did when they were younger. As a consequence, their $\dot{V}O_2$ max values have remained relatively constant, as shown in Table 18.3. Although their maximal oxygen uptake decreased from 69.0 to 64.3 ml · kg^{-1} · min^{-1}, most of that was due to a 2.1-kg increase in body weight. Thus, the actual change

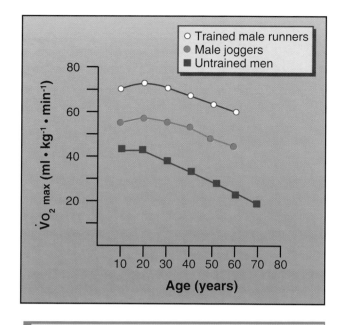

Figure 18.5 Changes in $\dot{V}O_2$ max with age for trained and untrained males.

in $\dot{V}O_2$ max (L · min^{-1}) over the 25-year span of this study averaged −3.6%. This is a decrease of only 0.14% per year (1.4% per decade).

This rate of decrease in the older athletes' $\dot{V}O_2$ max values is significantly less than the rate of decrease in either sedentary people or those who are fitness trained at levels and intensities below those of older athletes. In fact, one of these older runners performed a 4 min 11 s mile and a 2 hr 29 min marathon in 1992 at the age of 46! Both of these performances were significantly faster than his best in 1966. Similar findings have been reported for other athletes who have continued to train with the same relative intensity and volume as they did in college.

Are these performances exceptions to the natural rules of aging? Can other athletes reduce the effects of aging on their endurance by continuing to train intensely? Much depends on the training adaptability of the individual athlete, a factor that might be determined as much by heredity as by training regimen.

One of the most notable long-term studies with distance runners and aging was conducted by D.B. Dill and his colleagues from the Harvard Fatigue Laboratory.[9] Don Lash, world record holder for the 2-mi run (8 min 58 s) in 1936, was among those studied by the Harvard group. Although few of the former runners continued to train after leaving college, Lash was still running about 45 min per day at age 49. Despite this activity, his $\dot{V}O_2$ max had declined from 81.4 ml · kg^{-1} · min^{-1} at age 24 to 54.4 ml · kg^{-1} · min^{-1} at age 49, a 33% decline. As expected, runners who

Table 18.3 Changes in Aerobic Capacity ($\dot{V}_{O_2}$ max) and Maximal Heart Rates During Aging in a Group of Highly Trained Masters Distance Runners ($n = 10$)

Age (years)	Weight (kg)	$\dot{V}_{O_2}$ max ($L \cdot min^{-1}$)	$\dot{V}_{O_2}$ max ($ml \cdot kg^{-1} \cdot min^{-1}$)	HR max (beats $\cdot$ min^{-1})
21.3 (±1.6)	63.9 (±2.2)	4.41 (±.09)	69.0 (±1.4)	189 (±6)
46.3 (±1.3)	66.0 (±0.6)	4.25 (±.05)	64.3 (±0.8)	180 (±6)

Note. Values are ± SE.

did not continue to train during middle age showed much larger declines. On the average, their aerobic capacities declined by about 43% from age 23 to age 50 (70 to 40 ml $\cdot$ kg^{-1} $\cdot$ min^{-1}). These data suggest that prior training offers little advantage to endurance capacity in later life unless a person continues to engage in some form of vigorous activity.

But again questions must be asked: How much of the observed decrease in $\dot{V}_{O_2}$ max is a result of biological aging? How important is the habitual level of physical activity in determining the rate of decline? Norwegian studies provided insight into these questions when they compared the $\dot{V}_{O_2}$ max values for a group of 63 cross-country skiers, ages 50 to 66, with groups of office workers and industrial workers of similar ages, and with a group of 20- to 30-year-old students.[1] Their findings are shown in Table 18.4. This study supports the contention that the decline in $\dot{V}_{O_2}$ max with age is not strictly a function of age, although the possibility that heredity might be an important factor cannot be discounted.

IN REVIEW . . .

1. Much of the decline in endurance performance associated with aging can be attributed to decrements in central and peripheral circulation.
2. Aerobic capacity generally decreases by about 10% per decade in relatively sedentary men.
3. When evaluating decreases in $\dot{V}_{O_2}$ max with aging in men and women, comparisons per unit of body weight might not be accurate, because we tend to gain weight as we age, which falsely lowers the $\dot{V}_{O_2}$ max per unit of body weight, and these values do not account for a person's initial $\dot{V}_{O_2}$ max.
4. Instead, comparison should be based on the percentage of change in $\dot{V}_{O_2}$ max.
5. Studies with older athletes and less active people of the same age group indicate that the decrease in $\dot{V}_{O_2}$ max is not strictly a function of age. Athletes who continue to train have significantly less of a decrease in $\dot{V}_{O_2}$ max as they age.

KEY POINT

Because of their similarities, it is often difficult to differentiate between biological aging and physical inactivity. With aging, there is a natural deterioration in physiological function, but this is compounded by the fact that we also become more sedentary as we age.

Respiratory Changes With Aging

What are the underlying physiological causes for the decrease in cardiorespiratory endurance with aging? Lung function might be partly to blame because it can change considerably in sedentary people during aging. Both vital capacity (VC, the total volume of air expelled after maximal inhalation) and forced expiratory volume in 1 s (FEV$_{1.0}$, the volume of air exhaled in the first second after maximal inhalation) decrease linearly with age, starting at age 20 to 30. While these decrease, residual volume (RV, the amount that cannot be exhaled) increases and the total lung capacity remains unchanged. As a result, the ratio of the residual volume to total lung capacity (RV:TLC) increases, meaning that less air can be exchanged. In the early 20s, residual volume accounts for 18% to 22% of the total lung capacity, but this increases to 30% or more as we reach age 50. Smoking appears to accelerate this increase.

Table 18.4 Comparison of Aerobic Capacities for Four Groups of Norwegians

Group	Age range (years)	$\dot{V}_{O_2}$ max ($ml \cdot kg^{-1} \cdot min^{-1}$)
Skiers	50 – 66	48
Office workers	50 – 60	36
Industrial workers	50 – 60	34
Students	20 – 30	44

These changes are matched by changes in maximal ventilatory capacity during exhaustive exercise. Maximal expiratory ventilation ($\dot{V}_E$ max, the maximal volume of air that can be breathed in 1 min) increases until physical maturity, then decreases with aging. For males, $\dot{V}_E$ max values average about 40 L · min^{-1} for 4- to 6-year-old boys, increase to 110 to 140 L · min^{-1} at full maturity, then decrease to 60 to 80 L · min^{-1} for 60- to 70-year-olds. Females follow the same general pattern, although their absolute values are considerably lower at each age, primarily because of smaller stature.

These changes in pulmonary function among physically inactive men and women are probably the result of several factors. The most important of these is loss of elasticity of the lung tissue and chest wall as we age, which increases the work involved in breathing. The resulting stiffening of the chest wall appears to be responsible for most of the reduction in lung function. But despite all these changes, the lungs still hold a remarkable reserve and maintain an adequate diffusion capacity to permit maximal exertion.

During middle and older age, endurance training reduces the loss of elasticity from the lungs and chest wall. As a result, endurance-trained older athletes have only slightly decreased pulmonary ventilation capacities. Decreased aerobic capacity among these older athletes cannot be attributed to changes in external respiration. Also, during strenuous exercise, both normally active people and Masters athletes can reach near-maximal arterial oxygen saturation (97% saturation).[27] Thus neither changes in the lungs nor in the blood's oxygen-carrying capacity appear to be responsible for the observed drop in $\dot{V}O_2$ max reported in aging athletes.

Rather, the primary limitation is apparently linked with oxygen transport to the muscles. The maximum a-$\bar{v}O_2$ diff is lower in these athletes than in younger people, suggesting that less oxygen is extracted by our muscles as we age.

Cardiovascular Changes With Aging

As shown in Figure 18.6, cardiovascular function also changes as we age. One of the most notable changes that accompanies aging is a decrease in maximum heart rate (HR max). Whereas these values in children frequently exceed 200 beats per minute, the average 60 year old has a HR max of approximately 160 beats per minute. Maximum heart rate is estimated to decrease slightly less than one beat per minute per year as we age. The average HR max for any age can be estimated from the following equation:

$$HR \text{ max} = 220 - age$$

The reduction in HR max with age appears to be similar in both sedentary and highly trained adults. At age 50, for example, normally active men have the same HR max values as former and still-active distance runners of the same age. This reduction in maximum heart rate might be attributed to morphological and electrophysio-

---

■■■ IN REVIEW . . . ■■■

1. Both vital capacity and forced expiratory volume decrease linearly with age. Residual volume increases, and total lung capacity remains unchanged. This increases the RV:TLC ratio, meaning that less air can be exchanged with each breath.
2. Maximal expiratory ventilation also decreases with age.
3. Pulmonary changes that accompany age are primarily caused by a loss of elasticity in the lung tissue and the chest wall. However, older athletes have only slightly decreased pulmonary ventilation capacity. For them, the primary limiter of $\dot{V}O_2$ max appears to be decreased oxygen transport to the muscles. Furthermore, a-$\bar{v}O_2$ diff is decreased, indicating that less oxygen is extracted by their muscles.

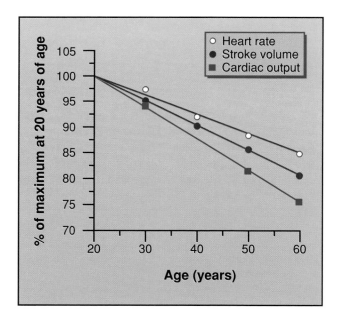

Figure 18.6 Effects of aging on maximal values for cardiac output, stroke volume, and heart rate.

The equation used to estimate HR max is:

$$HR_{max} = 220 - age$$

However, this only estimates the average value for a given age. Individual values can deviate by ±20 beats per minute or more from the predicted value. For example, the equation predicts that a 60 year old would have a HR max of 160 beats per minute, but actual HR max might be as low as 140 beats per minute or as high as 180 beats per minute.

logical alterations in the cardiac conduction system, specifically in the SA node and in the bundle of His, that could slow cardiac conduction.[19] There also appears to be down-regulation of the beta-1 receptors in the heart, decreasing the heart's sensitivity to catecholamine stimulation.

Maximum stroke volume and cardiac output also appear to decrease with age. Unfortunately, research in this area is limited. Studies on endurance runners have shown that the lower $\dot{V}O_2$ max observed in older athletes results from a reduction in maximal cardiac output, despite the fact that heart volumes of older athletes are similar to those of young athletes. Saltin has reported that 51-year-old orienteers (distance runners) have a maximal cardiac output that is about 5 L · min⁻¹ (21%) lower than young orienteers.[26] This difference is due to the older athletes' lower maximum heart rates and reduced maximal stroke volumes (recall that cardiac output = heart rate × stroke volume). Lower stroke volumes in older athletes are caused primarily by increased peripheral resistance. But when compared to sedentary men of the same age, these active older orienteers had markedly higher maximal oxygen uptake values, primarily because they had greater stroke volumes and thus also greater maximal cardiac outputs than their sedentary peers.

Stroke volume can be maintained well among middle-aged and older adults who continue to train intensely.[26] The heart size in older orienteers, for example, is similar to that in younger endurance athletes.[28] Heath et al. observed that left ventricular end-diastolic volumes were greater in trained older athletes than in sedentary men of the same body size and age.[12] This suggests that these athletes' stroke volumes are well maintained with aging, but are still less than those of younger athletes.

Peripheral blood flow, such as to the leg, decreases with aging, even though capillary density in the muscles

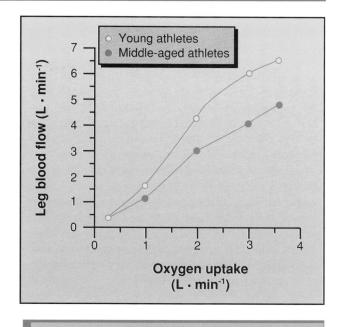

Figure 18.7   Leg blood flow during cycling exercise in young athletes and middle-aged athletes (data are from orienteers). Adapted from Saltin (1986).

is unchanged. Studies reveal a 10% to 15% reduction in blood flow to the exercising muscles in middle-aged athletes at any given work rate when compared to well-trained young athletes (Figure 18.7).[17,32] But the reduced blood flow to the legs of middle-aged endurance runners appears to be compensated for by a greater a-$\bar{v}O_2$ diff (more oxygen is extracted by the muscles). As a result, though the blood flow is different, oxygen uptake by the exercising muscles is similar at a given submaximal work intensity in both age groups.

Why, then, do maximal cardiac output and $\dot{V}O_2$ max decrease with age? One explanation is that aging causes increased peripheral resistance. With age, arteries and arterioles begin to lose their elasticity and become less capable of vasodilation. This increases peripheral resistance, and as a result, blood pressure is increased at rest and during exercise. Although older athletes have slightly lower mean arterial pressures than most sedentary men, they still have more peripheral resistance than younger athletes, which limits their stroke volume capacity.

Thus the gradual decline in maximal cardiac output and oxygen uptake among aging Masters athletes appears to be the result of restrictions placed on both the heart's pumping capacity and peripheral blood flow. It is hard to determine whether the age-related decreases in stroke volume, cardiac output, and peripheral blood flow result from the aging process or from cardiovascular deconditioning that accompanies reduced activity. Recent studies suggest that both are

KEY POINT

The decrease in $\dot{V}O_2$ max with aging and inactivity is largely explained by a decrease in HR max, SV max, and a-$\bar{v}O_2$ diff. The decrease in HR max is due largely to decreases in sympathetic nervous system activity and alterations in the cardiac conduction system. The decrease in SV max is due primarily to increased total peripheral resistance due to a reduced compliance in the arteries with aging and to possible reductions in left ventricular contractility. The decrease in a-$\bar{v}O_2$ diff is related to the reduction in blood flow to the active muscles, which is possibly due to the reduced cardiac output (both HR and SV are reduced, so cardiac output must also be reduced).

IN REVIEW . . .

1. Maximum heart rate decreases slightly less than one beat per minute per year as we age. The average HR max for a certain age can be estimated by the following equation: HR max = 220 − age.
2. Maximal stroke volume and cardiac output also appear to decrease with age. Stroke volume can be well maintained in older athletes who have continued to train, but it will still be less than in younger athletes.
3. Peripheral blood flow also decreases with age; however, in trained older athletes this is offset by an increased submaximal a-$\bar{v}O_2$ diff.
4. It is unclear how much of the decrease in cardiovascular function with aging is due to physical aging alone and how much is due to deconditioning because of decreased activity. However, many studies indicate that these changes are minimized in older athletes who continue to train, which seems to indicate that inactivity might play a larger role than physical aging.

involved, but the relative contribution of each is unknown. However, even the Masters athlete trains less than a 20-year-old athlete. Aging alone might decrease cardiorespiratory function and endurance less than the deconditioning that accompanies inactivity or decreased activity.

Thus, the decline in endurance performance, aerobic capacity, and cardiovascular function are likely more the result of a decrease in activity than of aging. Decreased physical activity, weight gain, and age-related changes in the respiratory and cardiovascular systems combine to decrease $\dot{V}O_2$ max in men by about 10% per decade after age 25. If body composition and physical activity are kept constant, deterioration due to the aging process per se results in a $\dot{V}O_2$ max decrease of only about 5% per decade. Some research indicates that Masters athletes who train with the same intensity and volume as their younger counterparts can have as little as a 1% to 2% decrease in aerobic capacity per decade until age 50. Nevertheless, in later life, after around ages 55 to 65, cardiovascular capacity will be reduced as a result of a lower maximum heart rate.

Changes in Strength With Aging

The level of strength needed to meet the daily demands of living remains unchanged throughout life. However, a person's maximal strength, generally well above the daily demands early in life, decreases steadily with aging. For example, the ability to stand from a sitting position is compromised at age 50, and by age 80 this task becomes impossible for some people. Older adults are typically able to engage in activities that require only moderate amounts of muscle strength. As an example, opening the cap on a jar that has a set resistance is a task that can easily be accomplished by 92% of

men and women in the age range of 40 to 60. But after age 60 the failure rate for this task increases dramatically.[27] By the time these individuals reach the age of 71 to 80, only 32% will be able to open the jar.

Similar data, shown in Figure 18.8, describe leg strength changes in aging adults. Knee extension strength in normally active men and women decreases rapidly after age 45 to 50. But strength training the knee extensor muscles enables the older adult male to perform better at age 60 than most normally active men at half that age.

Age-related losses of muscle strength result primarily from the substantial loss of muscle mass that accompanies aging or decreased physical activity. Sedentary older adults can show both a large loss in muscle mass and an increase in subcutaneous fat. Figure 18.9 shows a computerized tomographic (CT) scan of the upper arm in three 57-year-old men of similar body weight (about 78 to 80 kg). Note that the sedentary subject had substantially less muscle and more fat than the others. The swimming-trained subject had less fat and a markedly larger triceps muscle than the untrained subject, but his biceps muscle, which is seldom used during swimming, was not much different. Strength training, however, enlarged both of these muscles in the strength-trained subject.

There are conflicting results about the effects of aging on the composition of slow- and fast-twitch fibers. Cross-sectional studies that have examined the entire vastus lateralis (quadriceps) muscle in postmor-

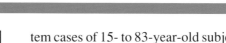

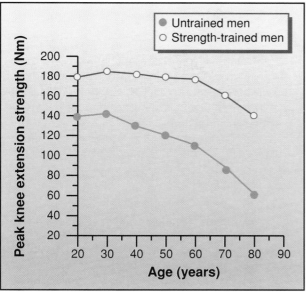

Figure 18.8   Changes in peak knee extension strength in untrained and trained men at various ages.

tem cases of 15- to 83-year-old subjects have suggested that fiber type remains unchanged throughout life.[16] In addition, cross-sectional studies with younger and older elite distance runners support this finding. However, measurements from the same people over an 18-year period indicate that amount or intensity of activity or perhaps both might play an important role in fiber-type distribution with aging.[30] Muscle biopsy samples from the gastrocnemius (calf) muscles of a group of previously elite distance runners obtained in 1974 and again in 1992 demonstrated that if training intensity and duration were maintained, fiber-type composition remained unchanged over the 18-year period (Figure 18.10). On the other hand, if a person's activity had decreased to a recreational level or ceased completely, the percentage of slow-twitch fibers was increased. Though the influence of aging on muscle fiber composition remains a bit unclear, it is generally agreed that normally active individuals have a shift toward a higher percentage of slow-twitch fibers with advancing age. These data indicate that the stimulus to the muscle (activity) plays a role in the distribution of fiber type with aging.

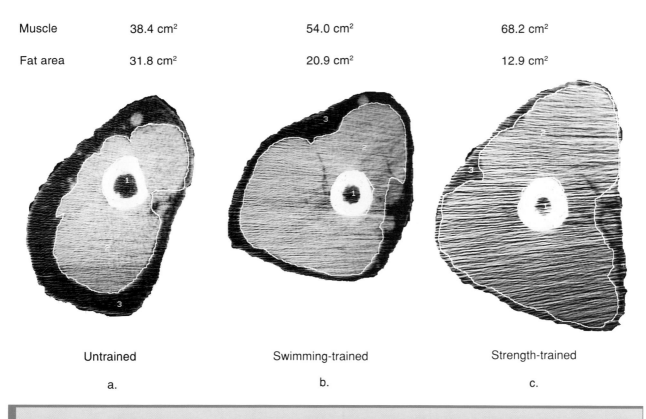

Muscle	38.4 cm²		54.0 cm²	68.2 cm²
Fat area	31.8 cm²		20.9 cm²	12.9 cm²

Untrained	Swimming-trained	Strength-trained
a.	b.	c.

Figure 18.9   CT scans of the upper arm of three 57-year-old males with similar body weights. The scans show (1) bone, (2) muscle, and (3) subcutaneous fat. Note the difference in the muscle area when the person is (a) untrained, (b) swimming-trained, and (c) strength-trained.

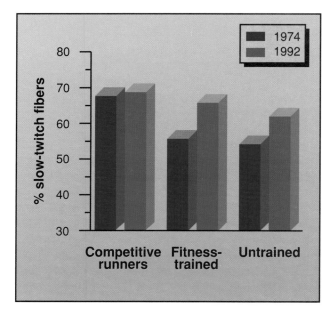

Figure 18.10 Changes in muscle fiber–type composition of the gastrocnemius in elite distance runners who remained competitive, stayed fitness-trained, or became untrained.

It has been suggested that the apparent increase in slow-twitch fibers is probably due to an actual decrease in the number of fast-twitch fibers, resulting in a greater proportion of slow-twitch fibers. Although the precise cause of this fast-twitch-fiber loss is unclear, it has been suggested that the number of fast-twitch motor neurons decreases during aging, which eliminates innervation of these muscle fibers. Fibers that cannot be activated gradually atrophy and eventually are absorbed by the body.

Documentation from numerous investigations has shown that a decrease in both the number and size of muscle fibers occurs with aging. Research indicates that approximately 10% of the total number of muscle fibers are lost per decade after age 50.[20] This might explain, in part, the muscle atrophy that occurs as we get older. Additionally, it appears that the size of both slow-twitch and fast-twitch fibers decreases with aging. But this seems to be offset by training, because the decline in fiber cross-sectional area is not as dramatic in physically active subjects.

Studies have also shown that aging is accompanied by substantial changes in the nervous system's capacity to process information and to activate muscles. Specifically, aging affects the ability to detect a stimulus and process the information to produce a response. Simple and complex movements are slowed

with aging, though people who remain physically active are only slightly slower than younger, active individuals.

These neuromuscular changes during aging are at least partially responsible for decreased strength and endurance, but active participation in sports tends to lessen aging's impact on performance. This doesn't mean that biological aging can be arrested by regular physical activity, but many of the decrements in physical work capacity can be markedly reduced by an active lifestyle.

Saltin has noted that despite the loss of muscle mass in aging men, the quality of the remaining muscle mass is well maintained.[26] The number of capillaries per unit area is similar in young and old endurance runners. Oxidative enzyme activities in the muscles of endurance-trained older athletes is only 10% to 15% lower than in young athletes. Thus oxidative capacity of skeletal muscle of older endurance-trained runners is only slightly less than in young elite runners, which suggests that aging has little effect on skeletal muscle's adaptability to endurance training.

Environmental Stress and Aging

Because a variety of physiological control processes become less effective with aging, we can logically assume that older people will be less tolerant of environmental stress than their younger counterparts. In the following discussion, we will compare the responses of younger and older adults during exposure to altitude and heat stress. Unfortunately, no specific studies have been done to examine the tolerance of older athletes to these environmental conditions, so only responses in healthy untrained adults can be reported here.

Exposure to Altitude

With the strenuous demands of exercise at moderate or high altitude, we might assume that normally active older adults would be at a disadvantage during exposure to the hypobaric conditions of altitude. Surprisingly, the opposite might be true. Many anecdotal stories have detailed the mountain climbing exploits of people who range in age from 70 to 90 years.[4] Though most of these efforts have been at less than 4,500 m, a 52-year-old American was able to climb to the top of Mt. Everest (8,848 m, or 29,030 ft).

As we saw in chapter 12, acute altitude sickness is the major problem confronting most trained and untrained mountain climbers. Onset of acute altitude sickness occurs within 6 to 96 hr after ascent and is characterized by such symptoms as headache, insomnia, loss of appetite, nausea, dizziness, and lassitude. A small percentage of cases rapidly progress into life-threatening high-altitude pulmonary edema (HAPE) or cerebral edema (HACE). Surprisingly, people below age 20 are more prone to HAPE than are older people.[15,29] The incidence of HAPE is generally about 50 cases per 100,000 people, but for those under age 14 it is 140 per 100,000.[29] Some evidence indicates that we might tend to outgrow this predisposition to develop HAPE, so increased age alone should not deter healthy adults from activities at altitude. In fact, aging might provide some protection against the symptoms of acute altitude sickness and high-altitude pulmonary edema.

Exposure to Heat

Exposure to heat stress presents a problem for older people. Considerable evidence indicates that older adults are more susceptible to fatal heat injuries than are younger people.[2,13] Measurements of heat stress in older and younger subjects show that aging reduces thermal tolerance. Even when matched for body size, body composition, $\dot{V}O_{2\,max}$, and degree of acclimatiza-tion, these age-related differences still persist. Both at rest and during submaximal exercise, older subjects develop a higher internal body temperature when exposed to heat than their younger counterparts. Part of the explanation for this is that older adults produce less sweat, decreasing their capacity for heat loss via evaporation.

KEY POINT

Aging does not appear to reduce our capacity to perform normal activity at high altitude. In fact, it might enhance our capacity! However, aging reduces our ability to adapt to exercise in the heat. This is largely because sweating capacity decreases as we age.

Most of these observations were made with normally active subjects. Thus we can't determine what influence varying lifestyles and activity levels might have had on these results. Unfortunately, no comparable data exist for highly trained young and old athletes. Knowing the positive influence that regular exercise, heat exposure, and endurance training have on heat tolerance, we can only assume that the negative effects of environmental heat stress would be reduced in these older athletes.

IN REVIEW . . .

1. Older people are generally less tolerant of environmental stress.
2. Some cases of acute altitude sickness progress to life-threatening conditions of high-altitude pulmonary edema or high-altitude cerebral edema. But these conditions are more common in young people. Aging might provide some protection against acute altitude sickness and high-altitude pulmonary or cerebral edema.
3. Aging reduces thermal tolerance partly because aging reduces sweat production; consequently, less heat can be lost via evaporation.

Body Composition and Aging

How much fat our bodies accumulate as we grow and age depends on our individual dietary and exercise habits, in addition to our heredity. As we saw in chapter 16, although heredity is unchangeable, our fat stores can be altered through diet and exercise. Figure 18.11 illustrates the relationship between percent body fat and age, showing that the amount of relative body fat increases with age after physical maturity. This is largely due to three factors that occur with aging:

1. Increased dietary intake
2. Decreased physical activity
3. Reduced ability to mobilize fat

Beyond age 30, fat-free mass also decreases progressively. This results primarily from the decreased muscle mass discussed earlier and from bone mineral loss. Both of these conditions result, at least partially, from decreased physical activity.

Normally active and sedentary men and women gradually gain body weight from age 20 to age 70, despite a gradual reduction in fat-free body tissue—muscle and bone. But this age-related tendency for greater fatness and less fat-free body mass is not constant throughout life. Figure 18.12 illustrates the changes in one man's fat-free mass, body weight, and relative body fat from age 35 to age 75.

As one might anticipate, the body fat content of physically active people is significantly lower than that of age-matched sedentary men and women. Highly trained runners at an average age of 45 years, for example, have been reported to average 11% body fat in men and 18% body fat in women. These values are considerably lower than those reported for sedentary people of similar age: 19% in men and 26% in women. Interestingly, older competitive swimmers (average age 50 for men and 43 for women) have less body fat than age-matched but sedentary people, yet these athletes are fatter on the average than a group of equally fit distance runners, with the swimmers averaging 15% body fat in men and 23% in women.

Although these values for both the runners and swimmers are lower than those for normal, sedentary adults of similar ages, older athletes have substantially more body fat than younger competitors. Nevertheless, compared to age-matched sedentary people, the older athletes' lower body fat levels undoubtedly result from their higher caloric expenditure rate and, often, conscious monitoring of their dietary habits.

KEY POINT

With age, body fat content increases, while at the same time fat-free mass decreases. Much of this can be attributed to the reduction in general activity levels that occurs with aging.

Trainability of the Older Athlete

Despite the decrements associated with aging, middle-aged and older athletes are capable of exceptional per-

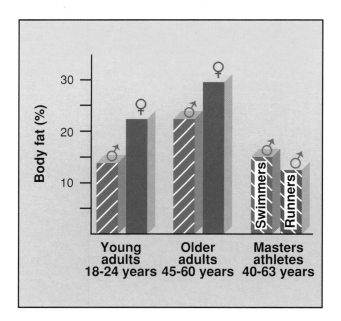

Figure 18.11 Changes with age in relative body fat for normally active young adults and for normally active older adults, compared to values for Master-level runners and swimmers.

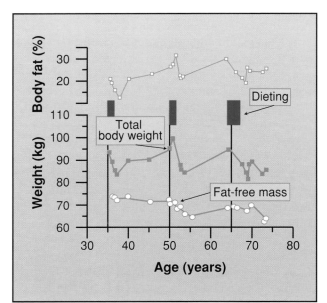

Figure 18.12 Variations in one man's relative body fat, total body weight, and fat-free mass throughout his adult life.

IN REVIEW . . .

1. The amount of relative body fat increases as we age, primarily because of

   - increased dietary intake,
   - decreased physical activity, and
   - a reduced ability to mobilize fat.

2. Beyond age 30, fat-free mass decreases, primarily because of decreased muscle mass and decreased bone mass, both resulting at least partly from decreased activity.

3. Training can help delay these changes in body composition.

formances. Their ability to adapt to endurance and strength training is well documented. Recent studies have shown that improvements in $\dot{V}O_{2\,max}$ with training are similar for younger (age 21 to 25) and older (age 60 to 71) men and women.[18,22] Although the pretraining $\dot{V}O_{2\,max}$ values were, on the average, lower for the older subjects, the absolute increase of 5.5 to 6.0 ml · kg^{-1} · min^{-1} was similar in both groups. Additionally, older men and women experienced similar increases in $\dot{V}O_{2\,max}$, averaging 21% for men and 19% for women, when they trained for 9 to 12 months by walking, running, or both about 4 mi (about 6 km) per day. This research indicates that endurance training produces similar gains in aerobic capacity in healthy people throughout the age range of 20 to 70 years, and this adaptation is independent of age, gender, and initial fitness level. However, this does not mean that endurance training can enable older athletes to achieve the performance standards established by younger athletes.

The precise mechanisms that trigger the body's adaptations to training at any age are not fully understood, so we don't know if improvements from training are achieved in the same way throughout life. For example, much of the improvement in $\dot{V}O_{2\,max}$ seen in younger subjects is associated with an increase in maximal cardiac output. But older subjects show significantly greater gains in muscle oxidative enzyme activities, which suggests that peripheral factors in older subjects' muscles might play greater roles in aerobic adaptations to training than in younger subjects.

As noted earlier, loss of strength might be attributed to a combination of aging and reduced physical activity that produces a decline in muscle function. But, although it is difficult to compare the adaptations to strength training in younger and older people, aging appears neither to impair the ability to improve muscle

strength nor to prevent muscle hypertrophy. For example, when older men (ages 60 to 72) strength trained for 12 weeks at 80% of their one repetition maximum for extension and flexion of both knees, their extension strength increased by 107% and flexion strength increased by 227%.[10] This improvement was attributed to muscle hypertrophy, as determined from midthigh CT scans. Biopsies of the vastus lateralis muscle (in the quadriceps) revealed that the cross-sectional area of slow-twitch fibers increased by 33.5% and that of fast-twitch fibers increased by 27.6%.

A study with older women (average age 72) who performed an aerobic-resistance program for 50 weeks found a 6% increase in leg strength at the end of the period. This was accompanied by a significant increase (29%) in cross-sectional area of only the FT fibers.[7] Many people believe that the degree of strength gains and muscle hypertrophy might be less in older women than in older men, but there are too few data to reinforce such a claim.

KEY POINT

The ability to adapt to training has been thought to greatly decrease with aging. Recent studies, however, where older subjects were trained at relatively high intensities indicate that older people have considerable ability to increase their endurance capacity or strength with training.

Regular physical activity is an important contributor to good health, so we can logically ask, "Does training throughout adulthood affect longevity?" Because the aging rate in rats is more rapid than in humans, they have been used as subjects in studies conducted to determine the influence of chronic exercise (training) on longevity. A study by Goodrick demonstrated that rats who exercised freely lived about 15% longer than sedentary rats did.[11] But an investigation at Washington University in St. Louis showed no significant increase in the life span of rats who voluntarily ran on an exercise wheel.[14] More of the active rats lived to old age, but, on the average, they still died at the same age as their sedentary counterparts. Interestingly, the rats that had a restricted food intake and maintained a lower body weight lived 10% longer than the freely eating sedentary rats.

Of course, we cannot simply apply these findings to humans, but these results raise some interesting questions that might be relevant to our health and longevity. Although it is true that an endurance exercise program can reduce a number of the risk factors associated with cardiovascular disease, there is only limited information to support the contention that you will live longer if you exercise regularly. Data collected from the alumni at Harvard University and the University of Pennsylvania, and from participants at the Aerobic Center in Dallas suggest that there is a decrease in the mortality rate and a small increase in longevity (about 2 years) among people who remain physically active throughout life. Perhaps future longitudinal studies will shed more light on the relationship between lifelong exercise and longevity.

IN REVIEW . . .

1. Endurance exercise training produces similar gains in healthy people, regardless of their age, gender, or initial level of fitness.
2. With endurance training, older individuals show greater improvement in their muscles' oxidative enzyme activities, whereas improvement in younger people is largely due to increased maximal cardiac outputs.
3. It appears that aging does not impair a person's ability to increase muscle strength or muscle hypertrophy.

In Closing . . .

In this chapter we have examined the effects of aging on physical performance. We have evaluated changes in cardiorespiratory endurance and in strength. We have considered the effect of aging on body composition, which we know can affect performance. And yet, throughout our discussion, it became clear that much of the change that occurs with aging is to a great extent due to the inactivity that often accompanies aging. When older people participate in training, most of the changes associated with aging are lessened. Thus we have dispelled many of the myths about the capacity for physical activity in older people.

In the next chapter, we turn our attention to another group that is often considered less capable of physical activity than young males are. We will consider the unique physiology of women, how this uniqueness affects their athletic ability, and how performances of women athletes compare to those of men.

Key Terms

cardiovascular deconditioning
forced expiratory volume ($FEV_{1.0}$)
longevity
maximal expiratory ventilation ($\dot{V}E_{max}$)
percentage of change in $\dot{V}O_{2\,max}$
peripheral blood flow
residual volume (RV)
total lung capacity (TLC)
vital capacity (VC)

Study Questions

1. Describe the changes in strength and endurance performance records with aging.
2. What cardiovascular changes occur during aging? How do these changes affect maximal oxygen uptake?
3. Describe the changes in $\dot{V}O_{2\,max}$ with age. How do trained individuals differ from untrained subjects?
4. How does the respiratory system change with aging? What happens to VC, $FEV_{1.0}$, RV, RV:TLC, and $\dot{V}E_{max}$?
5. Describe the changes in HR_{max} with age. How does training alter this relationship?
6. How does aging affect maximal stroke volume and maximal cardiac output? What mechanisms can potentially explain these changes?
7. What muscular changes occur with aging? How do they affect athletic performance?
8. How does training alter the biology of aging?
9. Differentiate between biological aging and physical inactivity.
10. What influence does aging and training have on body composition?
11. Describe the trainability of the older individual for both strength and endurance.

References

1. Anderson, K., & Hermansen, L. (1965). Aerobic work capacity in middle-aged Norwegian men. *Journal of Applied Physiology*, **20**, 432-436.

2. Applegate, W.B., Runyan, J.W., Brasfield, L., Williams, M.L., Konigsberg, C., & Fauche, C. (1981). Analysis of the 1980 heat wave in Memphis. *Journal of the American Geriatrics Society*, **29**, 337-342.

3. Åstrand, I., Åstrand, P.-O., Hallback, I., & Kilbom, A. (1973). Reduction in maximal oxygen intake with age. *Journal of Applied Physiology*, **35**, 649-654.

4. Balcomb, A.C., & Sutton, J.R. (1986). Advanced age and altitude illness. In J.R. Sutton & R.M. Brock (Eds.), *Sports medicine for the mature athlete*. Indianapolis, IN: Benchmark Press.

5. Buskirk, E.R., & Hodgson, J.L. (1987). Age and aerobic power: The rate of change in men and women. *Federation Proceedings*, **46**, 1824-1829.

6. Cempla, J., & Szopa, J. (1985). Decrease of maxi-

mum oxygen consumption in men and women during the fourth to sixth decades of life, in the light of cross-sectional studies of Cracow population. *Biology in Sport*, **2**, 45-59.

7. Cress, M.E., Thomas, D.P., Johnson, J., Kasch, F.W., Cassens, R.G., Smith, E.L., & Agre, J.C. (1991). Effect of training on V̇O₂ max, thigh strength, and muscle morphology in septuagenarian women. *Medicine and Science in Sports and Exercise*, **23**, 752-758.

8. Dill, D.B., Alexander, W.C., Myhre, L.G., Whinnery, J.E., & Tucker, D.M. (1985). Aerobic capacity of D.B. Dill, 1928-1984. *Federation Proceedings*, **44**, 1013 (abst).

9. Dill, D.B., Robinson, S., & Ross, J.C. (1967). A longitudinal study of 16 champion runners. *Journal of Sports Medicine and Physical Fitness*, **7**, 4-27.

10. Frontera, W.R., Meredith, C.N., O'Reilly, K.P., Knuttgen, W.G., & Evans, W.J. (1988). Strength conditioning in older men: Skeletal muscle hypertrophy and improved function. *Journal of Applied Physiology*, **64**, 1038-1044.

11. Goodrick, C.L. (1980). Effects of long-term voluntary wheel exercise on male and female Wistar rats l. Longevity, body weight and metabolic rate. *Gerontology*, **26**, 22-33.

12. Heath, G.W., Hagberg, J.M., Ehsani, A.A., & Holloszy, J.O. (1981). A physiological comparison of young and older endurance athletes. *Journal of Applied Physiology: Respiratory Environmental Exercise Physiology*, **51**, 634-640.

13. Henschel, A., Burton, L., & Morgalies, L. (1969). An analysis of the deaths in St. Louis during July 1966. *American Journal of Public Health*, **59**, 2232-2240.

14. Holloszy, J.O., Smith, E.K., Vining, M., & Adams, S. (1985). Effect of voluntary exercise on longevity of rats. *Journal of Applied Physiology*, **59**, 826-831.

15. Hultgren, H.N., & Marticorena, E.M. (1978). High altitude pulmonary edema: Epidemiologic observations in Peru. *Chest*, **74**, 372-376.

16. Johnson, M.A., Polgar, J., Weihtmann, D., & Appleton, D. (1973). Data on the distribution of fiber types in thirty-six human muscles: An autopsy study. *Journal of Neurological Science*, **1**, 111-129.

17. Jorfeldt, L., & Wahren, J. (1971). Leg blood flow during exercise in man. *Clinical Science*, **41**, 459-473.

18. Kohrt, W.M., Malley, M.T., Coggan, A.R., Spina, R.J., Ogawa, T., Ehsani, A.A., Bourey, R.E., Martin, W.H. III, & Holloszy, J.O. (1991). Effects of gender, age, and fitness level on response of V̇O₂ max to training in 60-71 yr olds. *Journal of Applied Physiology*, **71**, 2004-2011.

19. Lakatta, E.G. (1979). Alterations in the cardiovascular system that occur in advanced age. *Federation Proceedings*, **38**, 163-167.

20. Lexell, J., Taylor, C.C., & Sjostrom, M. (1988). What is the cause of the aging atrophy? Total number, size, and proportion of different fiber types studied in whole vastus lateralis muscle from 15- to 83-year-old men. *Journal of Neurological Science*, **84**, 275-294.

21. McKeen, P.C., Rosenberger, J.L., Slater, J.S., Nicholas, W.C., & Buskirk, E.R. (1985). A 13-year follow-up of a coronary heart disease risk factor screening and exercise program for 40- to 59-year-old men: Exercise habit maintenance and physiologic status. *Journal of Cardiac Rehabilitation*, **5**, 10-599.

22. Meredith, C.N., Frontera, W.R., Fisher, E.C., Hughes, V.A., Herland, J.C., Edwards, J., & Evans, W.J. (1989). Peripheral effects of endurance training in young and old subjects. *Journal of Applied Physiology*, **66**, 2844-2849.

23. Meusel, H. (1984). *Health and well-being for older adults through physical exercises and sports—Outline of Giessen model. Sports and aging.* Champaign, IL: Human Kinetics.

24. Pollock, M.L., Foster, C., Knapp, D., Rod, J.L., & Schmidt, D.H. (1987). Effect of age and training on aerobic capacity and body composition of master athletes. *Journal of Applied Physiology*, **62**, 725-731.

25. Robinson, S. (1938). Experimental studies of physical fitness in relation to age. *Arbeitsphysiologie*, **10**, 251-323.

26. Saltin, B. (1986). The aging endurance athlete. In J.R. Sutton & R.M. Brock (Eds.), *Sports medicine for the mature athlete*. Indianapolis, IN: Benchmark Press.

27. Saltin, B. (1990). *Aging, health and exercise performance*. Provost Lecture Series, Muncie, IN: Ball State University.

28. Saltin, B., & Grimby, G. (1968). Physiological analysis of middle-aged and old former athletes. *Circulation*, **38**, 1104-1115.

29. Scoggin, E.H., Meyers, T.M., Reeves, J.T., & Grover, R.F. (1977). High-altitude edema in young adults of Leadville, Colorado. *New England Journal of Medicine*, **297**, 1269-1272.

30. Trappe, S.W., Costill, D.L., Fink, W.J., Pearson, D.R, & Vukovich, M.D. (1993). Effects of aging on muscle atrophy morphology: A longitudinal analysis. *Medicine and Science in Sports and Exercise*, **25**, S161.

31. von Dobeln, W. (1957). Human standard and maximal metabolic rate in relation to fat-free body mass. *Acta Physiologica Scandinavica*, (Suppl. 126), 37-79.

32. Wahren, J., Saltin, B., Jorfeldt, L., & Pernow, B. (1974). Influence of age on the local circulatory adaptation to leg exercise. *Scandinavian Journal of Clinical Laboratory Investigation*, **33**, 79-86.

Selected Readings

Aniansson, A. (1980). *Muscle function in old age with special reference to muscle morphology, effect of training and capacity in activities of daily living.* Unpublished doctoral dissertation, University of Goteborg, Goteborg.

Åstrand, I. (1960). Aerobic work capacity in men and women with special reference to age. *Acta Physiologica Scandinavica*, **49**(Suppl. 169), 11.

Benestad, A. (1965). Trainability of old men. *Acta Medica Scandinavica*, **178**, 321.

Blair, S.N., Kohl, H.W. III, Paffenbarger, R.S., Clark, D.G, Cooper, K.H., & Gibbons, L.W. (1989). Physical fitness and all-cause mortality: A prospective study of healthy men and women. *JAMA*, **262**, 2395-2401.

Child, J.S., Barnard, R.J., & Taw, R.L. (1984). Cardiac hypertrophy and function in master endurance runners and sprinters. *Journal of Applied Physiology: Respiratory Environmental Exercise Physiology*, **57**, 176-181.

Coggan, A.R., Spina, R.J., Rogers, M.A., King, D.S., Brown, M., Nemeth, P.M., & Holloszy, J.O. (1990). Histochemical and enzymatic characteristics of skeletal muscle in master athletes. *Journal of Applied Physiology*, **68**, 1896-1901.

Costill, D.L. (1986). *Inside running: Basics of sports physiology.* Indianapolis, IN: Benchmark Press.

Costill, D.L., King, D., Hargreaves, M., & Holdren, A. (1984). The facts are in: Stress those sprint muscles and increase performance. *Swim Swim*, **6**, 13-14.

deVries, H.A. (1970). Physiological effects of an exercise training regimen upon men aged 52 to 88. *Journal of Gerontology*, **25**, 325-336.

deVries, H.A. (1980). *Physiology of exercise for physical education and athletics* (3rd ed.). Dubuque, IA: Brown.

Drinkwater, B.L., Bedi, J.F., Loucks, A.B., Roche, S., & Horvath, S.M. (1982). Sweating sensitivity and capacity of women in relation to age. *Journal of Applied Physiology*, **53**, 671-676.

Drinkwater, B.L., Horvath, S.M., & Wells, C.L. (1975). Aerobic power of females, ages 10 to 68. *Journal of Gerontology*, **30**, 385-394.

Ehsani, A.A., Ogawa, T., Miller, T.R., Spina, R.J., & Jilka, S.M. (1991). Exercise training improves left ventricular systolic function in older men. *Circulation*, **83**, 96-103.

Hagberg, J.M. (1987). Effect of training on the decline of $\dot{V}O_{2\ max}$ with aging. *Federation Proceedings*, **46**, 1830-1833.

Kenny, M.J., & Gisolfi, C.V. (1986). Thermal regulation: Effects of exercise and age. In J.R. Sutton & R.M. Brock (Eds.), *Sports medicine for the mature athlete.* Indianapolis, IN: Benchmark Press.

Kenny, W.L. & Hodgson, J.L. (1987). Heat tolerance, thermoregulation and aging. *Sports Medicine*, **4**, 446-456.

Larsson, L. (1978). Morphological and functional characteristics of the aging skeletal muscle in man. *Acta Physiologica Scandinavica*, (Suppl. 457), 36.

Ogawa, T., Spina, R.J., Martin, W.H. III, Kohrt, W.M., Schechtman, K.B., Holloszy, J.O., & Ehsani, A.A. (1992). Effects of aging, sex, and physical training on cardiovascular responses to exercise. *Circulation*, **86**, 494-503.

Orlander, J., & Aniansson, A. (1979). Effects of physical training on skeletal muscle metabolism and ultrastructure in 70 to 75-year-old men. *Acta Physiologica Scandinavica*, **109**, 149-154.

Paffenbarger, R.S., Hyde, R.T, Wing, A.L., & Hsieh, C.-C. (1986). Physical activity, all-cause mortality, and longevity of college alumni. *New England Journal of Medicine*, **314**, 605-613.

Pollock, M.L., Miller, H.S., Linnerud, A.C., & Cooper, K.H. (1975). Frequency of training as a determinant for improvement in cardiovascular function and body composition of middle-aged men. *Archives of Physical Medicine and Rehabilitation*, **56**, 141-145.

Pollock, M.L., Miller, H.S., & Wilmore, J.H. (1974). Physiological characteristics of champion American track athletes 40 to 75 years of age. *Journal of Gerontology*, **29**, 645-649.

Roberts, M.A., King, D.S., Hagberg, J.M., Ehsani, A.A., & Holloszy, J.O. (1990). Effect of 10 days of physical inactivity on glucose tolerance in master athletes. *Journal of Applied Physiology*, **68**, 1833-1837.

Rogers, M.A., Hagberg, J.M., Martin, W.H., Ehsani, A.A., & Holloszy, J.O. (1990). Decline in $\dot{V}O_{2\ max}$ with aging in master athletes and sedentary men. *Journal of Applied Physiology*, **68**, 2195-2199.

Seals, D.R., Hagberg, J.M., Hurley, B.F., Ehsani, A.A. & Holloszy, J.O. (1984). Endurance training in older men and women. I. Cardiovascular responses to exercise. *Journal of Applied Physiology: Respiratory Environmental Exercise Physiology*, **57**, 1024-1029.

Shephard, R.J. (1984). Physiological aspects of sport and physical activity in the middle and later years of life. In B. McPherson (Ed.) *Sport and Aging*. Champaign, IL: Human Kinetics Publishers.

Siegel, W., Blomquist, G., & Mitchell, J.H. (1970). Effects of a quantitated physical training program on middle-aged sedentary men. *Circulation*, **41**, 19-29.

Spirduso, W.W. (1975). Reaction and movement time as a function of age and physical activity level. *Journal of Gerontology*, **30**, 435.

Sutton, J.R., & Brock, R.M. (1986). *Sports medicine for the mature athlete*. Indianapolis, IN: Benchmark Press.

Young, K., & Young, J.H. (1985). *Running records by age: 1985*. Tuscon, AZ: National Running Data Center.

Chapter 19

Gender Issues
and the Female Athlete

■

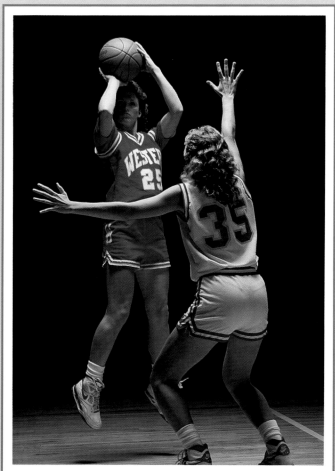

© F-Stock/Brian Drake

Chapter Overview

In the not-so-distant past, young girls were typically encouraged to play with dolls, play house, and play dress up while young boys climbed trees, raced against each other, and became active in various sports. The underlying notion was that boys were meant to be athletic but girls were weaker, frailer, and less well suited to physical activity. Physical education classes furthered this idea by having the girls exercise differently than the boys—by running shorter distances, performing modified push-ups, and doing fewer chin-ups. Less physical activity was expected of girls. And indeed, as they progressed through school, most girls could not compete on an equal basis with boys of their same age, even if given the opportunity.

But times have changed and more athletic activities are accessible to girls and women than in the past, and the results have often been surprising. This has led researchers to ask how much of the difference in the performance capabilities of females and males is due to biological differences. In this chapter, we will try to answer this question. We will probe the similarities and differences between females and males in physique and body composition as well as in physiological responses to acute exercise and to training. We will also consider gender differences in motor skills and athletic ability. Finally, we will review several areas of concern that are unique to female athletes, including menstruation and menstrual dysfunction, pregnancy, osteoporosis, eating disorders, and interaction with the environment, and we will consider how these factors affect the performance of female athletes.

Chapter Outline

Girls and women were prohibited from running any race longer than 800 m until the 1960s. They were also barred from official participation in the marathon until 1970. Both of these restrictions resulted from a misconception that women were physiologically unsuited for endurance activity. Yet at the 1984 Los Angeles Olympic Games, American runner Joan Benoit won the gold medal in the first-ever Olympic marathon for women, with a time of 02:24:52. Her time would have won 11 of the previous 20 men's Olympic marathons![22]

On the basis of world records in 1991, the female, compared to her male counterpart,

- ran 6.4% slower in the 100-m dash and 11.0% slower in the 1,500-m run,
- jumped 14.3% lower in the high jump, and
- swam 8.4% slower in the 400-m free-style swim.

Do these performance differences result from biological differences? Or do they reflect social and cultural restrictions placed on females during preadolescent and adolescent development? Our focus in this chapter is the extent to which biological differences between females and males affect performance capacity. Let's begin by considering basic physical differences and their impact on performance.

Body Size and Composition

Until age 12 to 14—around puberty—males and females do not differ substantially in

- height,
- weight,
- girth,
- bone width, and
- skinfold thickness.

A study of 609 normal boys and girls ages 7.5 to 20.5 found no gender differences in fat-free mass (FFM) prior to adolescence when FFM was expressed per unit of height.[15] At ages 12 to 13, the fat-free mass to height ratio in females begins to plateau, but in males it continues to increase to age 20. Female FFM peaks at age 15 to 16, but male FFM doesn't peak until age 18 to 20. The peak FFM attained by females is 72% of the FFM attained by males. These changes in FFM with age are illustrated in Figure 19.1.

Body density data are somewhat inconsistent with these findings. Females typically have lower total body density values at all ages, including preadolescence, which would normally indicate a higher relative body fat. But from age 7 to age 25, the density of the fat-free mass in females is consistently lower than in males.[25] The calculations used to determine relative body fat typically assume that these densities are the same in both sexes. As a result, most existing data on females in this age range overestimate their true relative body fat.

At puberty, the body compositions of the sexes begin to differ markedly, primarily because of endocrine changes. Prior to puberty, the anterior pituitary gland does not secrete gonadotropic hormones—follicle-stimulating hormone (FSH) and luteinizing hormone (LH). These hormones stimulate the gonads (ovaries and testes). During puberty, however, the anterior pituitary begins to secrete both of these hormones. In females, when sufficient quantities of FSH

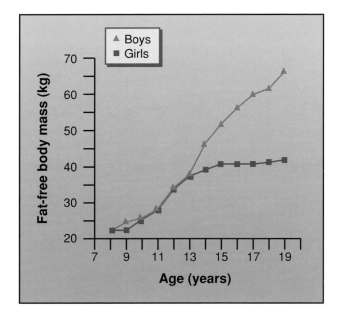

Figure 19.1 Gender differences with aging in fat-free body mass changes. Data from Forbes (1972).

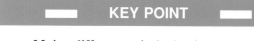

KEY POINT

Major differences in body size and composition between girls and boys do not start to appear until the time of puberty.

and LH are secreted, the ovaries develop and estrogen secretion begins. In males, these same hormones trigger development of the testes and, in turn, testosterone secretion. Testosterone causes increased bone formation, which leads to larger bones, as well as increased protein synthesis, which leads to increased muscle mass. As a result, adolescent males are larger and more muscular than females, and these characteristics continue into adulthood.

Estrogen also has a significant influence on body growth by broadening the pelvis, stimulating breast development, and increasing fat deposition, particularly in the thighs and hips. This increase in fat deposition in the thighs and hips is the result of increased lipoprotein lipase activity in these areas. This enzyme is considered the gatekeeper for storing fat in adipose tissue. Lipoprotein lipase is produced in the fat cells (adipocytes) but is bound to the walls of the capillaries where it exerts its influence on the chylomicrons, which are the major transporters of triglycerides in the blood. When lipoprotein lipase activity in any area of the body is high, chylomicrons are trapped and their triglycerides are hydrolyzed and transported into the adipocytes in that area for storage.

Many women are constantly fighting fat deposition on the thighs and hips, but they are usually fighting a losing battle. Lipoprotein lipase activity is very high and lipolytic activity low in the hips and thighs of women, compared to their other fat storage areas and to the hips and thighs of men. This results in a rapid storage of fat in women's thighs and hips, and the decreased lipolytic activity makes it difficult for women to lose fat from these areas. During the last trimester of pregnancy and throughout lactation, the activity of lipoprotein lipase drops and lipolytic activity increases dramatically, which suggests that fat is stored in the hips and thighs for reproductive purposes.

Estrogen also increases the growth rate of bone, allowing the final bone length to be reached within 2 to 4 years following the onset of puberty. As a result, females grow very rapidly for the first few years following puberty, then cease to grow. Males have a much longer growth phase, allowing them to attain a greater height. Because of these differences, compared to fully mature males, fully mature females are on average nearly

- 13 cm (5 in.) shorter,
- 14 to 18 kg (30 to 40 lb) lighter in total weight,
- 18 to 22 kg (40 to 50 lb) lighter in FFM,
- 3 to 6 kg (7 to 13 lb) heavier in fat mass, and
- 6% to 10% higher in relative body fat.

Anthropometric measurements at maturity differ substantially between the sexes, as indicated in Table 19.1. Women have narrower shoulders, broader hips, and smaller chest diameters and tend to have more fat in the hips and lower body, whereas men carry more fat in the abdomen and upper body.

With aging, both women and men tend to accumulate fat and lose fat-free body mass starting in their mid-20s. In one of the few longitudinal studies conducted, FFM was found to decrease by approximately 3 kg per decade (more than 0.6 lb per year).[16] This data is similar to cross-sectional data that indicated a loss in FFM of 0.1 to 0.2 kg (0.3 to 0.5 lb) per year. This loss is associated with lower levels of physical activity and testosterone. Apparently, the increase in total body fat is associated with a general decline in physical activity without an equal decrease in caloric intake. Table 19.2 illustrates the changes with aging in relative body fat for both sexes.

The average difference in relative body fat between young women and men ages 18 to 24 is about 6% to 10% (20% to 25% for women versus 13% to 16% for men). At first, this difference was thought to reflect sex-specific differences in fat deposit (namely, the breasts, hips, and thighs). But female athletes, particularly distance runners, can be exceptionally lean—well below the relative fat value for the average young woman and even below that for the average young man. Many of the better female runners are below 10% body fat (chapter 16). Such low values could result from either a genetic predisposition toward leanness or from the high weekly training distance these women run, sometimes exceeding 160 km (100 mi) per week. Thus we know that women can reduce fat stores well below what is considered normal for their age. In fact, there is increasing concern that some women are becoming too lean. This will be discussed in greater detail later in this chapter.

IN REVIEW . . .

1. Until puberty, females and males do not differ significantly in most measurements of body size and composition.
2. At puberty, due to the influences of estrogen and testosterone, body composition begins to change markedly. Estrogen causes increased fat deposition in females, particularly in the hips and thighs, and an increased rate of bone growth, such that bones in females reach their final length earlier than in males.
3. Although women tend to accumulate more body fat than men, research shows that some female distance runners are exceptionally lean.

Table 19.1 Anthropometric Measurements for Young and Middle-Aged Men and Women

	Women			Men		
	Young		Middle-aged	Young		Middle-aged
	Wilmore and Behnke[a] (n = 128)	Pollock et al[b] (n = 83)	Pollock et al[b] (n = 60)	Wilmore and Behnke[a] (n = 133)	Pollock et al[b] (n = 95)	Pollock et al[b] (n = 84)
Skinfolds (mm)						
Scapula	13.2	15.3	17.3	14.1	13.9	20.2
Triceps	12.8	18.8	22.2	7.9	13.6	18.5
Midaxillary	10.7	13.3	16.9	11.7	15.5	24.8
Chest		14.0	14.0		11.4	20.6
Suprailiac	17.2	15.3	17.3	19.3	15.2	22.0
Abdominal	15.1	22.8	29.6	16.0	20.6	30.0
Thigh	31.8	28.8	33.1	14.9	17.4	22.2
Knee	7.0	17.4	17.3	5.3		
Circumferences (cm)						
Head	55.0			57.5		
Neck	31.8			38.5		
Shoulders	101.9	99.7	100.9	117.0	112.5	114.8
Chest	85.2	84.6	87.1	97.4	91.4	96.3
Bust	87.8	87.7	90.8			
Abdomen	75.3	75.0	82.7	84.0	81.0	91.1
Hips	95.9	93.1	97.5	96.9	94.4	98.4
Thigh	57.0	56.5	57.6	58.0	57.1	59.0
Knee	36.1			37.7		
Calf	35.1	33.9	34.4	37.6	36.5	36.9
Ankle	21.1	20.8	20.8	22.7	22.1	22.1
Deltoid	30.7			36.3		
Biceps, flexed	27.2	27.0	28.6	33.2	32.6	34.0
Biceps, extended	25.0			29.1		
Forearm	23.5	23.8	24.4	27.6	28.3	29.2
Wrist	14.9	14.8	15.1	17.0	16.7	17.4
Diameters (cm)						
Head length	19.0			19.9		
Head width	14.9			15.5		
Biacromial	36.5	36.8	36.7	40.4	41.1	41.5
Bideltoid	42.1	41.4	41.8	47.6	46.9	47.4
Chest	25.8	27.8	28.6	29.3	31.8	33.0
Bi-iliac	28.4	29.9	31.2	28.4	29.6	31.4
Bitrochanteric	32.1	34.0	35.3	32.9	33.6	35.1
Knee	8.9	9.3	9.6	9.5	9.8	10.1
Ankle	6.3			7.1		
Elbow	6.0			7.0		
Wrist	4.9	5.1	5.2	5.6	5.9	6.0
Arm span	165.8			181.7		
Foot length	24.1			26.7		
Hand length	17.3			19.1		

[a]Data from Wilmore and Behnke (1969 and 1970).

[b]Data from Pollock et al. (1975 and 1976).

Physiological Responses to Acute Exercise

When females and males are exposed to an acute bout of exercise, whether an all-out run to exhaustion on the treadmill or a single attempt to lift the maximum weight, characteristic responses differentiate the sexes. Differences between prepubescent and adolescent boys and girls were discussed in chapter 17. Here we will briefly discuss these differences in adults, focusing on the following types of responses:

Table 19.2 Relative Body Fat Values for Women and Men of Various Ages

Age group (years)	Relative body fat (%)	
	Women	Men
15-19	20-24	13-16
20-29	22-25	15-20
30-39	24-30	18-26
40-49	27-33	23-29
50-59	30-36	26-33
60-69	30-36	29-33

- Neuromuscular
- Cardiovascular
- Respiratory
- Metabolic

Neuromuscular Responses

In terms of strength, women have typically been regarded as the weaker sex. In previous studies, women have been found to be 43% to 63% weaker than men in upper body strength, but only 25% to 30% weaker in lower body strength. Because of the considerable size difference between the sexes, several studies have expressed strength either relative to body weight (absolute strength / body weight) or relative to FFM, as a reflection of muscle mass (absolute strength / FFM). When lower body strength is expressed relative to body weight, women are still 5% to 15% weaker than men, but when expressed relative to FFM, this difference disappears, as shown in Figure 19.2. This indicates that the innate qualities of muscle and its mechanisms of motor control are similar for women and men.

Although differences in upper body strength are reduced somewhat when expressed relative to total body weight and FFM, substantial differences remain. There are at least two possible explanations for this. Women have a higher percentage of FFM below the waist, which implies that they have more muscle there as well. In addition and probably related to this FFM distribution, women use the muscle mass of their lower bodies much more than they use their upper-body muscle mass, particularly when compared to use patterns in men. Some average-sized women have remarkable strength, exceeding even that of an average man. This indicates the importance of neuromuscular recruitment and synchronization of motor unit firing in the ultimate determination of strength (chapter 4).

In the past few years, muscle biopsies have become more common among female athletes. From these biopsy data we have learned that men and women in the same sport or event have similar fiber-type distributions, as shown in Figure 19.3, although men in one

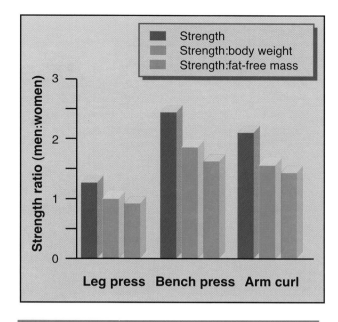

Figure 19.2   The ratio of men's strength values to women's strength values comparing absolute values with values scaled for body weight and for fat-free body mass.

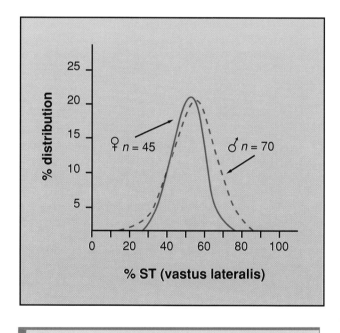

Figure 19.3   Distribution of slow-twitch fibers in the vastus lateralis muscle in women and men. Adapted from Saltin et al. (1977).

study reached greater extremes (> 90% ST or > 90% FT). However, different results were found in two studies of elite female and male distance runners.[7,14] With these elite runners the extremes for percentages of ST fibers were similar (90% to 96% for women and 92% to 98% for men) even though the mean values were different—women had a mean value of 69% ST fibers compared to a mean value of 79% for the men. However, the women had much smaller fiber areas for both ST and FT fibers (mean values of < 4,500 μm^2 in women and > 8,000 μm^2 in men).

Cardiovascular Responses

When placed on a cycle ergometer, where the power output can be precisely controlled independent of body weight, women generally have a higher heart rate response for any absolute level of submaximal exercise. However, maximum heart rate (HR max) is generally the same in both sexes. Cardiac output ($\dot{Q}$) for the same absolute power output is nearly identical in women and men. Because of this, recalling that cardiac output is the product of heart rate and stroke volume, the higher HR response in women is a compensation for a lower stroke volume (SV), which primarily results from at least three factors:

1. Women have smaller hearts and therefore smaller left ventricles because of their smaller body size, and possibly due to lower testosterone concentrations.
2. Women have a smaller blood volume, which is also related to their size.
3. The average woman is typically less active and therefore less well conditioned.

When power output is controlled to provide the same relative level of exercise, usually expressed as a fixed percentage of maximal oxygen uptake ($\dot{V}O_2$ max), the heart rate in women is still elevated compared to that in men. At 50% of $\dot{V}O_2$ max, for example, a woman's cardiac output, stroke volume, and oxygen consumption are generally less, and her heart rate is slightly higher, than a man's. These differences also are seen at maximal levels of exercise.

Women also have less potential for increasing their a-$\bar{v}O_2$ diff. This is likely due to their lower hemoglobin content, which results in a lower arterial oxygen content and a reduced muscle oxidative potential. Lower hemoglobin content is an important contributor to gender differences in $\dot{V}O_2$ max, because less oxygen is delivered to the active muscle for a given volume of blood.

Respiratory Responses

The differences between men's and women's respiratory responses to exercise are also due largely to body size differences. Breathing frequency when working at the same relative power output differs little. However, when you instead consider the same absolute power output, women tend to breathe more rapidly than men, probably because when both subjects are at the same absolute power output the woman is working at a higher percentage of her $\dot{V}O_2$ max.

Tidal volume and ventilatory volume are generally smaller in women at the same relative and absolute power outputs, up to and including maximal levels. Most highly trained female athletes have maximal ventilatory volumes below 125 L · min^{-1}, but highly trained men have maximal values of 150 L · min^{-1} and higher, some exceeding 250 L · min^{-1}! Again, these differences are closely associated with body size.

Metabolic Responses

The $\dot{V}O_2$ max is regarded by most exercise scientists as the single best index of a person's cardiorespiratory endurance capacity. Recall that $\dot{V}O_2$ is the product of cardiac output and a-$\bar{v}O_2$ diff. This means that $\dot{V}O_2$ max represents that point during exhaustive exercise where the subject has maximized oxygen delivery and utilization capabilities. The average female tends to reach her peak $\dot{V}O_2$ max between ages 13 and 15, but the average male does not reach his peak until ages 18 to 22. Beyond puberty, the average woman's $\dot{V}O_2$ max is only 70% to 75% that of the average man's.

$\dot{V}O_2$ max differences between women and men must be interpreted carefully. A classic study published in 1965 found considerable variability in $\dot{V}O_2$ max within each sex, and considerable overlap of values between sexes.[21] The study involved a group of women and men 20 to 30 years of age. The investigators divided the group into subgroups:

- Female athletes
- Female nonathletes
- Male athletes
- Male nonathletes

They compared the subjects' physiological responses to submaximal and maximal exercise. This study revealed that 76% of the female nonathletes overlapped 47% of the male nonathletes and that 22% of the female athletes overlapped 7% of the male athletes.[10] These data demonstrate the importance of looking beyond mean values to consider both the subjects' levels of physical conditioning and the extent of overlap between the groups being compared.

Although the $\dot{V}_{O_2 \, max}$ values of females and males are similar until puberty, many comparisons of $\dot{V}_{O_2 \, max}$ values of normal nonathletic females and males beyond puberty might not be valid. Such data likely reflect an unfair comparison of relatively sedentary females with relatively active males. Thus reported differences would reflect the level of conditioning as well as possible gender differences. To overcome this potential problem, investigators began to examine highly trained female and male athletes, with the assumption that the level of training would be similar for both sexes and allow a more accurate evaluation of true gender differences.

Saltin and Åstrand compared $\dot{V}_{O_2 \, max}$ values of female and male athletes from Swedish national teams.[33] In comparable events, the women had 15% to 30% lower $\dot{V}_{O_2 \, max}$ values. However, more recent data from the United States suggests a smaller difference. The $\dot{V}_{O_2 \, max}$ values for a group of elite and good female distance runners are illustrated in Figure 19.4 and are compared to values for elite male distance runners and for normal, nonathletic women and men. The elite female runners had substantially higher values than untrained men and women. Some women's values were even higher than a few of the elite male runners' values, but when you consider the average for each elite group, the women's values were still 8% to 12% lower than those of the elite male runners.

The highest $\dot{V}_{O_2 \, max}$ value reported in the literature for a female athlete is 77 ml · kg^{-1} · min^{-1}, reported in a Russian cross-country skier. The highest value for men was reported in a Norwegian cross-country skier who achieved a value of 94 ml · kg^{-1} · min^{-1}!

Several studies have attempted to scale $\dot{V}_{O_2 \, max}$ values relative to height, weight, FFM, or limb volume in an attempt to more objectively compare women's and men's values. Several of these studies have shown that differences between the sexes disappear when $\dot{V}_{O_2 \, max}$ is expressed relative to FFM or active muscle mass, yet some studies continue to demonstrate differences, even when adjusted for differences in body fat.

In one study, researchers employed a novel approach to this problem.[9] They studied the submaximal and maximal responses to treadmill runs under various

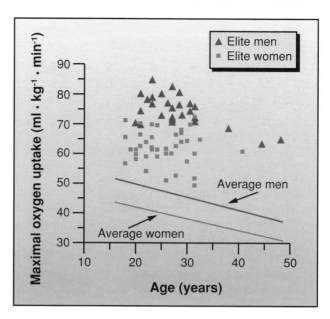

Figure 19.4 Maximal oxygen uptake values for elite female and male distance runners compared to average values in untrained women and men. Data from Robinson (1938); Åstrand (1960); Costill and Winrow (1980); Pollock (1977); Pate et al., (1987); and Wilmore and Brown (1984).

conditions in 10 women and 10 men who regularly engaged in distance running. The women exercised only under normal weight conditions, but the men exercised both at normal weight and with external weight added to their trunks so that the total percent of excess weight, defined as the men's fat weight plus the added weight, equaled the percent fat of the matched women. Equating the sexes for excess weight reduced mean gender differences in

- treadmill run time (32%),
- the amount of oxygen required per unit of fat-free mass for running at various submaximal speeds (38%), and
- $\dot{V}_{O_2 \, max}$ (65%).

The researchers concluded that women's greater sex-specific essential body fat stores are major determinants of gender differences in metabolic responses to running.

Women have lower hemoglobin levels than men, and this has also been proposed as a contributing factor to their lower $\dot{V}_{O_2 \, max}$ values. One study attempted to equate the hemoglobin concentrations of a group of 10 men and 11 women who were active but not highly trained.[8] An amount of blood was withdrawn from men to equalize their hemoglobin concentrations to those of the women subjects. This significantly reduced the men's $\dot{V}_{O_2 \, max}$ values, but these reductions accounted for only a relatively small portion of the gender differences in $\dot{V}_{O_2 \, max}$.

KEY POINT

Women generally have lower $\dot{V}O_2$ max values when expressed in ml · kg^{-1} · min^{-1}. A major part of the difference in $\dot{V}O_2$ max values between women and men is related to the extra body fat carried by women and, to a lesser extent, to their lower hemoglobin levels, which result in a lower oxygen content in the arterial blood.

If, instead of looking at $\dot{V}O_2$ max, we consider submaximal oxygen consumption ($\dot{V}O_2$), little if any difference is found between women and men for the same absolute power output. But remember that at the same absolute submaximal work rate, women are usually working at a higher percentage of their $\dot{V}O_2$ max. As a result, their blood lactate levels are higher and lactate threshold occurs at a lower absolute power output. Peak blood lactate values are generally lower in active but untrained women than in active but untrained men. Also, limited data suggest that elite female middle-distance and long-distance runners have peak lactate values that are approximately 45% lower than similarly trained elite male runners (8.8 mmol · L^{-1} versus 12.9 mmol · L^{-1}).[28,29] Such gender differences in peak blood lactate values are unexpected and unexplained.

With respect to anaerobic or lactate threshold, values appear to be similar between equally trained men and women if the values are expressed in relative, not absolute, terms. Anaerobic or lactate threshold appears to be closely related to the mode of testing and to the individual's state of training. Thus, gender differences are not expected.

Physiological Adaptations to Exercise Training

As we have seen in earlier chapters, basic physiological function both at rest and during exercise changes substantially with physical training. In this section, we will investigate how women adapt to chronic exercise, emphasizing areas in which their responses might differ from those of men.

Body Composition

With either cardiorespiratory endurance training or strength training, both women and men experience

- losses in total body mass,
- losses of fat mass,

IN REVIEW . . .

1. The innate qualities of muscle and the mechanisms of motor control are similar for women and men.
2. In lower body strength, when expressed relative to body weight or to fat-free mass, women and men do not differ. But women show less upper body strength, when expressed relative to body weight or fat-free mass, than men, largely because more of women's muscle mass is below the waist and women use their lower body muscles more.
3. At submaximal exercise levels, women have higher heart rates than men, but women's submaximal cardiac outputs are the same for the same rate of work. This indicates that women have lower stroke volumes, primarily because they have smaller hearts, less blood volume, and are generally less well conditioned than men.
4. Women also have a lower capacity to increase a-$\bar{v}O_2$ diff, probably because of their lower hemoglobin content, so less oxygen is delivered to their active muscles per unit of blood.
5. Differences in women's and men's respiratory responses are due primarily to body size differences.
6. Beyond puberty, the average woman's $\dot{V}O_2$ max is only 70% to 75% that of the average man's. However, much of this difference might be due to women's less active lifestyles. Research with highly trained athletes reveals that much of the difference is due to women's greater fat mass.
7. Little or no difference in anaerobic threshold is found between the sexes.

- losses of relative fat, and
- gains in fat-free mass (FFM).

Women generally gain much less in fat-free mass than men do. With the exception of FFM, the magnitude of the change in body composition appears to be related more to the total energy expenditure associated with the training activities than to the participant's sex. As for FFM, significantly more is gained in response to strength training than with endurance training, and the magnitude of these responses is much less in women, due primarily to hormonal differences.

Bone and connective tissue undergo alterations with training, but these are not well understood. In general, animal studies and limited human studies find an increase in the density of the weight-bearing long bones. This adaptation appears to be independent of sex, at least in young and middle-aged populations. We will discuss some exceptions to this later in this chapter.

Connective tissue appears to be strengthened with endurance training, and gender differences in this response have not been identified. The possibility that women are more susceptible to injury than men while participating in physical activity and sport has led to concerns about sex-specific differences in joint integrity and the strength of ligaments, tendons, and bones. Unfortunately, the research literature contributes little to confirming or denying the validity of such concerns. Where differences in the rate of injury have been observed, the injury could likely be more related to the level of conditioning than to the participant's gender. Those who are less fit are more prone to injury. This is an extremely difficult area in which to obtain objective data but is nevertheless an important area that needs to be better defined.

Neuromuscular Adaptations

Until the 1970s, prescribing strength training programs for girls and women was not considered appropriate. Women were not believed capable of gaining strength due to their extremely low levels of the male anabolic hormones. Paradoxically, many people also generally feared that strength training would masculinize women. During the 1960s and 1970s, however, it became evident that many of the United States' better female athletes were not doing well in international competition, largely because they were weaker than their competitors. Slowly, research demonstrated that women can gain considerably from strength training programs and that strength gains are usually not accompanied by large increases in muscle bulk.

One study compared the training responses of 47 women and 26 men who volunteered to participate in identical progressive resistance weight-training programs. The program was conducted twice each week, 40 min per day, for a total of 10 weeks. The strength gains were as follows:

Bench-press strength: 29% in women, 17% in men
Leg-press strength: 30% in women, 26% in men

Muscle girth increased only slightly in the women, but the men exhibited classic muscle hypertrophy.[39] Thus, hypertrophy is neither a necessary consequence of nor a prerequisite to gains in muscle strength. Several studies have confirmed these results.

Women have the potential to develop substantially greater strength than that normally identified in the average, typically sedentary woman. But will women ever be able to attain the same strength as men for all major regions of the body? As discussed earlier in this chapter, the leg strength to weight ratios between the sexes are similar, suggesting that the histological and biochemical qualities of muscle are the same, irrespective of gender. This was confirmed by computer tomography scans of the upper arms and thighs of physical education majors of both sexes and of male bodybuilders.[35] Although both groups of men had much greater absolute levels of strength than the women, no differences between the groups were found when strength was expressed per unit of muscle cross-sectional area (Figure 19.5).

Because of their lower levels of testosterone, women have less total muscle mass. If muscle mass is the major determinant of strength, then women have a distinct disadvantage. But if neural factors are as important, or even more important, than size, women's potential for absolute strength gains is considerable. Also, women can attain significant muscle hypertrophy. This has been demonstrated in women bodybuilders who have remained free of anabolic steroids. The basic mechanisms allowing greater levels of strength have not yet been clearly defined, so we cannot draw any conclusions at this time. Overall, though, women generally exhibit substantially less muscle hypertrophy to a given training stimulus than men do, but some women have more hypertrophy than some men. Similar to aerobic capacity, as discussed earlier,

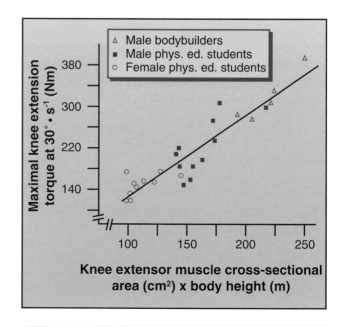

Figure 19.5   No gender differences in strength (maximal knee extension torque) are seen when strength is expressed per unit of muscle cross-sectional area.

some overlap occurs between female and male responses to the same training stimuli.

Cardiovascular and Respiratory Adaptations

Major cardiovascular and respiratory adaptations accompany cardiorespiratory endurance training, and these adaptations do not appear to be sex specific. Major increases in maximal cardiac output ($\dot{Q}$ max) accompany training. Maximum heart rate does not change with training, so this increase in $\dot{Q}$ max is the result of a large increase in stroke volume, which results from two factors. End-diastolic volume (the amount of blood in the ventricles before contraction) increases with training, because blood volume is increased and venous return is more efficient. In addition, end-systolic volume (the amount of blood remaining in the ventricles after contraction) is reduced with training, because the stronger myocardium produces a stronger contraction, ejecting more blood.

At submaximal work rates, cardiac output shows little or no change, although stroke volume is considerably higher for the same absolute rate of work. Consequently, heart rate for any given rate of work is reduced after training. Resting heart rate can be reduced to 50 beats per minute or less. Several female distance runners have had resting heart rates below 36 beats per minute. This is considered a classic training response and corresponds to an exceptionally high stroke volume.

The increases in $\dot{V}O_2$ max that accompany cardiorespiratory endurance training, which will be discussed momentarily, primarily result from the large increases in maximal cardiac output, with only small increases in a-$\bar{v}O_2$ diff. However, Saltin and Rowell state that the major limitation to $\dot{V}O_2$ max is oxygen transport to the working muscles.[34] Although cardiac output is important in this respect, these researchers believe that the increases in maximal aerobic power that accompany training are due primarily to increased maximal muscle blood flow and muscle capillary density. These changes are firmly established in men, and we have

no reason to suspect that women differ in this response to training. In fact, one study has demonstrated that endurance-trained women have considerably higher capillary-to-fiber ratios (1.69 capillaries per fiber) than untrained women (1.11 capillaries per fiber).[23] Elite female distance runners in one study had a mean capillary-to-fiber ratio of 2.50 capillaries per fiber![7] These values are similar to what has been reported in men of similar training status. Although women also experience considerable increases in maximal ventilation, reflecting increases in both tidal volume and breathing frequency, these changes are thought to be unrelated to the increase in $\dot{V}O_2$ max.

Metabolic Adaptations

With cardiorespiratory endurance training, women experience the same relative increase in $\dot{V}O_2$ max that has been observed in men. The magnitude of this increase is highly related to the initial level of fitness—those with low initial fitness generally experience a greater percentage increase. We each have a genetically established upper limit of $\dot{V}O_2$ max, which we cannot exceed, irrespective of the duration or intensity of our training. Consequently, the closer we are to this upper limit, the more difficult it is for us to obtain large improvements with subsequent training. Most women should experience substantial improvements in $\dot{V}O_2$ max with endurance training because they have relatively low initial values due to their comparatively less-active lifestyle. Women can improve their $\dot{V}O_2$ max by 10% to 40% with cardiorespiratory endurance training. These percentages are similar to improvements seen in men. The magnitude of change noted depends on

- the initial level of fitness,
- the intensity and duration of training sessions,
- the frequency of training, and
- the length of the study.

After cardiorespiratory endurance training, women's oxygen uptake at the same absolute submaximal work rate does not appear to change, although several studies have reported decreases. Blood lactate levels are reduced for the same absolute submaximal rates of work, peak lactate levels are generally increased, and the lactate threshold increases with training. Finally, endurance training also improves women's ability to utilize free fatty acids for fuel, an adaptation that, as we have seen, is very important for glycogen sparing.

From this discussion, we can see that women respond to physical training in the same manner as men do. Although the magnitude of their adaptations to training might differ somewhat from those of their male counterparts, the overall trends appear identical. This is an important consideration when prescribing exercise to females.

■ IN REVIEW . . . ■

1. With training, women generally gain less fat-free mass than men do, but other changes in body composition seem more related to total energy expenditure than to gender.
2. Women can gain considerable strength through strength training, and it is usually not accompanied by large increases in muscle bulk.
3. Cardiovascular and respiratory changes that accompany cardiorespiratory endurance training do not appear to be sex specific.
4. Women experience the same relative increase in $\dot{V}O_2\text{ max}$ that men experience with cardiorespiratory endurance training.
5. Women respond to physical training in the same manner as men do.

Athletic Ability

Women are outperformed by men in almost all sports, events, or activities. This is quite obvious in activities such as the shot put in track and field, where high levels of upper body strength are crucial to successful performance. In the 400-m freestyle swim, however, the winning time for women in the 1924 Olympic Games was 16% slower than that for men, but this difference decreased to 11.6% in the 1948 Olympics, and to only 6.9% in the 1984 Olympics. The fastest women's 800-m freestyle swimmer in 1979 swam faster than the world-record-holding man for the same distance in 1972! Therefore in this particular event the gap between the sexes is narrowing, and this is also true for other events and for other sports. Unfortunately, making valid comparisons through the years has been difficult because the degree to which an activity has been emphasized, or its popularity, is not constant, and other factors, such as opportunities to participate,

coaching, facilities, and training techniques, have differed considerably between the sexes over the years.

As noted at the beginning of this chapter, large numbers of girls and women didn't start entering competitive sport until the 1970s. Even then, there was an initial reluctance to train women as hard as men. Once girls and women started training as hard as boys and men, their performance improved dramatically. This is illustrated in Figure 19.6, which shows world records from 1975 to 1991 for women and men in six running events in track and field. For distances of 400 m through the marathon, women's present world records are consistently 10% to 13% slower than men's. Furthermore, the improvement in women's records, which was initially quite dramatic, is beginning to level off and parallel the curves for men's records.

Special Considerations

Although the sexes respond to acute exercise and adapt to chronic exercise in much the same manner, several additional areas that are unique to females must be considered. Specifically, we will look at

- menstruation and menstrual dysfunction,
- pregnancy,
- osteoporosis,
- eating disorders, and
- environmental factors.

Menstruation and Menstrual Dysfunction

Two questions that are foremost in the minds of exercising women, particularly female athletes, are "How does my menstrual cycle or pregnancy influence my exercise capacity and performance?" and "How does my physical activity and competition influence my menstrual cycle or pregnancy?" Let's try to answer these questions, beginning by focusing on the relationship between menstruation and physical performance.

The three major phases of the menstrual (uterine) cycle are illustrated in Figure 19.7. The first is the menstrual (flow) phase, which lasts 4 to 5 days during which time the uterine lining (endometrium) is shed and menstrual flow occurs. The second is the proliferative phase, which prepares the uterus for fertilization and lasts about 10 days. During this phase, the endometrium begins to thicken and some of the ovarian follicles that house the ova mature. These follicles secrete estrogen. The proliferative phase ends when a mature follicle ruptures, releasing its ovum (ovulation). The menstrual and proliferative phases correspond to the

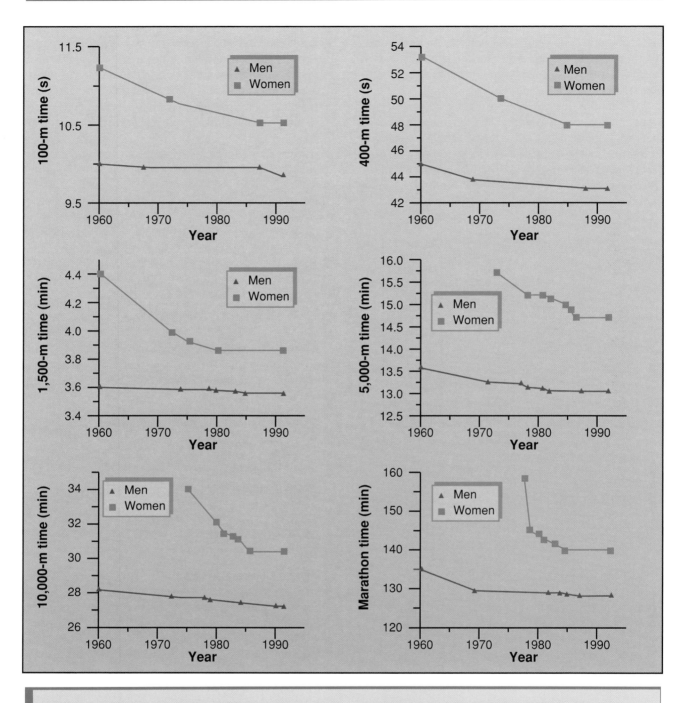

Figure 19.6   Women's and men's world records in six running events in track and field between 1960 and 1991.

follicular phase of the ovarian cycle. The third and final phase of the menstrual cycle is the secretory phase, which corresponds to the luteal phase of the ovarian cycle. This phase lasts 10 to 14 days during which the endometrium continues to thicken, its blood and nutrient supply increases, and the uterus prepares itself for pregnancy. During this time, the empty follicle (now termed a corpus luteum, hence the term luteal

phase) secretes progesterone, and estrogen secretion also continues. The complete menstrual cycle averages 28 days.

Menstruation and Performance

Alterations in athletic performance experienced during different phases of the menstrual cycle are subject to

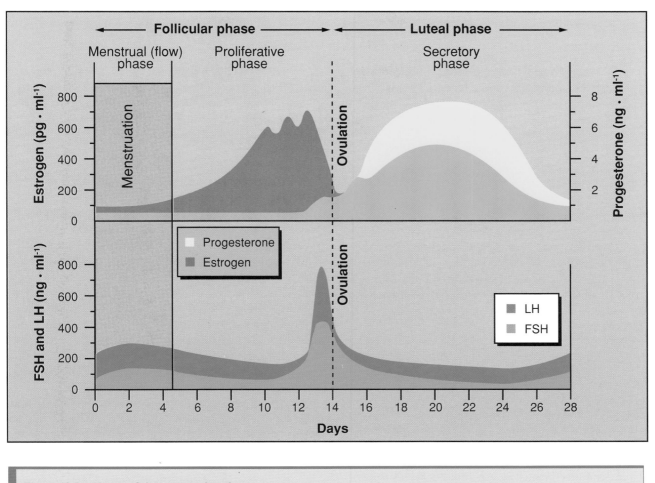

Figure 19.7   Phases of the menstrual cycle.

considerable individual variability. Some women have absolutely no noticeable change in their performance ability at any time during their menstrual cycle, yet others have considerable difficulty in either the pre-flow or the early-flow phases or during both. The number of women who report impaired performance during the flow phase is approximately the same as those who experience no difficulty. In fact, some female athletes have reportedly set world records during the flow phase. Adding to the confusion, much of the information available on this topic is based on anecdotes or subjective statements made by athletes during informal surveys.

Very little information is available from well-designed and well-controlled research studies. Several studies have suggested that athletic performance is best during the immediate post-flow period up to the 15th day of the cycle, with the first day of the cycle corresponding to the initiation of the flow, or menses, and ovulation occurring on about the 14th day. However, other studies have reported that performance is best during the flow phase. The confused state of research in this area is illustrated by three studies conducted on swimmers. Swimming is an excellent sport for studying this issue, because performance can be objectively measured with a stop watch. Of these three studies,

- one showed that swimmers had faster times during the flow phase,[3]
- one showed that swimmers swam fastest during the post-flow phase,[1] and
- one study found slightly faster times in the pre-flow phase, although the differences in times were not statistically significant.[31]

Such divergent results are perplexing. The disagreement between these studies could be due to the small number of subjects tested, to large individual variations among the swimmers, or to inadequately controlled experimental designs. Several studies have been conducted in research laboratories using physiological measures to gauge performance changes. These have generally found no performance differences in the various phases of the menstrual cycle.

From currently available information, we can conclude that performance in some women can be affected by the phase of their menstrual cycle, but that many, if not most, women are not affected. Any woman who experiences premenstrual syndrome (PMS) or dysmenorrhea (pain or abdominal cramping with menstruation) will likely not perform as well while she is experiencing symptoms. For these women, some degree of control over their menstrual cycle is possible through the use of low-dose oral contraceptives. This was discussed in chapter 14.

Menarche

Delayed menarche (the first menses) has been reported in young athletes involved in certain sports and activities, such as gymnastics and ballet. The median age of menarche for American girls is 12.8 years. For gymnasts, the median age appears to be closer to 15 years. Frisch has hypothesized that menarche is delayed 5 months for each year of training prior to menarche, implying that training causes delayed menarche.[17] Malina, however, has postulated that late maturers, such as those with delayed menarche, are more likely to be successful in sports such as gymnastics because of their small, lean bodies.[27] This implies that those who naturally experience delayed menarche have an advantage in, and thus are likely to be involved in, certain sports, rather than that their sport involvement causes delayed menarche.

These opposing viewpoints can be summarized by the following questions: Does intense training to achieve the level of an elite performer delay menarche, or does delayed menarche provide an advantage that contributes to the success of the elite performer? Stager et al., using computer modeling to analyze this issue, have concluded that it would be most appropriate to state that the age of menarche in athletes is later rather than delayed.[38] At this time, evidence is insufficient to support the theory that training delays menarche, so Malina's statement that menarche occurs later in the trained athlete is appropriate.

Menstrual Dysfunction

Female athletes can experience disruptions of their normal menstrual cycle. These disruptions are collectively referred to as menstrual dysfunction, of which there are several types. Eumenorrhea is the term for normal menstrual function. Oligomenorrhea refers to abnormally infrequent or scant menstruation. Primary amenorrhea refers to the absence of menarche in women 18 years of age and older—women who never began menstruating. Some athletes with previously normal menstrual function have reported the absence of menstruation for months or even years when they have trained and competed intensely in sports such as figure skating, ballet, gymnastics, bodybuilding, cycling, and distance running. This phenomenon is referred to as secondary amenorrhea.

The prevalence of secondary amenorrhea and oligomenorrhea among athletes is not well documented, but is estimated to vary from approximately 5% to 40% or higher, depending on the sport or activity and the level of competition. This is considerably higher than the estimated 2% to 3% prevalence for amenorrhea and 10% to 12% prevalence for oligomenorrhea in the general population. The prevalence appears to be greater in those who train many hours each day and in those who train at very high intensities.

Many women who become amenorrheic are relieved to be free of menstruation each month. Most also assume that they have developed a simple but effective form of birth control. However, athletes have become pregnant while amenorrheic, which indicates that ovulation, and thus fertility, is not always influenced by the absence of menstruation. This latter point needs to be stressed among female athletes prone to amenorrhea to reduce the possibility of unexpected pregnancy.

Neither the causes nor the long-term consequences of secondary amenorrhea or oligomenorrhea are known. We are tempted to surmise that high-level training leads to menstrual dysfunction, but the true cause might involve one or more factors associated with high-level training. Some factors that have been proposed include the following:

- Previous history of menstrual dysfunction
- Acute effects of stress
- High quantity and intensity of training
- Low body weight and body fat
- Inadequate nutrition and disordered eating
- Hormonal alterations

Let's briefly discuss each of these.

Prior History of Menstrual Dysfunction. The association between secondary amenorrhea and prior menstrual dysfunction was demonstrated in one study that found that 54.5% of amenorrheic runners had a prior history of irregular menstruation, compared to only 15.5% of eumenorrheic runners and 13.3% of nonrunners. Other studies, however, have been unable to confirm these results. Most likely, a previous history of menstrual dysfunction can be one of a number of factors, but is probably not the primary factor, in the development of secondary amenorrhea.

Stress. Stress is also a likely factor. One study showed that amenorrheic runners associated more stress with their training than did eumenorrheic runners.[36] Interestingly, formal psychological tests failed to detect any differences in the amenorrheic runners' levels of anxiety, depression, and other states that reflect stress.

High Quantity and Intensity of Training. Several studies have shown that quantity of training is associated with secondary amenorrhea. In runners, a direct relationship has been reported between the distance run per week and the prevalence of secondary amenorrhea. High mileage runners report more amenorrhea. But other studies have been unable to confirm this relationship. Researchers have tried to induce amenorrhea by increasing the quantity of the women's training.[2,4] In one study, none of the runners became amenorrheic, but 18 developed significant menstrual cycle changes, mainly oligomenorrhea.[2] In another study, only 4 of the 28 runners maintained normal menstrual cycles during the increased training period. The most significant menstrual dysfunctions noted were delayed menstruation, abnormal luteal function, and a loss of luteinizing hormone (LH) surge.[4] Within 6 months of completing this study, all runners returned to normal menstrual cycles. Fortunately, athletically induced amenorrhea is usually reversible during periods of reduced training, injury, or vacation.

The effect of training intensity on menstrual function has not been well documented. Training at a high intensity, because of the high physical stress placed on the body, might be more closely linked with secondary amenorrhea. Future studies need to focus on this aspect of training.

Low Body Weight or Body Fat. Excessive leanness, undernutrition, or both, have long been associated with amenorrhea. Some researchers have suggested that the loss of one third of a woman's body fat or a 10% to 15% decrease in her total body weight (mass) will induce amenorrhea. The reason for this is that androgens are converted into estrogens in adipose tissue, particularly breast and abdominal fat, and this conversion accounts for nearly one third of the estrogen in premenopausal women.[18] Any decrease in adipose tissue influences the storage and metabolism of estrogen. In other words, fat is an important estrogen source, necessary for normal menstrual function. At one time a certain minimal weight for height was believed necessary for achieving menarche and remaining eumenorrheic.[19] This later evolved into a hypothesis that girls need to attain a relative minimum body fat of 17% to achieve menarche, and after that females need a minimum of 22% relative body fat to maintain normal menstrual function.[37] More recently, however, investigators have challenged this theory. Numerous studies have now been published in which the relative body fat levels of eumenorrheic and amenorrheic athletes were identical. This strongly suggests that low body weight or body fat are not primary triggers of menstrual dysfunction.

Inadequate Nutrition and Disordered Eating. Current evidence indicates that inadequate nutrition is a potential cause of secondary amenorrhea. Studies have shown that inadequate intake of total calories, protein, fat, or specific vitamins and minerals might be implicated.

The relationship between disordered eating and menstrual dysfunction is a more recent concern, because several studies have shown a strong relationship between the two. In one study, 8 of 13 amenorrheic distance runners reported eating disorders, compared to 0 of 19 eumenorrheic distance runners.[20] In another study, 7 of 9 amenorrheic elite middle-distance and distance runners were diagnosed with either anorexia nervosa, bulimia nervosa, or both, compared to 0 of 5 eumenorrheic runners.[41] Most of the research in the area of nutrition and disordered eating is preliminary and more research will be necessary before definite conclusions can be drawn.

KEY POINT

A high percentage of female athletes in endurance and appearance sports experience secondary amenorrhea, where normal menstrual function is lost for months or even years. This appears to be reversible with reductions in the intensity and volume of training and an increase in caloric intake.

Hormonal Alterations. Numerous hormonal changes occur with acute bouts of exercise (transient changes) as well as with chronic periods of training (long-term changes). Recall from basic physiology the normal endocrine control of the menstrual cycle. We have discussed the importance of the gonadotropic hormones—luteinizing hormone (LH) and follicle-stimulating hormone (FSH). These hormones are released from the anterior pituitary gland in response to gonadotropin-releasing hormone (GnRH), which is produced by the hypothalamus. In athletes with menstrual dysfunction, the normal episodic secretion pattern of LH appears to undergo subtle changes. These might be caused by increased secretion of corticotropin-releasing hormone (CRH) from the hypothalamus. This hormone inhibits GnRH release, which would in turn inhibit the release of LH and FSH.[24] Cross-sectional studies of amenorrheic athletes have shown abnormal reproductive hormone patterns that suggest that the normal secretion of GnRH by the hypothalamus is disrupted and thus fails to initiate normal hypothalamic-pituitary-ovarian function.[26]

Pregnancy

Four major physiological concerns are associated with exercise during pregnancy:[42,43]

1. The acute risk associated with reduced blood flow to the uterus (blood is diverted to mother's active muscles), leading to fetal hypoxia (insufficient oxygen)
2. Fetal hyperthermia (elevated temperature) associated with the increase in the mother's internal body temperature during prolonged aerobic-type exercise, or exercise under conditions of heat stress
3. Reduced carbohydrate availability to the fetus as the mother's body uses more carbohydrate to fuel her exercise
4. The possibility of miscarriage and the final outcome of pregnancy

Let's discuss each of these.

Reduced Uterine Blood Flow and Hypoxia

There have been reports that uterine blood flow in sheep was reduced approximately 25% during exercise. Whether this reduction in uterine blood flow leads to fetal hypoxia is less clear. Apparently, an increase in the uterine a-$\bar{v}O_2$ diff at least partially compensates for any reduced blood flow. Increases in fetal heart rate, although not always observed during maternal exercise, have been interpreted as an index of hypoxia in the fetus. Although increased fetal heart rate might reflect hypoxia to a certain degree, it more likely represents the fetal heart's response to increased catecholamine levels in the blood resulting from the mother's exercise.

Hyperthermia

Fetal hyperthermia is a distinct possibility if the mother's core temperature is elevated substantially during and immediately following exercise. In animals, teratogenic effects (abnormal fetal development) have been documented with chronic exposure to thermal stress, and in humans, these effects have been documented with maternal fever. Central nervous system defects are the most common result.[43] Although fetal temperature has been shown to increase with exercise in animal

studies, it is unclear if this increase is sufficient to warrant concern.

Carbohydrate Availability

The potential for reduced carbohydrate availability for the fetus during exercise is also not well understood. We know that endurance athletes who train or compete for long durations reduce both liver and muscle glycogen stores and that blood glucose concentrations can also be reduced. But whether this is a potential problem in pregnant women is less clear. One study demonstrated small reductions in blood glucose levels of from 5.3 to 4.6 mmol · L^{-1} following steady-state treadmill running in recreational runners studied at 32 weeks into pregnancy.[6]

Miscarriage and Pregnancy Outcome

Concerns have also been expressed regarding the potential of exercise to induce miscarriage during the first trimester, to induce premature labor, and to alter the normal course of fetal development. Unfortunately, little information is available concerning the risk for miscarriage and premature labor. Regarding pregnancy outcome, data are scarce and conflicting. Although there are some indications of lighter birth weights, most studies have shown either favorable effects of exercise (such as reduced maternal weight gain, shorter postdelivery hospital stays, and fewer cesarean sections) or no differences between the control and exercise groups.

Recommendations

To summarize, exercise during pregnancy can have associated risks (see Table 19.3), but the benefits will far outweigh the potential risks if caution is taken in designing the exercise program. Wolfe et al. have provided a set of guidelines that should be followed when prescribing aerobic exercise during pregnancy.[43] These are presented in Table 19.4. It is important that the pregnant woman coordinate her exercise program with her obstetrician so sound medical judgment can be used to determine the most appropriate mode of activity, as well as frequency, duration, and intensity.

■— KEY POINT —■

Although there are several concerns over the health of the fetus during maternal exercise, the risk to the fetus from women performing aerobic exercise during pregnancy appears to be low, particularly if guidelines for exercising during pregnancy are followed.

Table 19.3 Hypothetical Risks and Postulated Benefits of Exercise During Pregnancy

<u>**Hypothetical risks**</u>

Maternal

    Acute hypoglycemia

    Chronic fatigue

    Musculoskeletal injury

Fetal

    Acute hypoxia

    Acute hyperthermia

    Acute reduction in glucose availability

    Miscarriage in the first trimester

    Induction of premature labor

    Altered fetal development

    Shortened gestation

    Reduced birth weight

<u>**Postulated benefits**</u>

Maternal

    Increased energy level (aerobic fitness)

    Reduced cardiovascular stress

    Prevention of excessive weight gain

    Facilitation of labor

    Faster recovery from labor

    Promotion of good posture

    Prevention of low back pain

    Prevention of gestational diabetes

    Improved mood state and body image

Fetal

    Fewer complications of a difficult labor

Adapted from Wolfe et al. (1989).

Table 19.4 Guidelines for the Prescription of Aerobic Exercise During Pregnancy

1. Obtain medical clearance prior to exercise.

2. Non-weightbearing exercise (e.g., cycling, swimming) is preferable to weightbearing exercise (e.g., jogging).

3. Exertion levels should be determined on an individual basis.

4. Avoid strenuous exertion during the first trimester.

5. Increases in exercise quantity and quality should be very gradual for previously inactive women.

6. Avoid exercise or positioning of the individual in the supine posture, particularly in late gestation.

7. Avoid exercise in warm/humid environments.

8. Drink liquids before and after exercise to ensure adequate hydration.

9. Do not exercise when fatigued, particularly in late gestation.

10. Periodic rest intervals may be helpful to minimize hypoxia or thermal stress to the fetus.

11. Know reasons to discontinue exercise and consult a physician immediately if they occur.

Adapted from Wolfe et al. (1989).

▬ IN REVIEW ... ▬

1. The effects of different phases of the menstrual cycle on performance are subject to considerable individual variation. In general, the number of women reporting impaired performance during the flow phase is about the same as the number reporting no difficulty. Any woman who experiences PMS or dysmenorrhea is likely to not perform as well while experiencing those symptoms.

2. Menarche can be delayed in some young athletes in certain sports. However, the most likely explanation for this is that late maturers, because of lean body build, are more likely to participate in these activities, not that these activities cause delayed menarche.

3. Female athletes can experience menstrual dysfunction, most often secondary amenorrhea or oligomenorrhea. The cause of these conditions in athletes is unknown, but current evidence implicates inadequate nutrition as a primary cause of secondary amenorrhea. In addition, hormonal changes from exercise and training might disrupt GnRH secretion, which is needed to direct the normal cycle.

4. During exercise, major concerns for the pregnant athlete include the risk of

   - fetal hypoxia,
   - fetal hyperthermia, and
   - reduced carbohydrate supply to the fetus.

5. The benefits of a properly prescribed exercise program during pregnancy outweigh the potential risks. Such an exercise program must be coordinated with the woman's obstetrician.

Osteoporosis

Maintaining a healthy lifestyle might retard one detrimental aging process that is a major health concern for women: osteoporosis. Osteoporosis is characterized by decreased bone mineral content, which causes increased bone porosity (see Figure 19.8). These changes lead to greater risk of fractures that typically begin to occur in the late 30s. The occurrence rate for these fractures increases by 2 to 5 times starting with the onset of menopause. Much remains to be learned about the etiology of osteoporosis; however, three major contributing factors common to postmenopausal women are

- estrogen deficiency,
- inadequate calcium intake, and
- inadequate physical activity.

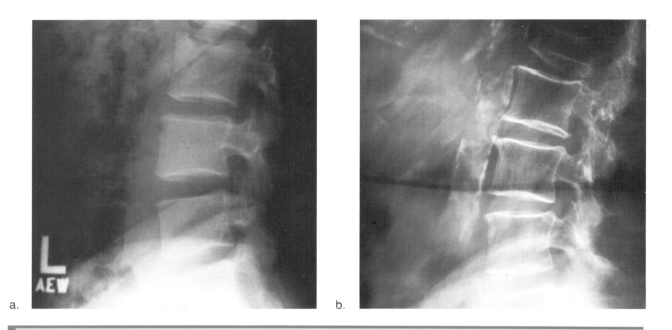

a.   b.

Figure 19.8   (a) Healthy bone and (b) bone showing increased porosity (decreased density, appearing darker) resulting from osteoporosis.

Although the first of these is a direct result of menopause, the last two reflect dietary and exercise patterns throughout life.

In addition to postmenopausal women, women with amenorrhea and those with anorexia nervosa also suffer from osteoporosis due to either insufficient calcium intake or low serum estrogen levels, or possibly both. In a study of women with anorexia, the investigators found that their bone densities were reduced significantly compared to controls.[32] Cann and associates were the first to report a substantially lower than normal bone mineral content in physically active women classified as having hypothalamic amenorrhea.[5]

In a second study, the radial and vertebral bone densities of fourteen athletic women with amenorrhea were compared to those of fourteen athletic women with normal menstruation (eumenorrhea).[12] Investigators discovered that physical activity did not protect the group with amenorrhea from significant bone density losses. This group's bone density values at a mean age of 24.9 were equivalent to those of women at a mean age of 51.2. In a follow-up study, increases in vertebral bone mineral density were found in the women who had previously been amenorrheic but had resumed menstruation.[13] However their bone mineral densities remained well below the average for their age group, even 4 years after they resumed normal menses.[11] Decreased spinal bone density might be more closely related to disturbances of ovulation than to either amenorrhea or physical activity.[30]

Bone mineral contents of normally menstruating runners tend to be higher than those of normally menstruating nonrunning controls, as is illustrated in Figure 19.9. This figure demonstrates that female runners have higher bone mineral contents than untrained

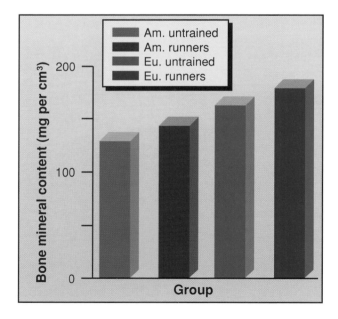

Figure 19.9   Bone mineral content of female runners and untrained females who are amenorrheic (Am) and eumenorrheic (Eu).

women when matched by menstrual status. Changes associated with amenorrhea or ovulation disturbances are the most likely to influence bone mineral status. Also, caution should be used when interpreting data such as those presented in this section because the results can be confounded by such factors as body composition, age, height, weight, and diet.

KEY POINT

Athletes with secondary amenorrhea are at increased risk for loss of bone mineral. This does not appear to be totally reversible with the resumption of normal menstrual function.

Although the precise mechanism is unknown, estrogen deficiency appears to play a major role in the development of osteoporosis. In the past, estrogen has been prescribed in an effort to reverse the degenerative effects of osteoporosis, but this therapy can have serious side effects, such as an increased risk of endometrial cancer. Increasing calcium intake to 1.5 to 2.0 g per day has also been proposed for decreasing the risk of osteoporosis. This approach, however, might not be as effective as once hoped, and an increased RDA for calcium remains controversial.

As of yet, a lack of sufficient data precludes drawing any firm conclusions on the effects of exercise and amenorrhea on osteoporosis. However, evidence certainly suggests that increased physical activity and adequate calcium intake combined with adequate caloric intake is a sensible approach to preserving the integrity of bone at any age, providing normal menstrual function is maintained.

Eating Disorders

Eating disorders in girls and women became the focus of considerable attention beginning in the 1980s. Men constitute less than 10% of the reported cases. Anorexia nervosa has been considered a clinical syndrome since the late 19th century, but bulimia nervosa was first described in 1976.

Anorexia nervosa is a disorder characterized by

- refusal to maintain more than the minimal normal weight based on age and height,
- distorted body image,
- intense fear of fatness or gaining weight, and
- amenorrhea.

Females age 12 to age 21 are at greatest risk for this disorder. Its prevalence in this group is likely less than

Table 19.5 Diagnostic Criteria for Anorexia Nervosa

1. Refusal to maintain body weight over a minimal normal weight for age and height, for example, weight loss leading to maintenance of body weight 15% below that expected, or failure to make expected weight gain during period of growth, leading to body weight 15% below that expected.

2. Intense fear of gaining weight or becoming fat, even though underweight.

3. Disturbance in the way in which one's body weight, size, or shape is experienced, for example, the person claims to "feel fat" even when emaciated, believes that one area of the body is "too fat" even when obviously underweight.

4. In females, absence of at least three consecutive menstrual cycles when otherwise expected to occur (primary or secondary amenorrhea). (A woman is considered to have amenorrhea if her periods occur only following hormone, e.g, estrogen, administration.)

Adapted from American Psychiatric Association (1987).

1%. The diagnostic criteria for anorexia nervosa are listed in Table 19.5.

Bulimia nervosa, originally termed bulimarexia, is characterized by

- recurrent episodes of binge eating,
- a feeling of lack of control during these binges, and
- purging behavior, which can include self-induced vomiting, laxative use, and diuretic use.

The diagnostic criteria for bulimia nervosa are listed in Table 19.6. Using these criteria, the prevalence of bulimia in the population at greatest risk, again adolescent and young adult females, is generally considered to be less than 5% and might be closer to 1%.

Table 19.6 Diagnostic Criteria for Bulimia Nervosa

1. Recurrent episodes of binge eating (rapid consumption of a large amount of food in a discrete period of time).

2. A feeling of lack of control over eating behavior during the eating binges.

3. The person regularly engages in either self-induced vomiting, use of laxatives or diuretics, strict dieting or fasting, or vigorous exercise in order to prevent weight gain.

4. A minimum average of two binge eating episodes a week for at least three months.

5. Persistent overconcern with body shape and weight.

Adapted from American Psychiatric Association (1987).

It is important to realize that a person might have disordered eating and yet not meet the strict diagnostic criteria for either anorexia or bulimia. As an example, the diagnosis of bulimia requires that the individual average a minimum of two binge-eating episodes a week for at least 3 months. What about the person who meets all the criteria, except that bingeing occurs only once per week? Though this person cannot technically be diagnosed as having bulimia, her or his eating is certainly disordered and is a potential cause for concern.

The prevalence of eating disorders in athletes is not well understood. Numerous studies have used either self-report or at least one of two inventories developed to diagnose disordered eating: the Eating Disorders Inventory (EDI) and the Eating Attitudes Test (EAT). Results have varied because not all studies used the strict standard diagnostic criteria for either anorexia or bulimia. As in the general population, female athletes are typically at a much higher risk than male athletes, and certain sports carry higher risks than others. The high-risk sports can generally be grouped into one of three categories:

1. Appearance sports, such as diving, figure skating, gymnastics, bodybuilding, and ballet
2. Endurance sports, such as distance running and swimming
3. Weight-classification sports, such as horse racing (jockeys), boxing, and wrestling

Self-reports or inventories do not always provide accurate results. In a study of 110 elite female athletes representing seven sports, EAT test results showed that no athlete fell within the disordered eating range of the inventory. But in the subsequent 2-year period, 18 of these athletes received either inpatient or outpatient treatment for eating disorders. In a second study of 14 nationally ranked middle-distance and distance runners who completed the EDI, only three were shown to have possible problems with disordered eating, and none were shown to have eating disorders.[41] In follow-up, seven subjects were subsequently diagnosed as having an eating disorder: four with anorexia nervosa, two with bulimia nervosa, and one with both. Eating disorders, by their very nature, are secretive. We cannot realistically expect those with eating disorders to identify themselves, even when anonymity is assured. For the athlete, this need for secrecy might be heightened by fear that a coach or a parent will learn of the eating disorder and not allow the athlete to compete.

Even though research is limited, it seems appropriate to conclude that athletes are at higher risk for eating disorders than the general population. Existing evidence likely does not reflect the seriousness of this problem in athletic populations. Although research data are not yet available, the prevalence might be as high as 50% or more in the specific high-risk athletic populations listed earlier.

KEY POINT

Disordered eating has become a major concern in female athletes. Some researchers have estimated the prevalence to be as high as 50% for elite athletes in certain sports.

Eating disorders are generally considered to be addictive disorders and are extremely difficult to treat. The physiological consequences are considerable and can include death. Considering this, along with the emotional distress suffered by the athlete, the extraordinary costs of treatment (from $5,000 to $25,000 per month for hospital inpatient treatment), and the effect on those closest to the athlete, eating disorders must be considered among the most serious problems facing female athletes today, paralleling the seriousness of anabolic steroid use in male athletes. The NCAA has become concerned about the problem of eating disorders and in 1990 released a three-part videotape series on eating disorders with accompanying written materials, articles, and posters for distribution to athletic administrators, coaches, trainers, and athletes. Among these materials is a list of warning signs designed specifically for athletes. These are presented in Table 19.7.

Female athletes are at higher risk for disordered eating for several reasons. Perhaps most importantly, there is tremendous pressure on athletes, particularly female athletes, to get weight down to very low levels, often below what is appropriate. This weight limit can be imposed by the coach, trainer, parent, or the athlete. In addition, the personality of the typical female athlete matches closely with the profile of the female at high risk for an eating disorder (competitive, perfectionistic, under the tight control of a parent or other significant figure, such as a coach). Furthermore, the nature of the sport or activity largely dictates those at high risk. As we mentioned, three categories are at high risk: appearance sports, endurance sports, and weight-classification sports. Finally, added to these are the normal pressures on young women, independent of whether they are athletes or not.

Environmental Factors

Exercise in the heat, in the cold, or at altitude provides additional stress or challenge to the body's adaptive

Table 19.7 Warning Signs for Anorexia Nervosa and Bulimia Nervosa

Warning signs for anorexia nervosa
1. Dramatic loss in weight
2. A preoccupation with food, calories, and weight
3. Wearing baggy or layered clothing
4. Relentless, excessive exercise
5. Mood swings
6. Avoiding food-related social activities

Warning signs for bulimia nervosa
1. A noticeable weight loss or gain
2. Excessive concern about weight
3. Bathroom visits after meals
4. Depressive moods
5. Strict dieting followed by eating binges
6. Increasing criticism of one's body

Note. The presense of one or two of these signs does not necessarily indicate an eating disorder. Absolute diagnosis should be done by appropriate health professionals.

Adapted from National Collegiate Athletic Association (1990).

future heat stress more efficiently. Recent evidence suggests that, after acclimatization, the internal temperature at which sweating and vasodilation begin is similarly lowered in women and men. Also, the sensitivity of the sweating response per unit increase in internal temperature increases by a similar amount in both sexes following both physical training and heat acclimatization. Any differences noted between the women and men were attributed to initial differences in their physical conditioning and not to the subjects' gender.

■ KEY POINT ■

Women generally have lower sweat rates than men for the same heat stress, and this appears to be the result of a lower sweat production per sweat gland. However, this reduced sweating capacity does not appear to affect women's ability to tolerate heat.

---

abilities (chapters 11 and 12). Many early studies indicated that women are less tolerant to heat than men are, particularly when physical work is involved. Much of this difference, however, is the result of lower fitness levels in the women included in these studies, as the men and women were tested at the same absolute rate of work. When the rate of work is adjusted relative to individual $\dot{V}O_2$ max, women's responses are almost identical to men's. Women generally have lower sweat rates for the same exercise and heat stress, although they possess a larger number of active sweat glands than men do.

Research shows that, when exposed to repeated bouts of heat stress, the body undergoes considerable adaptation (acclimatization) that enables it to survive

Women have a slight advantage over men during cold exposure because they have more subcutaneous body fat. But their smaller muscle mass is a disadvantage in extreme cold because shivering is the major adaptation for generating body heat. The greater the active muscle mass, the greater the subsequent heat generation. Muscle also provides an additional insulative layer.

Several studies have reported gender differences in response to altitude hypoxia, both at rest and during submaximal exercise. Maximal oxygen consumption decreases during hypoxic work in both sexes, but these decreases do not seem to adversely affect women's ability to work at high altitude. Studies of maximal

---

Female Athlete Triad

In the early 1990s, it became apparent that there is a reasonably strong association between

- disordered eating,
- secondary amenorrhea, and
- bone mineral disorders.

This has been termed the female athlete triad.[40] From the limited research available at this time, it appears that the triad might start with disordered eating. Over a period of time, the length of which has not been well established and might vary considerably from one athlete to another, an athlete who

has disordered eating starts to experience disordered menstrual function, which eventually leads to secondary amenorrhea. Following an additional period of time, again the length of which has not been defined, secondary amenorrhea leads to bone mineral disorders. A number of researchers are becoming interested in these intriguing relationships, and considerable research is now under way. We should know much more about this important sequence of events when the results of these research efforts are known.

exercise at altitude demonstrate no difference in response between the sexes.

■ IN REVIEW . . . ■

1. Three major contributing factors to osteoporosis are estrogen deficiency, inadequate calcium intake, and inadequate physical activity.
2. Postmenopausal women, amenorrheic women, and those who have anorexia nervosa have greater risk of osteoporosis.
3. Eating disorders, such as anorexia nervosa and bulimia nervosa, are more common in women than in men and, for athletes, are especially common in appearance sports, endurance sports, and weight-classification sports. Athletes seem to be at a higher risk for eating disorders than the general population.
4. When work rate is adjusted relative to individual $\dot{V}O_{2\,max}$, women and men respond almost identically to heat stress. Any differences noted are likely due to different initial levels of conditioning.
5. Because they have more insulative subcutaneous fat, women have a slight advantage over men during cold exposure, but their smaller muscle mass limits their ability to generate body heat.
6. Studies indicate that responses during exercise at altitude do not differ in women and men.

In Closing . . .

In this chapter, we discussed gender differences in performance. Most true differences between the sexes result from women's smaller size and greater body fat. We also considered how women's relatively more sedentary lifestyle, an artifact from a society that traditionally frowned on women's participation in physical activity, has affected their performance through the years. Finally, we have found that female and male athletes are not as different as many people believe.

With this chapter, we conclude our examination of special populations in sport and exercise. In the next part, we turn our attention from athletics to a different application of exercise physiology: the use of physical activity for health and fitness. We begin with its role in the prevention and treatment of cardiovascular disease.

■ Key Terms

anorexia nervosa
bulimia nervosa
disordered eating
eating disorders
estrogen
eumenorrhea

gender differences
lipoprotein lipase
menstrual cycle
menstrual dysfunction
oligomenorrhea
osteoporosis
pregnancy
primary amenorrhea
secondary amenorrhea
sex-specific differences
teratogenic effects
testosterone

■ Study Questions

1. How do females compare with males with respect to body composition? How do comparisons of athletes differ from those of nonathletes?
2. What is the role of testosterone in the development of strength and fat-free mass?
3. How do women and men compare relative to upper body strength? Lower body strength? Relative to fat-free weight? Can women gain strength with resistance training?
4. What differences in $\dot{V}O_{2\,max}$ exist between normal females and males? Between highly trained females and males?
5. What cardiovascular differences exist between females and males with respect to submaximal exercise? Maximal exercise?
6. Why are female and male performances in motor skills similar up to the age of puberty, and yet considerably different once puberty has been attained?
7. How does the menstrual cycle influence athletic performance?
8. What are some of the possible reasons that women athletes in intensive training will, in some cases, stop menstruating for intervals of several months to several years or more?
9. What are the risks associated with training during pregnancy? How can these be avoided?
10. What are the effects of amenorrhea on bone mineral? How does exercise training affect bone mineral?
11. What are the two major eating disorders, and what is the level of risk of elite female athletes for these eating disorders? How does this vary by sport?
12. How do women differ from men in their exercise response when exposed to intense heat and humidity? To altitude?

■ References

1. Bale, P., & Nelson, G. (1985). The effects of menstruation on performance of swimmers. *Australian Journal of Science and Medicine in Sport*, **19**, 19-22.

2. Boyden, T.W., Pamenter, R.W., Stanforth, P., Rotkis, T., & Wilmore, J.H. (1983). Sex steroids and endurance running in women. *Fertility and Sterility*, **39**, 629-632.

3. Brooks-Gunn, J., Gargiulo, J.M., & Warren, M.P. (1986). The effect of cycle phase on the adolescent swimmers. *Physician and Sportsmedicine*, **14**(3), 182-192.

4. Bullen, B.A., Skrinar, G.S., Beitins, I.Z., von Mering, G., Turnbull, B.A., & McArthur, J.W. (1985). Induction of menstrual disorders by strenuous exercise in untrained women. *New England Journal of Medicine*, **312**, 1349-1353.

5. Cann, C.E., Martin, M.C., Genant, H.K., & Jaffe, R.B. (1984). Decreased spinal mineral content in amenorrheic women. *Journal of the American Medical Association*, **251**, 626-629.

6. Clapp, J.F. III, Wesley, M., & Sleamaker, R.H. (1987). Thermoregulatory and metabolic responses to jogging prior to and during pregnancy. *Medicine and Science in Sports and Exercise*, **19**, 124-130.

7. Costill, D.L., Fink, W.J., Flynn, M., & Kirwan, J. (1987). Muscle fiber composition and enzyme activities in elite female distance runners. *International Journal of Sports Medicine*, **8**(Suppl. 2), 103-106.

8. Cureton, K., Bishop, P., Hutchinson, P., Newland, H., Vickery, S., & Zwiren, L. (1986). Sex differences in maximal oxygen uptake: Effect of equating haemoglobin concentration. *European Journal of Applied Physiology*, **54**, 656-660.

9. Cureton, K.J., & Sparling, P.B. (1980). Distance running performance and metabolic responses to running in men and women with excess weight experimentally equated. *Medicine and Science in Sports and Exercise*, **12**, 288-294.

10. Drinkwater, B.L. (1973). Physiological responses of women to exercise. *Exercise and Sport Sciences Reviews*, **1**, 125-153.

11. Drinkwater, B.L., Bruemner, B., & Chesnut, C.H. III. (1990). Menstrual history as a determinant of current bone density in young athletes. *Journal of the American Medical Association*, **263**, 545-548.

12. Drinkwater, B.L., Nilson, K., Chesnut, C.H. III, Bremner, W.J., Shainholtz, S., & Southworth, M.B. (1984). Bone mineral content of amenorrheic and eumenorrheic athletes. *New England Journal of Medicine*, **311**, 277-281.

13. Drinkwater, B.L., Nilson, K., Ott, S., & Chesnut, C.H. III. (1986). Bone mineral density after resumption of menses in amenorrheic athletes. *Journal of the American Medical Association*, **256**, 380-382.

14. Fink, W.J., Costill, D.L., & Pollock, M.L. Submaximal and maximal working capacity of elite distance runners. Part II. Muscle fiber composition and enzyme activities. *Annals of the New York Academy of Sciences*, **301**, 323-327.

15. Forbes, G.B. (1972). Growth of the lean body mass in man. *Growth*, **36**, 325-338.

16. Forbes, G.B. (1976). The adult decline in lean body mass. *Human Biology*, **48**, 161-173.

17. Frisch, R.E. (1983). Fatness and reproduction: Delayed menarche and amenorrhea of ballet dancers and college athletes. In *Anorexia nervosa: Recent developments in research* (pp. 343-363). New York: Liss.

18. Frisch, R.E. (1988). Fatness and fertility. *Scientific American*, **255**, 88-95.

19. Frisch, R.E., & McArthur, J.W. (1974). Menstrual cycles: Fatness as a determinant of minimum weight for height necessary for their maintenance or onset. *Science*, **185**, 949-951.

20. Gadpaille, W.J., Sanborn, C.F., & Wagner, W.W. (1987). Athletic amenorrhea, major affective disorders, and eating disorders. *American Journal of Psychiatry*, **144**, 939-942.

21. Hermansen, L., & Andersen, K. L. (1965). Aerobic work capacity in young Norwegian men and women. *Journal of Applied Physiology*, **20**, 425-431.

22. Hult, J.S. (1986). The female American runner: A modern quest for visibility. In B.L. Drinkwater (Ed.), *Female endurance athletes*. Champaign, IL: Human Kinetics.

23. Ingjer, F., & Brodal, P. (1978). Capillary supply of skeletal muscle fibers in untrained and endurance-trained women. *European Journal of Applied Physiology*, **38**, 291-299.

24. Keizer, H.A., & Rogol, A.D. (1990). Physical exercise and menstrual cycle alterations: What are the mechanisms? *Sports Medicine*, **10**, 218-235.

25. Lohman, T.G. (1986). Application of body composition techniques and constants for children and youths. *Exercise and Sport Sciences Reviews*, **14**, 325-357.

26. Loucks, A.B. (1990). Effects of exercise training on the menstrual cycle: Existence and mechanisms. *Medicine and Science in Sports and Exercise*, **22**, 275-280.

27. Malina, R.M. (1983). Menarche in athletes: A synthesis and hypothesis. *Annals of Human Biology*, **10**, 1-24.

28. Pate, R.R., Sparling, P.B., Wilson, G.E., Cureton, K.J., & Miller, B.J. (1987). Cardiorespiratory and metabolic responses to submaximal and maximal exercise in elite women distance runners. *International Journal of Sports Medicine*, **8**(Suppl. 2), 91-95.

29. Pollock, M.L. (1977). Submaximal and maximal working capacity of elite distance runners. Part I: Cardiorespiratory aspects. *Annals of the New York Academy of Sciences*, **301**, 310-322.

30. Prior, J.C. (1988). Reproductive changes with exercise: When and how to evaluate, who and why to treat. In J.L. Puhl, C.H. Brown, & R.O. Voy (Eds.), *Sport science perspectives for women* (pp. 131-150). Champaign, IL: Human Kinetics.

31. Quadagno, D., Faquin, L., Lim, G.-N., Kuminka, W., & Moffatt, R. (1991). The menstrual cycle: Does it affect athletic performance? *Physician and Sportsmedicine*, **19**, 121-124.

32. Rigotti, N.A., Nussbaum, S.R., Herzog, D.B., & Neer, R.M. (1984). Osteoporosis in women with anorexia nervosa. *New England Journal of Medicine*, **311**, 1601-1606.

33. Saltin, B., & Åstrand, P.-O. (1967). Maximal oxygen uptake in athletes. *Journal of Applied Physiology*, **23**, 353-358.

34. Saltin, B., & Rowell, L.B. (1980). Functional adaptations to physical activity and inactivity. *Federation Proceedings*, **39**, 1506-1513.

35. Schantz, P., Randall-Fox, E., Hutchison, W., Tyden, A., & Åstrand, P.-O. (1983). Muscle fibre type distribution, muscle cross-sectional area and maximal voluntary strength in humans. *Acta Physiologica Scandinavica*, **117**, 219-226.

36. Schwartz, B., Cumming, D.C., Riordan, E., Selye, M., Yen, S.S.C., & Rebar, R.W. (1981). Exercise-associated amenorrhea: A distinct entity? *American Journal of Obstetrics and Gynecology*, **141**, 662-670.

37. Sinning, W.E., & Little, K.D. (1987). Body composition and menstrual function in athletes. *Sports Medicine*, **4**, 34-45.

38. Stager, J.M., Wigglesworth, J.K., & Hatler, L.K. (1990). Interpreting the relationship between age of menarche and prepubertal training. *Medicine and Science in Sports and Exercise*, **22**, 54-58.

39. Wilmore, J.H. (1974). Alterations in strength, body composition and anthropometric measurements consequent to a 10-week weight training program. *Medicine and Science in Sports*, **6**, 133-138.

40. Wilmore, J.H. (1991). Eating and weight disorders in the female athlete. *International Journal of Sports Nutrition*, **1**, 104-117.

41. Wilmore, J.H., Wambsgans, K.C., Brenner, M., Broeder, C.E., Paijmans, I., Volpe, J.A., & Wilmore, K.M. (1992). Is there energy conservation in amenorrheic compared to eumenorrheic distance runners? *Journal of Applied Physiology*, **72**, 15-22.

42. Wolfe, L.A., Hall, P., Webb, K.A., Goodman, L., Monga, M., & McGrath, M.J. (1989). Prescription of aerobic exercise during pregnancy. *Sports Medicine*, **8**, 273-301.

43. Wolfe, L.A., Ohtake, P.J., Mottola, M.F., & McGrath, M.J. (1989). Physiological interactions between pregnancy and aerobic exercise. *Exercise and Sport Sciences Reviews*, **17**, 295-351.

▮ Selected Readings

Artal, R., & Wiswell, R.A. (Eds.) (1986). *Exercise in pregnancy*. Baltimore: Williams & Wilkins.

Åstrand, I. (1960). Aerobic work capacity in men and women with special reference to age. *Acta Physiologica Scandinavica*, **49**(Suppl. 169).

Åstrand, P.-O. (1952). *Experimental studies of physical working capacity in relation to age and sex*. Copenhagen: Munksgaard.

Drinkwater, B.L. (1984). Women and exercise: Physiological aspects. *Exercise and Sport Sciences Reviews*, **12**, 21-51.

Drinkwater, B.L. (Ed.) (1986). *Female endurance athletes*. Champaign, IL: Human Kinetics.

Highet, R. (1989). Athletic amenorrhoea: An update on aetiology, complications and management. *Sports Medicine*, **7**, 82-108.

Lotgering, F.K., Gilbert, R.D., & Longo, L.D. (1985). Maternal and fetal responses to exercise during pregnancy. *Physiological Reviews*, **65**, 1-36.

McMurray, R.G., & Katz, V.L. (1990). Thermoregulation in pregnancy: Implications for exercise. *Sports Medicine*, **10**, 146-158.

McMurray, R.G., Mottola, M.F., Wolfe, L.A., Artal, R., Millar, L., & Pivarnik, J.M. (1993). Recent advances in understanding maternal and fetal responses to exercise. *Medicine and Science in Sports and Exercise*, **25**(2), 1305-1321.

Puhl, J.L., Brown, C.H., & Voy, R.O. (Eds.) (1988). *Sport science perspectives for women*. Champaign: Human Kinetics.

Rutherford, O.M. (1993). Spine and total body bone mineral density in amenorrheic endurance athletes. *Journal of Applied Physiology*, **74**(6), 2904-2908.

Shangold, M. M. (1984). Exercise and the adult female: Hormonal and endocrine effects. *Exercise and Sport Sciences Reviews*, **12**, 53-79.

Shangold, M., & Mirkin, G. (Eds.) (1988). *Women and exercise: Physiology and sports medicine*. Philadelphia: Davis.

Sparling, P.B. (Ed.) (1987). A comprehensive profile of elite women distance runners. *International Journal of Sports Medicine*, **8**(Suppl. 2), 71-136.

Sundgot-Borgen, J. (1993). Prevalence of eating disorders in elite female athletes. *International Journal of Sport Nutrition*, **3**, 29-40.

Wells, C.L. (1991). *Women, sport & performance: A physiological perspective* (2nd ed.). Champaign, IL: Human Kinetics.

Physical Activity for Health and Fitness

In earlier parts of this book, we focused on the physiological bases of physical activity and how we can improve our performance. Now, in Part G, we shift our focus away from athletic performance and turn to a special area of exercise and sport physiology: the use of physical activity for health and fitness. As in Part F, we will concentrate on special populations, but now our interest is not in optimizing performance but rather in optimizing health and fitness. We begin in chapter 20, Cardiovascular Disease and Physical Activity, by examining the major types of cardiovascular disease, their physiological bases, and how physical activity can benefit those who have these diseases. In chapter 21, Obesity, Diabetes, and Physical Activity, we examine the causes of obesity and diabetes, the health risks associated with each, and how physical activity can be used to control both disorders. Finally in chapter 22, Prescription of Exercise for Health and Fitness, we discuss how to design an exercise program that can improve health and fitness. We will consider the essential components, how to tailor the program to an individual's specific needs, and the unique role of physical activity for rehabilitation of ill patients.

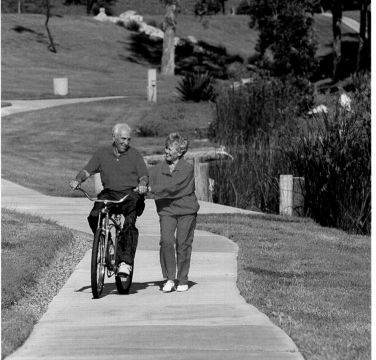

© Elaine Olsen/Photo Network

Chapter 20

Cardiovascular Disease and Physical Activity

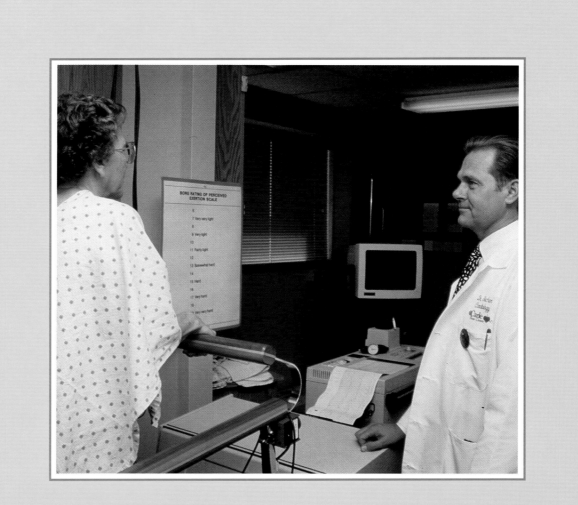

Chapter Overview

Most of us consider ourselves to be healthy until we experience some overt sign of illness. With chronic degenerative diseases, such as heart disease, most people are unaware that the disease process is smoldering and progressing to where it could cause major complications, including death. Fortunately, early detection and proper treatment of various chronic diseases can substantially reduce their severity and often avert death. Even more important, decreasing the risk factors for a disease can often either prevent the disease or delay its onset. To do this, we should

- change our dietary habits;
- increase our regular physical activity;
- abstain from the use of tobacco and other drugs;
- consume alcohol only in moderation, if at all;
- get adequate rest and sleep; and
- improve our ability to cope with stress.

Though this list is familiar to most of us, physical activity is too often ignored because it takes time and effort. But its importance to our health cannot be overlooked. In this chapter we will consider different types of cardiovascular disease and their pathophysiology, and we will explore the impact of physical activity on both prevention and treatment of these diseases.

Chapter Outline

On July 3, 1993, professional baseball Hall of Famer Don Drysdale was found dead of a heart attack in his Montreal hotel room at age 56. Drysdale broke into the major leagues in 1956 as a 19-year-old pitcher for the Brooklyn Dodgers. This tragedy illustrates the important fact that being an outstanding athlete during youth and young adulthood does not confer lifelong immunity from coronary artery disease. Maintaining an active lifestyle throughout life, however, has now been shown to be one of the most important decisions that you can make to reduce your risk of a fatal heart attack.

Chronic and degenerative diseases of the cardiovascular system are the major cause of serious illness and death in the United States. Cardiovascular diseases[1]

- affect more than 70 million Americans each year,
- result in nearly 1 million deaths each year (based on 1990 data), and
- cost individuals, government, and private industry nearly $120 billion annually.

As shown in Figure 20.1, cardiovascular diseases, including heart disease and stroke, now kill almost as many Americans each year as all other causes of death combined, including cancer, AIDS, infant mortality, and accidents!

From the early 1900s to the mid-1960s, the relative number of heart disease deaths, expressed per 100,000 people, increased threefold. The population of the United States more than doubled during that time, so the absolute number of heart disease deaths increased even more dramatically than the relative rate indicates. It was estimated that in 1993

- more than 1.5 million heart attacks would occur in America,
- about 500,000 Americans would die from heart attacks, and
- more than one out of every four Americans would suffer some form of cardiovascular disease.

Fortunately, the number of deaths from cardiovascular disease and heart attacks has steadily decreased since its peak in the mid-1960s (see Figure 20.2). The reasons for this decline have been heavily debated but likely include the following:

- Better and earlier diagnosis
- Better medical care
- Improved drugs for specific treatment
- Better emergency care and treatment for heart attack victims
- Improved public awareness
- Increased use of preventive measures, including lifestyle changes to reduce individual risk

---

KEY POINT

Cardiovascular diseases remain the number one cause of death in the United States, accounting for more than two out of every five deaths. However, from 1980 to 1990 there was a 26.7% decrease in the death rate from cardiovascular diseases, and the peak death rate from heart disease had, by 1990, declined by more than 50% from its peak in the mid-1960s.

Now that we have briefly discussed the extent of this health problem, let's turn our attention to some specific types of cardiovascular disease.

Forms of Cardiovascular Disease

There are several different cardiovascular diseases. In this section, we will focus primarily on those that are preventable and that affect the largest number of Americans each year.

Coronary Artery Disease

As humans age, their coronary arteries, which supply the heart muscle (myocardium) itself, become progressively narrower as a result of the formation of fatty plaque along the inner wall of the artery, as seen in Figure 20.3. This process of progressive narrowing of the arteries in general is referred to as atherosclerosis, and when the coronary arteries are involved, it is termed coronary artery disease. As the disease progresses and the coronary arteries become more narrowed, the capacity to supply blood to the myocardium is progressively reduced.

As the narrowing worsens, the myocardium eventually can't receive enough blood to meet all of its needs. When this occurs, the portion of the heart that is supplied by the narrowed arteries becomes ischemic, meaning it suffers a deficiency of blood. Ischemia of

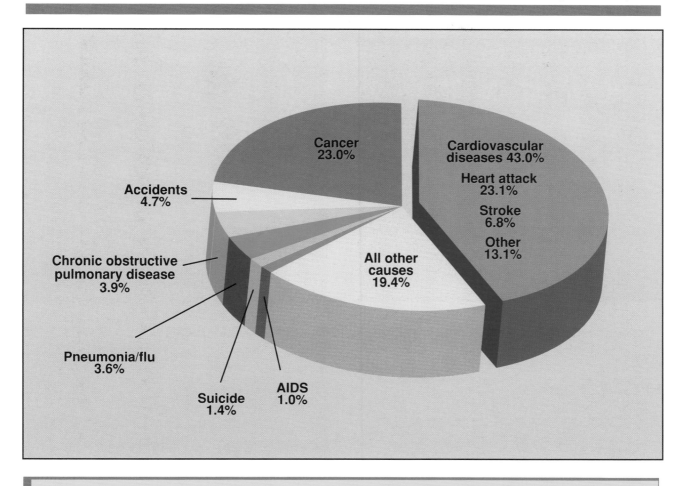

Figure 20.1   The leading causes of death in the United States in 1990. Data from American Heart Association (1993).

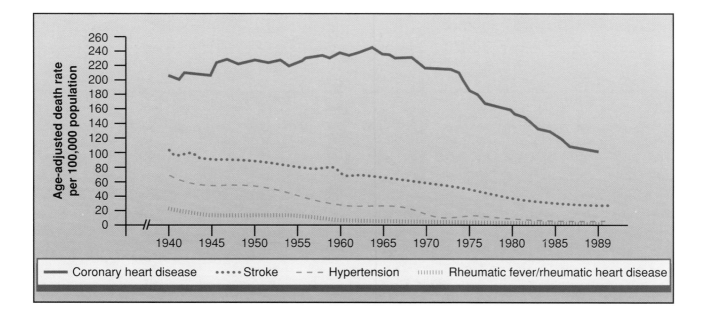

Figure 20.2   Age-adjusted death rates for major cardiovascular diseases, illustrating the marked decline in deaths from heart attacks, stroke, and hypertension. Data from American Heart Association (1993).

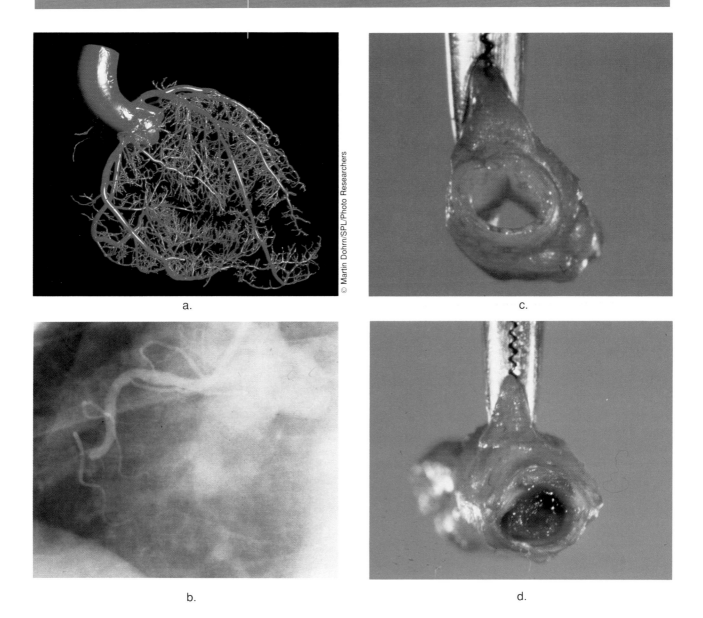

© Martin Dohrn/SPL/Photo Researchers

a.

b.

c.

d.

Figure 20.3   (a) A resin cast of the coronary arteries reveals the heart's extensive blood supply. (b) Occlusion of a coronary artery appears in an angiogram as an area of restricted blow flow. In coronary artery disease, (c) plaque may begin to build up in any of the coronary arteries, (d) eventually restricting circulation through that vessel.

the heart usually causes severe chest pain, referred to as angina pectoris. This is typically first experienced during periods of physical exertion or stress when the demands on the heart are greatest.

When blood supply to a part of the myocardium is severely or totally restricted, ischemia can lead to a heart attack, or myocardial infarction, because cardiac muscle cells that are deprived of blood for several minutes are also deprived of oxygen, which leads to irreversible damage and cellular death (necrosis). This can lead to mild, moderate, or severe disability or even death, depending on the location of the infarction and

the extent of the damage. Sometimes a heart attack is so mild that the victim is unaware that it has occurred. In such cases, discovery of the heart attack can come weeks, months, or even years later when an electrocardiogram is obtained during a routine medical examination.

Atherosclerosis is not a disease of the aged. Rather it is more appropriately classified as a pediatric disease because the pathological changes that lead to atherosclerosis begin in infancy and progress during childhood.[16] Fatty streaks, or lipid deposits, which are thought to be the probable precursors of atherosclerosis, are commonly found in the aortas of children by age 3 to 5. These fatty streaks start to appear in the coronary arteries during the early teens, can develop into fibrous plaques during the 20s, and can progress to complicated lesions during the 40s and 50s.

KEY POINT

Atherosclerosis is a pediatric disease, with its origin in childhood. The disease progresses at different rates, depending primarily on heredity and lifestyle choices.

The rate at which atherosclerosis progresses is largely determined by genetics and lifestyle factors, including smoking history, diet, physical activity, and stress. For some people, the disease progresses rapidly, with a heart attack occurring at a relatively young age—in the 30s or 40s. For others, the disease progresses very slowly, with few or no symptoms throughout their lives. Most people fall somewhere between these two extremes.

To illustrate this, a study of combat fatalities from the Korean War revealed that 77% of autopsied American soldiers, average age 22.1, already had some gross evidence of coronary atherosclerosis.[8] The extent of disease ranged from fibrous thickening to complete occlusion of one or more of the main branches of the coronary arteries. The autopsied Korean soldiers, however, were free of the disease. Evidence of coronary atherosclerosis was also found in 45% of the American fatalities from the Vietnam War, and 5% exhibited severe manifestations of the disease.[22]

Hypertension

Hypertension is the medical term for high blood pressure, a condition in which blood pressure is chronically elevated above levels considered desirable or healthy for a person's age and size. Blood pressure is primarily dependent on body size, so children and young adolescents have much lower blood pressures than adults. For this reason, determining what constitutes hypertension in the growing child and adolescent is difficult. Clinically, hypertension in these groups is defined as blood pressure values above the 90th or the 95th percentile for the youth's age. Hypertension is uncommon during childhood but can appear during midadolescence. For adults, the Joint National Committee on Detection, Evaluation, and Treatment of High Blood Pressure has established the guidelines, presented in Table 20.1, for diastolic blood pressure, which is the

Table 20.1 Adult Guidelines for Blood Pressure

Diastolic blood pressure (mmHg)	
< 85	Normal blood pressure
85 - 89	High-normal blood pressure
90 - 104	Mild hypertension
105 - 114	Moderate hypertension
> 114	Severe hypertension
Systolic blood pressure (mmHg), when diastolic pressure is <90 mmHg	
< 140	Normal blood pressure
140 - 159	Borderline isolated systolic hypertension
> 159	Isolated systolic hypertension

Note. Established by the Joint National Committee on Detection, Evaluation, and Treatment of High Blood Pressure.

lowest pressure in the arteries at any time, and for systolic blood pressure, which is the highest pressure in the arteries at any time.[15]

High blood pressure causes the heart to work harder than normal, as it has to expel blood from the left ventricle against a greater resistance. Furthermore, hypertension places great strain on the systemic arteries and arterioles. Over time, this stress can cause the heart to enlarge and the arteries and arterioles to become scarred, hardened, and less elastic. Eventually, this can lead to atherosclerosis, heart attacks, heart failure, stroke, and kidney failure.

In 1990, 63.6 million American adults and children were estimated to either have high blood pressure or to be undergoing treatment for it.[1] Approximately 25% of the United States' adult population has high blood pressure. Of those with hypertension, 46% are not aware of it and 67% are not on therapy to control it.[1] Even though the death rate from hypertension decreased by 21.6% from 1980 to 1990, it was estimated that nearly 33,000 Americans died as a result of hypertension in 1990. African-Americans, Puerto Ricans, Cuban-Americans, and Mexican-Americans are more likely to suffer from hypertension than Caucasians. This is clearly pointed out in the death rates from hypertension during 1989:[1]

- Caucasian men, 6.2 per 100,000
- Caucasian women, 4.6 per 100,000
- African-American men, 28.7 per 100,000
- African-American women, 21.4 per 100,000

KEY POINT

About one of every four adult Americans has hypertension.

Stroke

Stroke, also called cerebrovascular accident (CVA), is a form of cardiovascular disease that affects the cerebral arteries—those that supply the brain. Approximately 500,000 strokes occur in the United States each year, resulting in nearly 150,000 deaths per year.[1] Similar to coronary artery disease and hypertension, the number of deaths from strokes has also been decreasing significantly in recent years—a 32% reduction between 1980 and 1990.

The most common cause of stroke is cerebral infarction (see Figure 20.4a). This typically results from

- cerebral thrombosis, in which a thrombus (blood clot) forms in a cerebral vessel, often at the site of atherosclerotic damage to the vessel;
- cerebral embolism, in which an embolus (an undissolved mass of material, such as fat globules, bits of tissue, or a blood clot) breaks loose from another site in the body and lodges in a cerebral artery; or
- atherosclerosis that leads to narrowing of and damage to a cerebral artery.

In these cases, blood flow beyond the blockage is restricted and the part of the brain that relies on that supply becomes ischemic, is oxygen deficient, and can die.

Hemorrhage is the other major cause of stroke (Figure 20.4b). The two major types are cerebral hemorrhage, in which one of the cerebral arteries ruptures in the brain, and subarachnoid hemorrhage, in which one of the brain's surface vessels ruptures, dumping blood into the space between the brain and the skull. In both cases, blood flow beyond the rupture is diminished because the blood leaves the vessel at the site of injury. Also, as the blood accumulates outside of the vessel, it puts pressure on the fragile brain tissue, which can alter brain function. Brain hemorrhages often result from aneurysms, which arise from weak spots in the vessel wall that balloon outward, and aneurysms often arise because of hypertension or atherosclerotic damage to the vessel wall.

As with a heart attack, a stroke results in death of the affected tissue. The consequences depend largely on the location and extent of the stroke. Brain damage from a stroke can affect the senses, speech, body movement, thought patterns, and memory. Paralysis on one side of the body is common, as is the inability to verbalize thoughts. Most effects of a stroke are indicative of the side of the brain that was damaged. These are listed in Table 20.2.

Table 20.2 The Effects of Brain Damage on Either Side

Right brain damage	Left brain damage
Paralyzed left side	Paralyzed right side
Spatial, perceptual deficits	Speech, language deficits
Behavior style—quick, impulsive	Behavioral style—slow, cautious
Memory deficits—language	Memory deficits—performance

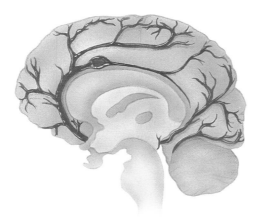

a. Cerebral infarction

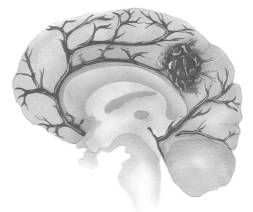

b. Cerebral hemorrhage

Figure 20.4   Two major causes of stroke are (a) cerebral infarction and (b) cerebral hemorrhage.

Congestive Heart Failure

Congestive heart failure is a clinical condition in which the heart muscle becomes too weak to maintain an adequate cardiac output to meet the body's oxygen demands. This usually results from the heart being either damaged or overworked. Hypertension, atherosclerosis, and heart attack are among the possible causes of this disorder.

When cardiac output is inadequate, blood begins to back up in the veins. This causes excess fluids to accumulate in the body, particularly in the legs and ankles. This fluid accumulation (edema) can also affect the lungs (pulmonary edema), disrupting breathing and causing shortness of breath. Congestive heart failure can progress to the point where there is irreversible damage to the heart and the patient becomes a candidate for a heart transplant.

Other Cardiovascular Diseases

Other cardiovascular diseases include

- peripheral vascular diseases,
- valvular heart diseases,
- rheumatic heart disease, and
- congenital heart disease.

Peripheral vascular diseases involve the systemic arteries and veins, as opposed to the coronary vessels. Arteriosclerosis refers to numerous conditions in which the walls of the arteries become thickened, hard, and less elastic. Atherosclerosis is a form of arteriosclerosis. Arteriosclerosis obliterans, in which the artery becomes completely occluded, is another form. Peripheral venous diseases include varicose veins and phlebitis. Varicose veins result from incompetency of the valves in the veins, allowing blood to back up in the veins and causing them to become enlarged, tortuous, and painful. Phlebitis is inflammation of a vein and is also very painful.

Valvular heart diseases involve one or more of the four valves that control the direction of blood flow into and out of the four heart chambers. Rheumatic heart disease is one form of valvular heart disease in which a streptococcal infection has caused acute rheumatic fever, typically in children between ages 5 and 15. Rheumatic fever is an inflammatory disease of the connective tissue and commonly affects the heart, specifically the heart valves. The damage to the valves usually causes difficulty in their opening, hindering blood flow out of that chamber, or difficulty in their closing, allowing blood to flow back into the previous chamber.

Congenital heart disease includes any heart defects that are present at birth and that are also appropriately termed congenital heart defects. These defects occur when the heart or the blood vessels near the heart do not develop normally before birth. These include coarctation of the aorta, in which the aorta is abnormally constricted; valvular stenosis, in which one or more heart valves are narrowed; and septal defects, in which the septum separating the right and left sides of the heart is defective, allowing blood from the systemic side to mix with that in the pulmonary side, and vice versa.

Now that we have considered various types of cardiovascular diseases, in the remainder of this chapter we will focus on the two major diseases in this category: coronary artery disease and hypertension.

■ IN REVIEW . . . ■

1. Atherosclerosis is a process in which arteries become progressively narrowed. Coronary artery disease is atherosclerosis of the coronary arteries.
2. When blood flow is sufficiently blocked, the part of the heart supplied by the diseased artery suffers from lack of blood (ischemia) and the resulting oxygen deprivation can cause myocardial infarction, which results in tissue death (necrosis).
3. Atherosclerotic changes in the arteries actually begin in young children, but the extent and progression of this disease process are quite variable.
4. Hypertension is the clinical term for high blood pressure.
5. Stroke, or cerebral vascular accident, affects the cerebral arteries so that the part of the brain they supply receives too little blood. The most common cause of stroke is cerebral infarction, usually resulting from a cerebral thrombosis or embolism, or from atherosclerosis. Another common cause of stroke is cerebral hemorrhage.
6. Congestive heart failure is a condition in which the cardiac muscle becomes too weakened to maintain an adequate cardiac output, causing blood to back up in the veins.
7. Peripheral vascular diseases involve systemic, rather than coronary, vessels and include arteriosclerosis, varicose veins, and phlebitis.
8. Congenital heart disease includes all heart defects present at birth.

Understanding the Disease Process

Pathophysiology refers to the physiology of a specific disease process or disordered function. Understanding the pathophysiology of a disease gives us insight into how physical activity might affect or alter the disease process. In the following sections we will examine the pathophysiology of coronary artery disease and hypertension.

Pathophysiology of Coronary Artery Disease

How does atherosclerosis develop in the coronary arteries? The coronary arteries, as shown in Figure 20.5, are composed of three distinct layers: the tunica intima or inner layer, the tunica media or middle layer, and the tunica adventitia or outer layer. More simply, these are referred to as the intima, the media, and the adventitia. The innermost layer of the intima is formed by a thin lining of cells that provide a smooth protective

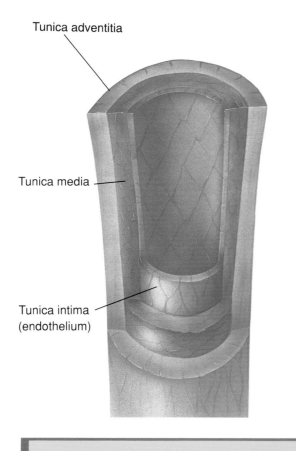

Tunica adventitia

Tunica media

Tunica intima (endothelium)

Figure 20.5   The wall of an artery has three layers: tunica intima, tunica media, and tunica adventitia.

coating between the blood flowing through the artery and the intimal layer of the vessel wall. Local injury to these cells, referred to as endothelial cells, can initiate the process of atherosclerosis.

This process is depicted in Figure 20.6. Early studies in primates have shown that scratching the inner lining of a coronary artery causes the endothelial cells to slough off, exposing the underlying connective tissue. Blood platelets are then attracted to the site of injury and adhere to the exposed connective tissue. These platelets release a substance referred to as platelet-derived growth factor (PDGF, see Figure 20.6b) that promotes migration of smooth muscle cells from the media into the intima. The intima normally contains few if any smooth muscle cells. A plaque, which is basically composed of smooth muscle cells, connective tissue, and debris, forms at the site of injury (see Figure 20.6c). Eventually, lipids in the blood, specifically low-density-lipoprotein cholesterol, are deposited in the plaque (see Figure 20.6d). This early theory of atherosclerosis evolved from the work of Dr. Russell Ross and his colleagues at the University of Washington.[33]

More recently, researchers have theorized that monocytes, which are effector cells of the immune system, attach between endothelial cells. These monocytes eventually become foam cells, or macrophages, and form fatty streaks. Smooth muscle cells then accumulate under these foam cells. When the endothelial cells separate or are sloughed off, the underlying connective tissue becomes exposed and platelets can attach to it.[33] In this modification of the original theory, endothelial injury is not always the precipitating event.

KEY POINT

The process of atherosclerosis appears to begin with injury to or disruption of the endothelial cells lining the intima. This leads to a chain of events that eventually develops into a full-blown atherosclerotic plaque.

Pathophysiology of Hypertension

The pathophysiology of hypertension is not well understood. In fact it is estimated that 90% or more of those identified with hypertension are classified as having idiopathic hypertension, which is hypertension of unknown origin. Idiopathic hypertension, also referred to as essential hypertension, can result from

- genetic factors,
- high sodium intake,

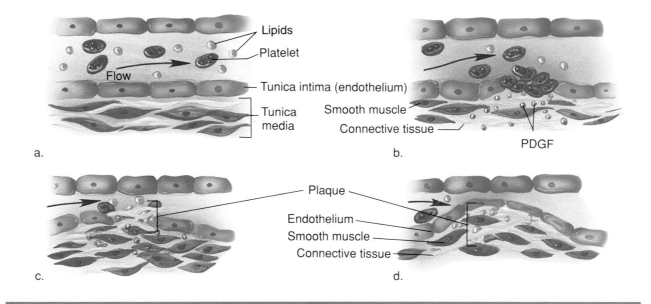

Figure 20.6   Changes in the arterial wall with injury, illustrating the disruption of the endothelium and the subsequent alterations that lead to atherosclerosis.

- obesity,
- insulin resistance,
- physical inactivity,
- psychological stress,
- a combination of these factors, or
- other factors yet to be substantiated or determined.

Determining Individual Risk

Over the years, scientists have attempted to determine the basic etiology, or cause, of both coronary artery disease and hypertension. Much of our understanding of these two diseases comes from the field of epidemiology, a science that studies the relationships of various factors to a specific disease or disease process. In several studies, selected members of various communities have been observed for extended periods of time. These observations have included periodic medical examinations and clinical tests.

Eventually, some of the participants in such studies become diseased and many die. All those who develop heart disease or hypertension or who die from heart attacks or hypertension are grouped accordingly. Then their previous medical and clinical tests are analyzed to determine shared attributes or factors. Although this approach does not define the causal mechanism of the disease, it does provide researchers with valuable insights into the disease process. As

IN REVIEW . . .

1. Pathophysiology refers to the physiology of a specific disease process or disordered function.
2. Early theories held that coronary artery disease can be initiated by damage to the smooth endothelial lining of the intimal layer of the arterial wall. This damage attracts platelets to the area which, in turn, release platelet-derived growth factor (PDGF). PDGF attracts smooth muscle cells, and a plaque, composed of smooth muscle cells, connective tissue, and debris, begins to form. Eventually lipids are deposited in the plaque.
3. More recent research indicates that monocytes, involved with the immune system, can attach between endothelial cells in the intima and begin forming fatty streaks; this then leads to plaque formation. According to this theory, endothelial damage is not necessary.
4. The pathophysiology of hypertension is poorly understood.
5. More than 90% of people with hypertension have idiopathic, or essential, hypertension, meaning its cause is unknown. Possible causes might be genetic factors, excessive sodium intake, obesity, insulin resistance, physical inactivity, and psychological stress.

identified in long-term longitudinal population studies, those factors that place individuals at risk for disease are referred to as risk factors. Let's examine the risk factors for heart disease and hypertension.

Risk Factors for Coronary Artery Disease

The factors associated with an increased risk for premature development of coronary artery disease can be classified into two groups: those over which a person has no control and those that can be altered through basic changes in lifestyle (see Table 20.3). Those that a person cannot control include heredity (family history of coronary artery disease), male gender, and advancing age. Factors that can be controlled or altered include

- elevated blood lipids (cholesterol and triglycerides),
- hypertension,
- cigarette smoking,
- physical inactivity,
- obesity,
- diabetes, and
- stress.

Primary risk factors are those that have been conclusively shown to have a strong association with coronary artery disease. These include smoking, hypertension, high blood lipid levels, and physical inactivity. The latter was added to this list in July 1992. Data from studies conducted in the 1980s suggest that obesity is also likely a primary risk factor. Table 20.4 lists the risk levels associated with actual values for these and other factors.

KEY POINT

Risk factors for a certain disease imply that when one or more of these factors are present, the individual is at increased risk for developing the disease or dying from it. The primary risk factors for coronary artery disease are smoking, hypertension, elevated blood lipids, and physical inactivity.

Lipoproteins

The inclusion of elevated blood lipids as a primary risk factor needs to be further defined. For many years, cholesterol and triglycerides were the only lipids observed in these epidemiologic studies. The public was confused by conflicting data and opinions about the role of lipids in the development of atherosclerosis. More recently, scientists have studied the manner in

Table 20.3 Coronary Artery Disease Risk Factors

Primary risk factors	Secondary risk factors
Smoking	**Alterable**
Hypertension	Obesity
Blood lipids	Diabetes
High LDL-cholesterol	Stress
Low HDL-cholesterol	**Unalterable**
High triglycerides	Heredity (family history)
Physical inactivity	Male gender
	Advancing age

which lipids are transported in the blood. Lipids by themselves are insoluble in blood, so they are packaged with a protein to allow transport through the body. Lipoproteins are the proteins that carry the blood lipids. Two classes of lipoproteins of major concern for coronary artery disease are low-density lipoprotein (LDL) and high-density lipoprotein (HDL). High levels of LDL-bound cholesterol (LDL-C) and low levels of HDL-bound cholesterol (HDL-C) place a person at an extremely high risk of having a heart attack at a relatively young age—under age 60. Conversely, a high level of HDL-C and a low level of LDL-C place a person at an extremely low risk. Yet a third class of lipoproteins, called very-low-density lipoproteins, or VLDL, is becoming increasingly implicated as a risk factor for coronary artery disease.

KEY POINT

High levels of HDL-C and low levels of LDL-C place the individual at the lowest risk for coronary artery disease. LDL-C has been implicated in plaque formation, whereas HDL-C is likely involved in plaque regression.

Merely looking at total cholesterol is not sufficient. A person might have moderately high levels of total cholesterol (Total-C) yet be at a relatively low risk because of a high concentration of HDL-C and low concentration of LDL-C. Conversely, a person might have moderately low levels of total cholesterol, yet be at a relatively high risk because of a high concentration of LDL-C and a low concentration of HDL-C.

Why are these two cholesterol carriers associated with different risk levels? The LDL-C is theorized to be responsible for depositing cholesterol in the arterial wall. The HDL-C, however, is regarded as a scavenger that removes cholesterol from the arterial wall and transports it to the liver to be metabolized. Because of these very different roles, it is essential to know

Table 20.4 Risk of Developing Coronary Artery Disease on the Basis of Specific Values for the Various Risk Factors

Risk factor	Relative level of risk				
	Very low	Low	Moderate	High	Very high
Blood pressure (mmHg)					
Systolic	<110	120	130-140	150-160	>170
Diastolic	<70	76	82-88	94-100	>106
Cigarettes (per day)	Never or none in 1 yr	5	10-20	30-40	>50
Cholesterol (mg • dl^{-1})	<180	<200	220-240	260-280	>300
Cholesterol ÷ HDL[a]	<3.0	<4.0	<4.5	>5.2	>7.0
Triglycerides (mg • dl^{-1})	<50	<100	130	200	>300
Glucose (mg • dl^{-1})	<80	90	100-110	120-130	>140
Body fat (%)					
Men	12	16	25	30	>35
Women	16	20	30	35	>40
Body Mass Index[b]	<25	25-30	30-40	>40	
Stress-tension	Never	Almost never	Occasional	Frequent	Nearly constant
Physical activity (min • wk^{-1})					
Above 6 kcal/min^{-1} (5 METs)[c]	240	180-120	100	80-60	<30
Above 60% HR$_{max}$[d] reserve	120	90	30	0	0
ECG abnormality (S-T–depression [mV])[e]	0	0	0.05	0.10	0.20
Family history of premature heart attack (blood relative)[f]	0	0	1	2	3+
Age	<30	40	50	60	>70

[a]HDL = high-density lipoprotein.

[b]Body Mass Index = weight (kg)/height^2 (m). Risk information from Bray, G.A.: Obesity and the heart. *Modern Concepts in Cardiovascular Disease*, 56:67–71, 1987.

[c]A MET is equal to the oxygen cost at rest. One MET is generally equal to 3.5 ml • kg^{-1} • min^{-1} of oxygen uptake or 1.2 kcal • min^{-1}

[d]HR$_{max}$ = maximal heart rate.

[e]Other ECG abnormalities are also potentially dangerous and are not listed here.

[f]Premature heart attack refers to persons younger than 60 years of age.

Adapted from Pollock and Wilmore (1990).

the specific levels of both of these lipoproteins when determining individual risk. The ratio of Total-C to HDL-C may be the best index of risk for coronary artery disease. Values of 3.0 or less place a person at low risk, but values of 5.0 or greater place a person at high risk. As an example, with a Total-C of 225 mg · dl^{-1}, an HDL-C of 45 mg · dl^{-1} would provide a ratio of 5.0 (225 ÷ 45 = 5.0), but an HDL-C of 75 mg · dl^{-1} would provide a ratio of 3.0 (225 ÷ 75 = 3.0).

Early Detection of Risk Factors

Evidence now suggests that coronary artery disease risk factors can be identified at an early age, and the

---

KEY POINT

The ratio of Total-C to HDL-C is possibly the most accurate lipid index of risk for coronary artery disease, with values of 5.0 or greater indicating increased risk, and values of 3.0 and lower representing low risk.

---

earlier they are identified, the earlier preventive treatment can begin. In a study of 96 boys ages 8 to 12,[41]

• 19.8% had total cholesterol values above the suggested high-normal value of 200 mg · dl^{-1},

- 5.2% exhibited abnormal resting electrocardiograms,
- 37.5% had more than 20% relative body fat, and
- none had elevated blood pressure.

Similar data were reported in a later study of 13- to 15-year-old boys.[40] Both studies are summarized in Table 20.5. Furthermore, those with an elevated risk during childhood generally remain at elevated risk as young adults.

In addition, the results of the Bogalusa Heart Study must be considered. This is a longitudinal study of cardiovascular disease risk factor development from birth through age 26. In 35 of the subjects who had died prematurely (from accidents, homicides, or suicides), the scientists found a strong relationship indicating that the higher the values of total cholesterol and LDL-C, the greater the development of aortic fatty streaks.[27] Fatty streaks in the coronary arteries were found to be related to VLDL-C levels.

Risk Factors for Hypertension

The risk factors for hypertension, as with those for coronary artery disease, can be classified as ones we can control and ones we cannot. Those we cannot control are heredity (family history of hypertension), advancing age, and race (increased risk for people of African or Hispanic ancestry). Risk factors we can control are

- insulin resistance,
- obesity,
- diet (excess sodium intake),
- use of oral contraceptives, and
- physical inactivity.

Although heredity is a risk factor for hypertension, it probably plays a much smaller role than many of the other proposed factors. We must remember that lifestyle factors are often quite similar within a family.

Recently, scientists have shown great interest in a possible link between hypertension, obesity, Type II diabetes, and coronary heart disease through the common pathway of insulin resistance or impaired insulin action. But obesity has also been established as an independent risk factor for hypertension. Numerous studies have shown substantial reductions in blood pressure with weight loss in hypertensive patients. Also, although sodium intake has traditionally been linked to hypertension, this relationship is likely limited to those who are salt-sensitive.

Table 20.5 Coronary Artery Disease Risk Factor Prevalence in Boys, 8 Through 15 Years of Age

Risk factor	Percentage of boys with risk factor	
	8 to 12-year-olds ($n = 96$)	13 to 15-year-olds ($n = 308$)
Blood lipids		
Total cholesterol ≥ 200 mg per 100 ml	20.0	11.0
HDL-C ≤ 36 mg per 100 ml	no data	14.6
Triglycerides ≥ 100 mg per 100 ml	8.4	25.0
Blood pressure		
Systolic > 90th percentile	0.0	13.0
Diastolic > 90th percentile	0.0	4.9
Smoking ≥ 10 cigarettes per day	0.0	0.0
Diabetes	0.0	1.3
Obesity ≥ 25% relative body fat	12.6	14.9
Physical activity $\dot{V}O_2$ max ≤ 42 ml • kg⁻¹ • min⁻¹	3.2	18.8
Family history Heart attack ≤ 60 years of age	33.7	30.9
Presence of risk factors		
None	36.0	29.9
One	46.0	35.4
Two	14.0	22.1
Three	3.0	10.7
Four or more	1.0	1.9

Note. Values represent the percentage of the boys with the risk factor.

> ### KEY POINT
>
> **Although the pathways are complex, it is becoming increasingly clear that hypertension, coronary artery disease, obesity, and diabetes might be linked through the common pathway of insulin resistance.**

Physical inactivity might or might not be a risk factor for hypertension. Its role has not been conclusively established in epidemiologic studies, but substantial evidence indicates that increasing physical activity tends to reduce elevated blood pressure.[11,12,34,37,38]

IN REVIEW . . .

1. Risk factors for coronary artery disease that we cannot control are heredity (and family history), male gender, and advancing age. Those that we can control are elevated blood lipids, hypertension, cigarette smoking, physical inactivity, obesity, diabetes, and stress. Primary risk factors are those that have been proven to be strongly associated with the diseases. For coronary artery disease, these are smoking, hypertension, high blood lipids, and physical inactivity.

2. LDL-C is thought to be responsible for depositing cholesterol in the arterial walls. VLDL-C is increasingly implicated in the generation of coronary artery disease. However, HDL-C acts as a scavenger, removing built-up cholesterol from the vessel walls.

3. The ratio of total cholesterol to HDL-C might be the best indicator of personal risk for coronary artery disease. Values below 3.0 reflect a low risk, but values above 5.0 reflect a high risk.

4. Risk factors for hypertension that can't be controlled include heredity, advancing age, and race. Those we can control are insulin resistance, obesity, diet (excess sodium), use of oral contraceptives, and physical inactivity.

Prevention Through Physical Activity

What role physical activity might play in preventing or delaying the onset of coronary artery disease and hypertension has been of major interest to the medical community for many years. In the following sections, we will try to unravel this mystery by examining the following areas:

- Epidemiologic evidence
- Physiological adaptations with training that might reduce risk
- Risk factor reduction with exercise training

Prevention of Coronary Artery Disease

Physical activity has been proven effective in reducing the risk of coronary artery disease. In the following sections we will discover what is known about this topic and what physiological mechanisms are involved.

Epidemiologic Evidence

Well over 100 research papers have dealt with the relationship between physical inactivity and coronary artery disease. Generally, studies have found the risk of heart attack in sedentary male populations to be about two to three times that of men who are physically active, in either their jobs or their recreational pursuits.[32] The early studies of Dr. J.N. Morris and his colleagues in England in the 1950s were among the first to demonstrate this relationship.[25] In these studies, sedentary bus drivers were compared to active bus conductors who worked on double-decker buses, and sedentary postal workers were compared to active postal carriers who walked their routes. The death rate from coronary artery disease was about twice as high in the sedentary groups as in the active groups. Many studies published over the subsequent 20 years showed essentially the same results: those who were occupationally sedentary were at twice the risk for death from coronary artery disease than those who were active.

Most of these early epidemiologic studies focused exclusively on occupational activity. Not until the 1970s did researchers start looking at leisure time activity as well. Again, the studies by Dr. Morris and his colleagues were among the first to observe the relationship between leisure time activity and the risk of coronary artery disease, with the least active people being at two to three times greater risk.[24,26] Subsequent studies by epidemiologists such as Paffenbarger and Blair have provided similar results.[2,3,7,20,21,30] Physical inactivity approximately doubles the risk of having a fatal heart attack.[32]

Powell and his colleagues at the Centers for Disease Control in Atlanta conducted an extensive review of all epidemiologic studies published on physical inactivity and coronary artery disease up to the mid-1980s.[32] They used stringent criteria for including studies in their analysis, and the quality of each study was also assessed. They found that the average relative risk of coronary artery disease associated with inactivity ranged from 1.5 to 2.4, with a median value of 1.9, meaning that inactive people have about twice the risk as more active people. The researchers found that relative risk from physical inactivity is similar to the risk associated with the three other major risk factors for coronary artery disease. Furthermore, the percentage of the total population of the United States that is physically inactive far exceeds the percentage with the other three major risks: those who smoke, are hypertensive, or have elevated cholesterol levels. This is illustrated in Figure 20.7. The results of these epidemiologic studies played a major role in leading the

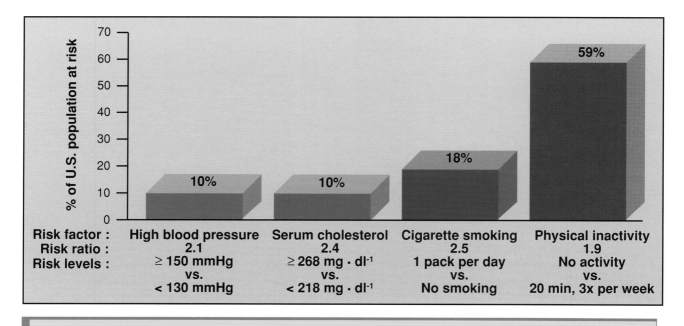

Figure 20.7   Percentages of the U.S. population at increased risk for coronary artery disease based on the primary risk factors. Adapted from Caspersen (1987).

American Heart Association in 1992 to declare physical inactivity a primary risk factor for coronary artery disease.

Another important concern was also raised in the mid-1980s: What level of physical activity or fitness is necessary to reduce one's risk of coronary artery disease?[19] It was not totally clear from the epidemiologic studies what level of fitness or activity was effective. In fact, during the mid-1980s scientists had just started to differentiate between activity level and fitness, defining personal fitness by a person's $\dot{V}O_{2 max}$. In retrospect, distinguishing these two terms was crucial because a person can be active yet unfit (low $\dot{V}O_{2 max}$), or be fit (high $\dot{V}O_{2 max}$) yet inactive. Dr. Ronald LaPorte and his colleagues at the University of Pittsburgh were instrumental in redirecting the thinking and subsequent

research in this area.[19] Dr. LaPorte pointed out that, based on various epidemiologic studies, the levels of activity associated with a lower risk for coronary artery disease were generally low and certainly not at the level that would increase aerobic capacity. Subsequent studies have supported this.[3,20,21] Low levels of activity, such as walking and gardening, can provide considerable benefit by reducing the risk for coronary artery disease.

Training Adaptations That Might Reduce Risk

The importance of regular physical activity in reducing the risk of coronary artery disease becomes apparent when we consider anatomical and physiological adaptations in response to exercise training. For example, as we learned in chapter 10, exercise training causes the heart to hypertrophy, primarily through an increase in left ventricular chamber size but also through increases in left ventricular wall thickness. This adaptation is possibly important for improved contractility and increased cardiac work capacity.

The capacity of the coronary circulation appears to increase with training. Studies have shown that the size of major coronary vessels increases, which implies an increased capacity for blood flow to all regions of the heart. In fact, several studies have demonstrated

---

KEY POINT

From epidemiologic studies, it has been established that physical inactivity doubles the risk of coronary artery disease. However, it is now equally clear that low-intensity activity is sufficient to reduce the risk of this disease. Health benefits do not require high-intensity exercise!

that the peak flow rate in the major coronary arteries is increased following an exercise training program. An important study was conducted at Boston University by Dr. Dieter Kramsch and his associates, who studied the effects of moderate exercise training on the development of coronary artery disease in monkeys.[18] The monkeys were divided into three groups:

1. A control group eating normal low-fat monkey chow
2. A nonexercising group eating an atherogenic (high fat) diet known to induce heart disease
3. An exercising group also eating the atherogenic diet

The sedentary group that consumed the atherogenic diet developed atherosclerosis. However, the coronary arteries of the exercising monkeys on this same diet had an increased internal diameter and substantially less atherosclerosis, as shown in Figure 20.8.

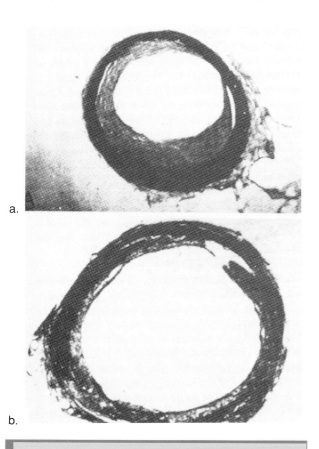

a.

b.

Figure 20.8 Comparison of the left main coronary artery in (a) sedentary and (b) exercising monkeys on atherogenic diets. Reprinted from Kramsch et al. (1981).

For this group, the cross-sectional area of the lumen of all of the major coronary vessels was two to three times larger than in the sedentary monkeys.

Some evidence also suggests that the heart's collateral circulation improves with exercise training. The collateral circulation is a system of small vessels that come off of the major coronary vessels and are important in providing blood to all regions of the heart, particularly when there are blockages in the major coronary arteries.

Risk Reduction With Exercise Training

Many studies have investigated the role of exercise in altering risk factors associated with heart disease. Let's consider the major risk factors and how exercise might affect them.

Little direct evidence is available to indicate that exercise leads to smoking cessation or a reduction in the number of cigarettes smoked. However, a great deal of anecdotal information suggests that this is true. Relatively strong data support the effectiveness of exercise in reducing blood pressure in those with mild to moderate hypertension. Endurance training can reduce both systolic and diastolic blood pressures by approximately 10 mmHg in individuals with moderate essential hypertension.[11,12,34,37,38] But exercise appears to have little or no effect in those with severe hypertension. The specific mechanisms responsible for the decreases in blood pressure with endurance training have yet to be determined.

■■ KEY POINT ■■

Aerobic training produces favorable physiological changes that decrease the risk of heart attack, including larger coronary arteries and increased heart size and pumping capacity. Aerobic training also has a favorable effect on most of the other risk factors for coronary artery disease.

Exercise possibly exerts its most beneficial effect on blood lipid levels.[10,13,14,39] Although the decreases in Total-C and LDL-C with endurance training are relatively small (generally less than 10%), there appear to be relatively major increases in HDL-C and major decreases in triglycerides. Cross-sectional studies of athletes and nonathletes alike show unequivocally that people with greater levels of aerobic activity or higher aerobic capacities have higher HDL-C and lower triglyceride levels. Results of longitudinal training studies, however, are much less clear. Many studies have reported increases in HDL-C and decreases in triglycerides from training, yet others have reported little or no change. Several have even reported decreased HDL-C levels. Almost all studies, however, have shown that the ratios LDL-C:HDL-C and Total-C:HDL-C are decreased following endurance training. This implies a reduced risk.

Two confounding factors must be considered when evaluating lipid changes with exercise training, because they can have a marked independent effect on such changes. Because plasma lipids are expressed as a concentration (mg lipid per dl blood), any change in plasma volume will affect plasma concentrations independent of the change in total lipid. Recall that training typically results in increased plasma volume (chapter 10). With this plasma expansion, the absolute amount of HDL-C could increase, yet the HDL-C concentration might not change or could even be lowered. In addition, plasma lipid levels are tightly coupled with changes in body weight. When evaluating the effects of exercise training, the independent effects that a change in body weight could have on plasma lipids must be considered.

With respect to the remaining risk factors, exercise plays an important role in weight reduction and control and in the control of diabetes. These will be discussed in detail in chapter 21. Exercise has also been reported to be effective in stress reduction and control and for reducing anxiety.[17,31] Some research supports the use of exercise training in the treatment of depression, although the results are not yet conclusive.[5]

Prevention of Hypertension

Physical activity's role in reducing the risk of hypertension has not been as well established as it has been in coronary artery disease. Let's consider what is known.

Epidemiologic Evidence

Very few epidemiologic studies have investigated the relationship between physical inactivity and hypertension. In the Tecumseh Community Health Study, 1,700 males (age 16 and older) completed questionnaires and interviews to provide estimates of their average daily energy expenditures, their peak daily energy expenditures, and the hours they spent in particular activities. The more active men had significantly lower systolic and diastolic blood pressures, irrespective of age.[23] Similar results were found when resting blood pressure was analyzed by fitness level in nearly 3,000 adult

men and more than 3,900 adult women tested at the Cooper Clinic in Dallas.[4,9] The more-fit individuals exhibited lower systolic and diastolic blood pressures. In a follow-up of the participants from the Cooper Clinic study, the investigators reported a relative risk of 1.5 for the development of hypertension in people with low levels of fitness compared with highly fit people.[2] From these limited studies, active people and fit people are at reduced risks for developing hypertension.

Training Adaptations That Might Reduce Risk

A number of physiological adaptations that accompany endurance training could affect blood pressure both at rest and during exercise. One of the most important changes associated with endurance training is the previously mentioned plasma volume increase. We might logically assume that any increase in plasma volume would increase blood pressure, particularly because one of the first lines of drug treatment for hypertension is the prescription of a diuretic to reduce total body water and thus plasma volume. However, recall from chapter 10 that trained muscle has a notable increase in capillaries. Also, the venous system in a trained person has a greater capacity, allowing it to contain more blood. For these reasons, the increased plasma volume following exercise training does not result in increased blood pressure.

Specific mechanisms responsible for reductions in resting blood pressure with endurance training have not been established. Some studies show that resting cardiac output is reduced and that the body's oxygen demands are met by an increased a-$\bar{v}O_2$ diff. But other studies have found cardiac output to remain unchanged. Without a decrease in cardiac output, the observed reductions in resting blood pressure that follow training must result from reductions in peripheral vascular resistance, which may be due to an overall reduction of sympathetic nervous system activity.

═══ KEY POINT ═══

Aerobic training reduces blood pressure in those who have moderate hypertension, but seems to have little effect on those with severe hypertension. The mechanisms by which exercise reduces blood pressure have not been completely determined.

Risk Reduction With Exercise Training

Not only does exercise itself reduce high blood pressure in those who are moderately hypertensive, but it also affects other risk factors. Exercise is important in reducing body fat and it can increase muscle mass, which may be important in reducing blood glucose levels, thus assisting in better glycemic, or blood sugar, control. This latter effect could reduce insulin resistance, another risk for hypertension. Exercise training has also been associated with stress reduction.

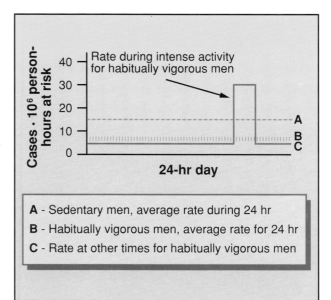

A - Sedentary men, average rate during 24 hr

B - Habitually vigorous men, average rate for 24 hr

C - Rate at other times for habitually vigorous men

Figure 20.9   The risk of primary cardiac arrest during vigorous exercise and at other times throughout a 24-hour day, comparing sedentary men with habitually active men. Data from Siscovick et al. (1984).

IN REVIEW . . .

1. Epidemiologic studies have generally found that the risk of coronary artery disease in sedentary male populations is about two to three times that of men who are physically active, and physical inactivity about doubles a person's risk of a fatal heart attack.
2. The levels of activity associated with a reduced risk for coronary artery disease are generally lower than those needed to increase aerobic capacity.
3. Physical training improves the heart's contractility, work capacity, coronary circulation, and collateral circulation.
4. Exercise may have its major impact on blood lipid levels. Studies show that endurance training decreases the ratios of LDL-C to HDL-C and of Total-C to HDL-C.
5. Exercise also can help control hypertension, weight, and diabetes; can help alleviate stress; and might decrease cigarette smoking.
6. People who are active and those who are fit have reduced risk for developing hypertension.
7. Increased plasma volume that accompanies physical training does not increase blood pressure because trained people have increased capillaries and greater venous capacity.
8. Resting blood pressure is decreased by training in people with moderate hypertension, probably due to decreased peripheral resistance, but the actual mechanisms are unknown.
9. Exercise also reduces body fat and blood glucose levels, which could reduce insulin resistance. Exercise can also reduce stress, which is another risk factor for hypertension.

KEY POINT

There is an increased risk of heart attack during the actual period of exercise. However, over the course of a 24-hour day, those who exercise on a regular basis have a much lower risk of a heart attack than those who do not exercise.

Risk of Heart Attack and Death During Exercise

Whenever a person dies while exercising, the incident usually makes newspaper headlines. Deaths during exercise don't happen often, but they are highly publicized. How safe, or how dangerous, is exercise? It is estimated that there will be approximately one death for every 7,620 middle-aged joggers per year.[36] Although the risk of death is increased during the period of vigorous exercise, habitual vigorous exercise is associated with an overall decreased risk of heart attack.[35] This is illustrated in Figure 20.9.

When death during exercise occurs in people age 30 or older, it usually results from a cardiac arrhythmia caused by atherosclerosis of the coronary arteries. On the other hand, those under age 30 are most likely to die from hypertrophic cardiomyopathy (enlarged diseased heart, usually genetically transmitted), an aortic aneurysm, or myocarditis (inflammation of the myocardium).

Exercise Training and Rehabilitating Patients With Heart Disease

Can active participation in a cardiac rehabilitation program that has a strong aerobic exercise component help a heart attack survivor to either survive or avoid altogether a subsequent attack? Endurance training leads to many physiological changes that reduce the work of the heart. As we have seen, many of these are peripheral, not involving the heart directly. To recap, training causes an increased capillary-to-muscle-fiber ratio and an increased plasma volume. Because of these changes, blood flow increases to the muscles. In some cases, as mentioned earlier, this allows a reduction in cardiac output, with the body's oxygen demands being met by an increased a-$\bar{v}O_2$ diff.

However, significant changes may also occur in the heart itself. Studies of heart disease patients at Washington University in St. Louis have provided dramatic evidence that intense aerobic conditioning can lead not only to substantial changes in peripheral factors, but also to changes in the heart itself, possibly including increases in blood flow to the heart and increases in left ventricular function.[6]

From our previous discussions in this chapter, it is clear that endurance exercise training can significantly reduce the risk of cardiovascular disease through its independent effect on the individual risk factors for coronary artery disease and hypertension. Favorable changes in blood pressure, lipid levels, body composition, glucose control, and stress have been reported in patients undergoing exercise training for cardiac rehabilitation. We have every reason to believe that these changes are just as important to the health of a patient who has had a heart attack as they are for a presumably healthy person.

Several studies have tried to determine if participation in a cardiac rehabilitation program reduces the risk of a subsequent heart attack or death from a subsequent heart attack. However, it is nearly impossible to design a study to resolve this issue, primarily because it would be necessary to enroll several thousand people into one study to have a large enough sample to prove a statistically significant effect. Consequently, two published reports have combined the results of the most highly controlled of these studies and have used special statistical analyses on the data.[28,29] Both reports concluded that exercise rehabilitation substantially reduces the risk of death from a subsequent heart attack, but has relatively little effect on reducing the risk for the recurrence of a nonfatal heart attack.

■■■ IN REVIEW . . . ■■■

1. Deaths during exercise are rare, though typically highly publicized.
2. Deaths during exercise in people over age 30 are usually caused by a cardiac arrhythmia resulting from atherosclerosis.
3. Deaths during exercise in people under age 30 are usually caused by hypertrophic cardiomyopathy, aortic aneurysm, or myocarditis.

In Closing . . .

In this chapter, we have seen how important physical activity is in preventing cardiovascular diseases, especially coronary artery disease and hypertension. We discussed the prevalence of these disorders, the risk factors associated with each, and how physical activity can help reduce our personal risks. In the next chapter, we continue examining the effects of exercise on our health, as we turn our attention to obesity and diabetes.

Key Terms

arteriosclerosis
atherosclerosis
blood lipids
cerebral infarction
congenital heart disease
congestive heart failure
coronary artery disease
diastolic blood pressure
fatty streaks
high-density-lipoprotein-
    bound cholesterol
    (HDL-C)
hypertension

ischemia
low-density-lipoprotein-
    bound cholesterol
    (LDL-C)
myocardial infarction
peripheral vascular
    disease
plaque
primary risk factors
rheumatic heart disease
stroke
systolic blood pressure
valvular heart diseases

Study Questions

1. What are the major causes of death in the United States at this time?
2. What is atherosclerosis, how does it develop, and at what age does it begin?
3. What is hypertension, how does it develop, and at what age does it begin?

4. What is stroke? How does stroke occur? What are the results of stroke?

5. What are the basic risk factors for coronary artery disease? For hypertension?

6. What is the risk of a sedentary lifestyle compared to that of an active lifestyle with respect to death from coronary artery disease? How has this been established?

7. What are three basic physiological alterations resulting from exercise training that would reduce the risk of death from coronary artery disease?

8. What changes occur in the heart disease risk factors resulting from endurance exercise training?

9. What is the risk of developing hypertension in a sedentary individual compared with an active individual?

10. What are three basic physiological alterations resulting from exercise training that would reduce the risk for developing hypertension?

11. What changes occur in blood pressure in moderately hypertensive individuals resulting from endurance exercise training?

12. Of what value is cardiac rehabilitation in treating the patient who has had a heart attack?

13. What is the risk of death with endurance exercise training?

References

1. American Heart Association. (1993). *1993 heart and stroke facts*. Dallas: American Heart Association.

2. Blair, S.N., Goodyear, N.N., Gibbons, L.W., & Cooper, K.H. (1984). Physical fitness and incidence of hypertension in healthy normotensive men and women. *Journal of the American Medical Association*, **252**, 487-490.

3. Blair, S.N., Kohl, H.W., Paffenbarger, R.S., Clark, D.G., Cooper, K.H., & Gibbons, L.W. (1989). Physical fitness and all-cause mortality: A prospective study of healthy men and women. *Journal of the American Medical Association*, **262**, 2395-2401.

4. Cooper, K.H., Pollock, M.L., Martin, R.P, White, S.R., Linnerud, A.C., & Jackson, A. (1976). Physical fitness levels vs. selected coronary risk factors: A cross-sectional study. *Journal of the American Medical Association*, **236**, 166-169.

5. Dunn, A.L., & Dishman, R.K. (1991). Exercise and the neurobiology of depression. *Exercise and Sport Sciences Reviews*, **19**, 41-98.

6. Ehsani, A.A. (1987). Cardiovascular adaptations to endurance exercise training in ischemic heart disease. *Exercise and Sport Sciences Reviews*, **15**, 53-66.

7. Ekelund, L.-G., Haskell, W.L., Johnson, J.L., Whaley, F.S., Criqui, M.H., & Sheps, D.S. (1988). Physical fitness as a predictor of cardiovascular mortality in asymptomatic North American men: The Lipid Research Clinics mortality follow-up study. *New England Journal of Medicine*, **319**, 1379-1384.

8. Enos, W.F., Holmes, R.H., & Beyer, J. (1953). Coronary disease among United States soldiers killed in action in Korea. *Journal of the American Medical Association*, **152**, 1090-1093.

9. Gibbons, L.W., Blair, S.N., Cooper, K.H., & Smith, M. (1983). Association between coronary heart disease risk factors and physical fitness in healthy adult women. *Circulation*, **67**, 977-983.

10. Goldberg, L., & Elliot, D.L. (1985). The effect of physical activity on lipid and lipoprotein levels. *Medical Clinics of North America*, **69**, 41-55.

11. Hagberg, J.M. (1990). Exercise, fitness and hypertension. In C. Bouchard, R.J. Shephard, T. Stephens, J.R. Sutton, & B.D. McPherson (Eds.), *Exercise, fitness, and health* (pp. 455-466). Champaign, IL: Human Kinetics.

12. Hagberg, J.M., & Seals, D.R. (1986). Exercise training and hypertension. *Acta Medica Scandinavica*, Suppl. 711, 131-136.

13. Haskell, W.L. (1984). The influence of exercise on the concentrations of triglyceride and cholesterol in human plasma. *Exercise and Sport Sciences Reviews*, **12**, 205-244.

14. Haskell, W.L. (1986). The influence of exercise training on plasma lipids and lipoproteins in health and disease. *Acta Medica Scandinavica*, Suppl. 711, 25-37.

15. Joint National Committee. (1988). The 1988 report of the Joint National Committee on Detection, Evaluation, and Treatment of High Blood Pressure. *Archives of Internal Medicine*, **148**, 1023-1038.

16. Kannel, W.B., & Dawber, T.R. (1972). Atherosclerosis as a pediatric problem. *Journal of Pediatrics*, **80**, 544-554.

17. Kirkcaldy, B. (1989). Exercise as a therapeutic modality. *Medicine and Sports Science*, **29**, 166-187.

18. Kramsch, D.M., Aspen, A.J., Abramowitz, B.M., Kreimendahl, T., & Hood, W.B. (1981). Reduction of coronary atherosclerosis by moderate conditioning exercise in monkeys on an atherogenic diet. *New England Journal of Medicine*, **305**, 1483-1489.

19. LaPorte, R.E., Adams, L.L., Savage, D.D., Brenes, G., Dearwater, S., & Cook, T. (1984). The spectrum

of physical activity, cardiovascular disease and health: An epidemiologic perspective. *American Journal of Epidemiology*, **120**, 507-517.

20. Leon, A.S., & Connett, J. (1991). Physical activity and 10.5 year mortality in the Multiple Risk Factor Intervention Trial (MRFIT). *International Journal of Epidemiology*, **20**, 690-697.

21. Leon, A.S., Connett, J., Jacobs, D.R., & Rauramaa, R. (1987). Leisure-time physical activity levels and risk of coronary heart disease and death. *Journal of the American Medical Association*, **258**, 2388-2395.

22. McNamara, J.J., Molot, M.A., Stremple, J.F., & Cutting, R.T. (1971). Coronary artery disease in combat casualties in Vietnam. *Journal of the American Medical Association*, **216**, 1185-1187.

23. Montoye, H.J., Metzner, H.L., Keller, J.B., Johnson, B.C., & Epstein, F.H. (1972). Habitual physical activity and blood pressure. *Medicine and Science in Sports*, **4**, 175-181.

24. Morris, J.N., Adam, C., Chave, S.P.W., Sirey, C., Epstein, L., & Sheehan, D.J. (1973). Vigorous exercise in leisure-time and the incidence of coronary heart-disease. *Lancet*, **1**, 333-339.

25. Morris, J.N., Heady, J.A., Raffle, P.A.B., Roberts, C.G., & Parks, J.W. (1953). Coronary heart-disease and physical activity of work. *Lancet*, **265**, 1053-1057, 1111-1120.

26. Morris, J.N., Pollard, R., Everitt, M.G., Chave, S.P.W., & Semmence, A.M. (1980). Vigorous exercise in leisure-time: Protection against coronary heart disease. *Lancet*, **2**, 1207-1210.

27. Newman, W.P., Freedman, D.S., Voors, A.W., Gard, P.D., Srinivasan, S.R., Cresanta, J.L., Williamson, G.D., Webber, L.S., & Berenson, G.S. (1986). Relation of serum lipoprotein levels and systolic blood pressure to early atherosclerosis. *New England Journal of Medicine*, **314**, 138-144.

28. O'Connor, G.T., Buring, J.E., Yusuf, S., Goldhaber, S.Z., Olmstead, E.M., Paffenbarger, R.S., & Hennekens, C.H. (1989). An overview of randomized trials of rehabilitation with exercise after myocardial infarction. *Circulation*, **80**, 234-244.

29. Oldridge, N.B., Guyatt, G.H., Fischer, M.E., & Rimm, A.A. (1988). Cardiac rehabilitation after myocardial infarction: Combined experience of randomized clinical trials. *Journal of the American Medical Association*, **260**, 945-950.

30. Paffenbarger, R.S., Hyde, R.T., Wing, A.L., & Hsieh, C.-C. (1986). Physical activity, all-cause mortality, and longevity of college alumni. *New England Journal of Medicine*, **314**, 605-613.

31. Petruzzello, S.J., Landers, D.M., Hatfield, B.D., Kubitz, K.A., & Salazar, W. (1991). A meta-analysis on the anxiety-reducing effects of acute and chronic exercise: Outcomes and mechanisms. *Sports Medicine*, **11**, 143-182.

32. Powell, K.E., Thompson, P.D., Caspersen, C.J., & Kendrick, J.S. (1987). Physical activity and the incidence of coronary heart disease. *Annual Reviews in Public Health*, **8**, 253-287.

33. Ross, R. (1986). The pathogenesis of atherosclerosis—an update. *New England Journal of Medicine*, **314**, 488-500.

34. Seals, D.R., & Hagberg, J.M. (1984). The effect of exercise training on human hypertension: A review. *Medicine and Science in Sports and Exercise*, **16**, 207-215.

35. Siscovick, D.S., Weiss, N.S., Fletcher, R.H., & Lasky, T. (1984). The incidence of primary cardiac arrest during vigorous exercise. *New England Journal of Medicine*, **311**, 874-877.

36. Thompson, P.D. (1982). Cardiovascular hazards of physical activity. *Exercise and Sport Sciences Reviews*, **10**, 208-235.

37. Tipton, C.M. (1984). Exercise, training, and hypertension. *Exercise and Sport Sciences Reviews*, **12**, 245-306.

38. Tipton, C.M. (1991). Exercise training and hypertension: An update. *Exercise and Sport Sciences Reviews*, **19**, 447-505.

39. Tran, Z.V., & Weltman, A. (1985). Differential effects of exercise on serum lipid and lipoprotein levels seen with changes in body weight. *Journal of the American Medical Association*, **254**, 919-924.

40. Wilmore, J.H., Constable, S.H., Stanforth, P.R., Tsao, W.Y., Rotkis, T.C., Paicius, R.M., Mattern, C.M., & Ewy, G.A. (1982). Prevalence of coronary heart disease risk factors in 13- to 15-year-old boys. *Journal of Cardiac Rehabilitation*, **2**, 223-233.

41. Wilmore, J.H., & McNamara, J.J. (1974). Prevalence of coronary heart disease risk factors in boys 8 to 12 years of age. *Journal of Pediatrics*, **84**, 527-533.

Selected Readings

American College of Sports Medicine (1993). Physical activity, fitness, and hypertension. *Medicine and Science in Sports and Exercise*, **25**(10), i-x.

Amsterdam, E.A., Wilmore, J.H., & DeMaria, A.N. (1977). *Exercise in cardiovascular health and disease.* New York: Yorke Medical Books.

Caspersen, C.J. (1987). Physical inactivity and coronary heart disease. *The Physician and Sportsmedicine*, **15**(11), 43-44.

Caspersen, C.J. (1989). Physical activity epidemiology: Concepts, methods, and applications to exercise science. *Exercise and Sport Sciences Reviews*, **17**, 423-473.

Dowell, R.T. (1983). Cardiac adaptations to exercise. *Exercise and Sport Sciences Reviews*, **11**, 99-117.

Eichner, E.R. (1983). Exercise and heart disease: Epidemiology of the ''exercise hypothesis.'' *American Journal of Medicine*, **75**, 1008-1023.

Grundy, S.M. (1986). Cholesterol and coronary heart disease. *Journal of the American Medical Association*, **256**, 2849-2858.

Harris, S.S., Caspersen, C.J., DeFriese, G.H., & Estes, E.H., Jr. (1989). Physical activity counseling for healthy adults as a primary preventive intervention in the clinical setting. *Journal of the American Medical Association*, **261**, 3590-3598.

Laughlin, M.H., & McAllister, R.M. (1992). Exercise training-induced coronary vascular adaptation. *Journal of Applied Physiology*, **73**, 2209-2225.

Morris, C.K., & Froelicher, V.F. (1993). Cardiovascular benefits of improved exercise capacity. *Sports Medicine*, **16**, 225-236.

Naughton, J.P., & Hellerstein, H.K. (Eds.) (1973). *Exercise testing and exercise training in coronary heart disease*. New York: Academic Press.

Pollock, M.L., & Schmidt, D.H. (Eds.) (1979). *Heart disease and rehabilitation*. Boston: Houghton Mifflin.

Pollock, M.L., & Wilmore, J.H. (1990). *Exercise in health and disease: Evaluation and prescription for prevention and rehabilitation* (2nd ed.). Philadelphia: Saunders.

Schaible, T.F., & Scheuer, J. (1985). Cardiac adaptations to chronic exercise. *Progress in Cardiovascular Disease*, **27**, 297-324.

Shephard, R.J. (1986). Exercise in coronary heart disease. *Sports Medicine*, **3**, 26-49.

Chapter 21

Obesity, Diabetes, and Physical Activity

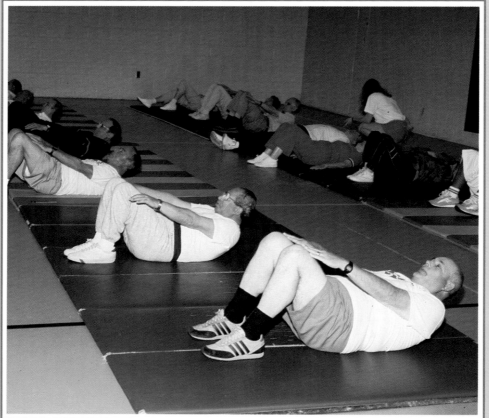

© Billy E. Barnes

While millions of people are dying of starvation each year in most parts of the world, many Americans are dying as an indirect result of overconsumption of food. Billions of dollars are spent each year overfeeding the American public, which in turn leads to the expenditure of billions of dollars more each year on various weight-loss methods. Another common disorder in America is diabetes mellitus, which affects about 12 million Americans. This disorder of carbohydrate metabolism centers on insulin. Interestingly, scientists have established a link between one type of diabetes and obesity, coronary artery disease, and hypertension.

As we saw in the previous chapter, exercise is essential for reducing our risk of coronary artery disease and hypertension. In this chapter, we will examine obesity and diabetes, keeping in mind the important link between the four disorders, and again exploring the role of physical activity in prevention and treatment.

William "the Refrigerator" Perry, defensive lineman for the Chicago Bears professional football team during the 1980s and early 1990s, reported to the 1988 summer training camp at a weight of 375 lb, some 55 lb over his mandated playing weight. Although there is an obvious concern regarding his ability to perform on the football field at this excessive weight, of greater concern are the health risks associated with obesity. Chris Taylor, as an Iowa State and U.S. Olympic team wrestler, competed at a weight of between 400 and 450 lb. He died in his sleep at age 29, most likely from obesity-related causes.

A sedentary lifestyle has been associated with an increased risk for two major metabolic and endocrine disorders: obesity and diabetes. Although neither disease by itself represents a major cause of death, both are strongly associated with other diseases that have high mortality rates, such as hypertension, coronary artery disease, and cancer. Furthermore, millions of Americans have obesity, diabetes, or both. The consequences of these diseases are debilitating, and the costs associated with their treatment are high.

In this chapter we will focus on obesity and diabetes, discussing

- their prevalence,
- their etiology,
- health problems associated with each disease, and
- general treatment options.

Finally, we will consider the role physical activity can play in prevention and treatment.

Obesity

The terms overweight and obesity are often used interchangeably, but technically they have different meanings. Overweight is defined as body weight that exceeds the normal or standard weight for a particular person based on height and frame size. These standard weights, presented in Table 21.1, were established in 1959 but are still the most widely used. New weight and height tables were introduced in 1983, but their introduction was controversial because many experts believed the weight allowances were too liberal. Many professional health organizations have refused to accept the newer tables.

Weight values in the standard tables are based solely on population averages. For this reason, a person can be overweight according to these standards yet have a lower-than-normal body fat content. For example, football players are frequently found to be overweight according to standard tables, yet they are typically much leaner than people of the same age, height, and frame size who are of normal weight or who are even underweight (see chapter 16). Still other people are within the normal range of body weights for their height and frame size by the standard tables yet are obese.

Obesity refers to the condition in which a person has an excessive amount of body fat. This implies that the actual amount of body fat or its percent of the total weight must be assessed or estimated (see chapter 16 for assessment techniques). Exact standards for allowable fat percentages have not been established. However, men with more than 25% body fat and women with more than 35% should be considered obese. Men with relative fat values of 20% to 25% and women with values of 30% to 35% should be considered borderline obese.

Most studies of large populations have used measurements of weight alone, weight combined with height, or skinfold thickness to estimate the prevalence of overweight and obesity. Relative weight is a term used to express the percentage by which an individual is either overweight or underweight. This value is generally determined by dividing the person's weight by the mean weight (from the standard weight tables) for the medium frame category, based on height. The result is then multiplied by 100 to express it as a percentage. For example, using Table 21.1, a man who weighs 230 lb (104 kg) at a height of 6 ft (183 cm) would have a relative weight of 142% [(230 lb ÷ 162 lb) × 100 = 142%]. The figure 162 lb (73 kg) is the mean value for the medium frame category for a 6-ft (183-cm) man (154 to 170 lb, or 70 to 77 kg).

Body mass index (BMI) is another frequently used standard to estimate obesity. A person's BMI is determined by dividing body weight in kilograms by the square of body height in meters. As an example, the man who weighs 230 lb (104 kg) and is 6 ft tall (183 cm), would have a BMI of 32 kg per m². Generally, the BMI is related to body composition. It is highly correlated with relative body fat and probably provides a better estimate of obesity than does relative weight.

Table 21.1 Standard Tables (1959) for Men's and Women's Weight for Height and Frame Size

| Men ages 25 years and over | | | | Women ages 25 years and over | | | | |
| Height with shoes 1-in. heels | | Desirable weight (lb) | | | Height with shoes 2-in. heels | | Desirable weight (lb) | | |
Ft	In.	Small frame	Medium frame	Large frame	Ft	In.	Small frame	Medium frame	Large frame
5	2	112-120	118-129	126-141	4	10	92-98	96-107	104-119
5	3	115-123	121-133	129-144	4	11	94-101	98-110	106-122
5	4	118-126	124-136	132-148	5	0	96-104	101-113	109-125
5	5	121-129	127-139	135-152	5	1	99-107	104-116	112-128
5	6	124-133	130-143	138-156	5	2	102-110	107-119	115-131
5	7	128-137	134-147	142-161	5	3	105-113	110-122	118-134
5	8	132-141	138-152	147-166	5	4	108-116	113-126	121-138
5	9	136-145	142-156	151-170	5	5	111-119	116-130	125-142
5	10	140-150	146-160	155-174	5	6	114-123	120-135	129-146
5	11	144-154	150-165	159-179	5	7	118-127	124-139	133-150
6	0	148-158	154-170	164-184	5	8	122-131	128-143	137-154
6	1	152-162	158-175	168-189	5	9	126-135	132-147	141-158
6	2	156-167	162-180	173-194	5	10	130-140	136-151	145-163
6	3	160-171	167-185	178-199	5	11	134-144	140-155	149-168
6	4	164-175	172-190	182-204	6	0	138-148	144-159	153-173

Note. Weights listed include indoor clothing. For nude weight, deduct 5 to 7 lb for men and 2 to 4 lb for women.

Prepared by Metropolitan Life Insurance Company, derived primarily from data of the Build and Blood Pressure Study, Society of Actuaries, 1959.

The prevalence of obesity and overweight in this country has increased dramatically over the past 30 years. On the basis of data from a large study conducted between 1976 and 1980 by the National Center for Health Statistics, 28.4% of American adults ages 25 to 74 are overweight.[13] Between 13% and 26% of the United States' adolescent population (ages 12 to 17) are obese, and an additional 4% to 12% are superobese (depending on gender and race, with the highest prevalence among white girls).[6] This represents a 39% increase in prevalence compared with data collected between 1966 and 1970. Equally alarming, the prevalence of obesity among children ages 6 to 11 has increased 54%!

KEY POINT

Over 25% of the adult population is overweight, and the prevalence of obesity in children has increased at an alarming rate.

The average person in the United States will gain approximately 1 lb (0.45 kg) of additional weight each year after age 25. Such a seemingly small gain, however, results in 30 lb (14 kg) of excess weight by age 55. At the same time, bone and muscle mass decrease by approximately 0.5 lb per year due to reduced physi-

cal activity. Taking this into account, an average person's body fat actually increases by 1.5 lb (0.7 kg) each year. This means a 45-lb (20-kg) fat gain over this 30-year period! It is no wonder that weight loss is an American obsession.

The Control of Body Weight

We must have a basic understanding of how body weight is controlled or regulated to better understand how a person becomes obese. Body weight regulation has puzzled scientists for years. The human body takes in an average of about 2,500 kcal per day, or nearly one million kcal per year. The average gain of 1.5 lb (0.7 kg) of fat each year represents an imbalance of only 5,250 kcal per year between energy intake and expenditure (3,500 kcal is the energy equivalent of 1 lb, or 0.45 kg, of adipose tissue). This translates into a surplus of less than 15 kcal per day. Even with a weight gain of 1.5 lb (0.7 kg) of fat per year, the body can balance caloric intake to within one potato chip per day of what is expended! That is truly remarkable.

The body's ability to balance its caloric intake and expenditure to within such a narrow range has led scientists to propose that body weight is regulated around a given set point similar to the way in which body temperature is regulated. Excellent evidence for this is found in the animal research literature.[10] When animals are force-fed or starved for various periods of time, their weights increase, or decrease, markedly. But when they go back to their normal eating patterns, they always return to their original weight or to the weight of the control animals (for animals that naturally continue to gain weight throughout their life span).

Similar results have been found in humans, although the number of studies is limited. Subjects placed on semistarvation diets have lost up to 25% of their body weight but regained that weight within months of returning to a normal diet.[11] In a study involving Vermont prisoners, overfeeding resulted in weight gains of 15% to 25%, yet their weights returned to original levels shortly after the experiment ended.[17]

How can the body do this? Let's consider energy expenditure. The total amount of energy expended each day can be expressed in three categories:

1. Resting metabolic rate
2. The thermic effect of a meal
3. The thermic effect of activity

These are depicted in Figure 21.1.

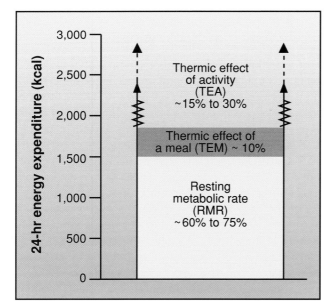

Figure 21.1   The three components of energy expenditure. Adapted from Poehlman (1989).

Resting metabolic rate (RMR) is your body's metabolic rate early in the morning following an overnight fast and 8 hr of sleep. The term basal metabolic rate (BMR) is also used but generally implies that the individual sleeps over in the clinical facility where the metabolic rate measurement will be made. Most research today uses resting metabolic rate. This value, as we learned in chapter 5, represents the minimum amount of energy expenditure needed to support basic physiological processes. It accounts for 60% to 75% of the total energy we expend each day.

The thermic effect of a meal (TEM) represents the increase in the metabolic rate that is associated with the digestion, absorption, transport, metabolism, and storage of ingested food. The TEM accounts for approximately 10% of our total energy expenditure each day. This value also includes some energy waste, because the body can increase its metabolic rate above that necessary for food processing and storage. The TEM component of metabolism might be defective in people with obesity, possibly due to a defect in the wastage component, leading to a surplus of calories.

The thermic effect of activity (TEA) is simply the energy expended above the resting metabolic rate to accomplish a given task or activity, whether it is combing your hair or running a 10-km race. The TEA accounts for the remaining 15% to 30% of our energy expenditure.

The body adapts to major increases or decreases in energy intake by altering the energy expended by each of these three components—RMR, TEM, and TEA. With very low calorie diets, all three decrease. The body appears to be attempting to conserve its energy stores. This is dramatically illustrated by decreases in resting metabolic rate of 20% to 30% or more, reported within several weeks after patients begin a very low calorie diet. Conversely, all three components of energy expenditure increase with overeating. In this case, the body appears to be trying to prevent unnecessary storage of the surplus calories. All of these adaptations may be under the control of the sympathetic nervous system and may play a major, if not the primary, role in maintaining weight around a given set point. This remains a most important area for future research.

IN REVIEW . . .

1. Overweight is a body weight that exceeds the standard weight for a certain height and frame size. Obesity refers to having excessive body fat, meaning greater than 25% body fat for men and greater than 35% body fat for women.
2. Relative weight refers to the percentage by which a person is either over- or underweight.
3. A person's body mass index (BMI) is calculated by dividing body weight in kilograms by the square of height in meters. This value is highly correlated with relative body fat and provides a better estimate of obesity than does relative weight.
4. Prevalence of obesity and overweight in the United States has increased dramatically, especially among children, in the past 30 years.
5. The average person gains 1 lb (0.45 kg) per year after age 25, but also loses 0.5 lb of fat-free mass per year, making a net gain of 1.5 lb (0.7 kg) of fat each year.
6. Body weight appears to be regulated around a given set point.
7. Daily energy expenditure is reflected by the sum of the resting metabolic rate (RMR), the thermic effect of a meal (TEM), and the thermic effect of activity (TEA). The body adapts to changes in energy intake by adjusting any or all of these components.

Etiology of Obesity

At various times throughout human history, obesity has been thought to be caused by basic hormonal imbalances resulting from failure of one or more of the endocrine glands to properly regulate body weight. At other times, it has been believed that gluttony, rather than glandular malfunction, was the primary cause of obesity. In the first case, a person is perceived as having no control over the situation, yet in the second, he or she is held directly responsible! Results of recent medical and physiological research show that obesity can be the result of any one or a combination of many factors. Its etiology is not as simple as was once believed.

Experimental studies on animals have linked obesity to hereditary (genetic) factors. Recent studies of humans by Dr. Albert Stunkard and his colleagues at the University of Pennsylvania have shown a direct genetic influence on height, weight, and BMI.[18,19,20] A study from Laval University in Quebec has provided

possibly the strongest evidence yet of a significant genetic component for obesity.[2] The investigators took 12 pairs of young adult male monozygotic (identical) twins and housed them in a closed section of a dormitory under 24-hr observation for 120 consecutive days. The subjects' diets were monitored during the initial 14 days to determine their baseline caloric intake. Over the next 100 days, the subjects were fed 1,000 kcal above their baseline consumption for 6 out of every 7 days. On the seventh day, the subjects were fed only their baseline diet. Thus they were overfed by 1,000 kcal per day for 84 out of the 100 days. Activity levels were also tightly controlled. At the end of the study period, as shown in Figure 21.2, the actual weight gained varied widely, from 4.3 to 13.3 kg—a three-fold variation in weight gain for overconsumption of the same calories. However, the response of both twins in any given twin pair was quite similar—the major variations occurred between different twin pairs. Similar results were found for gains in fat mass, percent body fat, and subcutaneous fat.

Obesity has also been experimentally and clinically linked with both physiological and psychological trauma. Hormonal imbalances, emotional trauma, and alterations in basic homeostatic mechanisms have all

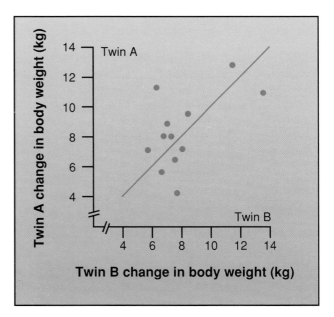

Figure 21.2 Similarity in weight gains among twins in response to a 1,000-kcal increase in dietary intake for 84 days of a 100-day study. A data point represents the weight gain for each twin in that pair; Twin A's value is shown on the y-axis, Twin B's on the x-axis. Adapted from Bouchard et al. (1990).

been shown to be either directly or indirectly related to the onset of obesity. Environmental factors, such as cultural habits, inadequate physical activity, and improper diets, also can contribute to obesity.

Thus obesity is of complex origin, and the specific causes undoubtedly differ from one person to the next. Recognizing this is important for treating existing obesity and for preventing its onset. To attribute their obesity solely to gluttony is unfair and psychologically damaging to people who are concerned about their problem and are attempting to correct it. In fact, several studies have shown that people with obesity actually eat less, although they get far less physical activity, than people of the same gender and similar age with average body fat contents.

Health Problems Associated With Excessive Weight and Obesity

For many years, researchers assumed that the major health risk associated with excess body weight was through an excess of body fat. Overweight, without being overfat, was generally not considered a significant health concern. Van Itallie conducted an analysis of the effects of overweight on health risk by classifying each person by[22]

- the degree of underweight or overweight, using relative body weight and body mass index, and
- the degree of leanness or obesity, using the sum of triceps and subscapular skinfold thickness measurements.

This analysis scheme is illustrated in Figure 21.3. In this figure, leanness–obesity is depicted in the upper bar, and the population is divided into three groups on the basis of the sum of the triceps and subscapular skinfolds: the lean group (< 15th percentile), the average group (15th to 85th percentile), and the obese group (> 85th percentile). Underweight–overweight is depicted in the side bar, with the population divided into three groups on the basis of the body mass index, using the same percentile breakdown for underweight, average, and overweight. Of note in this figure are the two rectangles (color coded), which indicate that there are some people who are overweight but not obese

(Rectangle 4), and there are others who are obese but not overweight (Rectangle 5). Both groups have been found to be at increased risk for certain diseases. Van Itallie found that there are health risks, primarily for hypertension, associated with being overweight, even in the absence of obesity.

Overweight and obesity are associated with an increased overall rate of death (general excess mortality). This relationship is curvilinear, as shown in Figure 21.4. A large jump in risk occurs when the body mass index exceeds 30 kg per m². Causes of the excess mortality associated with obesity and overweight include

- heart disease,
- hypertension,
- certain types of cancer,
- gallbladder disease, and
- diabetes.

Obesity has been directly related to

- changes in normal body function,
- increased risk for certain diseases,
- detrimental effects on established diseases, and
- adverse psychological reactions.

Changes in Normal Body Function

The prevalence and extent of changes in body function vary with the individual and with the degree of obesity. Respiratory problems are quite common among people with obesity. These lead to some other common consequences of obesity, such as lethargy (sluggishness) because of increased carbon dioxide levels in the blood, and polycythemia (increased red blood cell production) in response to lower arterial blood oxygenation. These can lead to abnormal blood clotting (thrombosis), enlargement of the heart, and congestive heart failure. Those with obesity typically have a lower exercise tolerance because of these respiratory problems and also due to the increased body mass that must be moved during exercise. Additional weight gains further reduce activity levels, and exercise tolerance decreases even more.

Increased Risk for Certain Diseases

An increased risk of developing certain chronic degenerative diseases is also associated with obesity. Both hypertension and atherosclerosis have been directly linked to obesity (see chapter 20). So have various metabolic and endocrine disorders, such as impaired carbohydrate metabolism and diabetes. For the latter, obesity is particularly a problem associated with the onset of Type II (late-onset, noninsulin-dependent) diabetes.

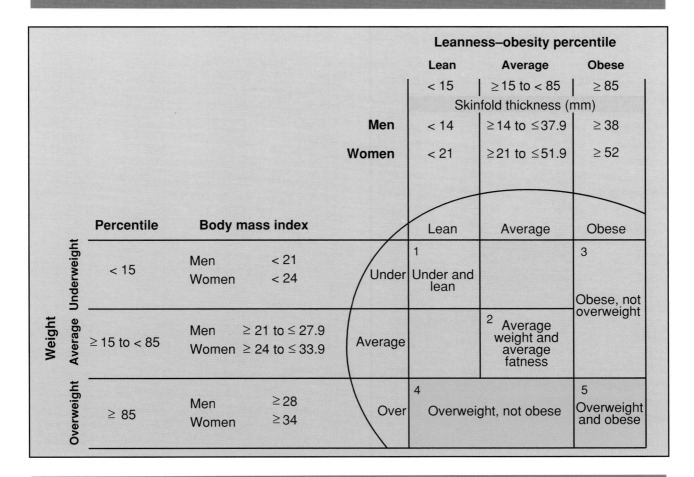

Figure 21.3   Cross-classification of the distribution of relative weight and body mass versus triceps plus subscapular skinfold measurements. Adapted from Van Itallie (1985).

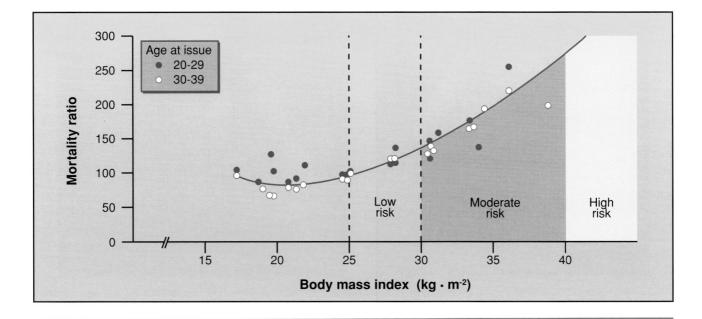

Figure 21.4   The relationship of body mass index to excess mortality. Adapted from Bray (1985).

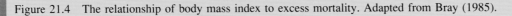

A major research breakthrough has enabled us to better understand the role of obesity as a risk factor for most of these diseases. Since the 1940s, major gender differences in the way in which fat is stored or patterned on the body have been recognized. Males tend to pattern fat in the upper body, particularly the abdominal area, whereas females tend to pattern fat in the lower body, particularly the hips, buttocks, and thighs, as shown in Figure 21.5. When obese, the male pattern is referred to as upper body, apple-shaped, or android obesity, and the female pattern is referred to as lower body, pear-shaped, or gynoid obesity.

Research beginning in the late 1970s and early 1980s established upper body obesity as a risk factor for[1]

- coronary artery disease,
- hypertension,
- stroke,
- elevated blood lipids, and
- diabetes.

Furthermore, upper body obesity appears to be more important than total body fatness as a risk factor for these diseases. Waist and hip circumference, or girth, measurements can be used to identify people with increased risk. A waist:hip girth ratio greater than 1.0 for men and greater than 0.8 for women indicates increased risk. With upper body obesity, the increased risk may result from visceral fat depots' close proximity to the portal circulatory system.

Detrimental Effects on Established Diseases

The effects of obesity on existing diseases are not clear at the present time. Obesity can contribute to further development of certain diseases and medical conditions, and weight reduction is usually prescribed as an integral part of treatment. Conditions that generally benefit from weight reduction include

- angina pectoris,
- hypertension,
- congestive heart disease,
- myocardial infarction (reduced risk of recurrence),
- varicose veins,
- diabetes, and
- orthopaedic problems.

■ ━━ KEY POINT ━━ ■

Obesity places you at significantly increased risk for hypertension, diabetes, coronary artery disease, and metabolic and digestive diseases. The health risks associated with obesity are most likely associated with the manner in which the fat is distributed on the body, with upper body obesity, representing high levels of visceral fat, being of significantly greater risk.

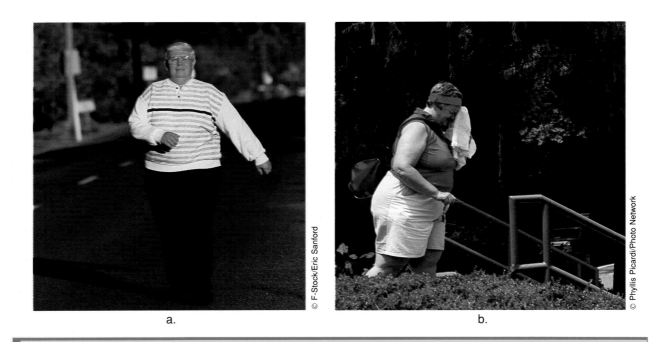

a.   b.

© F-Stock/Eric Sanford

© Phyllis Picardi/Photo Network

Figure 21.5   (a) Upper body (android) obesity; (b) lower body (gynoid) obesity.

Adverse Psychological Reactions

Emotional or psychological problems might be the cause of obesity in a substantial percentage of people with that disorder. Furthermore, emotional or psychological problems can arise from the condition itself. In our society, obesity carries a social stigma that contributes substantially to the problems of those who have it. Even our media typically glamorize only people with near-perfect bodies. Consequently, some people who have obesity might need psychiatric or professional counseling assistance in their efforts to lose weight.

General Treatment of Obesity

In theory, weight control seems to be a simple matter. The energy consumed by the body in the form of food must equal the total energy expended, which is the sum of the RMR, TEM, and TEA. The body normally maintains a balance between caloric intake and caloric expenditure, but when this balance is upset weight will be lost or gained. Both weight losses and weight gains appear largely dependent on just two factors: dietary intake and physical activity. This is now recognized as an oversimplification, considering the results of the overfeeding study of monozygotic twins discussed earlier, in which considerable variation in weight gains occurred for the same amount of overfeeding.[2] Not everyone responds to the same intervention in the same way. This difference in response must be considered when designing treatment programs for individuals attempting to lose weight, and people trying to lose weight must understand this difference so that they won't be discouraged.

Weight loss should generally not exceed 1 to 2 lb (less than 1 kg) per week. Losses greater than this should not be attempted without direct medical supervision. Losing just 1 lb (0.45 kg) of fat a week will result in the loss of 52 lb (24 kg) of fat in only a year! Few people become obese that rapidly. Weight loss should also be considered a long-term project. Research and experience have proven that rapid weight losses are usually short lived and the lost weight is usually quickly regained because rapid weight losses are generally the result of large losses of body water. The body has built-in safety mechanisms to prevent an imbalance in body fluid levels, so the lost water eventually will be replaced. Thus a person wishing to lose 20 lb (9 kg) of fat is advised to attempt to attain this goal in a minimum of 2-1/2 to 5 months.

Many special diets have achieved popularity over the years, such as the Drinking Man's Diet, the Beverly Hills Diet, the Cambridge Diet, the California Diet, Dr. Stillman's Diet, and Dr. Adkin's Diet. Each claims to be the ultimate in effective and comfortable weight loss. Some more recent diets have been developed for use either in the hospital or at home under the supervision of a physician. These are often referred to as very low calorie diets, as they allow only 350 to 500 kcal of food per day. Most of these have been formulated with a certain amount of protein and carbohydrate to minimize the loss of fat-free body mass. Research has shown that many of these are effective, but no single diet has been shown to be more effective than any other. Again, the important factor is the development of a caloric deficit while maintaining a complete, balanced diet that meets the body's vitamin and mineral requirements. The best diet is the one that meets these criteria and is best suited to individual comfort and personality.

Generally, improper eating habits are at least partially responsible for most weight problems, so no diet should be viewed as a quick fix. The person should learn to make permanent changes in dietary habits, especially reducing the intake of fat and simple sugars. For most people, simply eating a low-fat diet will gradually reduce weight to a desirable level without their needing to worry about restricting the quantity of food they eat. Also, for most people, simply reducing total caloric intake by 250 to 500 kcal per day would be sufficient to accomplish their desired weight loss goals.

Hormones and drugs have also been used to assist patients in weight loss by increasing their RMR. Surgical techniques are also used in the treatment of extreme obesity, but only as a last resort when other treatment procedures have failed and the obesity is life threatening. Intestinal bypass surgery involves surgically bypassing a large segment of the small intestine, thus reducing food absorption. This procedure is seldom used today because of associated complications. Gastric bypass surgery, which involves surgically reducing the size of the patient's stomach, is also seldom used today because of risks. More recently, gastric stapling to partition off part of the stomach, and the insertion of gastric balloons to reduce the capacity of the stomach, have been proposed as safer and more effective surgical techniques.

Behavior modification has been proposed as one of the most effective techniques for helping people with weight problems. Major weight losses have been achieved by changing basic behavior patterns associated with eating. Furthermore, these weight losses appear much more permanent. This approach appeals to most people because the techniques seem to make sense and are often easy to incorporate into a normal daily routine. For example, an individual might not have to consciously reduce the amount of food eaten, but simply agree that all eating will be done in one location, which often cuts down on snacking. Or an individual might be allowed to take as much food as desired with the first helping, but no second helpings are allowed. Many such simple changes can help regulate eating behavior and result in substantial weight loss.

■ IN REVIEW . . . ■

1. The etiology of obesity is not simple; it can be caused by any one or a combination of many factors.
2. Studies of twins indicate that there is a genetic component to obesity. The disorder has also been linked to hormonal imbalances, emotional trauma, homeostatic imbalances, cultural influences, physical inactivity, and improper diets.
3. Overweight and obesity are associated with increased risk of general excess mortality.
4. Respiratory problems are quite common among people with obesity. These, in turn, can lead to lethargy and polycythemia.
5. Obesity increases the risk of certain chronic degenerative diseases. Upper body obesity increases the risk of developing coronary artery disease, hypertension, stroke, elevated blood lipids, and diabetes. Also, obesity can worsen pre-existing health conditions and diseases.
6. Emotional or psychological problems may contribute to obesity, and the disorder itself, with the stigma it carries, can be psychologically damaging.
7. In treatment of obesity, it is important to remember that people respond differently to the same intervention.
8. Weight loss generally should not exceed 1 to 2 lb (less than 1 kg) per week. Simple diet modification, reducing intake of fat and simple sugars, is sufficient to help most people achieve their weight-loss goals.

The Role of Physical Activity in Weight Control

Inactivity is a major cause of obesity in the United States. In fact, inactivity may be a far more significant factor in the development of obesity than overeating! Thus exercise must be recognized as an essential component in any program of weight reduction or control. Let's examine why physical activity is so important.

Changes in Body Composition With Exercise Training

Physical training can substantially alter body composition. Many people have believed that physical activity has only a limited influence on changing body composition, and that even vigorous exercise burns too few calories to lead to substantial body fat reductions. Yet research has conclusively demonstrated the effectiveness of exercise training in promoting major alterations in body composition. How do we account for this apparent conflict?

A person who jogs 3 days a week for 30 min each day at a 7 mph (11 kph) pace (slightly over 8.5 min · mi^{-1}, or 5.3 min · km^{-1}) will expend about 14.5 kcal · min^{-1}, or 435 kcal for the 30-minute run each day. This results in a total expenditure per week of about 1,305 kcal, the equivalent of slightly over 0.33 lb (0.14 kg) of fat loss each week just from the exercise period alone. This might lead some people to believe that exercise is a painfully slow way to significantly reduce body fat levels, and that there are better and easier ways to lose fat. However, in 52 weeks, providing energy intake remained constant, this person would lose 17 lbs (8 kg)!

When estimating an activity's energy cost, typically the average or steady-state rate of energy expenditure for that activity is multiplied by how many minutes the activity is performed. For example, if the steady-state rate for shoveling snow is 7.5 kcal · min^{-1}, 1 hr of shoveling would require a total of only 450 kcal. This would allow an approximate loss of 0.13 lb (0.06 kg) of adipose tissue (450 kcal ÷ 3,500 kcal per lb of adipose tissue = 0.13 pounds).

But examining the energy expended only during exercise does not give us the full picture. Metabolism remains temporarily elevated after exercise ends. This phenomenon was at one time referred to as the oxygen debt but is now referred to as the excess post-exercise oxygen consumption (EPOC). Returning the metabolic rate back to its pre-exercise level can require several minutes following light exercise, such as walking; several hours following very heavy exercise, such as playing a football game; and up to 12 to 24 hr or even longer for prolonged, exhaustive exercise, such as running a marathon.

The EPOC can require a substantial energy expenditure when considered over the entire recovery period. If, for example, the oxygen consumption following exercise remains elevated by an average of only 0.05 L · min^{-1}, this will amount to approximately 0.25 kcal · min^{-1} or 15 kcal · hr^{-1}. If the metabolism remains elevated for 5 hr, this would provide an additional expenditure of 75 kcal that would not normally be included in the calculated total energy expenditure for that particular activity. This additional energy expenditure is ignored in most calculations of the energy costs of various activities. The person in this example, by exercising 5 days per week, would expend 375 kcal, or lose the equivalent of about 0.1 lb (0.05 kg) of fat in one week, or 1.0 lb (0.45 kg) in 10 weeks, from the additional caloric expenditure during the recovery period alone!

KEY POINT

Physical activity is important in both weight maintenance and weight loss. In addition to the calories that are expended during exercise, a substantial expenditure of calories occurs during the post-exercise period (EPOC).

Studies have shown major changes in both weight and body composition with exercise training. One study examined the changes in body composition with[26]

- diet alone,
- exercise alone, and
- a combination of diet and exercise.

Each of three groups of adult women maintained a caloric deficit of 500 kcal per day during a 16-week period of weight loss. The diet-only subjects reduced their daily caloric intake by 500 kcal per day but did not alter their activity level. The exercise-only subjects did not alter their diet but increased their daily activity by 500 kcal. The subjects who combined diet and exercise reduced their daily caloric intake by 250 kcal and increased their daily activity by 250 kcal. Results of this study are illustrated in Figure 21.6. Although the three groups had similar body weight losses, the two groups that exercised lost substantially more body fat. A major difference between the two exercise groups and the diet-only group was that fat-free body mass was gained with exercise, but lost with weight reduction through diet only.

Figure 21.7 illustrates the results of a second study in which 72 male subjects with mild obesity were assigned to one of several treatment programs that included either exercise or nonexercise in combination with different dietary treatments. Again, although the exercise and nonexercise groups lost similar amounts of weight, the exercise group lost significantly more fat and did not lose fat-free mass. The nonexercising group lost a significant amount of fat-free mass.[15]

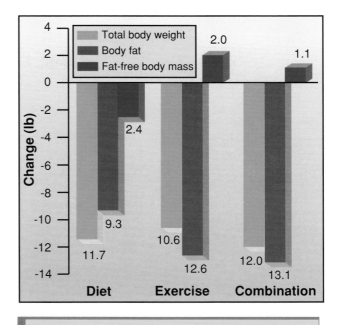

Figure 21.6 Changes in total body weight, body fat, and fat-free body mass as a result of using only diet, only exercise, and a combination of diet and exercise. Adapted from Zuti and Golding (1976).

Not all studies have been able to demonstrate such dramatic changes in weight and body composition with exercise training. But most studies have found similar trends:

- Total weight decreases.
- Fat mass and relative body fat decrease.
- Fat-free mass is either maintained or increases.

Although most of these studies have used aerobic training, several other studies have now used resistance training and have shown impressive decreases in body fat and increases in fat-free mass. The evidence shows that exercise is an important part of any weight loss program. But to maximize losses in body weight and body fat, it is necessary to combine exercise with decreased caloric intake.

KEY POINT

Attempts to lose weight are much more successful when you lose only 1 to 2 lb (slightly less than 1 kg) per week, and when you combine dietary restriction with moderate exercise (300 to 500 kcals per day). This will minimize loss of fat-free mass and maximize loss of fat mass.

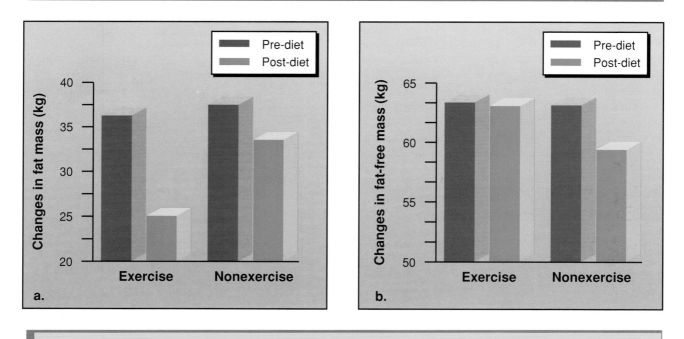

Figure 21.7   Changes in (a) fat mass and (b) fat-free mass resulting from a combined diet and exercise program and from dieting alone. Adapted from Pavlou et al. (1985).

Mechanisms for Change in Body Weight and Composition

When attempting to explain how exercise causes such changes in body weight and composition, we must consider both sides of the energy balance equation. Evaluating energy expenditure requires that we consider each of the three components of energy expenditure: the resting metabolic rate, the thermic effect of a meal, and the thermic effect of activity. Evaluating energy intake requires that we also consider the energy that is lost in the feces (energy excreted), which is generally less than 5% of the total caloric intake. Keeping this balance in mind, let's examine some of the possible mechanisms through which exercise might affect body weight and body composition.

KEY POINT

The Energy Balance Equation:

**Energy Intake − Energy Excreted
= RMR + TEM + TEA**

Exercise and Appetite.   Some believe that exercise stimulates the appetite to such an extent that food intake is unconsciously increased to at least equal that expended during exercise. In 1954, Jean Mayer, a world-famous nutritionist, reported that animals exercising for periods of from 20 min to 1 hr per day had a lower food intake than nonexercising control animals.[12] He concluded from this and other studies that when activity is less than a certain minimum level, food intake does not decrease correspondingly and the animal (or human) begins to accumulate body fat. This led to the theory that a certain minimum level of physical activity is necessary for the body to precisely regulate food intake to balance energy expenditure. A sedentary lifestyle may reduce this regulatory ability, resulting in a positive energy balance and weight gain.

Exercise does, in fact, appear to be a mild appetite suppressant, at least for the first few hours following intense exercise training. Furthermore, studies have shown that the total number of calories consumed per day does not change when a person begins a training program. Although some people interpret this as evidence that exercise does not affect appetite, a more accurate conclusion might be that appetite was affected, in fact suppressed, because caloric intake did not increase in proportion to the additional caloric expenditure from the exercise program. In studies conducted on rats, the food intake of male rats appears to be reduced with exercise training, while female rats tend to eat the same or even more than nonexercising control rats.[14] There is no obvious explanation for this gender difference, and so far similar results have not been reported in humans.

The decrease in appetite might occur only with intense levels of exercise in which the resulting increased catecholamine (epinephrine and norepinephrine) levels might suppress the appetite. The increased body temperature that accompanies either high-intensity activity or almost any activity performed under hot and humid conditions might also suppress appetite. We all know from experience that we desire less food when the weather is hot or when our body temperatures are elevated due to illness. This might also explain why a hard running workout results in little or no desire to eat, yet a hard swimming workout elicits a relatively strong craving for food. In the pool, providing the water temperature is well below core temperature, the heat generated by exercise is lost very effectively so core temperature is typically not elevated to the same extent.

KEY POINT

Regular physical activity may assist in better controlling your appetite so that caloric intake balances caloric expenditure.

Exercise and Resting Metabolic Rate.   The effects of exercise on the components of energy expenditure became a major topic of interest among researchers in the late 1980s and early 1990s. Of obvious interest is how exercise training might affect the resting metabolic rate, because it represents 60% to 75% of the total calories expended each day. For example, if a 25-year-old male's total daily caloric intake was 2,700 kcal and his RMR accounted for just 60% of that total ($0.60 \times 2,700 = 1,620$ kcal RMR), a mere 1% increase in his RMR would require an extra 16 kcal expenditure each day, or 5,840 kcal per year. This small increase in RMR alone would account for the equivalent of a 1.7 lb (0.8 kg) fat loss per year!

The role of physical training in increasing RMR has not been totally resolved. Several cross-sectional studies have found that highly trained runners have higher RMRs than untrained people of similar age and size. But other studies have not been able to confirm this.[16] Few longitudinal studies have been conducted to determine the change in RMR in untrained people who undergo training for a period of time. Those that have been conducted suggest that RMR might increase following training, but the data are not conclusive.[3] Because RMR is closely related to the fat-free mass of the body (fat-free tissue is more metabolically active), interest has increased in the use of resistance training to increase fat-free mass in an attempt to increase RMR.

Exercise and the Thermic Effect of a Meal.   Several studies have examined the role of individual bouts of exercise and exercise training in increasing the thermic effect of a meal. A single bout of exercise, either before or after a meal, increases the thermic effect of that meal.

Less clear is the role of exercise training on the TEM. Some studies have shown increases, others have shown decreases, and yet others have shown no effect at all. As with measuring changes in RMR accompanying exercise training, measurement of the TEM must be timed carefully with the last exercise bout. When measurements are made within 24 hr of the last bout, the TEM is typically lower than it is 3 days afterward.[21]

Exercise and Mobilization of Body Fat.   During exercise, fatty acids are freed from their storage sites to be burned for energy. Several studies suggest that human growth hormone may be responsible for this increased fatty acid mobilization. Growth hormone levels increase sharply with exercise and remain elevated for up to several hours in the recovery period. Other research has suggested that, with exercise, the adipose tissue is more sensitive to either the sympathetic nervous system or to the rising levels of circulating catecholamines. Either situation would increase lipid mobilization. More recent research suggests that this mobilization occurs in response to a specific fat-mobilizing substance that is highly responsive to elevated levels of activity. Thus, we cannot state with certainty which factors are of greatest importance in mediating this response.

Spot Reduction

Many people, including athletes, believe that by exercising a specific area of the body, the fat in that area will be utilized, reducing the locally stored fat. Results of several early research studies tended to support this concept of spot reduction. But later research suggests that spot reduction is a myth and that exercise, even when localized, draws from almost all of the fat stores of the body, not just from local depots.

One such study used outstanding tennis players, theorizing that they would be ideal subjects for studying spot reduction, because they could act as their own controls: Their dominant arms exercise vigorously for several hours every day, whereas their nondominant arms are relatively sedentary.[7] Researchers postulated that if spot reduction is a reality, the nondominant (inactive) arm should have substantially more fat than the dominant (active) arm. The players' dominant arms had substantially greater girths due to exercise-induced muscle hypertrophy. But the subcutaneous skinfold fat thicknesses in the active and inactive arms showed absolutely no differences.

Another study examined the localized effects of a 27-day intense sit-up training program. Researchers found no difference in the rate at which fat cell diameter changed in the abdomen, the subscapular region, and the gluteal region.[9] This indicates a lack of specific adaptation at the site of the exercise training (the abdomen). Researchers now theorize that fat is mobilized during exercise either mostly from those areas of highest concentration or equally from all areas, thus negating the spot reduction theory. Decreases in girth can occur with exercise training, but these result from increased muscle tone, not fat loss.

Low-Intensity Aerobics

As we have discussed in earlier chapters, the higher the exercise intensity, the greater the body's reliance on carbohydrate as an energy source. With high-intensity aerobic exercise, carbohydrate can supply 65% or more of the body's energy needs. During the latter 1980s, various professional exercise groups were promoting low-intensity aerobic exercise to increase the loss of body fat. These groups theorized that low-intensity aerobic training would allow the body to use more fat as the energy source, hastening the loss of body fat. Indeed, the body uses a higher percentage of fat for energy at lower exercise intensities. However, the total calories expended by the body's use of fat does not necessarily change.

━━ KEY POINT ━━

   Low-intensity aerobic activity does not necessarily lead to a greater expenditure of calories from fat. More importantly, the total caloric expenditure for a given period of time is much less when compared with high-intensity aerobic activity.

This is illustrated in Table 21.2. In this example, a 23-year-old woman with a maximal oxygen uptake of 3.0 L · min^{-1} exercises for 30 min at 50% of her $\dot{V}O_2$ max on one day, and for 30 min at 75% of her $\dot{V}O_2$ max on another. The total calories from fat do not differ between the low- and high-intensity aerobic workouts—in both cases she burns about 110 kcal of fat during 30 min. Most importantly, however, for the higher intensity workout she expends about 50% more total calories for the same time period!

Exercise Gadgets

We seldom get something for nothing. An effortless exercise program would be ideal, of course, but such a program would result in no significant changes in body composition or physical dimensions. With the increasing popularity of exercise, many gimmicks and gadgets have appeared on the market. Some of these are legitimate and effective, but unfortunately many are of no practical value for either exercise conditioning or weight loss. Three such devices were evaluated to determine the legitimacy of their claims: the Mark

II Bust Developer, the Astro-Trimmer Exercise Belt, and the Slim-Skins Vacuum Pants. The first device claimed to add 2 to 3 in. (5 to 8 cm) to the bust within 3 to 7 days, and the last two devices claimed to take inches off of the abdomen, hips, buttocks, and thighs in a matter of minutes. These devices are illustrated in Figure 21.8. All three devices failed to produce any changes whatsoever when evaluated in tightly controlled scientific studies.[24,25]

Those who are considering weight reduction often cringe at the thought of increasing their physical activity, and who wouldn't prefer immediate results over waiting for a payoff? But reality must be addressed. To gain the benefits from exercise it is necessary to actually do the work!

━━ IN REVIEW . . . ━━

1. Inactivity is a major cause of obesity in the United States, perhaps even more important than overeating.
2. The energy expended by activity includes the steady-state rate of energy expenditure during the activity and also the energy expended after the exercise, because the metabolic rate remains elevated (EPOC) for some time after the activity ends.
3. Diet alone causes fat loss, but fat-free mass is also lost. With exercise, either alone or with diet, fat is lost, but fat-free mass is either unchanged or increased.
4. Energy intake – energy excreted = RMR + TEM + TEA.
5. A certain amount of activity appears to be needed for the body to precisely balance energy intake and expenditure.
6. Research indicates that exercise can suppress appetite.
7. RMR can increase slightly following training, and even a single bout of exercise increases the TEM.
8. Exercise increases lipid mobilization from adipose tissue.
9. Spot reduction is a myth. Low-intensity aerobics burn no more fat than more vigorous exercise, and more total calories are spent in a more strenuous workout.

Diabetes

Diabetes, or more specifically diabetes mellitus, is a disorder of carbohydrate metabolism characterized by high blood sugar levels (hyperglycemia) and presence of sugar in the urine (glycosuria). It develops when there is inadequate production of insulin by the pancreas or inadequate utilization of insulin by the cells. Most cases of diabetes fall into two major categories:

1. Insulin-dependent diabetes mellitus (IDDM), also called Type I or juvenile-onset diabetes
2. Noninsulin-dependent diabetes mellitus (NIDDM), also called Type II or adult-onset diabetes

Approximately 12 million Americans have diabetes. About 10% to 15% of these people are classed as Type I, and the remaining 85% to 90% are classed as Type II. The prevalence of diabetes increases with aging, affecting more than 25% of the population age 85 and older.

Etiology of Diabetes

Heredity appears to play a major role in both Type I and Type II diabetes. With Type I diabetes, the beta

Table 21.2 Estimation of Kilocalories Used From Fat and Carbohydrate for a Low- and High-Intensity Aerobic Training Bout

			% kcal		kcal for 30 min		
Exercise intensity	Average $\dot{V}O_2$	Average RER	CHO	Fat	CHO	Fat	Total
Low—50%	1.50 L · min⁻¹	0.85	50	50	110	110	220
High—75%	2.25 L · min⁻¹	0.90	67	33	222	110	332

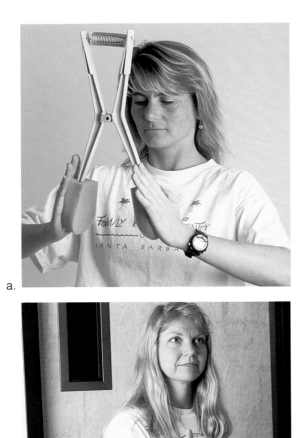

a.

b.

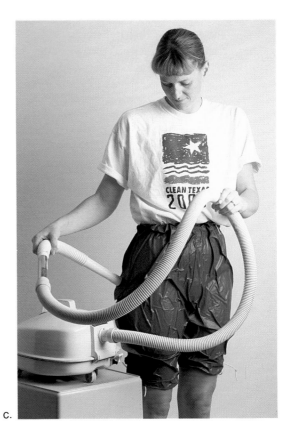

c.

Figure 21.8   Exercise devices once sold through the mail that supposedly would substantially alter body dimensions: (a) Mark II Bust Developer for increasing breast size and shape; (b) Astro-Trimmer Exercise Belt for reducing abdominal fat; (c) Slim-Skins Vacuum Pants for reducing fat in the abdomen, hips, buttocks, and thighs.

cells of the pancreas are destroyed. This destruction may be caused by

- the body's immune system,
- increased beta cell susceptibility to viruses, or
- beta cell degeneration.

Type I diabetes generally has a sudden onset during childhood or young adulthood. This leads to almost total insulin deficiency, and daily injections of insulin are usually required to control the disease.

In Type II diabetes, the onset of the disease is more gradual and the causes are more difficult to establish. Type II diabetes is often characterized by any of the following three major metabolic abnormalities:

1. Delayed or impaired insulin secretion
2. Impaired insulin action (insulin resistance) in the insulin-responsive tissues of the body, including muscle
3. Excessive glucose output from the liver

Obesity plays a major role in the development of Type II diabetes. With obesity, the beta cells of the pancreas often become less responsive to the stimulation of increased blood glucose concentrations. Furthermore, the target cells throughout the body, including muscle, often undergo a reduction in the number or activation of their insulin receptors, so the insulin in the blood is less effective in transporting glucose into the cell.

Health Problems Associated With Diabetes

Considerable health risks are associated with diabetes. People with this disease have a relatively high mortality rate. Diabetes places a person at increased risk for

- coronary artery disease,
- cerebrovascular disease,
- hypertension,
- peripheral vascular disease,
- toxemia during pregnancy,
- renal disorders, and
- eye disorders, including blindness.

During the late 1980s, scientists made the important association between coronary artery disease, hypertension, obesity, and Type II diabetes. Hyperinsulinemia (high blood levels of insulin) and insulin resistance appear to be the important threads linking these disorders, possibly through insulin-mediated sympathetic nervous system stimulation (increased insulin levels cause increased sympathetic nervous system activity).[5]

General Treatment of Diabetes

The major modes of treatment for diabetes are insulin administration, diet, and exercise. Not all patients need insulin, but for those who do, dosage is adjusted to allow normal carbohydrate, fat, and protein metabolism. The type of insulin injected—short-acting or long-acting—and the time of day at which the injections are administered are also individualized to maintain glycemic control throughout the day.

A well-balanced diet is generally prescribed for people with diabetes. In the past, patients were prescribed a low carbohydrate diet to better control blood sugar levels. However, a low carbohydrate diet necessitates an increase in dietary fat, which can have a major negative effect on blood lipid levels. Because people with diabetes are already at greater risk for coronary artery disease, this is not desirable. Maintenance of proper blood sugar levels is difficult in patients with obesity, so a reduced calorie diet is necessary for them to achieve major body fat losses. For many people with Type II diabetes, weight loss alone can bring blood sugar levels back into the normal range. This can be the most important aspect of the treatment plan for the overweight or obese person with diabetes.

The Role of Physical Activity in Diabetes

Although no conclusive evidence proves that a physically active lifestyle prevents diabetes, most physicians agree that physical activity is an important part of the treatment plan. Because there is such a disparity between the characteristics and responses of those with Type I and Type II diabetes, we will discuss each separately.

Type I Diabetes

The role of regular exercise and physical training in improving glycemic control (regulation of blood sugar levels) in patients with Type I diabetes has not been clearly defined and is controversial. The most distinguishing feature differentiating Type I and Type II diabetes is that those with Type I have low blood insulin levels due to the inability or reduced ability of the pancreas to produce insulin. Those with Type I diabetes are prone to hypoglycemia during and immediately after exercise because the liver fails to release glucose at a rate that can keep up with glucose utilization. For these people, exercise can lead to excessive swings in plasma glucose levels that are unacceptable for the management of the disease. The degree of glycemic control during exercise varies tremendously between individuals with Type I diabetes. As a result, exercise and exercise training can improve glycemic control in some patients, mainly those who are less prone to hypoglycemia, but not in others.[23]

Although glycemic control is generally not improved in most people with Type I diabetes, there are other potential benefits of exercise for these patients. Because these patients have a two to three times greater risk for coronary artery disease, exercise may be important to help reduce this risk. The same argument can be made for reducing the risk for cerebrovascular and peripheral arterial diseases.

People with uncomplicated Type I diabetes do not have to restrict physical activity, providing blood sugar levels are controlled appropriately. A number of athletes who have Type I diabetes have trained and competed successfully. Monitoring blood sugar levels in an exercising person with Type I diabetes is important so that diet and insulin dosages can be altered accordingly. Table 21.3 provides guidelines for avoiding hypoglycemia during and after exercise.

Special attention should also be given to the feet of people with diabetes, as it is common for them to experience peripheral neuropathy (diseased nerves) with some loss of sensation in the feet. Peripheral vascular disease is also more common in patients with diabetes, so the circulation to the extremities, especially the feet, is often impaired significantly. Ulcerations and other lesions on the feet account for more than half of all hospitalizations of diabetic patients.[4] Because weight-bearing exercise places additional stress on the feet, the proper selection of footwear and appropriate preventive foot care are important.

Diabetes and Exercise

To optimize treatment, whether through insulin, diet, or exercise, people with diabetes need to monitor their blood sugar levels, allowing them to make adjustments in one or more of these three treatment modalities. Home blood glucose monitoring kits (see Figure 21.9) are available that allow the individual to periodically take a finger-stick blood sample and determine its blood glucose concentration. This is particularly important when a person with diabetes is contemplating a change in insulin dosage, diet, or exercise patterns. As an example, people often need to reduce their insulin dosage once they start a regular exercise program. Furthermore, this monitoring can occur before, during, and following an exercise bout. This enables an exerciser to know if his or her blood sugar level has decreased to a critical level as a result of the exercise, in which case eating a high carbohydrate food would be required. Hypoglycemia is a potential risk during exercise, so a person with diabetes should always exercise in the company of another person who is familiar with the disease. A glucose drink or a source of simple sugar, such as jelly beans, should be available if needed to prevent insulin shock.

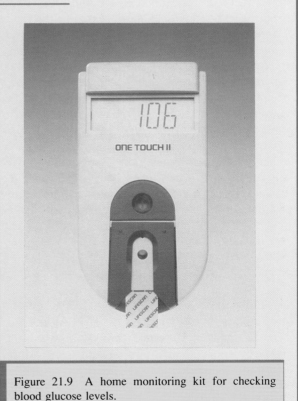

Figure 21.9 A home monitoring kit for checking blood glucose levels.

Table 21.3 Guidelines for Avoiding Hypoglycemia During and After Exercise in People With Type I Diabetes

1. Consume carbohydrates (15-30 g) for every 30 min of moderate intensity exercise.
2. Consume a snack of slowly absorbed carbohydrate following prolonged exercise sessions.
3. Decrease the insulin dose:
    a. *Intermediate-acting insulin*—decrease by 30-35% on the day of exercise.
    b. *Intermediate- and short-acting insulin*—omit the dose of short-acting insulin that precedes exercise.
    c. *Multiple doses of short-acting insulin*—reduce the dose prior to exercise by 30-35% and supplement carbohydrates.
    d. *Continuous subcutaneous infusion*—eliminate the mealtime bolus or increment that precedes or immediately follows exercise.
4. Avoid exercising muscle that underlies the injection site of short-acting insulin for 1 hr.
5. Avoid late evening exercise.

Adapted from Vitug et al. (1988).

Type II Diabetes

Exercise plays a major role in glycemic control for people with Type II diabetes. Insulin production is generally not of concern in this group, particularly during the early stages of the disease, so the major problem with this form of diabetes is the lack of target cell response to insulin (insulin resistance). Because the cells become resistant to insulin, the hormone cannot perform its function of facilitating glucose transport across the cell membrane. Ivy has demonstrated that muscle contraction has an insulin-like effect.[8] Membrane permeability to glucose increases with muscular contraction, possibly due to an increase in the number of glucose transporters associated with the plasma membrane. Thus acute bouts of exercise decrease insulin resistance and increase insulin sensitivity. This reduces the cells' requirements for insulin,

which means that people taking insulin must reduce their dosages. This decrease in insulin resistance and increase in insulin sensitivity may primarily be a response to each individual bout of exercise rather than the result of a long-term change associated with training.

▬ IN REVIEW . . . ▬

1. Diabetes is a disorder of carbohydrate metabolism characterized by hyperglycemia and glycosuria. It develops from inadequate insulin secretion or utilization.
2. Type I diabetes involves destruction of the beta cells in the pancreas, and it typically has a sudden, early onset. Type II diabetes typically involves impaired insulin secretion or action, excessive liver glucose output, or a combination of these.
3. Major modes of treatment for diabetes are insulin administration (if needed), diet, and exercise.
4. In people with Type I diabetes, glycemic control might or might not be improved with exercise. But these people have a greater risk for coronary artery disease, so exercise can certainly decrease that risk.
5. Blood sugar levels must be carefully monitored when exercising, particularly in people with Type I diabetes, so diet and insulin dosage can be altered as needed.
6. In people with Type I diabetes, feet deserve special attention, because peripheral neuropathy causes loss of sensation, and impaired peripheral circulation decreases blood flow. These people might not be aware of injuries to their feet, but these injuries can be very serious.
7. Type II diabetes responds well to exercise. Membrane permeability to glucose improves with exercise, which decreases the person's insulin resistance and increases insulin sensitivity.

▬ KEY POINT ▬

Physical activity has many desirable effects for people with diabetes, particularly those with Type II diabetes. Glycemic control is improved, primarily in people with Type II diabetes, possibly due to the insulin-like effect of muscle contraction on translocating glucose from the plasma into the cell.

In Closing . . .

In this chapter, we have concluded our look at the role of physical activity in the prevention and treatment of coronary artery disease, hypertension, obesity, and diabetes. We have seen that exercise can decrease individual risk and can also be an integral part of treatment, improving overall health as well as alleviating some symptoms.

Now that we know the importance of exercise in health maintenance, we are ready to put the theory into action. In the next chapter we turn our attention to the prescription of exercise for health and fitness.

Key Terms

beta cells
body mass index (BMI)
diabetes mellitus
excess post-exercise oxygen consumption (EPOC)
glycosuria
hyperglycemia
hyperinsulinemia
hypoglycemia
insulin
insulin resistance
lower body (gynoid) obesity
low-intensity aerobic exercise

obesity
overweight
relative weight
resting metabolic rate (RMR)
spot reduction
thermic effect of activity (TEA)
thermic effect of a meal (TEM)
Type I diabetes
Type II diabetes
upper body (android) obesity

Study Questions

1. What is the difference between overweight and obesity?
2. What is ideal body weight and how is it determined?
3. What is relative body weight? What is its significance?
4. What is body mass index? What is its significance?
5. What is the prevalence of obesity in the United States today? Is there a difference between men and women? Children and adults? Blacks and whites?
6. What are some of the health-related problems associated with obesity?
7. What is the association between obesity, coronary artery disease, hypertension, and diabetes?
8. Describe several methods for treating obesity. Which are the most effective?
9. What role does exercise play in the prevention and treatment of obesity?
10. By what mechanisms might exercise effect losses in total weight and fat weight?
11. How effective is spot reduction? Low-intensity aerobic exercise?
12. Describe the two major types of diabetes. How are they caused?
13. What are the health risks associated with diabetes?
14. Describe the role of exercise in treating patients with Type I diabetes.
15. Describe the role of exercise in treating patients with Type II diabetes.

References

1. Björntorp, P., Smith, U., & Lönnroth, P. (Eds.) (1988). *Health implications of regional obesity* (Acta Medica Scandinavica Symposium Series No. 4). Stockholm: Almqvist & Wiksell International.

2. Bouchard, C., Tremblay, A., Després, J.-P., Nadeau, A., Lupien, P.J., Thériault, G., Dussault, J., Moorjani, S., Pinault, S., & Fournier, G. (1990). The response to long-term overfeeding in identical twins. *New England Journal of Medicine*, **322**, 1477-1482.

3. Broeder, C.E., Burrhus, K.A., Svanevik, L.S., & Wilmore, J.H. (1992). The effects of either high intensity resistance or endurance training on resting metabolic rate. *American Journal of Clinical Nutrition*, **55**, 802-810.

4. Chisholm, D.J. (1992). Diabetes mellitus. In J. Bloomfield, P.A. Fricker, & K.D. Fitch (Eds.), *Textbook of science and medicine in sport* (pp. 555-561). Boston: Blackwell Scientific.

5. Daly, P.A., & Landsberg, L. (1991). Hypertension in obesity and NIDDM: Role of insulin and sympathetic nervous system. *Diabetes Care*, **14**, 240-248.

6. Gortmaker, S.L., Dietz, W.H., Jr., Sobol, A.M., & Wehler, C.A. (1987). Increasing pediatric obesity in the United States. *American Journal of Diseases of Children*, **141**, 535-540.

7. Gwinup, G., Chelvam, R., & Steinberg, T. (1971). Thickness of subcutaneous fat and activity of underlying muscles. *Annals of Internal Medicine*, **74**, 408-411.

8. Ivy, J.L. (1987). The insulin-like effect of muscle contraction. *Exercise and Sport Sciences Reviews*, **15**, 29-51.

9. Katch, F.I., Clarkson, P.M., Kroll, W., McBride, T., & Wilcox, A. (1984) Effects of sit up exercise training on adipose cell size and adiposity. *Research Quarterly for Exercise and Sport*, **55**, 242-247.

10. Keesey, R.E. (1986). A set-point theory of obesity. In K.D. Brownell & J.P. Foreyt (Eds.), *Handbook of eating disorders: Physiology, psychology, and treatment of obesity, anorexia, and bulimia* (pp. 63-87). New York: Basic Books.

11. Keys, A., Brozek, J., Henschel, A., Mickelsen, O., & Taylor, H.L. (1950). *The biology of human starvation*. Minneapolis: University of Minnesota Press.

12. Mayer, J., Marshall, N.B., Vitale, J.J., Christensen, J.H., Mashayekhi, M.B., & Stare, F.J. (1954). Exercise, food intake, and body weight in normal rats and genetically obese adult mice. *American Journal of Physiology*, **177**, 544-548.

13. National Center for Health Statistics. (1986). *Health, United States, 1986* (DHHS Publ. No. PHS 87-1232). Washington DC: U.S. Government Printing Office.

14. Oscai, L.B. (1973). The role of exercise in weight control. *Exercise and Sport Sciences Reviews*, **1**, 103-123.

15. Pavlou, K.N., Steffee, W.P., Lerman, R.H., & Burrows, V. (1985) Effects of dieting and exercise on lean body mass, oxygen uptake, and strength. *Medicine and Science in Sports and Exercise*, **17**, 466-471.

16. Poehlman, E.T. (1989). A review: Exercise and its influence on resting energy metabolism in man. *Medicine and Science in Sports and Exercise*, **21**, 515-525.

17. Sims, E.A.H. (1976). Experimental obesity, dietary-induced thermogenesis and their clinical implications. *Clinics in Endocrinology and Metabolism*, **5**, 377-395.

18. Stunkard, A.J., Foch, T.T., & Hrubec, Z. (1986). A twin study of human obesity. *Journal of the American Medical Association*, **256**, 51-54.

19. Stunkard, A.J., Harris, J.R., Pedersen, N.L., & McClearn, G.E. (1990). The body-mass index of twins who have been reared apart. *New England Journal of Medicine*, **322**, 1483-1487.

20. Stunkard, A.J., Sørensen, T.I.A., Hanis, C., Teasdale, T.W., Chakraborty, R., Schull, W.J., & Schulsinger, F. (1986). An adoption study of human obesity. *New England Journal of Medicine*, **314**, 193-198.

21. Tremblay, A., Nadeau, A., Fournier, G., & Bouchard, C. (1988). Effect of a three-day interruption of exercise-training on resting metabolic rate and glucose-induced thermogenesis in trained individuals. *International Journal of Obesity*, **12**, 163-168.

22. Van Italie, T.B. (1985). Health implications of overweight and obesity in the United States. *Annals of Internal Medicine*, **103**, 983-988.

23. Vitug, A., Schneider, S.H., & Ruderman, N.B. (1988). Exercise and Type I diabetes mellitus. *Exercise and Sport Sciences Reviews*, **16**, 285-304.

24. Wilmore, J.H., Atwater, A.E., Maxwell, B.D., Wilmore, D.L., Constable, S.H., & Buono, M.J. (1985a). Alterations in body size and composition consequent to Astro-Trimmer and Slim-Skins training programs. *Research Quarterly for Exercise and Sport*, **56**, 90-92.

25. Wilmore, J.H., Atwater, A.E., Maxwell, B.D., Wilmore, D.L., Constable, S.H., & Buono, M.J. (1985b). Alterations in breast morphology consequent to a 21-day bust developer program. *Medicine and Science in Sports and Exercise*, **17**, 106-112.

26. Zuti, W.B., & Golding, L.A. (1976). Comparing diet and exercise as weight reduction tools. *Physician and Sportsmedicine*, **4**, 49-53.

Selected Readings

Atkinson, R.L. (1989). Low and very low calorie diets. *Medical Clinics of North America*, **73**, 203-215.

Ballor, D.L., & Poehlman, E.T. (1994). Exercise-training enhances fat-free mass preservation during diet-induced weight loss: A meta-analytical finding. *International Journal of Obesity*, **18**, 35-40.

Behnke, A.R., & Wilmore, J.H. (1974). *Evaluation and regulation of body build and composition.* Englewood Cliffs, NJ: Prentice-Hall.

Björntorp, P. (1986). Fat cells and obesity. In K.D. Brownell & J.P. Foreyt (Eds.), *Handbook of eating disorders: Physiology, psychology, and treatment of obesity, anorexia, and bulimia* (pp. 88-98). New York: Basic Books.

Björntorp, P., & Brodoff, B.N. (Eds.) (1992). *Obesity.* Philadelphia: Lippincott.

Bray, G.A. (1985). Obesity: Definition, diagnosis and disadvantages. *Medical Journal of Australia*, **142**, S2-S8.

Brownell, K.D., & Foreyt, J.P. (Eds.) (1986). *Handbook of eating disorders: Physiology, psychology, and treatment of obesity, anorexia, and bulimia.* New York: Basic Books

Durak, E. (1989). Exercise for specific populations: Diabetes mellitus. *Sports Training, Medicine and Rehabilitation*, **1**, 175-180.

Gray, D.S. (1989). Diagnosis and prevalence of obesity. *Medical Clinics of North America*, **73**, 1-13.

Holloszy, J.O., Schultz, J., Kusnierkiewicz, J., Hagberg, J.M., & Ehsani, A.A. (1986). Effects of exercise on glucose tolerance and insulin resistance. *Acta Medica Scandinavica*, (Suppl. 711), 55-65.

Katch, F.I., & McArdle, W.D. (1988). *Nutrition, weight control, and exercise* (3rd ed.). Philadelphia: Lea & Febiger.

King, A.C., & Tribble, D.L. (1991). The role of exercise in weight regulation in nonathletes. *Sports Medicine*, **11**, 331-349.

National Institutes of Health. (1985). Health implications of obesity: National Institutes of Health Consensus Development Conference Statement. *Annals of Internal Medicine*, **103**, 1073-1077.

Pace, P.J., Webster, J., & Garrow, J.S. (1986). Exercise and obesity. *Sports Medicine*, **3**, 89-113.

Poehlman, E.T., & Horton, E.S. (1990). Regulation of energy expenditure in aging humans. *Annual Reviews in Nutrition*, **10**, 255-275.

Schneider, S.H., & Ruderman, N.B. (1990). Exercise and NIDDM. *Diabetes Care*, **13**, 785-789.

Segal, K.R., & Pi-Sunyer, F.X. (1989). Exercise and obesity. *Medical Clinics of North America*, **73**, 217-236.

Stefanick, M.L. (1993). Exercise and weight control. *Exercise and Sport Science Reviews*, **21**, 363-396.

Stunkard, A.J. (Ed.) (1980). *Obesity*. Philadelphia: Saunders.

Stunkard, A.J., & Wadden, T.A. (Eds.) (1993). *Obesity: Theory and therapy* (2nd ed.). New York: Raven Press.

Weinsier, R.L., Wadden, T.A., Ritenbaugh, C., Harrison, G.G., Johnson, F.S., & Wilmore, J.H. (1984). Guidelines for professional weight control programs. *American Journal of Clinical Nutrition*, **40**, 865-872.

Woo, R., Daniels-Kash, R., & Horton, E.S. (1985). Regulation of energy balance. *Annual Reviews in Nutrition*, **5**, 411-433.

Chapter 22

Prescription of Exercise for Health and Fitness

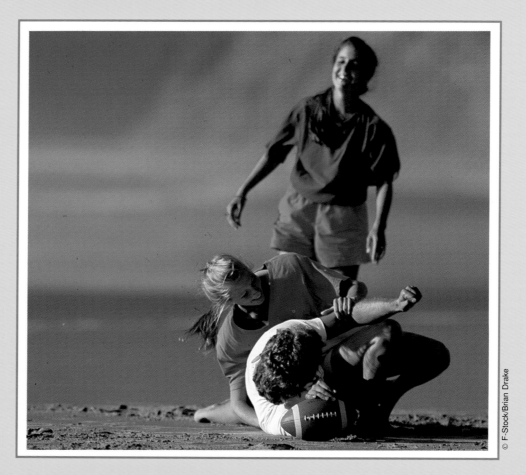

© F-Stock/Brian Drake

Chapter Overview

Patterns of today's living have channeled the average American into an increasingly sedentary existence. Humans, however, were designed and built for movement. Physiologically, we have not adapted well to this inactive lifestyle. In fact, during what appeared to be a fitness boom in the 1970s and 1980s, fewer than 10% of adult Americans were exercising at levels that would increase or maintain their aerobic fitness. Yet research has determined that, for most people, an individually prescribed exercise program to supplement normal daily activities is important for optimal health. We saw in the previous two chapters that exercise is beneficial to the prevention and treatment of cardiovascular diseases, obesity, and diabetes and that it can benefit people suffering from numerous other health problems.

In this chapter we will focus on the principles of exercise prescription. We will discuss the importance of obtaining medical clearance before beginning an exercise program, as well as what constitutes an appropriate medical screening. Then we will review the components that constitute the exercise prescription. Finally, we will examine the components of exercise programs for both healthy people as well as for those with diseases.

Chapter Outline

Jason Walker, a 35-year-old executive, went in for his annual physical examination with a vow to start a long overdue exercise program. Due to his high blood pressure and one-pack-a-day smoking habit, his physician decided to give Jason a graded exercise test to determine the normality of his electrocardiogram during the stress of exercise. As Jason was nearing exhaustion on the treadmill, his doctor noticed changes in the ST segment of his ECG, which are considered indicative of coronary artery disease. The following week, Jason, with fear and trepidation, underwent a coronary arteriogram procedure to check for coronary artery disease. His arteriogram was normal, indicating that his treadmill electrocardiogram was not accurate—it was a false positive test! Fortunately, Jason had been scared to the point that he stopped smoking and began an exercise program. He is now competing in 10 km-races, is very fit, and has his blood pressure under control.

The seeds for a fitness revolution were planted in the late 1960s with the publication of the book *Aerobics*, written by Dr. Kenneth Cooper (see Selected Readings). This book provided a sound medical basis for the importance of exercise, particularly aerobic exercise, to health and fitness. The fitness movement grew throughout the 1970s, possibly peaking in the early 1980s, at which time the media declared that America was in the midst of a fitness boom. This was an exciting time to be in the exercise sciences!

Then, in 1983, came a penetrating article by Kirshenbaum and Sullivan, published in *Sports Illustrated*, that brought everything into proper perspective.[14] The authors questioned the existence of the fitness boom, contending that involvement was basically limited to a small but highly visible segment of the total population. They maintained that the fitness boom included mostly high-income, executive-level, white, college-educated, young to middle-aged adults. The results of a survey by the Pacific Mutual Life Insurance Company confirmed this analysis.[10] Furthermore, additional national surveys reported that only 15% to 36% of the adult American population participated in regular vigorous activity.[11,12,20] Most importantly, recent estimates suggest that only 7.5% of all adult Americans meet the American College of Sports Medicine (ACSM) guidelines for cardiorespiratory fitness development and maintenance.[2,6]

In spite of the disappointing statistics, most Americans are aware that exercise is an integral part of preventive medicine. And yet people often equate exercise with jogging 5 mi (8 km) a day or lifting weights until their muscles can do no more. Many people decide that exercise is too difficult before they even try it, not realizing that the appropriate exercise type and intensity varies depending on individual characteristics, current fitness level, and specific health concerns. Knowing this, how can these people begin exercise programs to improve their general health and fitness? The first step is deciding to take action. The next step is getting medical clearance.

Medical Clearance

A medical evaluation is a useful and important part of the exercise prescription for many reasons:

- Some people either should not be exercising at all or are considered at high risk and should be restricted to exercising only under close medical supervision. A comprehensive medical evaluation will help identify these high-risk individuals.
- The information obtained in a medical evaluation can be used to develop the exercise prescription.
- The values obtained for certain clinical measures, such as blood pressure, body fat content, and blood lipid levels, can be used to motivate the person to adhere to the exercise program.
- A comprehensive medical evaluation, particularly of healthy people, can provide a baseline against which any subsequent changes in health status can be compared.
- Children and adults should establish the habit of periodic medical evaluations because many illnesses and diseases, such as cancer and cardiovascular diseases, can be identified in their earliest stages when the chances of successful treatment are much higher.

The Medical Evaluation

Unfortunately, although a comprehensive medical evaluation is useful and desirable before prescribing exercise, not all people will have one. Many people can't afford the cost of such an evaluation, and the medical system is not prepared to provide this service for the total population, even if money were available. Also, a medical evaluation prior to prescribing exercise in a presumed healthy population has not been proven to reduce the medical risks associated with exercise. For these reasons, guidelines or recommendations have been established that attempt to target the higher-risk populations.[2,3,8] People at high risk are those who have two or more major risk factors for coronary artery disease (Table 22.1) or symptoms of cardiopulmonary or metabolic disorders (Table 22.2).

In general, before beginning any exercise program that includes vigorous activity the following persons should have a complete medical examination by a physician:

- Men 40 years of age and older
- Women 50 years of age and older
- People of any age who are considered to be at high risk

Table 22.1 Major Coronary Risk Factors

1. Diagnosed hypertension or systolic blood pressure ≥ 160 or diastolic blood pressure ≥ 90 mmHg on at least 2 separate occasions, or on antihypertensive medication
2. Serum cholesterol ≥ 6.20 mmol $\cdot$ L^{-1} (≥ 240 mg $\cdot$ dl^{-1})
3. Cigarette smoking
4. Diabetes mellitus[a]
5. Family history of coronary or other atherosclerotic disease in parents or siblings prior to age 55
[a]Persons with insulin-dependent diabetes mellitus (IDDM) who are over 30 years of age, or have had IDDM for more than 15 years, and persons with non-insulin-dependent diabetes mellitus who are over 35 years of age should be classified as patients with disease.
Data from American College of Sports Medicine (1991).

Table 22.2 Major Symptoms or Signs Suggestive of Cardiopulmonary or Metabolic Disease

1. Pain or discomfort in the chest or surrounding areas that appears to be ischemic in nature
2. Unaccustomed shortness of breath or shortness of breath with mild exertion
3. Dizziness or syncope
4. Orthopnea/paroxysmal nocturnal dyspnea
5. Ankle edema
6. Palpitations or tachycardia
7. Claudication
8. Known heart murmur
Note. These symptoms must be interpreted in the clinical context in which they appear because they are not all specific for cardiopulmonary or metabolic disease.
Data from American College of Sports Medicine (1991).

The American College of Sports Medicine has published specific recommendations for each phase of the medical evaluation. This document should be consulted whenever there is any question as to what should be included.[2]

The physical examination should include discussion with the physician of the proposed exercise program in case any medical contraindications are associated with the proposed activity. For example, people with hypertension should be cautioned to avoid activities that use isometric actions. This is because these tend to increase blood pressure considerably and usually result in the Valsalva maneuver, in which intra-abdominal and intrathoracic pressures increase to the point of restricting blood flow through the vena cava, limiting venous return to the heart. Both responses can lead to serious medical complications, such as loss of consciousness or stroke. Also, as we have discussed previously, even dynamic resistance training can cause very high blood pressure during the activity.

The Exercise Electrocardiogram

The exercise electrocardiogram is obtained while you exercise, usually either on a treadmill or a cycle ergometer, as shown in Figure 22.1. The electrocardiogram is monitored as you progress from low-intensity exercise, such as slow walking, up to maximal intensity exercise. Maximal intensity might be brisk walking for an older, deconditioned subject, or running up a grade for a younger, fit individual. The rate of work is generally increased every 1 to 3 min until the maximal rate of work is achieved. This is referred to as a graded exercise test. The electrocardiogram is monitored for arrhythmias and for changes in the ST segment, the latter being predictive of existing coronary artery disease.

The exercise electrocardiogram is an extremely important part of the medical evaluation because a small but significant percentage of the adult population have abnormalities in electrocardiograms taken during or following exercise, even though they have normal resting electrocardiograms. These abnormalities often indicate the presence of coronary artery disease. Because of this, an exercise test is recommended primarily for disease detection. But the sensitivity, specificity, and predictive value of an exercise test must be considered. Sensitivity

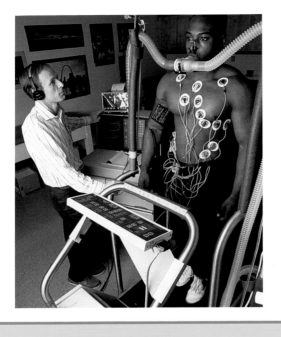

Figure 22.1   Obtaining an exercise electrocardiogram.

refers to the exercise test's ability to correctly identify people who have the disease in question, such as coronary artery disease. Specificity refers to the test's ability to correctly identify people who don't have the disease. And the predictive value of an abnormal exercise test refers to the accuracy with which abnormal test results reflect presence of the disease.

These concepts are illustrated in Table 22.3. The total population tested is divided into those who have documented coronary artery disease and those who don't. This is normally determined by a coronary arte-

riogram, where radiopaque dye is injected through a catheter into coronary arteries, allowing visualization of the insides of the arteries. Results from an exercise test are considered either positive, when there have been changes in the electrocardiogram that suggest the presence of coronary artery disease, or negative. A negative test implies that no disease was detected. The exercise electrocardiogram is not 100% accurate, so some people have a normal, or negative, exercise test, yet have coronary artery disease. These are false-negative tests. There are also people who do not have the disease, as determined by coronary arteriograms, yet who have a positive exercise electrocardiogram suggesting disease. These are false-positive tests. Table 22.3 illustrates how sensitivity, specificity, and the predictive value of an abnormal exercise test are calculated. A total of 100 subjects have been tested and 6 are true-positive, 10 are false-positive, 4 are false-negative, and 80 are true-negative. The prevalence of the disease in this population is 6% (6 true positives / 100 subjects).

Unfortunately, both the sensitivity and the predictive value of an abnormal exercise test for the detection of coronary artery disease are relatively low in healthy populations of people who have no symptoms for this disease. Past studies reveal that sensitivity averages from 50% to 80%, indicating that between 50% and 80% of those with coronary artery disease are correctly identified by exercise electrocardiograms as having the disease. Conversely, from 20% to 50% of those with the disease are incorrectly diagnosed as disease free, based on exercise electrocardiograms. Average specificity values range from 80% to 90%, indicating that 80% to 90% of those without disease are correctly identified by the exercise test as being

Table 22.3 Illustration of the Concept of Exercise Test Sensitivity (SN), Specificity (SP), and the Predictive Value (PV) of an Abnormal Test

Exercise test result	Those with coronary artery disease	Those without coronary artery disease	
Positive	True positive (TP)[a]	False positive (FP)[b]	$PV = [TP/(TP + FP)] \times 100$
Negative	False negative (FN)[c]	True negative (TN)[d]	
	$SN = [TP/(TP + FN)] \times 100$	$SP = [TN/(FP + TN)] \times 100$	

Note. An abnormal exercise test is defined as one in which the ST segment of the ECG is depressed, suggestive of myocardial ischemia.

[a]TP = those with disease that have an abnormal exercise test.

[b]FP = those without disease that have an abnormal exercise test.

[c]FN = those with disease that have a normal exercise test.

[d]TN = those without disease that have a normal exercise test.

disease free. Unfortunately, this means that 10% to 20% of the population is incorrectly identified as having the disease.

KEY POINT

The sensitivity and predictive value of an abnormal exercise test are generally low in a young, healthy population where there is a low prevalence of coronary artery disease. As a result, the value of using exercise electrocardiography to screen for coronary artery disease in this population is questionable.

The predictive value of an abnormal exercise test varies considerably with the prevalence of coronary artery disease in the population. This is illustrated in Table 22.4, comparing the predictive value of an abnormal test when the prevalence of coronary artery disease, per 1,000 people, is 5% versus 50%. In both cases, we assume an average sensitivity of 60% and an average specificity of 90%, based on past studies.

Table 22.4 Comparison of the Predictive Value of Exercise Testing Between Populations With 5% and 50% Prevalence of Coronary Artery Disease (CAD), Using a Sensitivity of 60% and a Specificity of 90%

Population subgroups	n (%) of subjects	n (%) abnormal exercise ECG	n (%) normal exercise ECG
5% prevalence			
Normal	950 (95)	95 (10%) FP[a]	855 (90%) TN[b]
CAD	50 (5)	30 (60%) TP[c]	20 (40%) FN[d]
Total	1,000 (100)	125 (12.5%)	875 (87.5%)
	Predictive value = [30/(30 + 95)] = 24.0%		
50% prevalence			
Normal	500 (50)	50 (10%) FP	450 (90%) TN
CAD	500 (50)	300 (60%) TP	200 (40%) FN
Total	1,000 (100)	350 (35%)	650 (65%)
	Predictive value = [300/(300 + 50)] = 85.7%		

[a]FP = false positive
[b]TN = true negative
[c]TP = true positive
[d]FN = false negative

Note. An abnormal exercise test is defined as one in which the ST segment of the ECG is depressed, suggestive of myocardial ischemia.

For the population with the 5% prevalence, the predictive value of an abnormal test is only 24.0%. This indicates that only 24% of those who have an abnormal exercise electrocardiogram actually have coronary artery disease. In other words, in this population, more than three out of every four people identified with abnormal exercise tests will be labeled as diseased but won't actually have identifiable coronary artery disease! But if we consider the population with a prevalence of 50%, the predictive value of an abnormal exercise test is much higher—85.7%.

In a 10-year study of YMCAs in the United States, investigators reported one sudden death during exercise per 3 million person-hours, and one cardiac arrest per 2 million person-hours.[19] Person-hours refers to the total amount of time the entire population exercises. For example, if each of 10 people exercised for 500 hr, that gives a total of 5,000 person-hours of exercise. Based on the uncertainties associated with positive and negative results from exercise tests in populations that have a low prevalence of disease and a relative scarcity of sudden deaths or cardiac arrests during exercise, they concluded that it is impractical to use exercise testing to prevent significant cardiovascular complications during exercise in asymptomatic individuals.

From this information, we can conclude that exercise testing is of limited value in screening young, apparently healthy individuals prior to giving them exercise prescriptions. The accuracy in interpreting the results of the exercise electrocardiogram is questionable, particularly in a population with such a low prevalence of disease. Also, the actual risk of death or cardiac arrest during exercise is relatively low. Another important consideration is the expense of conducting clinical exercise tests, generally around $150 to $350 per test. Finally, far too few clinical facilities are equipped to conduct these tests to accommodate testing everyone who should be involved in an exercise program. Fortunately, the American College of Sports Medicine and the American Heart Association have recommended this exercise test only for the at-risk groups mentioned earlier in this chapter.

From a medical-legal consideration, however, the question must be raised as to whether a recommendation within a set of national guidelines is tantamount to a standard of practice in the medical community. The most recent guidelines of the American College of Sports Medicine state that a medical examination and exercise test might not be necessary if moderate exercise is undertaken gradually, with appropriate guidance, and with no competitive participation.[2] Moderate exercise is defined as exercise that is well within the individual's current capacity and can be sustained comfortably for a prolonged period of time, such as 60 min. In contrast, vigorous exercise is defined as exercise at an intensity greater than 60% of the individual's $\dot{V}O_2$ max. This seems like a reasonable compromise, because moderate exercise is associated with considerable health benefits and few risks.[4,15,16,17] But, as mentioned earlier, exercise testing offers benefits other than diagnosing coronary artery disease—it can provide valuable physiological data, such as a person's blood pressure response to exercise, and much of the data obtained can be used in formulating the exercise prescription.

IN REVIEW . . .

1. Before beginning any exercise program, men over age 40, women over age 50, and anyone who is considered to be at a high risk for coronary artery disease should have a complete medical evaluation.
2. ACSM guidelines should be followed for each phase of the evaluation, and the physician should be consulted about the proposed exercise activity in case there are any medical contraindications.
3. Exercise electrocardiograms should be conducted for anyone in one of the previously mentioned high-risk categories. This test can detect undiagnosed coronary artery disease and other cardiac abnormalities.
4. Test sensitivity refers to the test's ability to correctly identify people with a given disease. Test specificity refers to its ability to correctly identify people who do not have the disease. The predictive value of an abnormal exercise test refers to the accuracy with which the test reflects presence of the disease.
5. The most recent ACSM guidelines state that a medical examination and exercise test might not be necessary if moderate exercise is undertaken gradually.

The Exercise Prescription

The exercise prescription involves four basic factors:

1. Mode or type of exercise
2. Frequency of participation
3. Duration of each exercise bout
4. Intensity of the exercise bout

In our discussion we will assume that the goal of the exercise program is to improve aerobic capacity in people who have not been exercising. The information contained in this section is not appropriate for designing training programs for elite endurance athletes, nor for those who simply wish to gain the health-related benefits of moderate activity but do not wish to improve aerobic capacity.

Before examining the components of the exercise prescription, we must consider how much exercise is effective. A minimum threshold for frequency, duration, and intensity of exercise must be reached before any aerobic benefits are obtained. But, as we have discussed elsewhere, individual response to any given training program is highly variable. Because of this, the threshold required differs from one person to the next. Using exercise intensity as an example, a position statement by the American College of Sports Medicine for developing and maintaining aerobic capacity recommends a training intensity of 60% to 90% of one's maximum heart rate (HR max), or 50% to 85% of $\dot{V}O_2$ max.[1] Although this recommendation is appropriate for most healthy adults, some could improve their aerobic capacities at, for example, intensities substantially below 50% of their $\dot{V}O_2$ max, whereas others would have to exercise at intensities greater than 85% of $\dot{V}O_2$ max to show improvement. Each individual's threshold for frequency, duration, and intensity must be exceeded to achieve gains in aerobic capacity, and this threshold is likely to increase as aerobic capacity improves.

KEY POINT

It is important to recognize that a minimal threshold must be reached for frequency, duration, and intensity of exercise to gain aerobic benefits from that exercise. Furthermore, minimal thresholds vary widely, making individualized exercise prescription necessary.

Mode of Exercise

The prescribed exercise program should focus on one or more cardiovascular endurance activities. Traditionally, the activities prescribed most frequently have been

- walking,
- jogging,
- running,
- hiking,
- cycling,
- rowing, and
- swimming.

Because these activities do not appeal to everyone, alternative activities have been identified that should promote similar cardiovascular endurance gains. Aerobic dance, box or bench stepping, and most racquet sports have also been shown to improve aerobic capacity (see Figure 22.2).

For most sport-type activities involving competition, preconditioning with one of the standard endurance activities, such as jogging, is advisable before undertaking serious competition. Some researchers, clinicians, and practitioners feel that for you to successfully compete in certain sports or activities, a basic preconditioning program is essential to bring you up to the level of conditioning needed for the sport or activity and to reduce your risk of injury. Rather than using the sport or activity to get in shape, you get in shape, or precondition, before participating in that sport or activity. For example, if the desired activity requires a moderate-to-high level of cardiovascular endurance, such as basketball, you might engage in a jogging, aerobic dance, or cycling program for several months until your endurance capacity increases to the necessary level. At that time, you switch over to the sport. The sport then acts as a maintenance activity through which you maintain your desired fitness level.

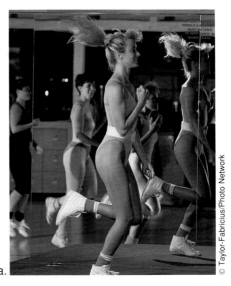
a.

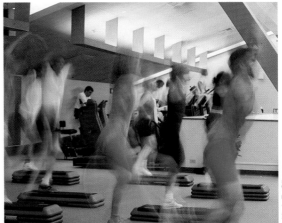
b.

KEY POINT

Sport and recreational activities are appropriate for maintaining desirable fitness levels, but they generally are not appropriate for developing fitness in unfit individuals. Use conditioning activities to reach the desired level of fitness, then switch to the sport and recreational activities.

When selecting activities, individuals must be matched with activities that they enjoy and are willing to continue throughout life. Exercise must be regarded as a lifetime pursuit, because, as we saw in chapter 13, the benefits are soon lost if participation stops. Motivation is probably the most important factor in a successful exercise program. Selecting an activity that is fun, provides a challenge, and can produce needed benefits is one of the most crucial tasks in exercise prescription. Other considerations include geographic location, climate, and availability of equipment and facilities. Home exercise has become more common as many people are homebound either because of responsibilities, such as child rearing, or due to weather considerations, such as heat, humidity, cold, rain, ice, and snow. Exercise videos and home exercise equipment have become popular, but they need to be selected carefully to avoid inappropriate exercise or faulty equipment. Seek professional advice and, when possible, give the video or equipment a trial period before purchase.

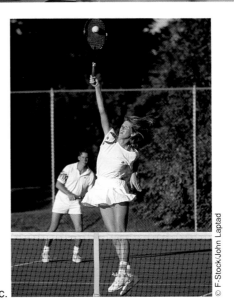
c.

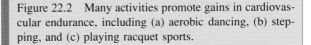
Figure 22.2   Many activities promote gains in cardiovascular endurance, including (a) aerobic dancing, (b) stepping, and (c) playing racquet sports.

Exercise Frequency

The frequency of participation, though certainly an important factor to consider, is probably less critical than either exercise duration or intensity. Research studies conducted on exercise frequency show that 3 to 5 days per week is an optimal frequency. This does not mean that 6 or 7 days per week won't give additional benefits, but simply for the health-related benefits, the optimal gain is achieved with a time investment of 3 to 5 days per week. Exercise should initially be limited to 3 or 4 days per week and frequency increased up to 5 or more days per week only if the activity is enjoyed and physically tolerated. All too often, a person starts out with great intentions, is highly motivated, and exercises every day for the first few weeks, only to stop from utter fatigue or injury. Obviously, additional days per week above the three-to four-day frequency are beneficial for weight loss, but this level should not be encouraged until the exercise habit is firmly established and the injury risk is reduced.

Exercise Duration

Several studies have demonstrated improvement in cardiovascular conditioning with endurance exercise periods as brief as 5 to 10 min per day. More recent research has indicated that 20 to 30 min per day is an optimal amount. Again, optimal is used here to reflect the greatest return for time invested, and the specified time refers to the time during which you are at your appropriate exercise intensity. In addition, exercise duration cannot be discussed appropriately without also discussing exercise intensity. Similar improvements in aerobic capacity are gained with either a short-duration–high-intensity program or a long-duration–low-intensity program if the minimal threshold is exceeded for both duration and intensity. Similar benefits are also gained whether the daily endurance training session is conducted in multiple shorter bouts or as a single long one, such as three 10-min bouts versus a single 30-min bout.

Exercise Intensity

The intensity of the exercise bout appears to be the most important factor. How hard must you push yourself to gain benefits? Ex-athletes immediately recall the exhaustive workouts they endured to condition themselves for their sport. Unfortunately, this concept also gets carried over into the exercise programs they pursue for health benefits. Evidence now suggests that a substantial training effect can be accomplished in some people by training at intensities of 45% or less of their aerobic capacities. For most, however, the appropriate intensity appears to be at a level of at least 60% of $\dot{V}O_2$ max.

As mentioned earlier, evidence now suggests that moderate levels of activity produce substantial health benefits. Dr. Ronald LaPorte, an epidemiologist from the University of Pittsburgh, was one of the first to observe that most studies reporting health-related benefits from regular physical activity involved relatively low-intensity exercise.[15] In fact, these benefits occurred at intensities substantially below the levels currently recommended for improving aerobic capacity. Lower intensities appear to have considerable health benefits without changing aerobic capacity. This important point must be more fully researched in the future. Less than 10% of adult Americans are meeting the guidelines, mentioned earlier, that are proposed for improving aerobic capacity.[6] Promoting lower intensity exercise might greatly increase our sedentary society's participation in activities that will provide health benefits, which should then reduce our nation's health care costs.

━━ IN REVIEW . . . ━━

1. The four basic factors in an exercise program are exercise mode, frequency, duration, and intensity. A minimum threshold for the last three must be met to attain any aerobic benefits, and this threshold is quite variable.
2. The program should include one or more cardiovascular endurance activities. If the activity involves competition, preconditioning with a standard endurance activity is recommended before sport participation begins to bring you up to an appropriate level of fitness.
3. Activities must be matched with individual needs and likes so that motivation can be maintained.
4. Optimal exercise frequency is 3 to 5 days of training each week, although greater frequency might provide additional benefits. Exercise should begin with three to four sessions per week, then more if desired.
5. Exercise duration of 20 to 30 min working at the appropriate intensity is optimal, but the key is reaching the threshold for both duration and intensity.
6. Exercise intensity appears to be the most important of these factors. For most people, intensity should be at least 60% of $\dot{V}O_2$ max. However, health benefits occur at intensities lower than those needed for aerobic conditioning.

Monitoring Exercise Intensity

Exercise intensity can be quantified on the basis of the training heart rate (THR), the metabolic equivalent (MET), or the rating of perceived exertion (RPE). Let's examine each of these, as well as their strengths and weaknesses in quantifying exercise intensity.

Training Heart Rate

The concept of training heart rate is based on the linear relationship between heart rate and $\dot{V}O_2$ with increasing rates of work, as shown in Figure 22.3. When you are tested, your heart rate and $\dot{V}O_2$ values are obtained each minute and plotted against each other. The THR is established by using the heart rate that is equivalent to a set percentage of your $\dot{V}O_2$ max. For example, if a training level of 75% of $\dot{V}O_2$ max is desired, the $\dot{V}O_2$ at 75% is determined ($\dot{V}O_2$ max $\times$ 0.75) and the heart rate corresponding to this $\dot{V}O_2$ is then selected as the THR. Importantly, the exercise intensity necessary to achieve a given percentage of $\dot{V}O_2$ max results in a much higher heart rate than that same percentage of HR max. As an example, a THR that is set at 75% of the $\dot{V}O_2$ max represents an intensity of 86% of the HR max (see Figure 22.3).

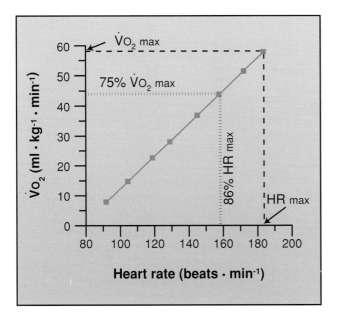

Figure 22.3   The linear relationship between heart rate and oxygen consumption with increasing rates of work, and the heart rate equivalent to a set percentage (75%) of $\dot{V}O_2$ max.

The Karvonen Method

The training heart rate can also be established by using what is known as the Karvonen concept of maximal heart rate reserve, or the Karvonen method.[13] Maximal heart rate reserve is defined as the difference between HR max and the resting heart rate (HR rest):

$$\text{Maximal heart rate reserve} = \text{HR max} - \text{HR rest}$$

By this method, the training heart rate is calculated by taking a given percentage of the maximal heart rate reserve and adding it to the resting heart rate. Let's consider an example. For 75% of maximal heart rate reserve, the equation would be as follows:

$$\text{THR}_{75\%} = \text{HR rest} + 0.75(\text{HR max} - \text{HR rest})$$

The Karvonen method adjusts the THR so that a specific percentage of the THR by the Karvonen method is identical to the HR equivalent of that same percentage of $\dot{V}O_2$ max.[7] Thus a THR computed at 75% of maximal heart rate reserve is approximately the same as the heart rate corresponding to 75% of the $\dot{V}O_2$ max.

Training Heart Rate Range

More recently, appropriate exercise intensity has been established by setting a THR range, rather than a single THR value. This is a more sensible approach because exercising at a set percentage of $\dot{V}O_2$ max can place you above your lactate threshold, making it difficult for you to train for any extended period. With the THR range concept, a low and high value are established that will ensure a training response. You start at the low end of the THR range and progress through the range as you feel comfortable. To illustrate this, using the Karvonen method for establishing the THR, consider the following example. A 40-year-old man has a resting heart rate of 75 beats per minute, a maximum heart rate of 180 beats per minute, and he is advised to exercise within a THR range of from 60% to 75% of his maximal heart rate reserve. His training heart rate range would be as follows:

$$\begin{aligned}
\text{THR}_{60\%} &= 75 + 0.60(180 - 75) \\
&= 75 + 63 = 138 \text{ beats per minute} \\
\text{THR}_{75\%} &= 75 + 0.75(180 - 75) \\
&= 75 + 79 = 154 \text{ beats per minute}
\end{aligned}$$

This same THR range method can be used by estimating HR max (220 − age) without losing much accuracy.

The concept of training heart rate is extremely valuable. Heart rate is highly correlated with the work done by the heart. Heart rate alone is a good index of myocardial oxygen consumption as well as coronary blood flow. By using the training heart rate method for monitoring your exercise intensity, your heart works at the same rate, even though the metabolic cost of the work might vary considerably. As an example, when exercising at high altitudes or in the heat, your heart rate will be elevated significantly if you attempt to maintain a set rate of work, such as running at a 9-min · mi⁻¹ (6-min · km⁻¹) pace. With the THR method, you simply train at a lower rate of work under these extreme environmental conditions to maintain the same heart rate (THR). This is a much safer approach to monitoring exercise intensity, particularly for high-risk patients in whom the work of the heart must be closely regulated. The THR method also allows for improvement in aerobic capacity with training. As you become better conditioned, your heart rate decreases for the same rate of work, which means that you must perform at a higher rate of work to reach your training heart rate.

KEY POINT

Heart rate is the preferred method for monitoring exercise intensity, because it is highly correlated to the work of the heart (or stress on the heart), and it allows for a progressive increase in the rate of training with improvements in fitness to maintain the same training heart rate.

When prescribing exercise intensity, it is appropriate to establish a training heart rate range, starting at the low end of the range and progressing to the upper end of the range over time.

Metabolic Equivalent

Exercise intensity has also been prescribed on the basis of the metabolic equivalent (MET) system. The amount of oxygen your body consumes is directly proportional to the energy you expend during physical activity. At rest, your body uses approximately 3.5 ml of oxygen per kilogram (2.2 lb) of body weight per minute (ml · kg⁻¹ · min⁻¹). This resting metabolic rate is referred to as 1.0 MET.

All activities can be classified by intensity according to their oxygen requirements. An activity that is rated as a 2.0 MET activity would require two times the resting metabolic rate, or 7 ml · kg⁻¹ · min⁻¹, and an activity that is rated at 4.0 MET would require approximately 14 ml · kg⁻¹ · min⁻¹. Some activities and their MET values are presented in Table 22.5. Please keep in mind that these values are only approximations, because metabolic efficiency varies considerably from one person to the next, and even in the same individual. Although the MET system is useful as a guideline for training, it fails to account for changes in environmen-

tal conditions and it does not allow for changes in physical conditioning, as illustrated in the previous section.

Ratings of Perceived Exertion

Ratings of perceived exertion (RPE) have also been proposed for use in the prescription of exercise intensity. With this method, individuals subjectively rate how hard they feel that they are working. A given numerical rating corresponds to the perceived relative intensity of exercise. When the RPE scale is used correctly, this system for monitoring exercise intensity has proven very accurate. Using the original Borg scale, which is a rating scale ranging from 6 to 20 (Table 22.6), your exercise intensity should be between an RPE of 12 to 13 (somewhat hard) and an RPE of 15 to16 (hard).

Finally, Table 22.7 provides a comparison of the various methods for rating exercise intensity. Let's use them to determine a moderate exercise intensity. As

---

IN REVIEW . . .

1. Exercise intensity can be monitored on the basis of training heart rate, metabolic equivalent, or rating of perceived exertion.
2. Training heart rate can be established by using the heart rate equivalent to a certain percent of $\dot{V}O_2$ max. It can also be determined using the Karvonen method, which takes a given percentage of maximal heart rate reserve and adds it to resting heart rate. With this method, the percent of maximal heart rate reserve that is used also reflects the percent of $\dot{V}O_2$ max that the person is working at when they are at the calculated training heart rate.
3. Rather than using a single THR, a more sensible approach is to establish THR ranges to work within, instead of a single THR.
4. The amount of oxygen consumed reflects the amount of energy expended during an activity. $\dot{V}O_2$ at rest is about 3.5 ml · kg⁻¹ · min⁻¹, which equals 1.0 MET. Activity intensities can be classified by their oxygen requirements as multiples of the resting metabolic rate.
5. The rating of perceived exertion method requires that a person subjectively rate how difficult the work is, using a numerical scale that is related to exercise intensity. The subject looks at the standard scale to determine the appropriate number.

Table 22.5 Selected Activities and Their Respective MET Values

Activity	METS	Activity	METS
Self-care		Level cycling, 6 mph (1 mi in 10 min)	3.5
Rest, supine	1.0	Level walking, 2.5 mph (1 mi in 24 min)	3.5
Sitting	1.0	Level walking, 3 mph (1 mi in 20 min)	4.5
Standing, relaxed	1.0	Calisthenics	4.5
Eating	1.0	Level cycling, 9.7 mph (1 mi in 6 min 18 s)	5.0
Conversation	1.0	Swimming, crawl, 1 ft $\cdot$ s^{-1}	5.0
Dressing and undressing	2.0	Level walking, 3.5 mph (1 mi in 17 min)	5.5
Washing hands and face	2.0	Level walking, 4.0 mph (1 mi in 15 min)	6.5
Propulsion, wheelchair	2.0	Level jogging, 5.0 mph (1 mi in 12 min)	7.5
Walking, 2.5 mph	3.0	Level cycling, 13 mph	
Showering	3.5	(1 mi in 4 min 37 s)	9.0
Walking downstairs	4.5	Level running, 7.5 mph (1 mi in 8 min)	9.0
Walking, 3.5 mph	5.5	Swimming, crawl, 2 ft $\cdot$ s^{-1}	10.0
Ambulation, braces and crutches	6.5	Level running, 8.5 mph (1 mi in 7 min)	12.0
		Level running, 10.0 mph (1 mi in 6 min)	15.0
Housework		Swimming crawl, 2.5 ft $\cdot$ s^{-1}	15.0
Handsewing	1.0	Swimming crawl, 3.0 ft $\cdot$ s^{-1}	20.0
Machine sewing	1.5	Level running, 12 mph (1 mi in 5 min)	20.0
Sweeping floor	1.5	Level running, 15 mph (1/4 mi in 1 min)	30.0
Polishing furniture	2.0	Swimming crawl, 3.5 ft $\cdot$ s^{-1}	30.0
Peeling potatoes	2.5		
Scrubbing, standing	2.5	**Recreational**	
Washing small clothes	2.5	Painting, sitting	1.5
Kneading dough	2.5	Playing piano	2.0
Scrubbing floors	3.0	Driving car	2.0
Cleaning windows	3.0	Canoeing, 2.5 mph	2.5
Making beds	3.0	Horseback riding, walk	2.5
Ironing, standing	3.5	Volleyball, 6-player recreational	3.0
Mopping	3.5	Billiards	3.0
Wringing wash by hand	3.5	Bowling	3.5
Hanging wash	3.5	Horseshoes	3.5
Beating carpets	4.0	Golf	4.0
		Cricket	4.0
Occupational		Archery	4.5
Sitting at desk	1.5	Ballroom dancing	4.5
Writing	1.5	Table tennis	4.5
Riding in automobile	1.5	Baseball	4.5
Watch repairing	1.5	Tennis	6.0
Typing	2.0	Horseback riding, trot	6.5
Welding	2.5	Folk dancing	6.5
Radio assembly	2.5	Skiing	8.0
Playing musical instrument	2.5	Horseback riding, gallop	8.0
Parts assembly	3.0	Squash rackets	8.5
Bricklaying and plastering	3.5	Fencing	9.0
Heavy assembly work	4.0	Basketball	9.0
Wheeling wheelbarrow 115 lb, 2.5 mph	4.0	Football	9.0
Carpentry	5.5	Gymnastics	10.0
Mowing lawn by handmower	6.5	Handball and paddleball	10.0
Chopping wood	6.5		
Shoveling	7.0		
Digging	7.5		
Physical-conditioning			
Level walking, 2 mph (1 mi in 30 min)	2.5		
Level cycling, 5.5 mph			
(1 mi in 10 min 54 s)	3.0		

Table 22.6 The Borg Scale of Perceived Exertion

Rating	15-point scale—A	15-point scale—B	Rating	10-point scale
6		No exertion at all	0	Nothing at all
7	Very, very light	Extremely light	0.5	Very, very weak
8			1	Very weak
9	Very light	Very light	2	Weak (light)
10			3	Moderate
11	Fairly light	Light	4	Somewhat strong
12			5	Strong (heavy)
13	Somewhat hard	Somewhat hard	6	
14			7	Very strong
15	Hard	Hard (heavy)	8	
16			9	
17	Very hard	Very hard	10	Very, very strong
18				
19	Very, very hard	Extremely hard		
20		Maximal exertion	—	Maximal

Adapted from Borg (1982), and Pollock and Wilmore (1990).

Table 22.7 Classification of Exercise Intensity Based on 20 to 60 Min of Endurance Activity

Relative intensity (%)		Rating of perceived exertion	Classification of intensity
HR_{max}	$\dot{V}O_2$ max or HR_{max} reserve		
<35%	<30%	<9	Very light
35-59%	30-49%	10-11	Light
60-79%	50-74%	12-13	Moderate
80-89%	75-84%	14-16	Heavy
≥90%	≥85%	>16	Very heavy

Adapted from Pollock and Wilmore (1990).

the first column shows, you would want to work within an HR_{max} range of 60% to 79%. If, instead, you were monitoring intensity by $\dot{V}O_2$ max or using the Karvonen method, this HR_{max} range is equivalent to 50% to 74% of either $\dot{V}O_2$ max or HR_{max} reserve, as shown in the second column. Using the rating of perceived exertion, shown in the third column, this is equivalent to an RPE value of 12 to 13. All of these values reflect moderate-intensity exercise.

The Exercise Program

Once the exercise prescription has been determined, it is integrated into a total exercise program, which is generally only part of an overall health improvement plan. Individual exercise capacity varies widely even between people of similar ages and physical builds. For this reason, each program must be individualized, based on results of physiological and medical tests and individual needs and interests.

KEY POINT

Physical activity must be considered a lifetime pursuit! The benefits of a sound exercise program are rapidly lost once that program is discontinued.

The total exercise program consists of the following activities:

- Warm-up and stretching activities
- Endurance training
- Cool-down and stretching activities
- Flexibility training
- Resistance training
- Recreational activities

Generally, the first three activities are performed three to four times each week. Flexibility training can be included as part of the warm-up, cool-down, and stretching exercises, or it can be done at a separate time during the week. Resistance training is usually done on alternate days when endurance training is not; however, the two can be combined into the same workout. Now, let's examine each of these activities.

Warm-Up and Stretching Activities

The exercise session should begin with low-intensity calisthenic-type and stretching exercises (see Figure 22.4). Such a warm-up period will increase both heart rate and breathing, preparing you for the efficient and safe functioning of your heart, blood vessels, lungs, and muscles during the more vigorous exercise that follows. A good warm-up also reduces the amount of muscle and joint soreness that you experience during the early stages of the exercise program and can decrease your risk of injury. An acceptable warm-up would begin with 5 to 10 min of stretching, followed by 5 to 10 min of low-intensity activity using the endurance-training mode of exercise. For example, if you train with running, you might start with stretching and follow it with 5 to 10 min of light jogging or jogging in place.

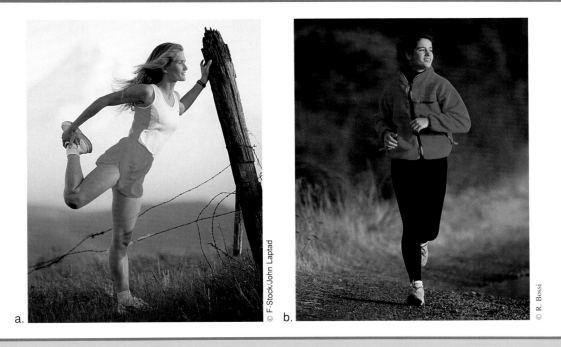

Figure 22.4   The warm-up period should include (a) stretching and (b) low-intensity activity, such as light jogging.

Endurance Training

Physical activities that develop cardiovascular endurance are the heart of the exercise program. They are designed to improve both the capacity and efficiency of your cardiovascular, respiratory, and metabolic systems. These activities also help you control or reduce your body weight. Activities such as walking, jogging, running, cycling, swimming, rowing, aerobic dancing, box stepping, and hiking are good endurance activities. Sports such as handball, racquetball, tennis, badminton, and basketball also have aerobic potential if they are pursued vigorously. Activities such as golf, bowling, and softball are generally of little value for developing aerobic capacity, but they are fun, have definite recreational value, and may have health-related benefits. For these reasons, such activities certainly have a place in the overall exercise program.

Cool-Down and Stretching Activities

Every endurance exercise session should conclude with a cool-down period. This is best accomplished by slowly reducing the intensity of the endurance activity during the last several minutes of your workout. After running, for example, a slow, restful walk for several minutes helps prevent blood pooling in your extremities. Stopping abruptly following an endurance exercise bout causes blood to pool in your legs and can result in dizziness or fainting. Also, catecholamine levels might be elevated during the immediate recovery

period, and this can lead to a fatal heart arrhythmia. After the cool-down period, stretching exercises can be performed to facilitate increased flexibility.

Flexibility Training

Flexibility exercises (see Figure 22.5) are usually supplementary to exercises performed during the warm-up period and are intended for those who have poor flexibility or muscle and joint problems, such as low back pain. These exercises should be performed slowly. Quick stretching movements are potentially dangerous and can lead to muscle pulls or spasms. At one time it was recommended that these exercises be performed before the endurance conditioning period. Now, though, it is hypothesized that the muscles, tendons, ligaments, and joints are more adaptable and responsive to flexibility exercises when they are done after the endurance conditioning phase. Research has yet to confirm this hypothesis.

Resistance Training

Increasing interest surrounds the use of resistance training as part of a general health and fitness exercise program. Indeed, many health-related benefits can be obtained from resistance training. The American College of Sports Medicine has recently included resistance training in its recommendations for a general health and fitness program.[1]

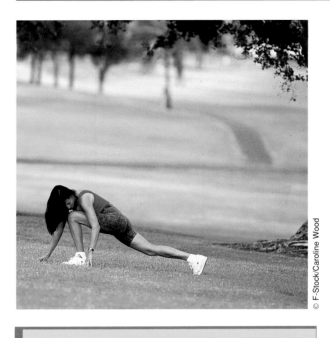

Figure 22.5 Flexibility exercises should be performed slowly to prevent injury.

© F-Stock/Caroline Wood

Starting a Resistance Training Program

Recall from chapter 1 that the maximum amount of weight you can lift successfully only one time is your one-repetition maximum, or 1-RM. When you begin a resistance training program, you should start with a weight that is exactly one half of your maximum strength, or 1-RM, for each lift. You should attempt to lift that weight 10 consecutive times. If you can lift the weight just 10 times before you reach fatigue, this is the proper starting point. If you could have done more, you should go to the next higher weight for your second set. If, instead, you were able to lift the weight less than eight times in your first set, the original weight was too heavy and should be reduced to the next lower weight for your second set.

When a given weight brings you to fatigue by the 8th to 10th repetition on your first set, this is your appropriate starting weight. You should try to achieve as many repetitions as possible during the second and third sets, but the number of repetitions you can complete in these last sets should decrease as your muscles become fatigued. You should perform two or three sets of each lift per day, 2 to 3 days per week.

As your strength increases, the number of repetitions you can complete per set will increase. When you reach 15 repetitions on the first set, you are ready to progress to the next higher weight. This training technique is referred to as progressive resistance exercise.

Health Benefits Associated With Resistance Training

Interest has surged in the use of resistance training for promoting improvements in general health. Unfortunately, research findings are not always consistent, and this is likely due to differences in the training programs used in different studies. The volume and intensity of the training, the rest interval between sets and exercises, and the selection of exercises all can greatly influence the results of a given study. With this in mind, let's briefly summarize some of the key findings from an extensive review, by Stone et al., of the health-related benefits of resistance training.[24]

Resistance training can have an impact on cardiorespiratory fitness, specifically on the risk factors associated with cardiovascular disease. With resistance training, the heart rate at submaximal rates of exercise is generally reduced, which typically reflects improved cardiorespiratory fitness. However, the resting heart rate has not been shown to be reduced consistently across studies. The heart can be enlarged by resistance training, likely because of increases in the thickness (hypertrophy) of the interventricular septum and the left ventricular wall. As we saw in earlier chapters, this can increase the contractility of the left ventricle and enhance stroke volume. These changes in the myocardium of the left ventricle are theorized to be adaptations to the heart contracting against an increased systemic arterial pressure during resistance training.

Some evidence indicates that resistance training can lead to reductions in the resting blood pressure of people with hypertension or borderline hypertension. Studies have also supported the use of resistance training to promote favorable alterations in blood lipid profiles, although the results have not always been consistent from one study to another. When blood lipid changes have been found, they generally reflect a decrease in the ratio of either total cholesterol to HDL-cholesterol, or of LDL-cholesterol to HDL-cholesterol. Resistance training may also increase insulin sensitivity and improve glucose tolerance, both of which are important factors in preventing diabetes. And diabetes is, as well as a disease entity itself, also a risk factor for cardiovascular disease.

Resistance training might reduce the risk of obesity. Good evidence indicates that a program of resistance training increases the participant's fat-free mass and decreases the fat mass. Some scientists speculate that this increased fat-free mass will increase the person's resting metabolic rate, because muscle is more metabolically active than fat. This would increase daily caloric expenditure.

Finally, the role of resistance training in preventing osteoporosis is currently under investigation. Preliminary results appear promising. Studies with re-

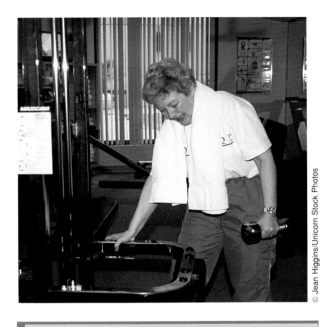

Figure 22.6   Resistance training in older women may decrease bone loss associated with menopause.

sistance training in older women (see Figure 22.6) suggest that the bone loss associated with menopause can be attenuated, or even reversed, with a resistance training program.

Recreational Activities

Recreational activities (see Figure 22.7) are important to any comprehensive exercise program. Although these activities are primarily engaged in for enjoyment and relaxation, many can also contribute to improving fitness. Activities such as hiking, tennis, handball, squash, and certain team sports fall into this category. Guidelines for selecting these activities include the following:

- Can you learn or perform the activities with at least a moderate degree of success?
- Do the activities include opportunities for social development, if that is desired?
- Are the costs associated with participation reasonable and within your budget?
- Are the activities varied enough to maintain your continued long-term interest?

Many excellent opportunities exist for people who have no recreational hobbies or activities but who would like to become involved. Local public recreation centers, park districts, YMCAs, YWCAs, and some public schools, community colleges, and universities

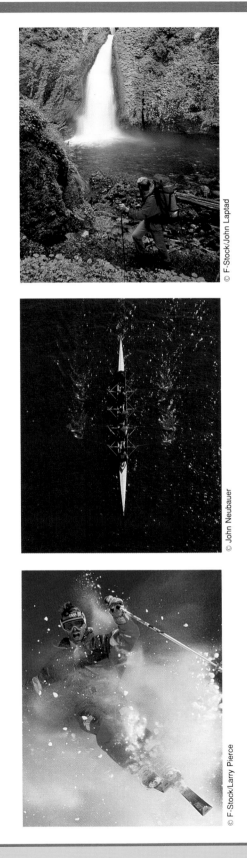

Figure 22.7   The recreational activities in which you can participate regularly may depend on your location, but many communities offer a wide variety of programs.

offer instructional classes in a wide variety of activities at little or no cost. Often the entire family can participate in these classes—an added bonus to a total health-improvement program! Also, the number of commercial fitness centers is rapidly growing and many now employ trained staff who can properly prescribe exercise programs and assist individuals in getting started.

KEY POINT

It is important to emphasize the whole exercise program and not focus on just one or two parts. This will assure that total body fitness needs are met.

IN REVIEW . . .

1. An exercise session should begin with a warm-up of low-intensity calisthenic-type and stretching exercises to prepare the cardiovascular, respiratory, and muscle systems to work more efficiently.
2. Endurance activities should be performed three to four times each week.
3. Each endurance session should be followed by cool-down and stretching to prevent blood pooling in the extremities and muscle soreness.
4. Flexibility exercise should be performed slowly, and this phase of the program might be best included immediately after the endurance component.
5. Resistance training should begin with a weight of one half your 1-RM. This is the proper weight if you can lift it about 10 times. If you lift it more than that, you need more weight, and if you lift it fewer than eight times, you need less.
6. Recreational activities should be included in your exercise program for enjoyment and relaxation.

Exercise and Rehabilitation of People With Diseases

Exercise has become a major component in rehabilitation programs for a number of diseases. Cardiopulmonary rehabilitation programs, which began in the 1950s, have become the most visible. Tremendous advances in cardiopulmonary rehabilitation have led to the formation of a professional association, The

American Association of Cardiovascular and Pulmonary Rehabilitation, and a professional research journal, the *Journal of Cardiopulmonary Rehabilitation*.

Exercise is also an important part of the rehabilitation of patients with

- cancer,
- obesity,
- diabetes,
- renal disease,
- arthritis, and
- cystic fibrosis.

Most recently, emphasis has increased on the use of exercise in the rehabilitation of transplant patients, including those with heart transplants, liver transplants, and kidney transplants, because it helps alleviate some drug side effects and improves general health.

KEY POINT

Exercise training has become an extremely important part of rehabilitation programs for a number of diseases. Although the specific physiological mechanisms explaining the benefits of exercise training for each of these diseases have not been clearly defined at this time, there are many general health benefits that appear to improve the patient's prognosis.

The manner in which exercise is used in the rehabilitation of people with disease is highly specific to the nature and extent of the disease. Because of this, it is beyond the scope of this chapter to go into specific details for any disease, but many of the references and selected readings listed at the end of this chapter provide more details about establishing exercise programs for specific disease states and the clinical values of these programs.[5,9,18,21,22,23]

IN REVIEW . . .

1. Exercise is a vital part of cardiopulmonary rehabilitation and is also essential in rehabilitating patients with such diseases as cancer, obesity, diabetes, renal disease, arthritis, and cystic fibrosis.
2. The type and details of the rehabilitation program depend on the patient, the specific disease involved, and its extent.

In Closing . . .

With this chapter, we conclude our journey to an understanding of exercise and sport physiology. We began by reviewing how various body systems function during exercise and how they respond to chronic training. We saw how physical activity and performance are affected by the environment, such as extremes of heat and cold, extremes of pressure, and even the unusual conditions of microgravity. We turned our attention to ways in which athletes can, or attempt to, optimize their performance. Then we considered the unique characteristics of special populations engaged in sport and exercise. And finally, we examined the role of exercise in the maintenance of health and the development of fitness.

It has been a long journey from cover to cover, but hopefully you will close this book with a new appreciation of physical activity. Perhaps you will leave this book with a new awareness of how your body performs physical activity. Maybe, if you have not yet done so, you will feel compelled to commit to a personal exercise program. And hopefully you now feel some excitement for exercise and sport physiology, realizing that these areas of study affect so many aspects of our lives.

Key Terms

Borg scale
exercise electrocardio-
  gram (ECG)
exercise prescription
Karvonen method
maximal heart rate
  reserve
metabolic equivalent
  (MET)
mode

predictive value of an abnormal exercise test
rating of perceived exer-
  tion (RPE)
rehabilitation programs
sensitivity
specificity
threshold
training heart rate (THR)

Study Questions

1. How active are adult Americans today? Are we in a fitness revolution?
2. What role does the graded exercise test to exhaustion play in the medical clearance? Is this test essential for all adults?
3. Discuss the concepts of sensitivity and specificity of exercise testing, and the predictive value of an abnormal test. Of what value is this information in the establishment of policy mandating who should be exercise tested?
4. How can we get our population to be more active? What levels of exercise do we need to promote to help people gain the health-related benefits associated with exercise?
5. What four factors must be considered in the exercise prescription? Which of these is the most important?
6. Discuss the concept of a minimal threshold for initiating physiological changes with exercise training as it relates to the exercise prescription.
7. Discuss the various ways of monitoring exercise intensity and give the advantages and disadvantages of each.
8. Describe the components of a good exercise program and their importance in the total program.
9. How do you effectively motivate individuals to maintain regular exercise habits?

References

1. American College of Sports Medicine. (1990). The recommended quantity and quality of exercise for developing and maintaining cardiorespiratory and muscular fitness in healthy adults. *Medicine and Science in Sports and Exercise*, **22**, 265-274.

2. American College of Sports Medicine. (1991). *Guidelines for exercise testing and prescription* (4th ed.). Philadelphia: Lea & Febiger.

3. American Heart Association. (1972). *Exercise testing and training of apparently healthy individuals: A handbook for physicians*. New York: American Heart Association.

4. Blair, S.N., Kohl, H.W., Paffenbarger, R.S., Clark, D.G., Cooper, K.H., & Gibbons, L.W. (1989). Physical fitness and all-cause mortality: A prospective study of healthy men and women. *Journal of the American Medical Association*, **262**, 2395-2401.

5. Bloomfield, J., Fricker, P.A., & Fitch, K.D. (1992). *Textbook of science and medicine in sport*. Boston: Blackwell Scientific.

6. Caspersen, C.J. (1987). Physical activity and coronary heart disease. *The Physician and Sportsmedicine*, **15**(11), 43-44.

7. Davis, J.A., & Convertino, V.A. (1975). A comparison of heart rate methods for predicting endurance training intensity. *Medicine and Science in Sports*, **7**, 295-298.

8. Fletcher, G.F., Froelicher, V.F., Hartley, L.H., Haskell, W.L., & Pollock, M.L. (1990). Exercise standards: A statement for health professionals from the American Heart Association. *Circulation*, **82**, 2286-2322.

9. Franklin, B.A., Gordon, S., & Timmis, G.C. (Eds.) (1989). *Exercise in modern medicine*. Baltimore: Williams & Wilkins.

10. Harris, Louis, & Associates, Inc. (1978). *Health maintenance*. Newport Beach, CA: Pacific Mutual Life Insurance Co.

11. Harris, Louis, & Associates, Inc. (1979). *The Perrier study: Fitness in America*. New York: Perrier-Great Waters of France, Inc.

12. Harris, Louis, & Associates, Inc. (1983). Prevention in America: Steps people take—or fail to take—for better health. *Prevention Magazine*, October-November.

13. Karvonen, M.J., Kentala, E., & Mustala, O. (1957). The effects of training heart rate: A longitudinal study. *Annales Medicinae Experimentalis et Biologiae Fenniae*, **35**, 307-315.

14. Kirshenbaum, J., & Sullivan, R. (1983). Hold on there America. *Sports Illustrated*, **58**(5), 60-74.

15. LaPorte, R.E., Adams, L.L., Savage, D.D., Brenes, G., Dearwater, S., & Cook, T. (1984). The spectrum of physical activity, cardiovascular disease and health: An epidemiologic perspective. *American Journal of Epidemiology*, **120**, 507-517.

16. Leon, A.S., & Connett, J. (1991). Physical activity and 10.5 year mortality in the Multiple Risk Factor Intervention Trial (MRFIT). *International Journal of Epidemiology*, **20**, 690-697.

17. Leon, A.S., Connett, J., Jacobs, D.R., & Rauramaa, R. (1987). Leisure-time physical activity levels and risk of coronary heart disease and death. *Journal of the American Medical Association*, **258**, 2388-2395.

18. Lowenthal, D.T., Bharadwaja, K., & Oaks, W.W. (1979). *Therapeutics through exercise*. New York: Grune & Stratton.

19. Malinow, M.R., McGarry, D.L., & Kuehl, K.S. (1984). Is exercise testing indicated for asymptomatic active people? *Journal of Cardiac Rehabilitation*, **4**, 376-380.

20. Miller Brewing Co. (1983). *The Miller Lite report on American attitudes towards sports*. Milwaukee, WI: Miller Brewing Co.

21. Pollock, M.L., & Schmidt, D.H. (Eds.) (1986). *Heart disease and rehabilitation* (2nd ed.). Boston: Houghton Mifflin.

22. Pollock, M.L., & Wilmore, J.H. (1990). *Exercise in health and disease: Evaluation and prescription for prevention and rehabilitation* (2nd ed.). Philadelphia: Saunders.

23. Skinner, J.S. (Ed.) (1993). *Exercise testing and exercise prescription for special cases: Theoretical basis and clinical application (2nd ed)*. Philadelphia: Lea & Febiger.

24. Stone, M.H., Fleck, S.J., Triplett, N.T., & Kraemer, W.J. (1991). Health and performance-related potential of resistance training. *Sports Medicine*, **11**, 210-231.

Selected Readings

Amsterdam, E.A., Wilmore, J.H., & DeMaria, A.N. (1977). *Exercise in cardiovascular health and disease*. New York: Yorke Medical Books.

Birk, T.J., & Birk, C.A. (1987). Use of ratings of perceived exertion for exercise prescription. *Sports Medicine*, **4**, 1-8.

Cooper, K.H. (1968). *Aerobics*. New York: Evans.

Gordon, N.F., Kohl, H.W., Scott, C.B., Gibbons, L.W., & Blair, S.N. (1992). Reassessment of the guidelines for exercise testing: What alterations to current recommendations are required? *Sports Medicine*, **13**, 293-302.

Karvonen, M.J., & Vuorimaa, T. (1988). Heart rate and exercise intensity during sport activities: Practical application. *Sports Medicine*, **5**, 303-312.

MacDougall, J.D., Tuxen, D., Sale, D.G., Moroz, J.R., & Sutton, J.R. (1985). Arterial blood pressure response to heavy resistance exercise. *Journal of Applied Physiology*, **58**, 785-790.

Swain, D.P., Abernathy, K.S., Smith, C.S., Lee, S.J., & Bunn, S.A. (1994). Target heart rates for the development of cardiorespiratory fitness. *Medicine and Science in Sports and Exercise*, **26**(1), 112-116.

Credits

Table 1.2: Data from ''Selective Persistence of Circadian Rhythms in Physiological Responses to Exercise'' by T. Reilly and G.A. Brooks, 1990, *Chronobiology International*, **7**, 59-67.

Figures 2.15 and 8.16 (data): From *Textbook of Work Physiology* by P.-O. Åstrand and K. Rodahl, 1985, New York: McGraw-Hill Book Co. Adapted by permission.

Table 4.1: From *Sensible Fitness* by J.H. Wilmore, 1986, Champaign, IL: Human Kinetics. Adapted by permission.

Table 4.2: From *Designing Resistance Training Programs* by S.J. Fleck and W.J. Kraemer, 1987, Champaign, IL: Human Kinetics. Adapted by permission.

Figure 4.3: From ''Neural Adaptation to Resistance Training'' by D.G. Sale, 1988, *Medicine and Science in Sport and Exercise*, **20**, S135-S145. Adapted by permission.

Figure 4.4: From ''Potential for Gross Muscle Hypertrophy in Older Men'' by T. Moritani and H.A. deVries, 1980, *Journal of Gerontology*, **35**, 672-682. Adapted by permission.

Figure 4.6: From ''Muscle Fiber Splitting in Trained and Untrained Animals'' by W.J. Gonyea, 1980, *Exercise and Sport Sciences Reviews*, **8**, 19-39. Adapted by permission.

Figure 4.7: From ''Skeletal Muscle, Fiber Splitting Induced by Weight-Lifting Exercise in Cats'' by W.J. Gonyea, G.C. Ericson, and F. Bonde-Petersen, 1977, *Acta Physiologica Scandinavica*, **19**, 105-109. Adapted by permission.

Figures 4.8 and 4.9: From ''Strength and Skeletal Muscle Adaptations in Heavy-Resistance Trained Women After Detraining and Retraining'' by R.S. Staron, M.J. Leonardi, D.L. Karapondo, E.S. Malicky, J.E. Falkel, F.C. Hagerman, and R.S. Hikida, 1991, *Journal of Applied Physiology*, **70**, 631-640. Adapted by permission.

Figures 5.17, 7.5, 7.6, 13.5, 13.6, and 18.2; Table 11.3: From *Inside Running: Basics of Sports Physiology* by D.L. Costill, 1986, Indianapolis: Benchmark Press. Adapted by permission.

Figure 7.3: From ''Adaptations in Skeletal Muscle Following Strength Training'' by D.L. Costill, E.F Coyle, W.F.Fink, G.R. Lesmes, and F.A. Witzmann, 1979, *Journal of Applied Physiology*, **46**, 96-99. Adapted by permission.

Figure 8.12: Data from ''Left Ventricular Performance in Normal Subjects: A Comparison of the Responses to Exercise in the Upright and Supine Position'' by L.R. Poliner, G.J. Dehmer, S.E. Lewis, R.W. Parkey, C.G. Blomqvist, and J.T. Willerson, 1980, *Circulation*, **62**, 528-534.

Figure 8.15: From ''Intraarterial Blood Pressure During Exercise With Different Muscle Groups'' by P.-O. Åstrand, B. Ekblom, R. Messin, B. Saltin, and J. Stenberg, 1965, *Journal of Applied Physiology*, **20**, 253-256. Adapted by permission.

Table 10.2: From ''Capillary Density of Skeletal Muscle in Well-Trained and Untrained Men'' by L. Hermansen and M. Wachtlova, 1971, *Journal of Applied Physiology*, **30**, 860-863. Adapted by permission.

Figure 10.2: Data from ''One- and Two-Dimensional Echocardiography in Body Builders and Endurance-Trained Subjects'' by A. Urhausen and W. Kindermann, 1989, *International Journal of Sports Medicine*, **10**, 139-144.

Figure 10.3: Data from ''Exercise Training Improves Left Ventricular Systolic Function in Older Men'' by A.A. Ehsani, T. Ogawa, T.R. Miller, R.J. Spina, and S.M. Jilka, 1991, *Circulation*, **83**, 96-103.

Figure 10.10: From ''Aerobic Performance in Brothers, Dizygotic and Monozygotic Twins'' by C. Bouchard, R. Lesage, G. Lortie, J.A. Simoneau, P. Hamel, M.R. Boulay, L. Pérusse, G. Thériault, and C. Leblanc, 1986, *Medicine and Science in Sports and Exercise*, **18**, 639-646.

Figure 10.11: Data from ''Effect of Age and Training on Aerobic Capacity and Body Composition of Master Athletes'' by M.L. Pollock, C. Foster, D. Knapp, J.L. Rod, and D.H. Schmidt, 1987, *Journal of Applied Physiology*, **62**, 725-731.

Figure 10.12: Data from ''Effects of Gender, Age, and Fitness Level on Response of $\dot{V}O_2$ max to Training in 60-70 yr Olds'' by W.M. Kohrt, M.T. Malley, A.R. Coggan, R.J. Spina, T. Ogawa, A.A. Ehsani, R.E. Bourey, W.H. Martin, III, and J.O. Holloszy, 1991, *Journal of Applied Physiology*, **71**, 2004-2011.

Figure 10.13: From ''Discussion: Heredity, Fitness, and Health'' by C. Bouchard, in C. Bouchard, R.J. Shephard, T. Stephens, J.R. Sutton, and B.D. McPherson (Eds.) *Exercise, Fitness, and Health* (pp. 147-153), 1990, Champaign, IL: Human Kinetics. Adapted by permission.

Figure 10.14: From ''Assessment of Maximal Aerobic Power in Specifically Trained Athletes'' by S.B. Strømme, F. Ingjer, and H.D. Meen, 1977, *Journal of Applied Physiology*, **42**, 833-837. Adapted by permission.

Table 11.4: From ''Prevention of Thermal Injuries During Distance Running'' by American College of Sports Medicine, 1987, *Medicine and Science in Sports and Exercise*, **19**, 529-533. Reprinted by permission.

Table 11.6: From 1973, Runner's World, **8**, 28. Adapted by permission.

Figure 11.6b: from ''Leg Muscle Metabolism During Exercise in the Heat and Cold'' by W. Fink, D.L. Costill, P.J. Van Handel, and L. Getchell, 1975, *European Journal of Applied Physiology*, **34**, 183-190. Adapted by permission.

Figure 11.9: From ''Muscle Metabolism During Exercise in the Heat in Unacclimatized and Acclimatized Humans'' by D.S. King, D.L. Costill, W.J. Fink, M. Hargreaves, and R.A. Fielding, 1985, *Journal of Applied Physiology*, **59**, 1350-1354. Adapted by permission.

Figure 11.10: From ''Metabolic Responses to Submaximal Exercise in Three Water Temperatures'' by D.L. Costill, P.J. Cahill, and D.O. Eddy, 1967, *Journal of Applied Physiology*, **22**(4), 628-632. Adapted by permission.

Figure 12.2: Data from E.R. Buskirk, J. Kollias, E. Piconreatique, R. Akers, E. Prokop, and P. Baker in R.F. Goddard (Ed.) *The Effects of Altitude on Physical Performance* (pp. 65-71), 1967, Chicago: Athletic Institute.

Figure 12.3: From ''Maximal Exercise at Extreme Altitude on Mt. Everest'' by J.B. West, S.J. Boyer, D.J. Graber, P.H. Hackett, K.H. Maret, J.S. Milledge, R.M. Peters, Jr., C.J. Pizzo, M. Samaja, F.H. Sarnquist, R.B. Schone, and R.M. Winslow, 1983, *Journal of Applied Physiology*, **55**, 688-698. Adapted by permission.

Tables 12.5 and 12.6: Data from ''Potential Benefits of Maximal Exercise Just Prior to Return From Weightlessness'' by V.A. Convertino, 1987, *Aviation, Space, and Environmental Medicine*, **58**, 568-572.

Figure 12.12: Data from ''Neuromuscular Aspects in Development of Exercise Countermeasures'' by V.A. Convertino, 1991, *The Physiologist*, **34**, S125-S128.

Figure 12.13: Data from ''Instrumented Personal Exercise During Long-Duration Space Flights'' by C.F. Sawin, J.A. Rummel, and E.L. Michel, 1975, *Aviation, Space, and Environmental Medicine*, **46**, 394-400.

Table 13.2: From ''Effects of Detraining on Cardiovascular Responses to Exercise: Role of Blood Volume'' by E.F. Coyle, M.K. Hemmert, and A.R. Coggan, 1986, *Journal of Applied Physiology*, **60**, 95-99. Adapted by permission.

Figure 13.12: From ''Response to Submaximal and Maximal Exercise After Bed Rest and Training'' by B. Saltin, G. Blomqvist, J.H. Mitchell, R.L. Johnson, Jr., K. Wildenthan, and C.B. Chapman, 1968, *Circulation*, **38**(Suppl. 7). Adapted by permission.

Opening case on p. 320 is reprinted courtesy of SPORTS ILLUSTRATED from the May 25, 1992 issue. Copyright © 1992, Time Inc. ''Died.'' by Sally Guard. All Rights Reserved.

Figure 14.1: From ''Anabolic Steroids: the Physiological Effects of Placebos'' by G. Ariel and W. Saville, 1972, *Medicine and Science in Sports and Exercise*, **4**, 124-126. Adapted by permission.

Table 14.2: From *The Physiological Basis of Physical Education and Athletics* (p. 632), by E.L. Fox, R.W. Bowers, and M.L. Foss, 1988, Philadelphia: Saunders College Publishing. Adapted by permission.

Table 14.3: From ''The Effect of Amphetamines On Selected Physiological Components Related to Athletic Success'' by J.V. Chandler and S.N. Blair, 1980, *Medicine and Science in Sports and Exercise*, **12**, 65-69. Adapted by permission.

Table 14.4: From *Drugs and the Athlete* (p. 84), by G.I. Wadler and B. Hainline, 1989, Philadelphia: F.A. Davis. Adapted by permission.

Figure 14.3: Adapted from ''Effects of Methadienone on the Performance and Body Composition of Men Undergoing Athletic Training'' by G.R. Hervey, A.V. Knibbs, L. Burkinshaw, D.B. Morgan, P.R.M. Jones, D.R. Chettle, and D. Vartsky, 1981, *Clinical Science*, **60**, 457-461.

Figure 14.4: From ''Anabolic Steroid Use Among Athletes: Changes in HDL-C Levels'' by D.L. Costill, D.R. Pearson, and W.J. Fink, 1984, *The Physician and Sportsmedicine*, **12**(6), 113-117. Adapted by permission.

Table 14.5, Figure 15.5 (data): From *Eating on the Run* (2nd ed.), by E. Tribole, 1992, Champaign, IL: Leisure Press. Copyight 1992 by Evelyn Tribole. Adapted by permission.

Figure 14.5: Adapted from ''Effect of Induced Erythrocythemia on Aerobic Work Capacity'' by F.J. Buick, N. Gledhill, A.B. Froese, L. Spreit, and E.C. Meyers, 1980, *Journal of Applied Physiology*, **65**, 1821-1826.

Figure 14.6: From ''Blood Doping and Oxygen Transport'' by L.L. Spriet, in D.R. Lamb and M.H. Williams (Eds.) *Ergogenics - Enhancement of Performance in Exercise and Sport* (p. 224), 1991, Dubuque, IA: Brown & Benchmark. Adapted by permission.

Figure 14.8: From ''Acid-Base Balance During Repeated Bouts of Exercise: Influence of HCO_3'' by D.L. Costill, F. Verstappen, H. Kuipers, E. Janssen, and W. Fink, 1984, *International Journal of Sports Medicine*, **5**, 228-231. Adapted by permission.

Figure 15.1: From ''Nutrition for Endurance Sport: Carbohydrate and Fluid Balance'' by D.L. Costill and J. Miller, 1980, *International Journal of Sportsmedicine*, **1**, 2-14. Adapted by permission.

Figure 15.4: From ''Effects of Elevated Plasma FFA and Insulin on Muscle Glycogen Usage During Exercise'' by D.L. Costill, E. Coyle, G. Dalsky, W. Evans, W. Fink, and D. Hoopes, 1977, *Journal of Applied Physiology*, **43**, 695-699. Adapted by permission.

Figure 15.8: Data from ''Fluid and Electrolyte Balance During Prolonged Exercise'' by B. Saltin and D.L. Costill. In *Exercise, Nutrition, and Energy Metabolism* (pp. 150-158) by E.S. Horton and R.L. Terjung (Eds.), 1988.

Figure 15.10: Data from ''Nutrition and Physical Performance'' by P.-O. Åstrand, in M. Rechcigl (Ed.), *Nutrition and the World Food Problem*, 1979, Basel, Switzerland: S. Karger; and ''Effects of Exercise-Diet Manipulation on Muscle Glycogen and Its Subsequent Utilization During Performance'' by W.M. Sherman, D.L. Costill, W.J. Fink, and J. Miller, 1981, *International Journal of Sport Medicine*, **2**, 1-15.

Figure 16.1: From ''Body Weight and Body Composition'' by J.H. Wilmore, in K.D. Brownell, J. Rodin, and J.H. Wilmore (Eds.), *Eating, Body Weight, and Performance in Athletes: Disorders of Modern Society*, 1992, Philadelphia: Lea & Febiger. Adapted by permission.

Table 16.3: Data from ''Relationships of Body Fat to Motor Fitness Test Scores'' by R.P. Riendeau, B.E. Welch, C.E. Crisp, L.V. Crowley, P.E. Griffin, and J.E. Brockett, 1958, *Research Quarterly*, **29**, 200-203.

Table 16.4: Data from ''The Iowa Wrestling Study: Lessons for Physicians'' by C.M. Tipton and R.A. Oppliger, 1984, *Iowa Medicine*, September, 381-385.

Figure 16.4: From ''Generalized Equations for Predicting Body Density in Men'' by A.S. Jackson and M.L. Pollock, 1978, *British Journal of Nutrition*, **40**, 497-504. Adapted with permission of Cambridge University Press.

Figure 16.8: Data from ''Body Physique and Composition of the Female Distance Runner'' by J.H. Wilmore, C.H. Brown, and J.A. Davis, 1977, *Annals of the New York Academy of Sciences*, **301**, 764-776.

Table 17.2: From *Designing Resistance Training Programs*, by S.J. Fleck and W.J. Kraemer, 1987, Champaign, IL: Human Kinetics. Reprinted by permission.

Figure 17.5: Data from the NHANES-I, National Center for Health Statistics.

Figure 17.6: Data from ''Growth of the Lean Body Mass in Man'' by G.B. Forbes, 1972, *Growth*, **36**, 325-338.

Figure 17.7: Data from the President's Council on Physical Fitness and Sports, 1985.

Figure 17.8: Data from *Physical and Motor Tests in the Medford Boys' Growth Study*, by H.H. Clarke, 1971, Englewood Cliffs, NJ: Prentice Hall.

Figure 17.11: From ''Anaerobic Characteristics in Male Children and Adolescents'' by O. Inbar and O. Bar-Or, 1986, *Medicine and Science in Sports and Exercise*, **18**, 264-269. Adapted by permission.

Figure 17.12: From *Pediatric Sports Medicine for the Practitioner: From Physiologic Principles to Clinical Applications*, by O. Bar-Or, 1983, New York: Springer-Verlag. Adapted by permission.

Figure 17.13: From *Strength Training for Young Athletes* (p. 12), by W.J. Kraemer and S.J. Fleck, 1993, Champaign, IL: Human Kinetics. Adapted by permission.

Figure 18.1: From J.O. Holloszy, 1985, *Journal of Applied Physiology*, **59**, 826-831. Adapted by permission.

Figure 18.7: From ''The Aging Endurance Athlete'' by B. Saltin. In *Sports Medicine for the Mature Athlete* by J.R. Sutton and R.M. Brock (Eds.), 1986, Indianapolis: Benchmark Press. Adapted by permission.

Figure 19.1: Data from ''Relation of Lean Body Mass to Height in Children and Adolescents'' by G.B. Forbes, 1972, *Pediatric Research*, **6**, 32-37.

Tables 19.3 and 19.4: From ''Prescription of Aerobic Exercise During Pregnancy'' by L.A. Wolfe, P. Hall, K.A. Webb, L. Goodman, M. Monga, and M.J. McGrath, 1989, *Sports Medicine*, **8**, 273-301. Adapted by permission.

Tables 19.5 and 19.6: From *Diagnostic and Statistical Manual of Mental Disorders, Third Edition - Revised (DSM-III-R)*, by the American Psychiatric Association, 1987, Washington, D.C. Reprinted by permission.

Figure 19.3: From ''Fiber Types and Metabolic Potentials of Skeletal Muscles in Sedentary Man and Endurance Runners'' by B. Saltin,

J. Henriksson, E. Nygaard, and P. Andersen, 1977, *Annals of the New York Academy of Sciences*, **301**, 3-29. Adapted by permission.

Figure 19.4: Normal values for males from "Experimental Studies of Physical Fitness in Relation to Age" by S. Robinson, 1938, *Arbeitsphysiologie*, **10**, 251-323; normal values for females from "Aerobic Work Capacity in Men and Women With Special Reference to Age" by I. Åstrand, 1960, *Acta Physiologica Scandinavica*, **49**(Suppl. 169); values for elite male distance runners from "Maximal Oxygen Intake Among Marathon Runners" by D.L. Costill and E. Winrow, 1980, *Archives of Physical Medicine and Rehabilitation*, **51**, 317-320 and "Submaximal and Maximal Working Capacity of Elite Distance Runners. Part I: Cardiorespiratory Aspects" by M.L. Pollack, 1977, *Annals of the New York Academy of Sciences*, **301**, 310-322; values for elite female distance runners from "Cardiorespiratory and Metabolic Responses to Submaximal and Maximal Exercise in Elite Women Distance Runners" by R.R. Pate, P.B. Sparling, G.E. Wilson, K.J. Cureton, and B.J. Miller, *International Journal of Sportsmedicine*, **8**(Suppl. 2), 91-95 and "Physiological Profiles of Women Distance Runners" by J.H. Wilmore and C.H. Brown, 1984, *Medicine and Science in Sports*, **6**, 178-181, and Wilmore, J.H. (unpublished).

Table 19.7: Data from the National Collegiate Athletic Association, 1990, Kansas City, Missouri.

Table 20.4: From *Exercise in Health and Disease: Evaluation and Prescription for Prevention and Rehabilitation (2nd ed.)*, by M.L. Pollock and J.H. Wilmore, 1990, Philadelphia: W.B. Saunders, Co. Adapted by permission.

Figures 20.1 and 20.2: Data from *Heart and Stroke Facts* by the American Heart Association, 1993, Dallas, Texas.

Figure 20.7: From "Physical Inactivity and Coronary Heart Disease" by C.J. Caspersen, 1987, *Physician and Sportsmedicine*, **15**(11), 43-44. Adapted by permission.

Figure 20.9: Data from "The Incidence of Primary Cardiac Arrest During Vigorous Exercise" by D.S Siscovik, N.S. Weiss, R.H. Fletcher, and T. Lasky, 1984, *New England Journal of Medicine*, **311**, 874-877.

Figure 21.1: Data from "A Review: Exercise and Its Influence on Resting Energy Metabolism in Man" by E.T. Poehlman, 1989, *Medicine and Science in Sports and Exercise*, **21**, 515-525.

Figure 21.2: From "The Response to Long-Term Overfeeding in Identical Twins" by C. Bouchard, A. Tremblay, J.-P. Després, A. Nadeau, P.J. Lupien, G. Thériault, J. Dussalt, S. Moorjani, S. Pinault, and G. Fournier, 1990, *New England Journal of Medicine*, **322**, 1477-1482. Adapted by permission.

Table 21.3: From "Exercise and Type I Diabetes Mellitus" by A. Vitug, S.H. Schneider, and N.B. Ruderman, 1988, *Exercise and Sport Sciences Reviews*, **16**, 292. Adapted by permission.

Figure 21.3: From "Health Implications of Overweight and Obesity in the United States" by T.B. Van Itallie, 1985, *Annals of Internal Medicine*, **103**, 983-988. Adapted by permission.

Figure 21.4: Data from "Obesity: Definition, Diagnosis, and Disadvantages" by G.A. Bray, 1985, *Medical Journal of Australia*, **142**, S2-S8.

Figure 21.6: From "Comparing Diet and Exercise as Weight Reduction Tools" by W.B. Zuti and L.A. Golding, 1976, *Physician and Sportsmedicine*, **4**, 49-53. Adapted by permission.

Figure 21.7: From "Effects of Dieting and Exercise on Lean Body Mass, Oxygen Uptake, and Strength" by K.N. Pavlou, et al., 1985, *Medicine and Science in Sports and Exercise*, **17**, 466-471. Adapted by permission.

Tables 22.1 and 22.2: Data from *Guidelines for Exercise Testing and Prescription Training*, by the American College of Sports Medicine, 1991, Philadelphia: Lea & Febiger.

Tables 22.6 and 22.7: From *Exercise in Health and Disease: Evaluation and Prescription for Prevention and Rehabilitation (2nd ed.)*, by M.L. Pollock and J.H. Wilmore, 1990, Philadelphia: W.B. Saunders, Co. Adapted by permission.

Photo Credits:

Figures 1.1, 1.2, 1.3, 1.5, 1.6, 1.7, 2.9, 2.10, 4.5, 4.10, 4.11, 5.18, 7.1, 7.4, 13.8, and 18.9: Provided courtesy of the authors.

Figures 1.4, 1.8, 1.9, 1.11, 4.14, 4.15, 5.11, 8.9, 11.8, 13.7, 16.3, 16.5, 16.6, 21.8, and 22.1: by Susan Allen Camp.

Chapter 2 Opening Photo: from *Visualizing Muscles, A New Ecorché Approach to Surface Anatomy*, by John Cody, M.D., 1990, Lawrence, Kansas: University Press of Kansas. Reprinted by permission.

Figures 2.1b, 2.3, 8.2, 10.1, and 20.3b-d; Chapter 5, 6, 8, and 9 Opening Photos: Special thanks to James Hawker, Coordinator of Photography; Biomedical Communications/SIU School of Medicine, Springfield, Illinois.

Figures 4.10 and 4.11: From "Muscle Damage in Marathon Runners" by F.C. Hagerman, R.S. Hikida, R.S. Staron, W.M. Sherman, and D.L. Costill, 1984, *Physician and Sportsmedicine*, **12**, 39-48. Reprinted by permission.

Figure 11.3: Courtesy of R.C. Purohit and D.D. Pascoe.

Figure 12.8: © Dennis Graver; recompression chamber courtesy of NOAA, Seattle, Wahington.

Figure 12.14: Courtesy of National Aeronautical and Space Administration.

Chapter 14 Opening Photo: Photo of packed red blood cells courtesy of Champaign County Blood Bank.

Figure 17.3: Courtesy of Murray Robertson, M.D., Tucson, AZ.

Figure 18.4a: Courtesy of CYBEX ®, a division of Lumex, Inc.

Figure 19.8: X-rays courtesy of Barbara A. Kammer, M.D.; Department of Radiology, Carle Clinic Association, Champaign, Illinois.

Chapter 20 Opening Photo: © Don Clegg, for the Carle Foundation Hospital.

Figure 20.3a: © Martin Dohrn/Royal College of Surgeons/Science Photo Laboratory/Photo Researchers.

Figure 20.8: From "Reduction of Coronary Atherosclerosis by Moderate Conditioning Exercise in Monkeys on an Atherogenic Diet" by D.M. Kramsch, A.J. Aspen, B.M. Abramowitz, T. Kreimendahl, and W.B. Hood, 1981, *New England Journal of Medicine*, **305**, 1483-1489. Reprinted by permission.

Figure 21.9: Courtesy of ONE TOUCH II Blood Glucose Monitoring System by LifeScan, Inc., a Johnson & Johnson company.

Part D Opening Photo: © R. Bossi / Rob Bossi, Portsmouth, New Hampshire.

Glossary

acclimation—Laboratory adaptation to an environmental stress.

acclimatization—Natural adaptation to an environmental stress.

acetyl coenzyme A (acetyl CoA)—The compound that forms the common entry point into the Krebs cycle for the oxidation of carbohydrate and fat.

actin—A thin protein filament that acts with myosin filaments to produce muscle action.

action potential—A large depolarization of the membrane of a neuron or muscle cell that is conducted through the cell.

acute altitude (mountain) sickness—Illness characterized by headache, nausea, vomiting, dyspnea, and insomnia. It typically begins 6 to 96 hr after one reaches high altitude and lasts several days.

acute muscle soreness—Pain felt during and immediately after an exercise bout.

acute response—A physiological response to an individual bout of exercise.

adenosine diphosphate (ADP)—A high-energy phosphate compound from which ATP is formed.

adenosine triphosphatase (ATPase)—An enzyme that splits the last phosphate group off ATP, releasing a large amount of energy and reducing the ATP to ADP and P_i.

adenosine triphosphate (ATP)—A high-energy phosphate compound from which the body derives its energy.

aerobic capacity—*See maximal oxygen consumption.*

aerobic interval training—Training with repeated bouts of moderate- to high-intensity activity separated by brief rest periods.

aerobic metabolism—A process occurring in the mitochondria that uses oxygen to produce energy (ATP). Also known as *cellular respiration.*

aerobic training—Training that improves the efficiency of the aerobic energy-producing systems and can improve cardiorespiratory endurance.

alcohol—A CNS depressant believed by some athletes to have ergogenic properties.

amenorrhea—The absence (primary) or cessation (secondary) of normal menstrual function.

amphetamine—A CNS stimulant believed by some athletes to have ergogenic properties.

anabolic steroids—Prescription drugs with the anabolic (growth-stimulating) characteristics of testosterone, taken by some athletes to increase body size and muscle mass.

anabolism—The building up of body tissue; the constructive phase of metabolism.

anaerobic—In the absence of oxygen.

anaerobic threshold—The point at which the metabolic demands of exercise can no longer be met by available aerobic sources and at which an increase in anaerobic metabolism occurs, reflected by an increase in blood lactate concentration.

anaerobic training—Training that improves the efficiency of the anaerobic energy-producing systems and can increase muscular strength and tolerance for acid-base imbalances during high intensity effort.

anorexia nervosa—A clinical eating disorder characterized by distorted body image, intense fear of fatness or weight gain, amenorrhea, and refusal to maintain more than the minimal normal weight based on age and height.

arterial-venous oxygen difference (a-$\bar{v}O_2$ diff)—The difference in oxygen content between arterial and mixed venous blood, which reflects the amount of oxygen removed by the tissues.

arteriosclerosis—A condition that involves loss of elasticity, thickening, and hardening of the arteries.

aspartates—Salts of aspartic acid, believed by some athletes to have ergogenic properties.

atherosclerosis—A form of arteriosclerosis that involves changes in the lining of the arteries and plaque accumulation, leading to progressive narrowing.

athlete's heart—A nonpathological enlarged heart, often found in endurance athletes, that results primarily from left ventricular hypertrophy in response to training.

ATP-PCr system—A simple anaerobic energy system that functions to maintain ATP levels. Breakdown of phosphocreatine (PCr) frees P_i, which then combines with ADP to form ATP.

atrophy—Loss of size, or mass, of body tissue, such as muscle atrophy with disuse.

autogenic inhibition—Reflex inhibition of a motor neuron in response to excessive tension in the muscle fibers it supplies, as monitored by the Golgi tendon organs.

autoregulation—Local control of blood distribution (through vasodilation) in response to a tissue's changing needs.

axon terminal—One of numerous branched endings of an axon. Also known as a *terminal fibril.*

basal metabolic rate—The lowest rate of body metabolism (energy use) that can sustain life, measured after an overnight sleep in a laboratory under optimal conditions of quiet, rest, and relaxation.

beta blockers—A class of drugs that block transmission of neural impulses from the sympathetic nervous system; believed by some athletes to have ergogenic properties.

beta (β) cells—Cells in the islets of Langerhans in the pancreas that secrete insulin.

beta oxidation (β oxidation)—The first step in fatty acid oxidation, breaking fatty acids into separate 2-carbon units of acetic acid, each of which is then converted to acetyl CoA.

bicarbonate loading—Ingesting bicarbonate to elevate blood pH, with hopes of delaying fatigue by increasing the capacity to buffer acids.

bioelectric impedance—A procedure for assessing body composition in which an electrical current is passed through the body. The resistance to current flow through the tissues reflects the relative amount of fat present.

blood doping—Any means by which a person's total volume of red blood cells is increased, typically via transfusion of red blood cells.

blood lipids—Blood-borne fats, such as triglycerides and cholesterol.

body build—The morphology (form and structure) of the body.

body composition—The chemical composition of the body. The model used in this book considers two components—fat-free mass and fat mass.

body density (D_{body})—Body weight divided by body volume.

body mass index (BMI)—A measurement of body weight determined by dividing weight (kg) by height (m) squared. BMI is highly correlated with body composition.

body size—A person's height and mass (weight).

Borg scale—A numerical scale for rating perceived exertion.

buffer—A substance that combines with either an acid or a base to maintain a constant acid-base (pH) balance.

bulimia nervosa—A clinical eating disorder characterized by recurrent episodes of binge eating, a feeling of lack of control during these binges, and purging behavior, which may include self-induced vomiting and use of laxatives and diuretics.

caffeine—A CNS stimulant believed by some athletes to have ergogenic properties.

calorimeter—A device for measuring the heat produced by the body (or by specific chemical reactions).

capillary to fiber ratio—The number of capillaries per muscle fiber.

cardiac cycle—The period that includes all events between two consecutive heart beats.

cardiac output ($\dot{Q}$)—The volume of blood pumped out by the heart per minute. $\dot{Q}$ = heart rate × stroke volume.

cardiorespiratory endurance—The ability of the body to sustain prolonged exercise.

cardiovascular deconditioning—A decrease in the cardiovascular system's ability to deliver sufficient oxygen and nutrients.

cardiovascular drift—An increase in heart rate during exercise to compensate for a decrease in stroke volume. This compensation helps maintain a constant cardiac output.

catabolism—The tearing down of body tissue; the destructive phase of metabolism.

catecholamines—Biologically active amines, such as epinephrine and norepinephrine, that have powerful effects similar to those of the sympathetic nervous system.

cerebral infarction—Death of brain tissue that results from insufficient blood supply due to blockage or damage of a cerebral vessel. *See also* **stroke**.

chronic adaptation—A physiological change that occurs when the body is exposed to repeated exercise bouts over weeks or months. These changes generally improve the body's efficiency at rest and during exercise.

chronic hypertrophy—An increase in muscle size that results from repeated long-term resistance training.

circuit resistance training—A combination of circuit training and resistance training, typically involving working at 40% to 60% of your maximum strength for about 30 s, with 15-s rest intervals between work bouts.

circuit training—Selected exercises or activities performed rapidly in a sequence.

cocaine—A so-called recreational drug that is a CNS stimulant and a sympathomimetic drug, believed by some athletes to have ergogenic properties.

concentric action—Muscle shortening.

conduction—Transfer of heat or cold through direct molecular contact. Also movement of an electrical impulse, such as through a neuron.

congenital heart disease—A heart defect present at birth that occurs from abnormal prenatal development of the heart or associated blood vessels. Also known as *congenital heart defect*.

congestive heart failure—A clinical condition in which the myocardium becomes too weak to maintain adequate cardiac output to meet the body's oxygen demands; usually results from the heart being damaged or overworked.

continuous training—Training with continuous activity and no rest intervals, varying from high-intensity continuous activity of moderate duration to low-intensity activity of extended duration.

convection—The transfer of heat or cold via the movement of a gas or liquid across an object, such as the body.

coronary artery disease—Progressive narrowing of the coronary arteries.

cross-innervation—The innervation of a fast-twitch motor unit by a slow-twitch motor neuron, or vice versa.

cross-sectional research design—A research design in which a cross-section of a population is tested at one specific time, then data from groups within that population are compared.

cross-training—Training for more than one sport at the same time, or training multiple fitness components (such as endurance, strength, and flexibility) within the same period.

cycle ergometer—An exercise device that uses cycling to measure physical work.

decompression sickness (bends)—A condition in which bubbles of nitrogen are trapped in the blood and tissues during a too-rapid ascent from depth during diving; characterized by severe discomfort and pain.

dehydration—Loss of body fluids.

delayed-onset muscle soreness (DOMS)—Muscle soreness that develops a day or two after a heavy bout of exercise.

densitometry—The measurement of body density.

depolarization—A decrease in the electrical potential across a membrane, such as when the inside of a neuron becomes less negative relative to the outside.

detraining—Changes the body undergoes in response to a reduction or cessation of regular physical training.

development—Changes that occur in the body starting at conception and continuing through adulthood; differentiation along specialized lines of function, reflecting changes that accompany growth.

diabetes mellitus—A disorder of carbohydrate metabolism characterized by high blood sugar levels (hyperglycemia) and presence of sugar in the urine (glycosuria). The disease develops when there is inadequate production of insulin by the pancreas or inadequate utilization of insulin by the cells.

diaphysis—The shaft of a long bone.

diastolic blood pressure—The lowest arterial pressure, resulting from ventricular diastole (the resting phase).

direct calorimetry—A method that gauges the body's rate and quantity of energy production by direct measurement of the body's heat production.

direct gene activation—The method of action for steroid hormones. They bind to receptors in the cell, then the hormone-receptor complex enters the nucleus and activates certain genes.

disordered eating—Abnormal eating behavior that ranges from excessive restriction of food intake to pathological behaviors, such as self-induced vomiting and laxative abuse; can lead to clinical eating disorders, such as anorexia nervosa and bulimia nervosa.

diuretics—Substances that promote water excretion.

diurnal variation—Fluctuations in physiological responses that occur during a 24-hr period.

down-regulation—Decreased cellular sensitivity to a hormone, likely the result of a decreased number of cell receptors available to bind with the hormone.

dynamic action—Any muscle action that produces joint movement.

dyspnea—Difficult breathing.

eating disorders—A group of clinical disorders involving eating. *See* anorexia nervosa, bulimia nervosa.

eccentric action—Muscle lengthening.

eccentric training—Training that involves eccentric action.

ejection fraction (EF)—The fraction of blood pumped out of the left ventricle with each contraction, determined by dividing stroke volume by end-diastolic volume, then multiplying by 100.

electrical stimulation training—Stimulation of a muscle by passing an electrical current through it.

electrocardiogram (ECG)—A recording of the heart's electrical activity.

electrolyte—A dissolved substance that can conduct an electrical current.

electron transport chain—A series of chemical reactions that converts the hydrogen ion generated by glycolysis and the Krebs cycle into water and produces energy for oxidative phosphorylation.

end-diastolic volume (EDV)—The volume of blood inside the left ventricle at the end of diastole, just before contraction.

endomysium—A sheath of connective tissue that covers each muscle fiber.

end-systolic volume (ESV)—The volume of blood remaining in the left ventricle at the end of systole, just after contraction.

endurance—The ability to resist fatigue; includes muscular endurance and cardiorespiratory endurance.

engram—A specific, learned, and memorized motor pattern, stored in both the sensory and motor portions of the brain, that can be replayed on request.

epimysium—The outer connective tissue that surrounds an entire muscle, holding it together.

epiphyseal plate—A plate of cartilage between the diaphysis and epiphysis. Also known as the *growth plate*.

epiphysis—An end of a long bone, which ossifies separately before uniting with the diaphysis.

ergogenic—Able to improve work or performance.

ergogenic aid—A substance or phenomenon that can improve athletic performance.

ergolytic—Able to impair work or performance.

ergometer—An exercise device that allows the amount and rate of a person's physical work to be controlled (standardized) and measured.

erythropoietin—The hormone that stimulates erythrocyte (red blood cell) production.

essential amino acids—The eight or nine amino acids necessary for human growth that the body cannot synthesize and are thus essential parts of our diets.

estrogen—A female sex hormone.

eumenorrhea—Normal menstrual function.

evaporation—Heat loss through the conversion of water (such as in sweat) to vapor.

exercise electrocardiogram—A recording of the heart's electrical activity during exercise.

excessive training—Training in which volume, intensity, or both are too great or are increased too quickly without proper progression.

excess post-exercise oxygen consumption (EPOC)—Elevated oxygen consumption above resting levels after exercise; at one time referred to as *oxygen debt*.

excitatory postsynaptic potential (EPSP)—A depolarization of the postsynaptic membrane caused by an excitatory impulse.

exercise physiology—The study of how body structure and function is altered by exposure to acute and chronic bouts of exercise.

exercise prescription—Individualization of an exercise program on the basis of the exercise duration, frequency, intensity, and mode.

expiration—The process by which air is forced out of the lungs through relaxation of the inspiratory muscles and elastic recoil of the lung tissue, which increases the pressure in the thorax.

external respiration—The process of bringing air into the lungs and the resulting exchange of gas between the alveoli and the capillary blood.

extracellular fluid—The 35% to 40% of the water in the body that is outside the cells; includes interstitial fluid, blood plasma, lymph, cerebrospinal fluid, and other fluids.

extrinsic neural control—Redistribution of blood at the system or body level, controlled by neural mechanisms.

Fartlek training (speed play)—Training in which an athlete's pace is varied at will, from a fast sprint to slow jogging; normally performed in the hilly countryside.

fasciculus—A small bundle of muscle fibers wrapped in a connective tissue sheath within a muscle.

fast-twitch (FT) fiber—A type of muscle fiber with a low oxidative capacity and a high glycolytic capacity; associated with speed or power activities.

fat-free mass—The mass (weight) of the body that is not fat, including muscle, bone, skin, and organs.

fatigue—An inability to continue work.

fat mass—The absolute amount of body fat.

fatty streaks—Early lipid deposits within blood vessels.

forced expiratory volume (FEV$_{1.0}$)—The volume of air exhaled in the first second after maximal inhalation.

Frank-Starling mechanism—The mechanism by which an increased amount of blood in the ventricle causes a stronger ventricular contraction to increase the amount ejected.

free fatty acids—The components of fat that are used by the body for metabolism.

frostbite—Tissue damage that occurs during cold exposure because circulation to the skin decreases, in an attempt to retain body heat, to the point that the tissue receives insufficient oxygen and nutrients.

gastric emptying—The movement of food mixed with gastric secretions from the stomach into the duodenum.

gender differences—Any differences between females and males.

gluconeogenesis—The conversion of protein or fat into glucose.

glycogen—The storage form of carbohydrate in the body, found predominantly in the muscles and liver.

glycogenesis—The conversion of glucose to glycogen.

glycogen loading—The manipulation of exercise and diet to optimize the body's glycogen storage.

glycogenolysis—The conversion of glycogen to glucose.

glycolysis—The breakdown of glucose to pyruvic acid.

glycolytic system—A system that produces energy through glycolysis.

glycosuria—The presence of glucose in the urine.

Golgi tendon organ—A sensory receptor in a muscle tendon that monitors tension.

graded potential—A localized change (depolarization or hyperpolarization) in the membrane potential.

growth—An increase in the size of the body or any of its parts.

heart rate recovery period—The time it takes for heart rate to return to the resting rate following exercise.

heat content—The total heat (kilocalories) contained in the body.

heat cramp—Cramping of the skeletal muscles as a result of excessive dehydration and the associated salt loss.

heat exhaustion—A heat disorder resulting from an inability of the cardiovascular system to meet all of the body's tissue needs while also shifting blood to the periphery for cooling, characterized by elevated body temperature, breathlessness, extreme tiredness, dizziness, and rapid pulse.

heat stroke—The most serious heat disorder, resulting from failure of the body's thermoregulatory mechanisms. Heat stroke is characterized by body temperature above 105 °F (40.5 °C), cessation of sweating, and total confusion or unconsciousness; and can lead to death.

hematocrit—The percentage of red blood cells in the total blood volume.

hemoconcentration—A relative (not absolute) increase in the red blood cell mass per unit of blood volume, resulting from a reduction in plasma volume.

hemodilution—An increase in blood plasma, resulting in a dilution of the blood's cellular contents.

hemoglobin—The iron-containing pigment in red blood cells that binds oxygen.

hemoglobin saturation—The amount of oxygen bound by each molecule of hemoglobin.

high-altitude cerebral edema (HACE)—A condition of unknown cause in which fluid accumulates in the cranial cavity at altitude, characterized by mental confusion that can progress to coma and death.

high-altitude pulmonary edema (HAPE)—A condition of unknown cause in which fluid accumulates in the lungs at altitude, interfering with ventilation and resulting in shortness of breath, fatigue, and characterized by impaired blood oxygenation, mental confusion, and loss of consciousness.

high-density-lipoprotein-bound cholesterol (HDL-C)—A cholesterol carrier regarded as a scavenger that removes cholesterol from the arterial wall and transports it to the liver to be metabolized.

high-intensity continuous training—A form of continuous training performed at work intensities representing 85% to 95% of an athlete's HR max.

hormonal agents—A group of hormones believed by some athletes to have ergogenic properties.

hormone—A chemical substance produced or released by an endocrine gland and transported by the blood to a specific target tissue.

human growth hormone—A hormone that promotes anabolism and is believed by some athletes to have ergogenic properties.

hydrostatic weighing—A method of measuring body volume in which the athlete is weighed while submerged underwater. The difference between the scale weight on land and the underwater weight (corrected for water density) equals body volume. This value must be further corrected to account for any air trapped in the body.

hyperbaric environment—An environment, such as that underwater, involving high atmospheric pressure.

hyperglycemia—An elevated blood glucose level.

hyperplasia—An increase in the number of cells.

hyperpolarization—An increase in the electrical potential across a membrane.

hypertension—Abnormally high blood pressure; in adults it is usually defined as systolic pressure above 140 mmHg or diastolic pressure above 90 mmHg.

hyperthermia—Elevated body temperature.

hypertrophy—Increase in the size or mass of an organ or body tissue.

hyperventilation—A breathing rate or tidal volume greater than necessary for normal function.

hypobaric environment—an environment, such as that at high altitude, involving low atmospheric pressure.

hypoglycemia—A low blood glucose level.

hyponatremia—A blood sodium concentration below the normal range of 136 to 143 mmol · L^{-1}.

hypothermia—Low body temperature.

hypoxia—A decreased concentration of oxygen.

hypoxic vasoconstriction—The constriction of blood vessels in response to low levels of oxygen.

indirect calorimetry—A method of estimating energy expenditure by measuring respiratory gases.

infrared interactance—A procedure for measuring body composition using a probe that emits electromagnetic radiation through the skin over the site to be measured. The amount of energy reflected back from the tissues indicates tissue composition.

inhibiting factors—Hormones transmitted from the hypothalamus to the anterior pituitary that inhibit release of some other hormones.

inhibitory postsynaptic potential (IPSP)—A hyperpolarization of the postsynaptic membrane caused by an inhibitory impulse.

inspiration—The active process involving the diaphragm and the external intercostal muscles that expands the thoracic dimensions and thus the lungs. The expansion causes decreased pressure in the lungs, allowing outside air to rush in.

insulin—A hormone produced by the beta cells in the pancreas that assists glucose entry into cells.

insulin resistance—A deficient target cell response to insulin.

internal respiration—The exchange of gases between the blood and tissues.

interval training—Repeated brief, fast-paced exercise bouts with short rest intervals in between.

intestinal absorption—The movement of nutrients through the intestinal wall into the blood.

intracellular fluid—The approximately 60% to 65% of total body water that is contained in the cells.

ischemia—A temporary deficiency of blood to a specific area of the body.

Karvonen method—The calculation of training heart rate by adding a given percentage of the maximal heart rate reserve to the resting heart rate. This method gives an adjusted heart rate that is equivalent to the desired percentage of $\dot{V}O_2$ max.

Krebs cycle—A series of chemical reactions that involve the complete oxidation of acetyl CoA and produce 2 moles of ATP (energy), and hydrogen and carbon, which combine with oxygen to form H_2O and CO_2.

lactate—A salt formed from lactic acid.

lactate threshold (LT)—The point during exercise of increasing intensity at which blood lactate begins to accumulate above resting levels.

lipoprotein lipase—The enzyme that breaks down triglycerides to free fatty acids and glycerol, allowing the free fatty acids to enter the cells for use as a fuel or for storage.

longevity—The length of a person's life.

longitudinal research design—A research design in which subjects are tested initially and then one or more times later to directly measure changes over time.

long, slow distance (LSD) training—A form of continuous training in which the athlete performs at a relatively low intensity (such as 60% to 80% of maximum heart rate), with the main objective of distance rather than speed.

lower body (gynoid) obesity—The typical pattern of fat storage in a female with obesity, in which fat is stored primarily in the lower body, particularly in the hips, buttocks, and thighs.

low-density-lipoprotein-bound cholesterol (LDL-C)—A cholesterol carrier theorized to be responsible for depositing cholesterol in the arterial wall.

low-intensity aerobic exercise—Aerobic exercise performed at low intensity, in theory to cause the body to burn a higher percentage of fat.

macrominerals—Those minerals that the body needs more than 100 mg of per day.

marijuana—A so-called recreational drug that is generally ergolytic.

maturation—The process by which the body takes on the adult form and becomes fully functional. It is often defined by the system or function being considered.

maximal expiratory ventilation ($\dot{V}E$ max)—The highest ventilation that can be achieved during exhaustive exercise.

maximal heart rate reserve—The difference between maximal heart rate and resting heart rate.

maximal oxygen uptake ($\dot{V}O_2$ max)—The maximal capacity for oxygen consumption by the body during maximal exertion. It is also known as *aerobic power*, *maximal oxygen intake*, *maximal oxygen consumption*, and *cardiorespiratory endurance capacity*.

maximum heart rate (HR max)—The highest heart rate value attainable during an all-out effort to the point of exhaustion.

mean body temperature (T_{body})—A weighted average of skin and internal body temperatures.

menarche—The onset of menstruation; the first menses.

menses—The menstrual or flow phase of the menstrual cycle.

menstrual (uterine) cycle—The cycle of uterine changes, averaging 28 days and consisting of the menstrual (flow) phase, the proliferative phase, and the secretory phase.

menstrual dysfunction—Disruption of the normal menstrual cycle; it includes oligomenorrhea, primary amenorrhea, and secondary amenorrhea.

metabolic equivalent (MET)—A unit used to estimate the metabolic cost (oxygen consumption) of physical activity. One MET equals the resting metabolic rate of approximately $3.5 \ ml \ O_2 \cdot kg^{-1} \cdot min^{-1}$.

microgravity—An environment in which the body experiences a reduced gravitational force.

microminerals—The minerals that the body needs less than 100 mg of per day. Also known as *trace elements*.

mode—Type of exercise.

morphology—The form and structure of the body.

motor reflex—An involuntary motor response to a given stimulus.

motor unit—The motor nerve and the group of muscle fibers it innervates.

muscle buffering capacity—The muscles' ability to tolerate the acid that accumulates in them during anaerobic glycolysis.

muscle fiber—An individual muscle cell.

muscle spindle—A sensory receptor located in the muscle that senses how much the muscle is stretched.

muscular endurance—The ability of a muscle to avoid fatigue.

myelination—The process of acquiring a myelin sheath.

myelin sheath—The outer covering of a myelinated nerve fiber, formed by a fatlike substance called myelin.

myocardial infarction—Death of heart tissue that results from insufficient blood supply to part of the myocardium.

myocardium—The muscle of the heart.

myofibrils—The contractile elements of skeletal muscle.

myoglobin—A compound similar to hemoglobin, but found in muscle tissue, that carries oxygen from the cell membrane to the mitochondria.

myosin—One of the proteins that forms filaments that produce muscle action.

myosin cross-bridge—The protruding part of a myosin filament. This includes the myosin head, which binds to an active site on an actin filament to produce a power stroke that causes the filaments to slide across each other.

needs analysis—An assessment of factors that determine what specific training program is appropriate for an individual.

negative feedback system—The primary mechanism through which the endocrine system maintains homeostasis. Some body change upsets homeostasis, which triggers release of a hormone to correct the change. Once that is accomplished, the hormone is no longer needed, so its secretion decreases.

nerve impulse—The electrical signal conducted along a neuron; it can be transmitted to another neuron or an end organ, such as a group of muscle fibers.

neuromuscular junction—The site at which a motor neuron communicates with a muscle fiber.

neurotransmitter—A chemical used for communication between a neuron and another cell.

nicotine—A CNS stimulant found in tobacco products. It is believed by some athletes to have ergogenic properties.

nitrogen narcosis—A condition caused by breathing air underwater at depths where the partial pressure of nitrogen increases until the central nervous system experiences a narcotic-like effect, leading to distortions in judgment and sometimes to serious injury or death. Also known as *rapture of the deep*.

nonessential amino acids—The 11 or 12 amino acids the body synthesizes.

nonresponders—Individuals who show little or no improvement compared to others who undergo the same training program.

nonshivering thermogenesis—The stimulation of metabolism by the sympathetic nervous system to generate more metabolic heat.

nonsteroid hormones—Hormones derived from protein, peptides, or amino acids and that cannot easily cross cell membranes.

obesity—An excessive amount of body fat, generally defined as greater than 25% in men and 35% in women.

oligomenorrhea—Abnormally infrequent or scant menstruation.

onset of blood lactate accumulation (OBLA)—a standard value set at either 2.0 or 4.0 mmol lactate · L^{-1} and used as a common reference point.

oral contraceptives—Drugs used for birth control and other medical purposes, and which are believed by some female athletes to have ergogenic properties.

osmolality—The ratio of solutes (such as electrolytes) to fluid.

ossification—The process of bone formation.

osteoporosis—Decreased bone mineral content that causes increased bone porosity.

overtraining—The attempt to do more work than can be physically tolerated.

overtraining syndrome—A condition brought on by overtraining and characterized by performance decrements.

overweight—Body weight that exceeds the normal or standard weight for a particular individual based on sex, height, and frame size.

oxidative capacity ($\dot{Q}O_2$)—A measure of the muscle's maximal capacity to use oxygen.

oxidative system—The body's most complex energy system, which generates energy by disassembling fuels with the aid of oxygen and has a very high energy yield.

oxygen diffusion capacity—The rate at which oxygen diffuses from one place to another.

oxygen poisoning—A condition caused by breathing concentrated oxygen for a long period, such as during a deep dive, characterized by visual distortion, confusion, rapid and shallow breathing, and convulsions.

oxygen supplementation—The breathing of supplemental oxygen, which is believed by some athletes to have ergogenic properties.

oxygen transport system—The components of the cardiovascular and respiratory systems involved in transporting oxygen.

partial pressures—The pressures exerted by individual gases in a mixture of gases.

percentage of change in $\dot{V}O_2$ max—% change = [(Final $\dot{V}O_2$ max - Initial $\dot{V}O_2$ max) / Initial $\dot{V}O_2$ max] × 100.

perimysium—The connective tissue sheath surrounding each muscle fasciculus.

periodization—Varying the training stimulus over discrete periods of time to prevent overtraining.

peripheral blood flow—Blood flow to the extremities and the skin.

peripheral vascular disease—Diseases of the systemic arteries and veins, especially those to the extremeties, that impede adequate blood flow.

pharmacological agents—A group of drugs believed by some athletes to have ergogenic properties.

phosphate loading—The practice of ingesting sodium phosphate, which is believed by some athletes to have ergogenic properties.

phosphocreatine (PCr)—An energy-rich compound that plays a critical role in providing energy for muscle action by maintaining ATP concentration.

physical maturity—The point at which the body has attained the adult physical form.

physiological agents—A group of agents normally present in the body that are believed by some athletes to have ergogenic properties.

placebo—An inactive substance usually provided in a manner identical to an active substance, typically to test for real versus imagined effects.

placebo effect—An effect produced by the subject's expectations after being administered an inactive substance (placebo).

plaque—A buildup of lipids, smooth muscle cells, connective tissue, and debris that forms at the site of injury to an artery.

plyometrics—A type of dynamic action resistance training based on the theory that use of the stretch reflex during jumping will recruit additional motor units.

power—The product of force and velocity.

power stroke—The tilting of the myosin head, caused by a strong intermolecular attraction between the myosin crossbridge and the myosin head.

predictive value of an abnormal exercise test—The accuracy with which abnormal test results reflect presence of a disease.

pregnancy—The state of carrying an embryo in the body.

primary amenorrhea—the absence of menarche (the beginning of menstruation) beyond age 18.

primary risk factors—Risk factors that have been conclusively shown to have a strong association with a certain disease. Primary risk factors for coronary artery disease include smoking, hypertension, high blood lipid levels, and physical inactivity.

principle of disuse—The theory that a training program must include a maintenance plan or the gains from training will be lost.

principle of individuality—The theory that any training program must consider the specific needs and abilities of the individual for whom it is designed.

principle of orderly recruitment—The theory that motor units are generally activated on the basis of a fixed order of recruitment, in which the motor units within a given muscle appear to be ranked.

principle of progressive overload—The theory that all training programs must include overload and progression.

principle of specificity—The theory that a training program must stress the physiological systems critical for optimal performance in a given sport in order to achieve desired training adaptations.

puberty—The point at which a person becomes physiologically capable of reproduction.

pulmonary diffusion—The exchange of gases between the lungs and the blood.

pulmonary ventilation—The movement of gases into and out of the lungs.

radiation—The transfer of heat through electromagnetic waves.

rating of perceived exertion (RPE)—A person's subjective assessment of how hard he or she is working.

recompression—Increasing the pressure exerted on the body, usually in a recompression chamber, to cause nitrogen bubbles to go back into solution. Recompression is used to treat decompression sickness.

rehabilitation programs—Programs designed to reestablish health or fitness following a disability or illness.

relative body fat—The ratio of fat mass to total body mass, expressed as a percentage.

relative weight—The percentage by which an individual is either overweight or underweight, generally determined by dividing the person's weight by the mean weight for the medium frame category for his or her height (from standard weight tables), then multiplying by 100.

releasing factors—Hormones transmitted from the hypothalamus to the anterior pituitary that promote release of some other hormones.

renin-angiotensin mechanism—The mechanism involved in renal control of blood pressure. The kidneys respond to decreased blood pressure or blood flow by forming renin, which converts angiotensinogen into angiotensin I, which is finally converted to angiotensin II. Angiotensin II constricts arterioles and triggers aldosterone release.

residual volume (RV)—The amount of air that cannot be exhaled from the lungs.

resistance training—Training designed to increase strength, power, and muscular endurance.

respiratory alkalosis—A condition in which increased carbon dioxide clearance allows blood pH to increase.

respiratory centers—Autonomic centers located in the medulla oblongata and the pons that establish breathing rate and depth.

respiratory exchange ratio (RER, or R)—The ratio of carbon dioxide expired to oxygen consumed at the level of the lungs.

respiratory membrane—The membrane separating alveolar air and blood, composed of the alveolar wall, the capillary wall, and their basement membranes.

responders—Individuals who show improvement in response to a training program.

resting heart rate—The heart rate at rest, averaging 60 to 80 beats per minute.

resting membrane potential (RMP)—The potential difference between the electrical charges inside a cell and outside the cell, caused by a separation of charges across the membrane.

resting metabolic rate (RMR)—The body's metabolic rate early in the morning following an overnight fast and 8 hr of sleep.

retraining—Recovery of conditioning after a period of inactivity.

saltatory conduction—The rapid means of nerve impulse conduction through myelinated fibers.

sarcolemma—A muscle fiber's cell membrane.

sarcomere—The basic functional unit of a myofibril.

sarcoplasm—The gel-like cytoplasm in a muscle fiber.

sarcoplasmic reticulum (SR)—A longitudinal system of tubules that is associated with the myofibrils and stores calcium for muscle action.

scuba—A self-contained underwater breathing apparatus.

secondary amenorrhea—The cessation of menstruation in a woman with previously normal menstrual function.

second messenger—A substance that acts as a messenger inside of a cell after a nonsteroid hormone binds to receptors outside the cell.

sensitivity—A test's ability to correctly identify subjects who fit the criteria being tested for, such as coronary artery disease.

sensory-motor integration—The process by which the sensory and motor systems communicate and coordinate with each other.

sex-specific differences—True physiological differences between females and males.

shivering—A rapid, involuntary cycle of contraction and relaxation of skeletal muscles that generates heat.

skinfold fat thickness—The most widely applied field technique used to estimate body density, relative body fat, and fat-free mass. It involves measurement of the skinfold fat with calipers at one or more sites.

sliding filament theory—A theory explaining muscle action: A myosin cross-bridge attaches to an actin filament, then the power stroke drags the two filaments past one another.

slow-twitch (ST) fiber—A type of muscle fiber that has a high oxidative and a low glycolytic capacity, associated with endurance-type activities.

specificity—A test's ability to correctly identify subjects who do not fit the criteria being tested for.

specificity of training—Physiological adaptations in response to physical training are highly specific to the nature of the training activity. To maximize benefits, training should be carefully matched to an athlete's specific performance needs.

spontaneous pneumothorax—The entrance of air into the pleural cavity, often caused by rupture of alveoli, and can lead to lung collapse.

sport physiology—The application of the concepts of exercise physiology to training athletes and enhancing sport performance.

spot reduction—The practice of exercising a specific area of the body to (theoretically) reduce locally stored fat.

sprint training—A form of anaerobic training involving very brief intense training bouts.

static action—Action in which the muscle contracts without moving, generating force while its length remains static (unchanged). Also known as isometric action.

static action resistance training—Resistance training that emphasizes static muscle action.

steady state heart rate—A heart rate that is maintained constant at submaximal levels of exercise when the rate of work is held constant.

steroid hormones—Hormones with chemical structures similar to cholesterol that are lipid-soluble and diffuse through cell membranes.

strength—The ability of a muscle to exert force.

stroke—A cerebral vascular accident; a condition in which blood supply to some part of the brain is impaired, typically due to infarction or hemorrhage, so the tissue is damaged.

stroke volume (SV)—The amount of blood ejected from the left ventricle during contraction; it is the difference between the end-diastolic volume and the end-systolic volume.

summation—The summing of all individual changes in a neuron's membrane potential.

swimming flume—A device that uses propeller pumps to circulate water past the swimmer, who attempts to maintain body position by swimming against the current.

synapse—The junction between two neurons.

systolic blood pressure—The greatest arterial blood pressure, resulting from systole.

tapering—A reduction in training intensity prior to a major competition to give the body and mind a break from the rigors of intense training.

taper period—A time during which training intensity is reduced, allowing time for tissue damage from intense training to heal and for the body's energy reserves to be fully replenished.

target cells—Cells that possess specific hormone receptors.

teratogenic effects—Effects that cause abnormal fetal development.

test specificity—Matching the type of ergometer used in testing to the type of activity an athlete usually performs to ensure the most accurate results.

testosterone—The predominant male androgen.

tethered swimming—A method of monitoring a swimmer in which the swimmer is attached to a harness connected to a rope, a series of pulleys, and a pan that contains weights that allow the swimmer to swim while maintaining a constant position in the pool.

thermal stress—Stress imposed on the body by external temperature.

thermic effect of activity (TEA)—The energy expended in excess of the resting metabolic rate to accomplish a given task or activity.

thermic effect of a meal (TEM)—The increase in the metabolic rate associated with digestion, absorption, transport, metabolism, and storage of ingested food.

thermoreceptors—Sensory receptors that detect changes in body temperature and external temperature and relay this information to the hypothalamus.

thermoregulation—The process by which the thermoregulatory center, located in the hypothalamus, readjusts body temperature in response to small deviations from the set point.

thermoregulatory center—An autonomic nervous center located in the hypothalamus that is responsible for maintaining normal body temperature.

thirst mechanism—A neural mechanism that triggers thirst in response to dehydration.

threshold—A minimum amount of stimulus needed to elicit a response. Also, the minimum depolarization required to produce an action potential in neurons.

tidal volume—The amount of air inspired or expired during a normal breathing cycle.

TLV:RV ratio—The ratio between total lung volume (TLV) and residual volume (RV).

total lung capacity—The sum of vital capacity and residual volume.

training heart rate (THR)—A heart rate goal established by using the heart rate equivalent to a set percentage of $\dot{V}O_2$ max. For example, if a training level of 75% $\dot{V}O_2$ max is desired, the $\dot{V}O_2$ at 75% is determined and the heart rate corresponding to this $\dot{V}O_2$ is selected as the THR.

transient hypertrophy—The "pumping-up" of muscle that happens during a single exercise bout, resulting mainly from fluid accumulation in the interstitial and intracellular spaces of the muscle.

transverse tubules (T tubules)—Extensions of the sarcolemma (plasma membrane) that pass laterally through the muscle fiber, allowing nerve impulses to be transmitted rapidly to individual myofibrils and transporting nutrients to them.

treadmill—An ergometer in which a motor and pulley system drives a large belt on which a person can either walk or run.

tropomyosin—A tube-shaped protein that twists around actin strands, fitting in the groove between them.

troponin—A complex protein attached at regular intervals to actin strands and tropomyosin.

Type I diabetes—Insulin-dependent diabetes mellitus (IDDM). Type I diabetes generally has a sudden onset during childhood or young adulthood and leads to almost total insulin deficiency, usually requiring daily insulin injections. Also known as *juvenile-onset diabetes.*

Type II diabetes—Non-insulin-dependent diabetes mellitus (NIDDM). In Type II diabetes, disease onset is more gradual and the causes are more difficult to establish than in Type I diabetes. Type II diabetes is characterized by impaired insulin secretion, impaired insulin action, or excessive glucose output from the liver. Also known as *adult-onset diabetes.*

upper body (android) obesity—The typical pattern of fat storage in a male with obesity, in which fat is stored primarily in the upper body, particularly in the abdomen.

up-regulation—An increased cellular sensitivity to a hormone, often caused by increased hormone receptors.

Valsalva maneuver—The process of holding the breath and attempting to compress the contents of the abdominal and thoracic cavities, causing increased intraabdominal and intrathoracic pressure.

valvular heart diseases—Diseases involving one or more of the heart valves. Rheumatic heart disease is one example.

ventilatory breakpoint—The point at which ventilation increases disproportionately compared to oxygen consumption.

ventilatory equivalent for carbon dioxide ($\dot{V}E/\dot{V}CO_2$)—The ratio of the volume of air ventilated ($\dot{V}E$) to the amount of carbon dioxide produced ($\dot{V}CO_2$).

ventilatory equivalent for oxygen ($\dot{V}E/\dot{V}O_2$)—The ratio between the volume of air ventilated ($\dot{V}E$) and the amount of oxygen consumed ($\dot{V}O_2$); it indicates breathing economy.

vital capacity (VC)—The maximal volume of air expelled from the lungs after maximal inhalation.

vitamins—A group of unrelated organic compounds that perform specific functions to promote growth and to maintain health. They act primarily as catalysts in chemical reactions.

wet bulb globe temperature (WBGT)—A system that simultaneously accounts for conduction, convection, evaporation, and radiation, providing a single temperature reading to estimate the cooling capacity of the surrounding environment. The apparatus consists of a dry bulb, a wet bulb, and a black globe.

windchill—A chill factor created by the wind's increase in the rate of heat loss via convection and conduction.

Index